INTRODUCTION TO PHYSICAL THERAPY AND PATIENT SKILLS

INTRODUCTION TO PHYSICAL THERAPY AND PATIENT SKILLS

Mark Dutton, PT

Allegheny General Hospital

West Penn Allegheny Health System (WPAHS)

Adjunct Clinical Instructor, Duquesne University

School of Health Sciences

Pittsburgh, Pennsylvania

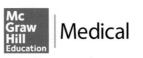

New York   Chicago   San Francisco   Athens   London   Madrid   Mexico City
New Delhi   San Juan   Singapore   Sydney   Toronto

Introduction to Physical Therapy and Patient Skills

1 2 3 4 5 6 7 8 9 0   CTP/CTP   18 17 16 15 14 13

Set ISBN 978-0-07-177243-3; MHID 0-07-177243-X
Book ISBN 978-0-07-177241-9; MHID 0-07-177241-3
DVD ISBN 978-0-07-177242-6; MHID 0-07-177242-1

This book was set in Minion by Aptara, Inc.
The editors were Michael Weitz and Brian Kearns.
The production supervisor was Catherine Saggese.
The illustration manager was Armen Ovsepyan.
Project management was provided by Indu Jawwad.
The cover designer was Thomas De Pierro.
China Translation & Printing Services, Ltd. was printer and binder.

This book is printed on acid-free paper.

Library of Congress Cataloging-in-Publication Data

Dutton, Mark, author.
    Introduction to physical therapy and patient skills / by Mark Dutton.
        p. ; cm.
    Includes bibliographical references.
    ISBN 978-0-07-177241-9 – ISBN 0-07-177241-3
    I. Title.
    [DNLM: 1. Physical Therapy Specialty. 2. Physical Therapists.
3. Physical Therapy Modalities. WB 460]
    RM701
    615.8′2–dc23
                                        2013026862

Please tell the author and publisher what you think of this book by sending your comments to pt@mcgraw-hill.com. Please put the author and title of the book in the subject line.

McGraw-Hill books are available at special quantity discounts to use as premiums and sales promotions, or for use in corporate training programs. To contact a representative please visit the Contact Us pages at www.mhprofessional.com.

Contents

Acknowledgments

From inception to completion, my books span almost 13 years. Such an endeavor cannot be completed without the help of many. I would like to take this opportunity to thank the following:

► My family, especially my daughters Leah and Lauren.

► My parents.

► The exceptional team at McGraw-Hill—Michael Weitz, Brian Kearns, Armen Ovsepyan, and Catherine Saggese.

► To the production crew of Aptara, Inc., especially the Senior Project Manager, Indu Jawwad.

Introduction

This book is designed to introduce a conceptual framework about the art of physical therapy and to give the entry-level physical therapy student a broad foundation to support their journey as they begin the in-depth study of a typical physical therapy curriculum. Included in this conceptual framework are a historical perspective on the physical therapy profession, an introduction to healthcare policy, and a definition of evidence-informed practice. In addition, various chapters describe how movement evolves, how that movement becomes skilled, and how movement dysfunction can occur or develop. Finally, the later chapters introduce the reader to the knowledge and practical skills that are necessary for the general practice of physical therapy as well as providing a foundation for the development of specific areas of clinical expertise, including how to enhance a patient's function in such tasks as bed mobility, transfers, and gait training.

Chapter 1 provides a historical perspective to the physical therapy profession.

Chapter 2 introduces the reader to healthcare policy.

Chapter 3 describes the importance of evidence-informed practice.

Chapter 4 describes all of the neuromuscular structures involved with movement, the physiology behind movement, and the development of skilled movement.

Chapter 5 outlines the sequence behind the typical interaction between a physical therapist and the patient/client.

Chapter 6 familiarizes the reader with all of the major causes of movement dysfunction.

Chapter 7 summarizes the various methods by which a physical therapist can correct movement dysfunction.

Once the reader has completed these chapters, the next step is to put these concepts into practice. Often, these concepts cannot be taught to, or practiced by, a patient without the clinician first taking and then monitoring the patient's vital signs (heart rate, blood pressure, and body temperature). All of these skills, techniques, and procedures will be used by the physical therapist throughout his or her professional career to varying degrees. With every patient interaction, the clinician should always ensure patient and clinician safety. Although patient safety is paramount, it must not be forgotten that clinician safety is also extremely important. The potential for injury or harm is a real threat to the practicing clinician, whether from incurring an injury while lifting a patient, or from contracting an infection or disease from a patient. Throughout the appropriate chapters, emphasis is placed on both patient and clinician safety through the use of correct body mechanics, the application of assistive and safety devices, and effective infection control procedures.

Chapter 8 helps prepare the clinician for patient care.

Chapter 9 describes the various methods by which a clinician can take a patient's vital signs and the significance of each of these vital signs.

Chapter 10 covers the various methods to drape a patient, position a patient, and teach a patient how to perform bed mobility skills.

Chapter 11 teaches the reader how to perform a range of motion assessment and how to apply range of motion techniques as a method of treatment.

Chapter 12 describes in detail the various methods to specifically test the strength of each of the patient's muscles.

Chapter 13 describes the various methods by which the clinician or clinical team can perform the transfer of a patient from and to a variety of surfaces. Wheelchair mobility skills are also described.

Chapter 14 details the various components of gait and how the clinician can train a patient to ambulate with or without an assistive device.

Physical therapy involves clinical decision making in a wide range of situations in order to enhance human movement and function, which is accomplished by a thorough assessment of movement dysfunction. Without the necessary background information, decision-making errors will be made that will affect patient safety, clinician safety, and the effectiveness of care. Clinical decision making is easier if there is a natural progression of basic principles to follow. Without the necessary tools, decision making is made more difficult. The progression of a patient from dependence to independence is often measurable. The simplest such measurements include strength and range of motion; at the other end of the continuum are measurements of function. Assessing function and dysfunction requires a working knowledge of the components of normal movement and how such factors as a lack of range of motion or muscle weakness can affect outcomes. Thus, the assessment of range of motion using goniometry, and strength using manual muscle testing, are critical skills for the physical therapist.

No two clinical situations are the same, as there are many internal and external factors to consider. Such factors include the environment, the patient, and the specific task being undertaken. Many aspects of this book draw from the theories and concepts put forward by Thelen and colleagues[1-3] and by Shumway-Cook and Woollacott.[4]

▶ Thelen and colleagues[1-3] expanded on the work of Bernstein on systems theory and introduced a dynamic systems perspective (see Chapter 4), in which human movement is thought to involve a highly intricate network of codependent subsystems (e.g., respiratory, circulatory, neuromusculoskeletal, and perceptual) composed of a large number of interacting components (e.g., blood cells, oxygen molecules, muscle tissue, connective tissue, and nervous tissue) within an individual that constrain or support movement. According to this theory, a small but critical change in one subsystem can cause the whole system to shift, resulting in a new motor behavior.

▶ Shumway-Cook and Woollacott's approach is related to dynamic systems theory, but also incorporates many of the concepts proposed by other theories of motor control. This theory emphasizes that movement emerges from interactions among the individual, the task, and the environment in which the task is being carried out. Thus, it is important that the student clinician be able to create an optimal environment, break down complex movements into manageable components, and relate to the patient in such a way that task performance is maximized.

It is important to remember that once a physical therapy intervention has been delivered, the continuum of patient care may involve a referral to, or consultation with, another healthcare professional if some of the barriers to attaining full function require expertise outside of the scope of physical therapy.

REFERENCES

1. Thelen E, Ulrich BD: Hidden skills: a dynamic systems analysis of treadmill stepping during the first year. Monogr Soc Res Child Dev 56:1-98, 1991.
2. Thelen E, Corbetta D: Exploration and selection in the early acquisition of skill. Int Rev Neurobiol 37:75-102, 1994.
3. Thelen E: Motor development. A new synthesis. Am Psychol. 50:79-95, 1995.
4. Shumway-Cook A, Woollacott MH: Motor control: issues and theories, in Shumway-Cook A, Woollacott MH (eds): Motor control – Translating research into clinical practice. Philadelphia, Lippincott Williams and Wilkins, 2007, pp 3-20.

CHAPTER 1

The Profession

OVERVIEW

The American Physical Therapy Association (APTA) is the organization that represents physical therapists and physical therapist assistants. It currently has a national office in Alexandria Virginia, as well as a chapter office in almost every state. APTA membership is voluntary and not mandatory for licensure. A number of APTA publications, including *The Guide to Physical Therapist Practice* ("the Guide")[1] and a monthly journal aptly named *Physical Therapy*, provide guidance for the physical therapy profession.

The Guide has defined physical therapy as follows:

Physical therapy includes diagnosis and management of movement dysfunction and enhancement of physical and functional abilities; restoration, maintenance, and promotion of optimal physical function, optimal fitness and wellness, and optimal quality of life as it relates to movement and health; and prevention of the onset, symptoms, and progression of impairment, functional limitations, and disabilities that may result from diseases, disorders, conditions, or injuries.

An APTA publication, *Today's Physical Therapist: A Comprehensive Review of a 21st-Century Health Care Profession*,[2] describes the practice of physical therapists in the following way:

Physical therapists are health care professionals who maintain, restore, and improve movement, activity, and health enabling an individual to have optimal functioning and quality of life, while ensuring patient safety and applying evidence to provide efficient and effective care. Physical therapists evaluate, diagnose, and manage individuals of all ages who have impairments, activity limitations, and participation restrictions. In addition, physical therapists are involved in promoting health, wellness, and fitness through risk factor identification and the implementation of services to reduce risk, slow the progression of or prevent functional decline and disability, and enhance participation in chosen life situations.

In addition to providing habilitation and rehabilitation services, as well as prevention and risk reduction services, physical therapists also collaborate with other healthcare professionals to address patient needs, increase communication, and provide efficient and effective care. Physical therapists also provide consulting, education, research, and administration services across the continuum of healthcare settings.

The APTA further defines physical therapists and physical therapy services as follows:

▶ Physical therapists are experts in how the musculoskeletal and neuromuscular systems function.

▶ Physical therapist services are cost effective. Early physical therapy intervention prevents more costly treatment later, can result in a fast recovery, and reduces costs associated with lost time from work.

▶ Patients pay less when they have direct access to physical therapy services.

As we move forward in the 21st century, the practice of physical therapy continues to evolve. Many of the challenges facing today's physical therapist are due to an increased prevalence to certain contemporary lifestyle conditions. These include hypertension, obesity, diabetes, ischemic heart disease, cerebrovascular accidents, and smoking-related diseases. In addition to having a primary focus of rehabilitating those individuals with impairments and dysfunction, today's physical therapists are becoming more involved in multi-pronged strategies to help reduce or prevent poor lifestyle choices. The evolution of physical therapy can best be appreciated through a historical perspective.

HISTORICAL PERSPECTIVE

Current physical therapy treatment methods, such as hydrotherapy, breathing exercises, positioning techniques, therapeutic massage, and therapeutic exercises, have been used since around 3000 BC for the relief of pain and the treatment of a variety of health problems.[3] From these rudimentary beginnings, therapeutic interventions began to emerge as various civilizations added advancements and adaptations (see Box 1-1).

Descriptions of the early years of the physical therapy profession in the United States begin between 1914 and 1916 and center mainly in the New England states. These descriptions portray the role of the physical therapist to include the assessment, prevention, and treatment of movement dysfunction and physical disability, with the overall goal of enhancing human movement and function. In essence, these descriptions contain many of the vital elements still used in the practice of physical therapy today.

CLINICAL PEARL

In the early 1900s, physical therapists were referred to as "educated trained assistants to the members of the established medical profession practicing only under the prescription of a licensed physician" in the following agencies:

- Muscle training
- Therapeutic massage
- Electrotherapy
- Light therapy
- Mechanotherapy
- Hydrotherapy

Much of the impetus behind the profession during these early years resulted from the high incidence of acute anterior poliomyelitis, referred to then as infantile paralysis, which occurred in 1916 (Figure 1-1). At that time, the primary modes of treatment for infantile paralysis included long-term splinting and casting to immobilize the limbs or the spine, combined with prolonged bed rest, while keeping the patient in quarantine and isolation. Predictably, these immobilizations and prolonged bed rests resulted in muscle atrophy and a loss of flexibility in the extremities of the patients. At this point in history, the majority of Americans regarded disability as irreversible, but that was about to change, as was the type of treatment offered.

Box 1-1

- Approximately 1000 BC: Taoist priests in China describe a type of exercise that involves body positioning and breathing routines to relieve pain and other symptoms.
- Approximately 500 BC: A Greek physician called Herodicus gives written descriptions about an elaborate system of exercises called Ars Gymnastica, which consisted of various gymnastic exercises.
- Approximately 400 BC: Hippocrates, who is considered the father of medicine, recommends the use of muscle strengthening exercises, an early form of transverse friction massage, and therapeutic massage. Hippocrates was also the first to use electrical stimulation.
- Approximately 180 BC: The ancient Romans introduce a series of therapeutic exercises that they called gymnastics.
- Approximately 200 AD: Galen, a renowned physician of ancient Rome, emphasizes the importance of moderate exercise to strengthen the body, increase body temperature, allow the pores of the skin to open, and to improve a person's spiritual well-being.
- Approximately 1400 AD: Therapeutic exercises are introduced into schools as physical education courses.

- Approximately 1500 AD: The first printed book on exercise is published in Spain.
- Approximately 1700 AD: Massage, hydrotherapy, and exercises performed en masse are first introduced in the United States.
- 1723 AD: Nicolas Andry, considered to be the grandfather of orthopedics, emphasizes the importance of exercise to cure many infirmities of the body.
- Mid-1700s AD: Exercise equipment appears on the market.
- 1800s AD: Introduction of Swedish exercise/gymnastics by Per Henrik Ling. These exercises are adapted by Dr. Johann Georg Mezger, who introduced the terms *effleurage*, *petrissage*, and *tapotement*, which became known as Swedish massage. In 1864, Gustav Zander introduced 71 different types of apparatus to assist in the performance of Swedish exercise/gymnastics and opened numerous Zander institutes throughout Europe and the United States. At the end of the 1800s, H. S. Frenkel introduced a series of neurological exercises and rehabilitation techniques to enhance coordination and gait in those patients with ataxia resulting from nerve cell destruction. Frenkel's exercises continue to be used today.

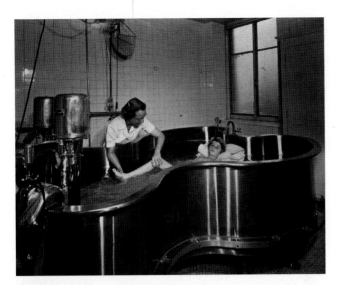

FIGURE 1-1 Early treatment approach to poliomyelitis

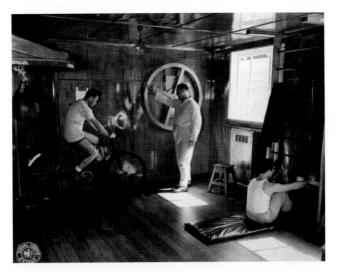

FIGURE 1-2 Exercises using machines

CLINICAL PEARL

Wilhelmine G. Wright developed the training technique of ambulation with crutches for patients who had paraplegia or paralysis caused by polio. She also introduced the concepts of manual muscle testing in physical therapy, which appeared in a book called *Muscle Function*. The book describes the systematic method of manual muscle testing using palpation, gravity, external manual resistance, and the arc of active movement. These concepts were later modified by clinicians, including Kendall, Brunnström, Dennen, and Worthingham, to include such variables as a patient's fatigue, body position, and incoordination.

The focus on different interventions for infantile paralysis resulted in a huge demand for muscle testing and muscle reeducation to restore function. Much of this emphasis on muscle testing and muscle reeducation was based on the work by Robert W. Lovett, a professor of orthopedic surgery at Harvard, who had discovered that muscle training exercises were the most important early therapeutic measures for polio treatment. Lovett organized teams of workers including physicians, nurses, and other nonphysician personnel. Included among the nonphysician personnel were three individuals—Wilhelmine Wright, Janet Merrill, and Alice Lou Plastridge—who received special training in massage, muscle training, and corrective exercises from Dr. Lovett.

The United States entered World War I by declaring war on Germany in 1917, and the Army recognized the need to rehabilitate soldiers injured in the war.[3] The U.S. Congress authorized the military draft and passed legislation to rehabilitate all servicemen permanently disabled from war-related injuries. Attention became focused on the use of multiple and combined methods to restore physical function in members of both the military forces and the civilian workforce under the umbrella term *physical reconstruction*. A report from the Division of Orthopedic Surgery called for the establishment of hospitals for the reconstruction of soldiers

with disabilities, and a national training corps for personnel (therapists). Physical reconstruction was defined as the "maximum mental and physical restoration of the individuals achieved by the use of medicine and surgery, supplemented by physical therapy, occupational therapy or curative workshop activities, education, recreation, and vocational training." Many of the exercises used were based on Ling's Swedish exercise/gymnastics and the use of Zander's exercise machines (Figure 1-2) (see Box 1-1). These exercise-based approaches and their subsequent outcomes began to change the belief that disability was irreversible.

CLINICAL PEARL

▶ Physical therapy practice in the United States evolved around two major historical events: the poliomyelitis epidemics of the 1800s through the 1950s and the effects of the ravages of several wars including World War I, World War II, and the Korean conflict.

▶ Historically, physical therapy emerged as a profession within the medical model, not as an alternative to medical care.[2]

The report from the Division of Orthopedic Surgery also suggested that standards be developed by the schools. In 1917, a special unit of the Army Medical Department, the Division of Special Hospitals and Physical Reconstruction, developed 15 "reconstruction aide" training programs to respond to the need for medical workers with expertise in rehabilitation to treat the more than 200,000 U.S. troops wounded in battle (Figure 1-3). Preference for applicants with high scholastic standing in the fundamentals of physical education demonstrated the importance that was placed on the knowledge of human movement. Individuals who completed the courses, and who worked in the Division of Special Hospitals and Physical Reconstruction in the Office of the Surgeon General, U.S. Army, were given the title Reconstruction Aide (those practitioners rendering similar service in civilian facilities were referred to as physical

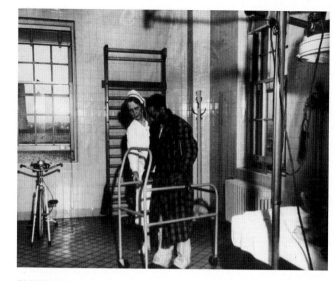

FIGURE 1-3 Gait training

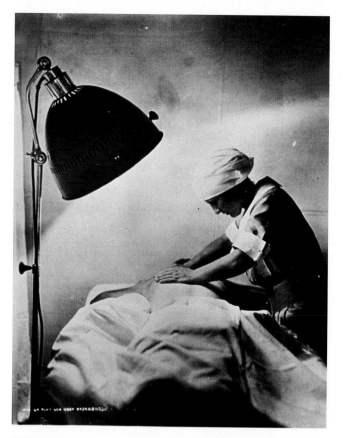

FIGURE 1-5 Massage therapy

therapy technicians, physiotherapy aides, and physiotherapy technicians). Two different groups of reconstruction aides were established.

1. Reconstruction aides/physical therapists who assisted physicians by providing exercise programs, hydrotherapy (Figure 1-4), and other modalities, and massage (Fig 1-5) for these patients.

2. Reconstruction aides/occupational therapists who had been working in alms houses and insane asylums and who were to provide training to patients in those vocational skills necessary for them to return to gainful employment.

Marguerite Sanderson and Mary McMillan were the first two individuals involved in the training of those reconstruction aides responsible for caring for individuals wounded during the war. Marguerite Sanderson was hired under this new division as director of the Reconstruction Aide Program in 1917 at Walter Reed General Hospital and was joined by Mary McMillan.

By 1918, outlines for a three-month course to be used in training programs had been developed to prepare practition-

ers who would serve, in a civilian capacity, as reconstruction aides in the recently established Division of Special Hospitals and Physical Reconstruction. The required subjects for this course included:

▶ Biological and physical sciences, including anatomy, physiology, chemistry, physics, and kinesiology

▶ Social sciences, including psychology and ethics

▶ Clinical sciences (physical therapy), including electrotherapy, exercise, hydrotherapy, light therapy, massage, thermotherapy, physical agents, tests and measures

▶ Clinical sciences (medical), including medicine, neurology, orthopedics, surgery, and pathology

CLINICAL PEARL

The terms *physiotherapy, physical therapy, physiotherapist,* and *physical therapist* were used in the United States until the 1950s to refer either to a medical specialty or to the physicians who practiced that specialty.

As World War I drew to a close, physical reconstruction practices, which had previously been directed toward preserving, restoring, and maintaining a fighting force, were directed toward preserving and maintaining a working force. Between 1919 in 1920, there was a major postwar decrease in large hospitals, whose numbers shrank from 748 to 49. The remaining hospitals had physiotherapy facilities and employed more than 700 reconstruction aides. Nearly 50,000 veterans, or almost half of those 125,000 Americans who were disabled during World War I, were treated at these facilities.[4]

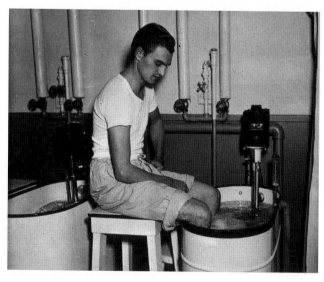

FIGURE 1-4 Early use of hydrotherapy

CLINICAL PEARL

The American Women's Physical Therapeutics Association (AWPTA) was founded in 1921.[5] Mary McMillan was elected the first president of the AWPTA by a mail-in vote. The first issue of the association's official publication, *The P.T. Review*, appeared on March 1, 1921. Today, the *P.T. Review* is called *Physical Therapy* and is the official publication of the APTA. The first edition of the P.T. Review reported the full text of the constitution and bylaws of the association, which promised:

▶ Professional and scientific standards for its members

▶ To increase competency among members by encouraging advanced studies

▶ To promulgate medical literature and articles of professional interest

▶ To make available efficiently trained members

▶ To sustain professional socialization

During the early years of the association, membership was open to nurses who had additional training in specific types of clinical experiences. From 1929 until 1933, an American Physical Therapy Association existed as an organization that was formed through the merger of two organizations of physicians, the Western Association of Physical Therapy and the American Electrotherapeutic Association. In 1922, at its first conference, the name of the American Women's Physical Therapeutics Association was changed to the American Physiotherapy Association (APA)[5] in recognition of the fact that men also practiced physiotherapy, and subsequently, in 1947, to its current name, the American Physical Therapy Association (APTA).[6]

In the early 1920s, the passage of the Rehabilitation Bill in New Jersey resulted in a growing enthusiasm about the future of rehabilitation and of "reconstruction aids or teachers of vocational and educational forms of work that are therapeutic in process." This resulted in a partnership of physical therapists with the medical and surgical communities and increased public recognition and validation of the profession of physical therapy.[3] In 1921, Mary McMillan published *Massage and Therapeutic Exercise*, the first textbook written by a physiotherapist.[7] McMillan referred to four distinct branches in physical therapeutics: massage, therapeutic exercise (Figure 1-6), electrotherapy, and hydrotherapy. Textbooks from the early years of the profession document the application of physical therapy for problems related to the musculoskeletal, neuromuscular, cardiovascular, pulmonary, integumentary, reproductive, renal, and psychogenic systems.

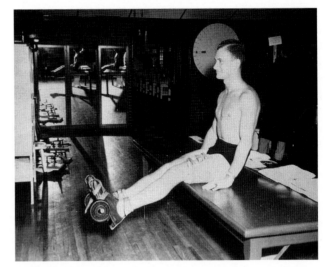

FIGURE 1-6 Therapeutic exercise

In 1924, Leo Buerger, a urologist, and Arthur W. Allen, a surgeon, created a series of exercises for patients with vascular disease, specifically arterial insufficiency in the legs, which used the application of the effects of gravity and posture on the vascular musculature and blood circulation.

Poliomyelitis continued to rage throughout the United States in the 1920s and 1930s, with the country witnessing an increase in both the incidence and magnitude of poliomyelitis outbreaks. During this period, the APA attempted to stay side-by-side with the medical profession. In 1925, a group of physical therapy physicians founded the American College of Physical Therapy (ACPT), and then established the American Registry of Physical Therapy Technicians for the purpose of conferring a registered title on physiotherapists who passed the test.[7] Under this arrangement, registered physiotherapists remained technicians under the supervision of physicians.[7] Later that year the ACPT joined the AMA and changed its name to the American Congress of Physical Therapy. By 1937, physical therapy physicians had achieved recognition as a medical specialty. At that time, in an effort to further distinguish themselves from physiotherapists, and in order to gain respect within the medical profession, the physical therapy physicians began to call themselves "physiatrists."[7] The AMA became concerned that the public might consider physiotherapists to be physicians. This concern led to a name change from physiotherapists to physical therapists in the early 1940s.

CLINICAL PEARL

Today, the APTA is the one national organization recognized as speaking for the profession of physical therapy. The association's members are physical therapists, physical therapist assistants, and students who voluntarily join. To join the association, an individual must be accepted, currently enrolled, or a graduate of an accredited physical therapy or physical therapist assistant program.

CLINICAL PEARL

Around 1934, Ernest A. Codman, a surgeon, introduced a series of shoulder exercises known as Codman pendulum exercises, which were based on the concept that a diseased supraspinatus muscle could relax if the shoulder is abducted in the stooping position. These exercises continue to be used today.

The advent of World War II resulted in an ever-increasing demand for physical therapy specialists. During this time, drastic improvements in medical management and surgical techniques led to increasing numbers of survivors, albeit with disabling war wounds.[8] Wounded veterans who returned home with amputations, burns, cold injuries, wounds, fractures, and nerve and spinal cord injuries required the attention of physical therapists in the first half of the 1940s, with World War II at its peak.[9] However, the principles of muscle training that had been used by reconstruction aides in World War I and for the treatment of polio were found to be ineffective for treating many of the problems associated with war-related injuries. The subsequent demand for more effective techniques propelled the practice of physical therapy through a major growth period as the attention switched to a focus on the application of neurophysiologic principles, which in turn prompted the advent of a number of techniques still used today, including progressive resistive exercise (PRE).

In 1945, Thomas DeLorme, a physician, first introduced the concept of PRE after using increasing resistance on himself following knee surgery.

CLINICAL PEARL

Immediately after World War II, $1 million was allocated by the U.S. government for the enhancement of prosthetic services, and physical therapists became integral elements of teaching and training programs for the management of patients with amputations.

The rehabilitation concepts introduced to treat those wounded in World War II fostered the growth of this new specialty of physical medicine, also referred to as rehabilitation medicine, or simply as rehabilitation.

The passage of the Hospital Survey and Construction Act of 1946, the "Hill–Burton Act," initiated a nationwide hospital-building program and increased public access to hospitals and healthcare facilities, which in turn led to an increase in hospital-based practice for physical therapists. To this day, the hospital has continued to be the primary setting for the services of therapeutic intervention provided by a physical therapist, with up to 50% of active physical therapists currently practicing in a hospital setting.

Because of the increased need for physical therapists and the discontinuation of the army-based schools, the Schools Section of the APTA, which recognized the need to educate more physical therapists, made recommendations about admissions, curricula, education, and administration of physical therapy programs, and the APTA embarked on an effort to encourage more universities and medical schools to create programs and expand existing programs, including creating opportunities for graduate-level education.[10]

CLINICAL PEARL

After World War II, a large number of patients who had sustained brain injuries sought the services of physical therapists. Signe Brunnström, a Swedish physical therapist, documented new approaches for the assessment and treatment of individuals with cerebrovascular accidents and, after observing thousands of patients, delineated the stages of stroke recovery.[11] Also, during this time, Berta Bobath and Dr. Karl Bobath began to develop their reflex-inhibiting postures for the management of children with cerebral palsy, which utilized specialized handling techniques to decrease tone and stiffness, to increase muscle control against gravity, and to help stabilize muscle activity.[12]

The role of the physical therapist progressed further in the 1950s from that of a technician to a professional practitioner.[7]

The outbreak of the Korean War in 1950 involved the United States in yet another war effort.[7] In addition, poliomyelitis continued to afflict thousands of Americans. As the practice of physical therapy evolved, aides, attendants, and volunteers began to provide valuable assistance in direct care of the large numbers of persons injured in the war and those who had poliomyelitis during the epidemics. These individuals assisted patients before and after treatment, performed general housekeeping duties, and were involved in the routine maintenance of equipment and supplies. It is during this time that Margaret Rood, a physical therapist and occupational therapist, broke new ground in the treatment of individuals with central nervous system (CNS) disorders.[13] In an effort to discover a vaccine that would prevent polio, massive national field trials were organized. These trials, from the research that had been initiated in earnest in the 1940s, bore fruit when, in 1955, Jonas Salk developed such a vaccine, and massive vaccination programs were initiated. In 1957, Albert Sabin developed an oral vaccine using attenuated poliovirus, which was licensed in 1962.

The 1950s decade was a pivotal time for the physical therapy profession in terms of gaining independence, autonomy, and professionalism.

CLINICAL PEARL

► In the beginning of the 1950s, a neurophysiologist named Herman Kabat introduced the neurological concepts of tonic neck reflex, flexion reflex, and stretch reflex and applied these concepts to develop neurological exercises called proprioceptive facilitation. In 1956, Margaret Knott and Dorothy Voss[14] expanded on this work, and similar work by Gessell, Hellebrandt, Hooker, Rabat, McGraw, and Sherrington, and established the concepts of proprioceptive neuromuscular facilitation (PNF) as a treatment for patients with paralysis.

► In 1953, Paul C. Williams introduced a series of postural exercises, known today as the Williams exercises, which were designed to strengthen the spine flexors and extensors and relieve back pain.

► In the 1950s and 1960s, Robin McKenzie pioneered a series of back extension exercises that complemented the Williams exercises.

Two events in the 1950s contributed to the progression of the physical therapist from technician to professional practitioner[10]:

▶ The Self-Employed Section formed as a component of the APTA in 1955 as private practice expanded.

▶ The Physical Therapy Fund, created in 1957, fostered science through research and education within the profession.

Pursuing a replacement to the system of registration that had been fashioned through the American Medical Association (AMA), which required a questionable assessment of professional competence in physical therapy, the APTA pressed its state chapters to seek licensure through the states, and by 1950, Connecticut, Maryland, and Washington had adopted physical therapy practice acts, joining New York and Pennsylvania, whose initial licensing efforts dated back to 1926 and 1913, respectively.[2,10]

CLINICAL PEARL

During the late 1950s and into the 1960s, increasing numbers of states enacted state licensure laws for physical therapists, and in 1954, a seven-hour professional competency exam was developed by the APTA in conjunction with the Professional Examination Service of the American Public Health Association.[7] By 1959, 45 states and the territory of Hawaii had physical therapy practice acts in place.[5]

The 1960s brought profound changes in the U.S. healthcare system as increasing numbers of states began to enact a number of practice acts.[5] In addition, the polio vaccines had virtually eradicated poliomyelitis in the United States by 1961. While some physical therapists continued to treat those patients with poliomyelitis, many others began focusing their efforts on the management of many other types of disabling conditions.

The earlier efforts to gain state licensure clearly influenced the Medicare program in 1967 and 1968 as the majority of states had licensure laws by this time, which regulated the practice of physical therapy and the services provided by physical therapists. Amendments to the Social Security Act (SSA) in 1967 added a definition of "outpatient physical therapy services." This meant that the Social Security organization recognized physical therapy services as a healthcare provider for reimbursement. This amendment also resulted in dramatic changes to the practice of physical therapy for patients with neuromuscular disorders. Influenced by the earlier work of Margaret Rood, Margaret Knott, Dorothy Voss, and Signe Brunnström, Berta and Karl Bobath developed techniques for adults with a cerebrovascular accident (stroke), cerebral palsy, and other disorders of the central nervous system.[9] Since that time, the physical therapy profession has continued to expand its treatment areas, which has led to the need for specializations.

CLINICAL PEARL

The APTA currently recognizes the following 18 specialty sections as part of the professional organization of physical therapy:

▶ Acute care
▶ Aquatic physical therapy
▶ Cardiopulmonary and pulmonary
▶ Clinical electrophysiology and wound management
▶ Education
▶ Federal physical therapy
▶ Geriatrics
▶ Hand rehabilitation
▶ Health policy and administration
▶ Home health
▶ Neurology
▶ Oncology
▶ Orthopedics
▶ Pediatrics
▶ Private practice
▶ Research
▶ Sports physical therapy
▶ Women's health

In the late 1960s and early 1970s, open-heart surgery became possible, and the physical therapy profession expanded the cardiovascular/pulmonary area of its practice with increasing chest physical therapy programs for pre- and postoperative patients. In the orthopedic practice arena, there was an expansion of joint replacements, resulting in the emergence of new avenues for orthopedic physical therapist practice through the introduction of new options for patients with severe joint restrictions to live more independent and pain-free lives. During this time, technological advances provided new testing methodologies and options to improve patient function, which allowed physical therapists new opportunities to develop more objective outcome measures, new intervention strategies, and an increase in the types of diseases and conditions that physical therapy could positively influence.

CLINICAL PEARL

▶ The APTA House of Delegates adopted the Physical Therapist Assistant (PTA) Policy, and affiliate membership was granted to PTAs in 1973.

▶ The APTA House of Delegates adopted its first Standards for Services and Practice in 1975.

▶ The first Combined Sections Meeting was held in Washington, DC, in 1976.

▶ The PT Fund became the Foundation for Physical Therapy in 1979.

The 1970s and 1980s saw an increase in opportunities for practice with the implementation of Occupational Safety and Health Administration (OSHA) rules and regulations, the passage of the Education for All Handicapped Children Act (PL 94-142), and the epidemic spread of acquired immunodeficiency syndrome (AIDS). OSHA was formed for the prevention, management, and compensation of on-the-job injuries. The AIDS epidemic resulted in physical therapists once again providing services to patients with multisystem involvement. In addition, physical therapists began providing services in the areas of women's health, oncology, and hand rehabilitation.

In the early 1980s, the APTA adopted a policy indicating that "physical therapy practice independent of practitioner referral was ethical as long as it was legal in the state."[9]

The first examinations for specialist certification were taken in 1985 by three physical therapists who became members of the American Board for Physical Therapy Specialties—certified cardiopulmonary specialists.[7] These specialist certifications were followed by clinical electrophysiology, pediatric, neurology, sports, and orthopedic certifications.[7] Also significant during this time was the formation of the Federation of State Boards of Physical Therapy (FSBPT) in 1986, providing an organization through which member licensing authorities could coordinate to promote and protect the health, welfare, and safety of American communities.[2]

Substantial changes in the healthcare delivery system in the United States required a major association focus in the 1990s, influencing the practice of physical therapy in ways that continue today.[2] The Americans with Disabilities Act (ADA) and the National Center for Medical Rehabilitation Research (NCMRR) led to new opportunities for practice. Physical therapists were faced with the challenges of increasing governmental cost savings, decreasing reimbursement, increasing governmental regulations, the influences of the insurance industry and corporate America, and the sudden personnel supply exceeding demand for services.[7]

In August 1997, President Clinton signed the Balanced Budget Act (BBA) to eliminate the Medicare deficit. The BBA, which took effect in January 1999, applied an annual cap of $1500 (for both physical therapy and speech therapy services) per beneficiary for all outpatient rehabilitation services. These changes had a dramatic effect, reducing rehabilitation services to Medicare patients. In November 1999, because of increasing pressure from the public, President Clinton signed the Refinement Act, which suspended the $1500 cap for two years in all rehabilitation settings starting on January 3, 2000.

CLINICAL PEARL

The 1990s introduced some major changes in the healthcare delivery system, including Managed Care, point-of-service plans, and other alternative organizational structures (see Chapter 2). In addition, skilled nursing facilities were affected by the following regulations[7]:

▶ *PPS:* Medicare Prospective Payment System. A PPS is a method of Medicare reimbursement that is intended to motivate providers to deliver patient care efficiently, effectively, and without an overutilization of services in hospitals, skilled nursing facilities (SNFs), and home health agencies. The payment is based on a unique assessment classification of each patient, and the payment amount for a particular service is derived based on a classification system (e.g., per diem or per stay).

▶ *MDS:* Minimum Data Set. MDS is part of a federally mandated process for all residents in Medicare- or Medicaid-certified nursing facilities regardless of the source of payment for the individual resident. The MDS is a comprehensive resident assessment instrument (RAI) that measures functional status, mental health status, and behavioral status to identify chronic-care patient needs and formalize a care plan in response to 18 Resident Assessment Protocols (RAPs). Under federal regulation, assessments are conducted at the time of admission into a nursing facility, on return from a 72-hour hospital admission, whenever there is a significant change in status, quarterly, and annually. In the majority of cases, participants in the assessment process are licensed health care professionals employed by the facility. Data collected from the MDS assessments are used for the Medicare reimbursement system, many state Medicaid reimbursement systems, and to monitor the quality of care provided to nursing facility residents.

▶ *RUGs (Resources Utilization Groups):* A RUG is a mutually exclusive category that reflects various levels of resource need in a long-term care (LTC) setting. These categories, which are assigned to individuals based on data elements derived from the LTC Minimum Data Set (MDS), are primarily used to facilitate Medicare and Medicaid payment. Each RUG, which is organized in a hierarchical fashion, is associated with relative weighting factors. A number of RUGs have evolved over the years:

  ▪ *RUG 34:* An initial set of RUGs that was developed primarily to support resource risk adjustment for Medicaid payment.

  ▪ *RUG 44:* An expanded version of RUG 34 that included 14 Rehab RUGs and a new hierarchical order primarily to support Medicare PPS starting in 1998.

  ▪ *RUG 53:* An expanded version of RUG 44 that included nine mixed Rehab and Extensive Service RUGs, which were used to support Medicare PPS since January 2006.

▶ *OBRA:* Omnibus Budget Reconciliation Act of 1987. OBRA requires a comprehensive assessment of all nursing facility residents within 14 days of admission, a quarterly assessment (within 92 days) thereafter, and an annual full assessment (within 366 days of prior full assessment).

Prompted by a need to formally define the role of the physical therapist and to describe the practice of physical therapy, the *Guide to Physical Therapist Practice* (the Guide) was created.[15] This model for physical therapist practice was adopted in 1997 and the *Guide to Physical Therapist Practice*, published in 1999 introduced the terminology of examination, evaluation, diagnosis, prognosis, intervention, reexamination, and the assessment of outcomes.[7]

CLINICAL PEARL

Physical therapy is one of the few healthcare professions that is integrated into the majority of the federal programs that provide healthcare services to U.S. veterans, members of the armed services, individuals with disabilities who have been harmed by natural disasters and public health threats, and Native Americans. Additionally, the Department of Veterans Affairs (VA) is one of the largest employers of physical therapists nationwide.[2]

Thus, throughout the 20th century, biomedicine was the dominant model of medical care with its focus on an impairment model. During this time, healthcare priorities shifted from the prevention, cure, and management of acute infectious conditions to the present-day focus on the prevention, cure, and management of lifestyle conditions such as hypertension, obesity, and metabolic syndrome (a group of risk factors that occur together and increase the risk for coronary artery disease, cerebrovascular accident, and type 2 diabetes).[16]

With the arrival of the 21st century, a vastly revised version of the *Guide to Physical Therapist Practice* was published in 2001.[1] Continued development of the Guide led to the development of an interactive CD-ROM version that included the specifics of all the tests and measures used in the physical therapist examination process.[7]

The Guide is divided into two parts:

▸ Part I delineates the physical therapist's scope of practice and describes patient management by physical therapists (PTs).
▸ Part II describes each of the diagnostic preferred practice patterns of patients typically treated by PTs.

That same year, the "Hooked on Evidence" project was developed to facilitate increasing practice based on evidence, when available. Legislation was introduced in 2001 in the House of Representatives to allow Medicare patients direct access to physical therapist services.[7]

The impetus behind these publications and legislations was driven by a combination of increased life expectancy, end-of-life morbidity, and thus prolonged disability. Unfortunately, it had also become apparent that many of the lifestyle conditions that had only affected adults, such as heart disease,

type 2 diabetes, and obesity, were now affecting the pediatric population. In an effort to combat these lifestyle conditions, it was necessary to shift the focus from symptom reduction with drugs and surgery to one that addressed their causes through prevention at both the individual and societal levels. It became clear that many of the most common lifestyle conditions were preventable, and in some cases reversible, with removal of their associated risk factors (Table 1-1).

The environment in which physical therapists practice continues to be subjected to the push and pull of multiple forces. These forces include[17]:

▸ Ethical considerations, including patient confidentiality and informed consent
▸ Societal and cultural beliefs and values
▸ Population demographics
▸ The economy
▸ Governmental legislation, rules, and regulations
▸ Public and private organizations and agencies
▸ Scientific and technological advances

Given that most people have one or more risk factors or adverse manifestations of lifestyle conditions, strategies to address these conditions in the 21st century have included multiple health behavior change strategies and evidence-informed interventions. These strategies are targeted at the individual based on an assessment of health and risk factors.[18] To be equipped to address present-day health issues, the contemporary physical therapist needs sufficient clinical competencies, knowledge, and expertise to serve as the primary caregiver with respect to smoking cessation, basic nutritional recommendations, weight control, regular physical activity guidelines, exercise prescription, stress and sleep management, and recommendations for moderate rather than excessive alcohol consumption.[16] These non-invasive interventions will play an increasingly important role as the profession progresses through the 21st century.

The growing responsibility for physical therapists in patient care has led the APTA to develop a vision statement known as Vision 2020, which states, "By 2020, physical therapy will be provided by physical therapists who are doctors of physical therapy, recognized by consumers and other healthcare professionals as practitioners of choice to whom consumers have direct access for the diagnosis of, interventions for, and prevention of impairments, functional limitations, and

TABLE 1-1	Six Major Risk Factors Related to Lifestyle Conditions				
Risk Factor	Cancer	Obstructive Lung Disease	Stroke	Diabetes	Cardiovascular Disease
Physical inactivity	■		■	■	■
Obesity	■	■	■	■	
Smoking	■	■	■	■	■
Hypertension			■	■	■
Dietary fat (saturated and trans-fats)	■		■	■	■
Alcohol			■	■	■

THE PROFESSION

9

disabilities related to movement, function, and health." The year 2020 is fast approaching, necessitating continual changes in the preparation of students to become physical therapists and physical therapist assistants. For Vision 2012 to be realized, there are six key elements:

1. *Autonomous practice.* The physical therapist is solely responsible for the patient's physical therapy diagnosis, evaluation, intervention, and outcomes from the treatment. It is important to note that with this autonomy comes accountability and increased liability exposure.

2. *Direct access.* This is a situation in which a state's licensure laws allow a physical therapist to evaluate and treat a patient without the requirement of the physician's referral or prescription. At the time of writing, 43 states now have some type of direct access. For this to be effective, physical therapists must recognize the parameters associated within the scope of practice.

3. *Doctor of physical therapy.* By the year 2020, practicing physical therapists will have obtained a doctorate degree in physical therapy. This doctoral degree can take two forms:

   ▶ An academic doctoral degree (PhD) in physical therapy

   ▶ A transitional doctoral degree (DPT or tDPT) in physical therapy

4. *Evidence-based practice.* The goal is to provide the most cost-effective and beneficial treatment based on research. The APTA's Hooked on Evidence program now provides a platform called "Open Door: APTA's Portal to Evidence-based Practice" to help members obtain this goal.

5. *Practitioner of choice.* The goal for this is that physical therapists and physical therapist assistants will be the consumer's first choice for treatment of movement dysfunction, dysfunction related to pain, and restoration of function lost to diseases and disabilities. As with autonomy of practice, this describes a situation in which there is no one overseeing the evaluation of services the physical therapist provides, which increases therapist liability.

6. *Professionalism.* The APTA has identified seven core values of professionalism in physical therapy:

   ▶ Accountability

   ▶ Altruism

   ▶ Compassion/caring

   ▶ Excellence

   ▶ Integrity

   ▶ Professional duty

   ▶ Social responsibility

THE EDUCATION OF THE PHYSICAL THERAPIST

Over more than a century, physical therapy education has evolved from early training programs for reconstruction aides to its current status as the doctor of physical therapy (DPT) degree.[19] As mentioned in the History section, the early beginnings of the profession emerged from the U.S. Army's Division of Special Hospitals and Physical Reconstruction, Office of the Surgeon General, which established an education program with focuses on anatomy and exercise. Graduates of this program were given the official title of "reconstruction aide."[20] By 1918, a number of educational institutions worked in partnership with the Army to expand the program to a 6-month, intensive, certificate-granting physical therapy program that focused more on the study of technical skills. Then, in 1928, the APA established the first Minimum Standards for an Acceptable School for Physical Therapy Technicians, which included a 9-month program of instruction. The prerequisite for admission to this program was graduation from a recognized school of physical education or nursing.[6]

CLINICAL PEARL

Physical therapist education programs have been reviewed and recognized in some manner since 1928, beginning with approval by the American Physiotherapy Association (APA).

These requirements continued for almost a decade until, in 1936, the AMA established the Essentials for an Acceptable School for Physical Therapy Technicians, and the first 13 institutions were accredited.[5] During the next 25 years, the various physical therapist programs offered certificates, a certificate or baccalaureate degree, or a baccalaureate degree. By the 1960s there were more patients with complex and multisystem dysfunctions that called for advanced problem-solving and analytical skills on the part of the physical therapist.[2] These requirements resulted in changes in the school curricula, with the addition of neuroanatomy, neurophysiology, psychology of individuals with disabilities, research, education, administration, and management classes, and resulted in the baccalaureate degree becoming the minimum required qualification.[5]

Postprofessional advanced degrees for physical therapists began to emerge in the 1960s, with schools offering a master's degree program, and by the mid-1960s a number of schools were offering postprofessional PhD programs.

Over the past few decades a number of legislative and healthcare industry changes have provided physical therapists with greater autonomy within their scope of practice, further expansion of settings in areas of practice, and greater autonomy for the physical therapist to practice without a physician referral to varying degrees.[8] To address the new demand for knowledge, skills, and professional behaviors, in 1979, the APTA adopted a resolution to require a postbaccalaureate degree to enter physical therapy beginning in 1990, although in reality, it took 23 years to complete the full transition.[8] To help augment this transition, two APTA documents were introduced[2]:

▶ The *Guide to Physical Therapist Practice* (*Volume I: A Description of Patient Management* published in August 1995 and *Volumes I and II: Preferred Practice Patterns* published in November 1997).[1] This document described the breadth, depth, and scope of physical therapist practice across the various systems and life span, and outlined the physical therapist's role in patient/client management.

▶ *A Normative Model of Physical Therapist Professional Education.*[3] This document defined the preferred curricular content in the foundation, behavioral, and clinical sciences; entry-level practice expectations and associated curricular content; clinical education; and noncurricular components (i.e., educational settings, admissions criteria, and qualifications and role of faculty and program administrators).

The rather quick transition to the Doctor of Physical Therapy (DPT) degree began to occur in 1995–1996. This transition is thought to have occurred for a number of reasons[2]:

▶ The expanding needs of society for physical therapy services in a broad range of settings

▶ Greater evidence available about physical therapy interventions

▶ Increased competition among programs for high-quality applicants

▶ Augmentation in required basic and applied science curricular coursework

▶ Lengthening of clinical internships

▶ To prepare for contemporary and future healthcare needs

The voluntary transition to the DPT degree has moved very rapidly, with 96.7% of accredited programs offering the DPT as of August 2010.[21]

Accreditation

Between 1933 and 1956, at the APA's invitation, the AMA Council on Medical Education reviewed and approved PT education programs. Between 1957 and 1976 the AMA and the APTA had first informal and then formal collaborative arrangements for accreditation based on the AMA's 1955 revision of the *Essentials of an Acceptable School of Physical Therapy.*[2] In 1977, the APTA severed their relationship with the AMA by creating a new accrediting body: the Commission on Accreditation in Physical Therapy Education (CAPTE). Since that time, CAPTE has been recognized by the U.S. Department of Education (USDE) to accredit physical therapy (physical therapist and physical therapist assistant) programs.[2] In the private sector, CAPTE has been recognized continuously since 1977, first by the Council for Post-Secondary Accreditation (COPA), then by the short-lived Council for Recognition of Post-Secondary Accreditation (CORPA), and currently by the Council for Higher Education Accreditation (CHEA).[2]

As of January 1, 2002, CAPTE took the step of no longer accrediting baccalaureate physical therapy programs. The rationale for this was that the amount of information that physical therapy students were required to learn was beyond the scope of a baccalaureate program.

The *Evaluative Criteria for Accreditation of Education Programs for the Preparation of Physical Therapists* used by CAPTE to assess the quality of physical therapist education programs are organized around two major components[2]:

1. *Integrity and capacity of the institution and program.* The evaluative criteria address a number of program characteristics, including institutional integrity and capacity, program integrity and capacity, curriculum, and outcomes.

2. *Curriculum content and outcomes.* CAPTE's Evaluated Criteria include a list of 98 skills that graduates of accredited physical therapist programs are expected to possess, which it subdivides into three groupings:

▶ Professional practice expectations

▶ Patient/client management expectations

▶ Practice management expectations

These competencies form the basis of CAPTE's evaluative criteria regarding curriculum content. In such competency-based curricula, the emphasis is less on the courses offered, or how the content is delivered, and more on the outcomes of the educational efforts.[2]

THE PRACTICE OF PHYSICAL THERAPY

The following descriptions of physical therapist practice are based on the *Guide to Physical Therapist Practice.*[22]

Role in Patient/Client Management

A physical therapist provides care to patients/clients of all ages who have impairments, activity limitations, and participation restrictions due to musculoskeletal, neuromuscular, cardiovascular/pulmonary, and/or integumentary disorders.

Following the patient/client management model (described in Chapter 5), a physical therapist designs an individualized plan of care (POC) based on clinical judgment and the patient/client goals.

To facilitate communication among healthcare disciplines, the APTA has adopted the World Health Organization's International Classification of Functioning, Disability and Health (ICF) to provide a standardized language and framework for the description of health and functioning (see Chapter 5).

Role in Prevention and Risk Reduction

A physical therapist provides prevention services and promotes health and fitness by helping prevent a targeted health condition in a susceptible or potentially susceptible population or individual through risk identification and mitigation strategies.

In such specific populations, a physical therapist can decrease the duration, severity, and the sequelae of health conditions through prompt intervention.

Finally, a physical therapist plays an important role in limiting a person's degree of disability, through the restoration and maintenance of function in patients/clients with chronic health conditions to allow optimal performance and participation.

Additional Clinical and Nonclinical Roles

A physical therapist may assume additional clinical and nonclinical roles, which can include consultation, education, research, and administration to health facilities, educational programs (e.g., public schools), colleagues, businesses, industries, third-party payers, families and caregivers, and community organizations and agencies.

A physical therapist may also provide education and other professional services to patients/clients, students, facility staff, communities, and organizations and agencies and may also engage in research activities, including those related to measuring and improving the outcomes of service provision.

A physical therapist administrates in practice, research, and education settings and is involved in shaping community services and policies.

Standards of Practice

It is the role of the primary representative body for the physical therapy profession, the APTA, to outline and promote the expected level of quality of care for that profession. The APTA's commitment to society is to promote optimal health and functioning in individuals by pursuing excellence in care.[2] To that end, the APTA has established the Standards of Practice for Physical Therapy (see Appendix A) and the corresponding Criteria for Standards of Practice in Physical Therapy (see Appendix B). These are the profession's statements of conditions and performances that are essential for high-quality professional service to individuals in society and the necessary foundation for the assessment of physical therapy.

Code of Ethics

It is generally recognized that a code of ethics is important to professions, professionals, and the public, such that every clinician–patient interaction should be performed with a high degree of professionalism.

CLINICAL PEARL

A profession is an occupation that regulates itself through systematic, required training and collegial discipline; that has a base in technical, specialized knowledge; and that has a service rather than a profit orientation, enshrined in its code of ethics.[23]

Professionalism enhances trust. Throughout the history of physical therapy, physical therapists have always been concerned about the ethics of their profession. A formal set of ethical principles was first adopted by members of the APA in 1935. The four principles listed covered professional practice, advertising, behavior, and discipline. In effect, the 1935 Code of Ethics sacrificed professional autonomy for stability in their relations with the medical profession.[24] Since then, the code of ethics has undergone a number of revisions and expansions. The Guide for Professional Conduct was issued by the Ethics and Judicial Committee of the American Physical Therapy Association in 1981 (last amended in January 2004) and published in the *Guide to Professional Conduct*, APTA.[22] In June 2009, the House of Delegates (HOD) of the APTA passed a major revision of the APTA Code of Ethics for physical therapists (see Appendix C) and the Standards of Ethical Conduct for the Physical Therapist Assistant (see Appendix D). The revised documents were effective July 1, 2010. It may be that the 2009 revision of the core ethics documents represents the culmination of an increasing awareness within the profession and the professional organization of the ethical implications of the maturation of the profession.[24]

A number of authors have elaborated on the purposes of a professional code of ethics, putting forth such descriptions as "providing a vocabulary for intraprofessional argument, self-criticism, and reform,"[25] and "a profession's code of ethics is perhaps its most visible and explicit enunciation of its professional norms."[26] A code not only embodies the collective conscience of a profession and is testimony to the group's recognition of its moral dimension,[24] but also serves as a set of broad moral guidelines and as a public document stating the moral commitments of a group at a period in time.

CLINICAL PEARL

Some professions and institutions distinguish between "codes of ethics" and "codes of conduct." When this distinction is made, the code of ethics typically outlines the general ethical principles or ideals, and the code of conduct provides specific rules for behavior.[24,27]

Two words that are commonly used when describing an individual's attitude and behavior are *morals* and *ethics*.

- *Morals.* Morals are the attitudes and behaviors that society agrees on as desirable and necessary for maximizing the realization of things cherished most in that society.[28] Within healthcare, the basic moral is to do no harm. Other examples include honesty, the rights of a patient to his or her life and autonomy, and character traits such as compassion, empathy, and conscientiousness.

- *Ethics.* Ethics is the study of morals and moral judgments. At its basic level, it is the study of right and wrong. An ethical dilemma is a situation in which there is no right answer.

CLINICAL PEARL

It is possible to act morally but still be confronted with ethical dilemmas.

Practice Settings

Physical therapists practice in a broad range of inpatient, outpatient, and community-based settings. At a fundamental level, healthcare is divided into three levels: primary, secondary, and tertiary.

- *Primary care.* This level of care, which accounts for 80% to 90% of visits to a physician or other caregiver, involves basic or entry-level healthcare, which includes diagnostic, therapeutic (e.g., diabetes, arthritis, or hypertension) or preventive services (e.g., vaccinations or mammograms) for common health problems. The care is provided on an outpatient basis by primary-care physicians (PCPs), including family practice physicians, internists, and pediatricians. These physicians often serve as *gatekeepers* to other subspecialists, such as physical therapy. The physical therapist serves a supportive role for the primary care teams by providing an examination, evaluation, physical therapy diagnosis, prognosis, and intervention for musculoskeletal and neuromuscular dysfunctions.

- *Secondary care.* Secondary care services are provided by medical specialists (e.g., orthopedists, cardiologists, urologists, or dermatologists) for problems that require more specialized clinical expertise. This second level of care may require inpatient hospitalization or ambulatory same-day surgery. Physical therapy involvement varies according to how much the patient's condition affects his or her function.

- *Tertiary care.* This level of care involves the management of rare and complex disorders (e.g., pituitary tumors, organ transplants, major surgical procedures, or congenital malformations) that require sophisticated technologies. At this level of care, physical therapy may be prescribed on an as needed basis.

Hospital

A hospital is an institution whose primary function is to provide inpatient diagnostic and therapeutic services for a wide variety of medical, surgical, and nonsurgical conditions. In addition, most hospitals provide some outpatient services, particularly emergency care. Hospitals may be classified in a number of ways, including by:

- Length of stay (short-term or long-term):
  - *Acute-care (short-term hospital).* An acute-care hospital can be defined as a facility that provides hospital care to patients who generally require a stay of up to 7 days, but less than 30 days, and whose focus is on a physical or mental condition requiring an immediate intervention and constant medical attention, equipment, and personnel. The goal of a hospital is for rapid discharge to the next level of care (to home or to another healthcare facility), and the physical therapist's recommendation is often very important in the discharge planning.
  - *Subacute (long-term).* Medical care is provided to medically unstable patients who cannot return home. Required services (medical, nursing, rehabilitative) are provided within a hospital or skilled nursing facility.

- Teaching or nonteaching hospital.
  - *Teaching:* A hospital that serves as a teaching site for medicine, dentistry, allied health, nursing programs, or medical residency programs
  - *Nonteaching:* A hospital that has no teaching responsibilities, or one that serves as an elective site for health-related programs

- *Major types of services:* psychiatric, tuberculosis, burn, general, and other specialties, such as maternity, pediatric, or ear, nose, and throat (ENT).

- *Type of ownership or control:* federal, state, or local government; for-profit or nonprofit.

Home Healthcare

Home healthcare involves the provision of medical or health-related care by a home health agency (HHA), which may be governmental, voluntary, or private; nonprofit or for-profit. Home care services were introduced to reduce the need for hospitalization and its associated costs. A HHA provides part-time and intermittent skilled and nonskilled services and other therapeutic services on a visiting basis to persons of all ages in their homes. Patient eligibility includes:

- Any patient who is homebound or who has great difficulty leaving the home. A person may leave home for medical treatment or short infrequent nonmedical absences such as a religious service, dialysis, or a hairdresser/barber.

- *Medicaid waiver clients.* The Medicaid Waiver for the Elderly and Disabled (E&D Waiver) program is designed to provide services to seniors and the disabled whose needs would otherwise require them to live in a nursing home. The goal is for clients to retain their independence by providing services that allow them to live safely in their own homes and communities for as long as it is appropriate.

- A patient who requires skilled care from one of the following disciplines: nursing, physical therapy, occupational therapy, or speech therapy. The home health services provided by intermittent skilled nursing (<7 days/wk; <8 hours a day) include:
  - Observation and assessment
  - Teaching and training

- Complex care plan management and evaluation
- Administration of certain medications
- Tube feedings
- Wound care, catheters and ostomy care
- Nasopharyngeal and tracheostomy aspiration/care
- Rehabilitation nursing

▶ *Physician certification.* In the case of an elderly patient, recertification by Medicare is required every 60 days. Medicare only pays for skilled home health services that are provided by a Medicare-certified agency. Medicare defines *intermittent* as skilled nursing care needed or given for less than 7 days each week or less than eight hours per day over a period of 21 days (or less), with some exceptions in special circumstances. A patient must have a face-to-face encounter in 90-days prior or 30-days after the start of home health care with a physician, advanced practice nurse, or a physician assistant related to the condition(s) that necessitate home health care

▶ Patients who continue to demonstrate the potential for progress.

The physical therapy focus includes:

▶ Environmental safety, including proper lighting, securing scatter rugs, handrails, wheelchair ramps, and raised toilet seats

▶ Early intervention (refer to the following section, School System)

▶ Addressing equipment needs:
  - Equipment ordered in the hospital is reimbursable.
  - Adaptive equipment ordered in the home is not reimbursable except for items such as wheelchairs, commodes, and hospital beds.

▶ Observing for any evidence of substance abuse, or physical abuse:
  - Substance abuse should be reported immediately to the physician.
  - Physical abuse should be immediately communicated to the proper authorities (varies from state to state).

School System

The major goal of physical therapy intervention in the school is to enhance the child's level of function in the school setting—the physical therapist serves as a consultant to teachers working with children with disabilities in the classroom. Recommendations are made for adaptive equipment to facilitate improved posture, head control, and function.

▶ *Early Intervention Program (EIP).* National program designed for infants and toddlers with disabilities and their families.

▶ The EIP was created by Congress in 1986 under the Individuals with Disabilities Education Act (IDEA). To be eligible for services, children must be less than 3 years of age and have a confirmed disability, or established developmental delay, as defined by the state, in one or more of the following areas of development: physical, cognitive, communication, social-emotional, and/or adaptive.

Therapeutic and support services include:

▶ Family education and counseling, home visits, and parent support groups
▶ Special instruction
▶ Speech pathology and audiology
▶ Occupational therapy
▶ Physical therapy
▶ Psychological services
▶ Service coordination
▶ Nursing services
▶ Nutrition services
▶ Social work services
▶ Vision services
▶ Assistive technology devices and services

Private Practice

Private practice settings are privately owned and freestanding independent physical therapy practices.

▶ Practice settings vary from physical therapy and orthopedic clinics, to rehabilitation agencies.

▶ Documentation is required every visit, and reevaluations are required by Medicare every 30 days for reimbursement purposes.

Other healthcare facilities in which a physical therapist can practice are described in Table 1-2.

THE HEALTHCARE TEAM

As a physical therapist begins a career in healthcare, he or she becomes part of the healthcare team, the extent of which depends on the type of facility. It is important that the student physical therapist has an understanding of the various members of the healthcare team in terms of their roles and capabilities.

Primary Care Physician (PCP)

A practitioner, usually an internist, general practitioner, or family medicine physician, providing primary care services and managing routine healthcare needs. Most PCPs serve as gatekeepers for the managed-care health organizations—they provide authorization for referrals to other specialty physicians or services, including physical therapy. State medical boards require that physicians applying for license should document a passing grade on national licensing examinations, certification of graduation from medical school, and, in most cases, completion of at least one year of residency training after medical school.

Physician Assistant (PA)

As the name suggests, a physician assistant (PA) works closely with physicians, especially in primary care fields and underserved communities. A PA can perform physical examinations, make a diagnosis, prescribe medications, and

TABLE 1-2	Physical Therapist Practice Settings	
Setting	**Characteristics**	**Physical Therapist Role**
Transitional care unit	▶ Non–medically based facility, which may be in a group home or part of a continuum of a rehabilitation center. ▶ Typical stay is 4–8 months with discharge to home, assisted living facility, or skilled nursing facility (SNF). ▶ Greater focus placed on compensation versus restoration.	Physical therapy emphasis is on improving functional skills for maximum independence to prepare a patient for community reentry or for transfer to an assisted-living/skilled nursing facility.
Skilled nursing/ Extended care facility (ECF)	▶ Freestanding facility or part of a hospital that is licensed and approved by the state (Medicare certified). ▶ Eligible individuals receive skilled nursing care and appropriate rehabilitative and restorative services. ▶ Accepts patients in need of rehabilitation and medical care that is of a lesser intensity than that received in the acute/subacute care setting of a hospital. ▶ Provides skilled services, including rehabilitation, and various other health services (nursing) on a daily basis (Medicare defines *daily* as seven days a week of skilled nursing care and five days a week of skilled therapy). ▶ Physician orders must be rewritten every 60 days.	A SNF must be able to provide 24-hour nursing coverage and the availability of physical, occupational and speech therapy.
Inpatient rehabilitation facility	▶ Usually based in a medical setting. ▶ Provides early rehabilitation, social, and vocational services once a patient is medically stable. ▶ Primary emphasis is to provide intensive physical and cognitive restorative services in the early months to disabled persons to facilitate their return to maximum functional capacity. ▶ Typical stay is 3–4 months.	Physical therapist involved in the coordinated services of medical, social, educational, vocational, and the other rehabilitative services (OT, Speech).
Chronic/Long-term care facility	▶ Long-term care facility that is facility- or community-based. ▶ Sometimes referred to as *extended rehabilitation*. ▶ Designed for patients with permanent or residual disabilities caused by a nonreversible pathological health condition. Also used for patients who demonstrate slower than expected progress. ▶ Used as a placement facility—60 days or longer, but not for permanent stays.	The facility has a full range of rehabilitation services (physical, occupational, and speech therapy) available.
Comprehensive outpatient rehabilitation facility (CORF)	▶ A nonresidential facility established and operated exclusively for the purpose of providing outpatient diagnostic, therapeutic, and restorative services for the rehabilitation of injured, disabled, or sick persons, at a single fixed location, by or under the supervision of a physician. Services include physician services; physical, occupational, and respiratory therapy; speech-language pathology services; prosthetic and orthotic devices, including testing, fitting, or training in the use of these devices; social and psychological services; nursing care provided by or under the supervision of a registered professional nurse; drugs and biologicals that cannot be self-administered; and supplies and durable medical equipment. ▶ CORFs are surveyed every six years at a minimum.	Physical therapy (and occupational therapy and speech-language pathology services) may be provided in an off-site location.

(continued)

TABLE 1-2	Physical Therapist Practice Settings (*continued*)	
Setting	**Characteristics**	**Physical Therapist Role**
Custodial care facility	▶ Provides medical or nonmedical services, which do not seek to cure, but which are necessary for the patient who is unable to care for him/herself. ▶ Provided during periods when the medical condition of the patient is not changing. ▶ Patient does not require the continued administration of medical care by qualified medical personnel. ▶ This type of care is not usually covered under managed-care plans.	Physical therapy involvement is minimal.

Hospice care	▶ A facility or program that is licensed, certified, or otherwise authorized by law, which provides supportive care for the terminally ill.
	▶ Focuses on the physical, spiritual, emotional, psychological, financial, and legal needs of the dying patient and the family.
	▶ Services provided by an interdisciplinary team of professionals and perhaps volunteers in a variety of settings, including hospitals, freestanding facilities, and at home.
	▶ Medicare and Medicaid require that at least 80% of hospice care be provided at home. Eligibility for reimbursement includes:
	  ▪ Medicare eligibility.
	  ▪ Certification of terminal illness (less than or equal to six months of life) by physician.
		Physical therapy may be consulted on an as-needed basis.

Personal care	Optional Medicaid benefit that allows a state to provide services to assist functionally impaired individuals in performing the activities of daily living (e.g., bathing, dressing, feeding, grooming).	Physical therapy may be consulted on an as-needed basis.
Ambulatory care (outpatient care)	▶ Includes outpatient preventative, diagnostic, and treatment services that are provided at medical offices, and surgery centers or outpatient clinics (including private practice physical therapy clinics, outpatient satellites of institutions or hospitals). ▶ Designed for patients who do not require overnight hospitalization. ▶ More cost-effective than inpatient care, and therefore favored by managed-care plans.	Physical therapy may be consulted on an as-needed basis.

administer therapies under the supervision of a physician (see also Registered Nurse). Studies of PAs in primary care settings have found that the scope overlaps with approximately 80% of the scope of work of primary care physicians. A PA is usually licensed by the same state boards that license physicians. To be eligible for licensure in most states, a PA must have graduated from an accredited training program and pass the Physician Assistant National Certifying Examination.

Physiatrist

A physiatrist is a physician specializing in physical medicine and rehabilitation, who has been certified by the American Board of Physical Medicine and Rehabilitation. The primary role of the physiatrist is to diagnose and treat patients with disabilities involving musculoskeletal, neurological, cardiovascular, or other body systems.

Nurse Practitioner

A nurse practitioner (NP) is an advanced practice registered nurse who has completed graduate-level education at either a Master of Nursing or Doctor of Nursing Practice level in addition to the basic nurse training. NPs can diagnose a wide range of acute and chronic diseases, provided that they are within their scope of practice, and can provide appropriate treatment for patients, including the prescribing of medications. Licensing and related regulations for NPs are less uniform across states than those for physicians, PAs, and RNs. In lieu of a single national licensing examination for all NPs, certification examinations are administered by different organizations and are specialty specific, similar to medical specialty board certification. State boards of nursing vary in the scope of practice they allow NPs, with most states requiring that NPs work in collaboration with the physician.

Physical Therapy Director

The director of physical therapy is responsible for the day-to-day running of the physical therapy department. The director is either promoted or hired because he or she has demonstrated the necessary education and experience in the field of physical therapy and is willing to accept the inherent responsibilities of the role.[22] The director of a physical therapy service must:

► Establish guidelines and procedures that will delineate the functions and responsibilities of all levels of physical therapy personnel in the service and the supervisory relationships inherent in the functions of the service and the organization.[22]

► Ensure that the objectives of the service are efficiently and effectively achieved within the framework of the stated purpose of the organization, and in accordance with safe physical therapist practice. This often includes the design of policies and procedures.

► Interpret administrative policies.

► Act as a liaison between line staff and administration.

► Foster the professional growth of the staff.

► Be responsible for the departmental budget.

Staff Physical Therapist

A physical therapist engages in the examination, evaluation, diagnosis, prognosis, and intervention in an effort to maximize patient outcomes. CAPTE serves the public by establishing and applying standards that ensure quality and continuous improvement in the entry-level preparation of physical therapists and physical therapist assistants. All physical therapists in the United States are licensed in all 50 states and the District of Columbia, Puerto Rico, and the Virgin Islands. State licensure is required in each state in which a physical therapist practices and must be renewed on a regular basis (typically every two years), with a majority of states requiring continuing education units (CEUs) or other continuing competency requirement for renewal. A physical therapist must practice within the scope of physical therapy practice defined by his or her state licensure law (physical therapy practice act), including supervision of physical therapist assistants (PTAs).

CLINICAL PEARL

Traditionally, to receive an evaluation and/or treatment from a physical therapist or physical therapist assistant, the patient had to have a physician's order, or referral. However, the practice of physical therapy today has evolved such that in some states, the physician referral for physical therapy is no longer necessary or is required only at certain stages in the physical therapy treatment process.

Physical Therapist Assistant

A physical therapist assistant (PTA) works under the direction and supervision of the physical therapist, who directs appropriate physical therapy interventions to the PTA. Care provided by a PTA may implement selected components

of patient/client interventions; obtain outcomes data related to the interventions provided; modify interventions either to progress the patient/client as directed by the physical therapist or to ensure patient/client safety and comfort; educate and interact with other healthcare providers, students, aides/technicians, volunteers, and patients/clients and their families and caregivers; and respond to patient/client and environmental emergency situations.

CLINICAL PEARL

A PTA may modify an intervention only in accordance with changes in patient status and within the established plan of care developed by the physical therapist.

PTAs currently are licensed or certified in 49 states (Hawaii is the only state that does not regulate PTAs.). Typically, a PTA has an associate's degree from an accredited PTA program and operates within the scope of work and supervision requirements defined by the physical therapy practice act in each state.

Physical Therapy Aide

A physical therapy aide is an individual who may be involved in support services under the direction and supervision of a physical therapist or physical therapist assistant. A physical therapy aide receives on-the-job training and is permitted to function only with continuous on-site supervision. The duties of a physical therapist aide are limited to those methods and techniques that do not require clinical decision making or clinical problem solving by a physical therapist or a physical therapist assistant.

Physical Therapist and Physical Therapist Assistant Student

The PT or PTA student can perform duties commensurate with their level of education.

CLINICAL PEARL

Patients, parents, or legal guardians can refuse treatment by a student practitioner.

Physical Therapy Volunteer

A volunteer is usually a member of the community who has an interest in assisting with departmental activities. Responsibilities of a voluntary include:

► Taking phone messages

► Basic nonclinical/secretarial duties

CLINICAL PEARL

Volunteers may not provide or set up a patient treatment, transfer patients, clean whirlpools, or maintain equipment.

Home Health Aide

A home health aide provides health-related services to the elderly, disabled, and unwell in their homes. Their duties include performing housekeeping tasks, assisting with ambulation or transfers, and promoting personal hygiene. The registered nurse, physical therapist, or social worker caring for the patient may assign specific duties to, and supervise, the home health aide.

Occupational Therapist

An occupational therapist (OT) assesses a patient's function in activities of daily living (ADLs), including dressing, bathing, grooming, meal preparation, writing, and driving, which are essential for independent living. In making treatment recommendations, the OT addresses a number of factors including, but not limited to, (1) fatigue management, (2) upper body strength, movement, and coordination, (3) adaptations to the home and work environment, including both structural changes and specialized equipment for particular activities, and (4) compensatory strategies for impairments in thinking, sensation, or vision. All states require an OT to obtain a license to practice.

Certified Occupational Therapy Assistant

A certified occupational therapy assistant (COTA) works under the direction of an OT. COTAs perform a variety of rehabilitative activities and exercises as outlined in an established treatment plan. The minimum educational requirements for the COTA are described in the current *Essentials and Guidelines of an Accredited Educational Program for the Occupational Therapy Assistant* (AOTA, 1991b).

Speech-Language Pathologist (Speech Therapist)

A speech-language pathologist evaluates speech, language, cognitive communication, and swallowing skills of children and adults. Speech-language pathologists are required to possess a master's degree or equivalent. The vast majority of states require a speech-language pathologist to obtain a license to practice.

Chiropractor

A Doctor of Chiropractic (DC), or chiropractor, is an individual trained in the science, art, and philosophy of chiropractic. A chiropractic evaluation and treatment is directed at providing a structural analysis of the musculoskeletal and neurological systems of the body because, according to chiropractic doctrine, abnormal function of these two systems may affect the function of other systems in the body. In order to practice, chiropractors are usually licensed by a state board. A patient may see a chiropractor and physical therapist concurrently.

Certified Orthotist

A certified orthotist (CO) designs, fabricates, and fits orthoses (braces, splints, collars, corsets), prescribed by physicians, to patients with disabling conditions of the limbs and spine. A CO must have successfully completed the examination by the American Orthotist and Prosthetic Association (AOPA).

Certified Prosthetist

A certified prosthetist (CP) designs, fabricates, and fits prostheses for patients with partial or total absence of a limb. A CP must have successfully completed the examination by the AOPA.

CLINICAL PEARL

An individual may be certified in both orthotics and prosthetics (CPO).

Respiratory Therapist

A respiratory therapist evaluates, treats, and cares for patients with breathing disorders. The vast majority of respiratory therapists are employed in hospitals. Patient care activities include performing bronchial drainage techniques, measuring lung capacities, administering oxygen and aerosols, and analyzing oxygen and carbon dioxide concentrations. Education programs for a respiratory therapist are offered by hospitals, colleges, and universities, vocational-technical institutes, and the military. The vast majority of states require a respiratory therapist to obtain a license to practice.

Respiratory Therapy Technician Certified (CRRT)

A CRRT is a skilled technician who:

► Holds an associate's degree from a two-year training program accredited by the Committee in Allied Health Education and Accreditation

► Has passed a national examination to become registered

► Administers respiratory therapy as prescribed and supervised by a physician, including:

■ Pulmonary function tests

■ Treatments consisting of oxygen delivery, aerosols, nebulizers

■ Maintenance of all respiratory equipment

Registered Nurse

A registered nurse is an individual who has graduated from a nursing program at a college or university and has passed a national licensing exam. Historically, many nurses received their education in vocational programs administered by hospitals and were awarded diplomas of nursing. Nowadays, most nurses are educated either in 2- to 3-year associate degree programs administered by community colleges or in baccalaureate programs administered by 4-year colleges. A registered nurse is licensed by the state to provide nursing services and is legally authorized or registered to practice as a registered nurse (RN) and use the RN designation. A registered nurse may:

- Make referrals to other services under a physician's direction
- Supervise other levels of nursing care
- Administer medication, but cannot change drug dosages
- Communicate to the supervising physician any change in the patient's medical or social condition

Rehabilitation (Vocational) Counselor

A rehabilitation counselor helps people deal with the personal, physical, mental, social, and vocational effects of disabilities resulting from birth defects, illness or disease, accidents, or the stress of daily life. The role of the rehabilitation counselor includes:

- An evaluation of the strengths and limitations of individuals
- Providing personal and vocational counseling
- Arranging for medical care, vocational training, and job placement

Audiologist

An audiologist evaluates and treats individuals of all ages with the symptoms of hearing loss and other auditory, balance, and related sensory and neural problems.

Athletic Trainer Certified (ATC)

The certified athletic trainer is a professional specializing in athletic healthcare. In cooperation with the physician and other allied health personnel, the athletic trainer functions as an integral member of the athletic healthcare team in secondary schools, colleges and universities, sports medicine clinics, professional sports programs, and other athletic healthcare settings.

Certified athletic trainers have, at minimum, a bachelor's degree, usually in athletic training, health, physical education, or exercise science.

Social Worker

A social worker helps patients and their families to cope with chronic, acute, or terminal illnesses and attempts to resolve problems that stand in the way of recovery or rehabilitation. A bachelor's degree is often the minimum requirement to qualify for employment as a social worker; however, in the health field, the master's degree is often required. All states have licensing, certification, or registration requirements for social workers.

Massage Therapist

Massage therapy is a regulated health profession with a growing number of states and provinces now requiring a license. Registered massage therapists must uphold specific standards of practice and codes of ethics in order to hold a valid license. In order to become a licensed or registered massage therapist, most states and provinces require the applicant to pass specific government board examinations, which consist of a written and a practical portion. A registered massage therapist is covered under most health insurance plans.

Acupuncturist

An acupuncturist treats symptoms by inserting very fine needles, sometimes in conjunction with an electrical stimulus, into the body's surface to, theoretically, influence the body's physiological functioning. Typical sessions last between 30 minutes and an hour. At the end of the session, the acupuncturist may prescribe herbal therapies for the patient to use at home. At the time of writing, 32 states and the District of Columbia use National Certification Commission for Acupuncture and Oriental Medicine (NCCAOM) certification as the main examination criterion for licensure; this takes three to four years to achieve. Each state may also choose to set additional eligibility criteria (usually additional academic or clinical hours). A small number of states have additional jurisprudence or practical examination requirements such as passing the CNT (Clean Needle Technique) exam.

The Patient

Although often overlooked, the patient is critical to the healthcare team. The population of patients evaluated and treated in physical therapy can vary in age from newborn to elderly.

WORKING IN HEALTHCARE

Despite the fact that working in healthcare is altruistic, caring for other individuals can prove stressful over time. These stresses can result in a condition known as *caregiver burnout*. The classic symptoms for this condition include the following:

- A depletion of physical energy
- Emotional exhaustion
- Physical withdrawal
- An increasingly pessimistic outlook
- Increased absenteeism from work
- Excessive use of alcohol, medications, or sleeping pills
- Difficulty concentrating

It is important for every clinician to put time into taking care of him- or herself emotionally and physically. Whenever possible, any caregiving responsibility should be varied or delegated. If necessary, the clinician should strongly consider finding a support group or speaking to someone about getting help. A number of activities have been shown to be beneficial to reduce stress. These include aerobic exercise, meditation, massage, and relaxation techniques.

REFERENCES

1. American Physical Therapy Association: Guide to Physical Therapist Practice (ed 2). Phys Ther 81:9-746, 2001.
2. American Physical Therapy Association: Today's Physical Therapist: A Comprehensive Review of a 21st-Century Health Care Profession. Alexandria, Va, American Physical Therapy Association, 2011.
3. American Physical Therapy Association: A Normative Model of Physical Therapist Professional Education: Version 2000. Alexandria, Va, American Physical Therapy Association, 2000.
4. U.S. Army Medical Services: Medical Department of the United States Army in the World War. Washington, DC, The Surgeon General's Office Government Printing Office, 1923.

5. Murphy W: Healing the Generations: A History of Physical Therapy and the American Physical Therapy Association. Lyme, Conn, Greenwich, 1995.

6. Pinkston D: Evolution of the practice of physical therapy in the United States, in Scully RM, Barnes MR (eds): Physical Therapy (ed 1). Philadelphia, JB Lippincott, 1989, pp 2-30.

7. Moffat M: The history of physical therapy practice in the United States. JOPTE 17:15-25, 2003.

8. Moffat M: Three quarters of a century of healing the generations. Phys Ther 76:1242-1252, 1996.

9. American Physical Therapy Association: Professionalism in Physical Therapy: Core Values. Alexandria, Va, American Physical Therapy Association, 2003.

10. Cary JR, Ness KK: Erosion of professional behaviors in physical therapist students. JOPTE 15:20-24, 2001.

11. Brunnstrom S: Associated reactions of the upper extremity in adult patients with hemiplegia; an approach to training. Phys Ther Rev 36:225-236, 1956.

12. Bobath K, Bobath B: The facilitation of normal postural reactions and movements in the treatment of cerebral palsy. Physiotherapy 50:246-262, 1964.

13. Rood MS: Neurophysiological reactions as a basis for physical therapy. Phys Ther Rev 34:444-449, 1954.

14. Knott M, Voss DE: Proprioceptive Neuromuscular Facilitation (ed 2). New York, Harper & Row, 1968.

15. American Physical Therapy Association: Guide to Physical Therapist Practice: Revisions. Phys Ther 79:623-629, 1999.

16. Dean E: Physical therapy in the 21st century (Part I): toward practice informed by epidemiology and the crisis of lifestyle conditions. Physiother Theory Pract 25:330-353, 2009.

17. Schmoll BJ: Physical therapy today and in the 21st century, in Scully RM, Barnes MR (eds): Physical Therapy (ed 1). Philadelphia, JB Lippincott, 1989, pp 31-35.

18. Greenland P, Knoll MD, Stamler J, et al: Major risk factors as antecedents of fatal and nonfatal coronary heart disease events. JAMA 290:891-897, 2003.

19. Plack MM, Wong CK: Evolution of the DPT: the current controversy. JOPTE 16:48-59, 2002.

20. Murphy W: Healing the Generations: A History of Physical Therapy Education and the American Physical Therapy Association. Alexandria, Va, American Physical Therapy Association, 1995.

21. Commission on Accreditation of Physical Therapy Education: Number of PT and PTA Programs, 2010. http://www.capteonline.org/home.aspx. Last accessed March 7, 2013.

22. Guide to physical therapist practice: Phys Ther 81:S13-S95, 2001.

23. Starr P: The Social Transformation of American Medicine. New York, NY, Basic Books, 1982.

24. Swisher LL, Hiller P: The revised APTA code of ethics for the physical therapist and standards of ethical conduct for the physical therapist assistant: theory, purpose, process, and significance. Phys Ther 90:803-824, 2010.

25. Fullinwider RK: Professional codes and moral understanding, in Coady M, Block S (eds): Codes of Ethics and the Professions. Victoria, Australia, Melbourne University Press, 1996, pp 72-87.

26. Frankel MS: Professional codes: why, how, and with what impact? J Bus Ethics 8:109-115, 1989.

27. Coady M, Block S: Codes of Ethics and the Professions. Victoria, Australia, Melbourne University Press, 1996.

28. Purtillo R: Ethical considerations in physical therapy, in Scully RM, Barnes MR (eds): Physical Therapy (ed 1). Philadelphia, JB Lippincott, 1989, pp 36-40.

CHAPTER 2

Healthcare Policy

CHAPTER OBJECTIVES

*At the completion of this chapter,
the reader will be able to:*

1. Describe the various methods by which healthcare services are reimbursed

2. List the challenges associated with obtaining appropriate access to healthcare within the United States

3. Describe the various associations and organizations that regulate the quality of healthcare

4. Define *malpractice* and provide examples of patient negligence

5. Describe the impact of the Balanced Budget Act of 1997

6. Have a good understanding of patient rights within healthcare

7. Describe how the Health Insurance and Portability and Accountability Act (HIPAA) is designed to protect a patient's privacy

8. Discuss the various legislation that protects a patient within the healthcare system

9. Describe the importance of the Americans with Disabilities Act (ADA) and its impact on society

10. List some of the considerations when assessing the home and work environments

OVERVIEW

There exists a paradox of excess and deprivation in the healthcare system of the United States, in which some individuals are deprived of adequate care because they cannot afford suitable insurance, while others receive an excess of care that is expensive and unnecessary. Healthcare in the United States encompasses a wide spectrum, ranging from the highest quality, most compassionate treatment of those with complex illnesses, to the turning away of the very ill because of an inability to pay; from well-designed protocols for prevention of illness

to inappropriate high-risk surgical procedures performed on uninformed patients.[1] For the physical therapist, embarking on a career in healthcare, an understanding of how healthcare works, including its strengths and inadequacies, is essential.

REIMBURSING HEALTHCARE PROVIDERS

Reimbursement to healthcare providers can occur in a number of ways, with each designed in an attempt to solve the problem of unaffordable care for certain groups while also trying to control healthcare costs.[2]

Units of Payment

The methods by which physicians and healthcare services have been reimbursed over the years have varied and range from the simplest to the most complex[3]:

▸ *Fee-for-service.* Reimbursement based on a fee-for-service mechanism, in which the physician or hospital is paid a fee for each office visit, procedure, or supply provided.

▸ *Payment by episode of illness.* The entity is paid one sum for all services delivered during one episode of illness. A diagnosis-related group (DRG) is a system of reimbursement designed to replace cost-based reimbursement that is based on ICD (International Classification of Diseases) diagnoses, procedures, age, sex, discharge status, and the presence of complications or comorbidities. For example, the federal Medicare program for the elderly typically pays a hospital a flat fee per hospital case, with a different per-case price for each DRG. Today, there are several different DRG systems that have been developed in the United States. They include:

- Medicare DRG (CMS-DRG & MS-DRG)
- Refined DRGs (R-DRG)
- All Patient DRGs (AP-DRG)
- Severity DRGs (S-DRG)
- All Patient Severity-Adjusted DRGs (APS-DRG)

21

- All Patient Refined DRGs (APR-DRG)
- International-Refined DRGs (IR-DRG)

▶ *Per diem payments.* A hospital is paid for all services delivered to a patient during one day of inpatient care. The levels of these payments are set unilaterally by the state governments or by private insurers. The per-diems that private insurers pay hospitals are negotiated annually between each hospital and each insurance carrier.

CLINICAL PEARL

Private insurers pay hospitals predominantly on the basis of per-diems or fee-for-service schedules. The profits built into these payments by the hospitals cover the losses incurred by serving Medicare and Medicaid patients, who are billed at high prices but are not reimbursed in full.

▶ *Capitation payment.* Capitation is one of several forms of prepaid medical care that differs from a fee-for-service arrangement. Capitation pays a hospital, physician, or group of physicians a set amount for each enrolled person assigned to them, per period of time, whether or not that person seeks care. In exchange for this fixed rate of reimbursement, physicians essentially become the enrolled patients' insurers, who resolve their patients' claims and assume the responsibility for their unknown future healthcare costs.

▶ *Payment for all services delivered to all patients within a certain time frame.* This includes a global budget payment of hospitals and salary payment for physicians. Facilities or systems that use a global budget have clear incentives to control costs and to operate efficiently. The major problem with this type of reimbursement is that providers who find themselves in danger of exceeding their budget may respond with "rationing by waiting," which in turn results in access problems for the patients.

▶ *Out-of-pocket payments.* This method is used by individuals who have no insurance, whether by choice or because of financial restrictions.

Types of Health Insurance

At present, individuals can have access to healthcare services through a number of insurance methods, which include:

▶ *Individual private insurance (generally for self-employed individuals).* In return for paying a monthly sum, people receive assistance in case of illness.

▶ *Employment-based private insurance.* Employers usually pay most of the premium to purchase health insurance for their employees as one of the benefits of employment. In most cases, employment-based plans now require employee contributions and copayments. The government does not treat the health insurance fringe benefits as taxable income to the employee, so the government is in essence subsidizing employer-sponsored health insurance. A new form of employment-based private insurance is

consumer-driven healthcare (CDH). Defined narrowly, CDH refers to health plans in which individuals have a personal health account, such as a health savings account (HSA) or a health reimbursement arrangement (HRA), from which they pay medical expenses directly. The phrase is sometimes used more broadly to refer to defined-contribution health plans, which allow employees to choose among various plans, often with a fixed dollar contribution from an employer. The characteristics of a CDH include:

- High benefit level options that involve significant employee contributions and deductibles in addition to an employer's contribution, *or* lower benefit level options that involve less employee contribution and deductibles.

- Greater choice and control over one's health plan.

- Economic incentives to better manage care—economic rewards for making good decisions and economic penalties for making ill-advised ones. These economic incentives make patients more likely to seek information about medical conditions and treatment options, including information about prices and quality.

▶ *Government financing.* This occurs through government-funded programs, such as Medicare, Medicaid, and the Federal Employees Health Benefit Plans.

- *Medicare.* Administered by the federal government—Center for Medicare and Medicaid services (CMS). CMS is an agency within the U.S. Department of Health and Human Services, through the extension of title XVIII of the Social Security Act, 1965 (the law that created Medicare, Medicaid, and other federal programs).

CLINICAL PEARL

Healthcare Financing Administration (HCFA) was the previous name for Center for Medicare and Medicaid services (CMS).

CLINICAL PEARL

Medicare currently covers physical therapy services in the following provider settings: skilled nursing facilities (SNFs), home health agencies (HHA), long-term care hospitals (LTCHs), inpatient rehabilitation facilities (IRFs), acute care hospitals, physical therapist private practice offices, physician's offices, rehabilitation agencies, and comprehensive outpatient rehabilitation facilities (CORFs).[4]

There are different varieties or parts to Medicare:

- *Part A.* On reaching the age of 65 years, people who are eligible for Social Security are automatically enrolled in Medicare Part A, whether or not they are retired. If a person has paid into the Social Security system for 10 years, his or her spouse is eligible for Social Security.[3] People who are not eligible for Social Security can enroll in Medicare Part A by paying a monthly premium. People under the age of 65 who are totally and permanently disabled may enroll

TABLE 2-1	Medicare Part A and Part B (2008)		
Medicare Part	**Method of Financing**	**Benefit**	**Medicare Pays**
A	Employers and employees each pay to Medicare 1.45% of wages and salaries into the social security system. Self-employed people pay 2.9%.	*Hospitalization* First 60 days	All but a $1024 deductible per spell of illness
		61st to 90th day	All but $256 per day
		91st to 150th day	All but $512 per day
		Beyond 90 days if lifetime reserve days are used up	Nothing
		Skilled Nursing Facility (SNF) First 20 days	All
		21st to 100th day	All but $128 per day
		Beyond 100 days	Nothing
		Home health care 100 visits per spell of illness	100% for skilled care as defined by Medicare regulations
		Hospice care Requires physician certification that individual has a terminal illness	100% of services, copays for outpatient drugs and coinsurance for inpatient respite care
B	In part by general federal revenues (personal income and other federal taxes) and in part by Part B monthly premium.	Medical expenses Physician services Physical, occupational, and speech therapy Medical equipment Diagnostic tests	80% of approved amount after a $135 annual deductible
		Preventative care (some Pap smears; some mammogram; hepatitis B, pneumococcal, and influenza vaccinations)	Included in medical expenses, with deductible and coinsurance waived for some services
		Outpatient medications. Partially covered under Medicare Part D	All except for premium, deductible, coinsurance
		Eye refractions, hearing aids, dental services	Not covered

Data from: Bodenheimer TS, Grumbach K: Paying for healthcare, in Bodenheimer TS, Grumbach K (eds): Understanding health policy: a clinical approach (ed 5). New York, McGraw-Hill, 2009, pp 5-16.

in Medicare Part A after they have received Social Security disability benefits for 24 months. People with chronic renal disease requiring dialysis or transplant may also be eligible for Medicare Part A without a two-year waiting period. Part A helps pay for medically necessary inpatient hospital care (limits the number of hospital days), and, after a hospital stay, limited inpatient care in a skilled nursing facility, or limited home healthcare or hospice care (Table 2-1).

CLINICAL PEARL

The Medicare modernization Act of 2003 made two major changes in the Medicare program:

▶ Medicare Advantage program: an expansion of the role of private health plans that rejuvenated the previous Medicare + Choice program by which Medicare beneficiaries could pay an additional premium to enroll in private Medicare health maintenance organization (HMO) plans.

▶ Medicare part D: a prescription drug benefit. This program has proved controversial:

■ There are major gaps in coverage.

■ Coverage has been farmed out to private insurance companies rather than administered by the federal Medicare program.

■ The government is not allowed to negotiate with pharmaceutical companies for lower drug prices.[3]

■ *Part B:* Part B (see Table 2-1) is for people who are eligible for Medicare Part A and who elect to pay the Medicare Part B premium of $99.90 per month (2012).[3] Some low-income persons are not required to pay the premium.

■ *Medicaid.* A federal program mandated by Title XIX of the Social Security Act, which is administered by the states, with the federal government paying between 50% and 76% of the total Medicaid costs. Benefits vary from state to state—the federal contribution is greater in states with lower per capita incomes. Medicaid pays for medical and other services on behalf of certain groups:

- Low-income families with children who meet certain eligibility requirements.
- Most elderly, disabled, and blind individuals who receive cash assistance under the federal Supplemental Security Income (SSI) program.
- Children younger than age 6 and pregnant women whose family income is at or below a percentage of the federal poverty level. In 2013, the federal poverty level was $23,550 for a family of four.
- School-age children (6–18) whose family income is at or below the federal poverty level.

CLINICAL PEARL

Medicaid services are provided in a variety of settings including but not limited to home care, intermediate-care facilities for people with mental retardation (ICF/MR), and schools.[4]

Because of a large expenditure growth, the federal government ceded enhanced control of the Medicaid programs to states through Medicaid waivers, which allow states to reduce the number of people on Medicaid, make alterations to the scope of covered services, require Medicaid recipients to pay part of their costs, and obligate Medicaid recipients to enroll in managed care plans.[3]

CLINICAL PEARL

Medicaid waivers are an exception to the usual requirements of Medicaid granted to a state by CMS. The waivers allow states to:

- ▶ Waive provisions of the Medicaid law to test new concepts that are consistent with the goals of the Medicaid program. System-wide changes are possible under this provision. Frequently used to establish Medicaid managed care programs.
- ▶ Waive freedom of choice. States may require that beneficiaries enroll in HMOs or other managed care programs, or select a physician to serve as their primary care case manager.
- ▶ Waive various Medicaid requirements to establish alternative, community-based services for (a) individuals who would otherwise require the level of care provided in a hospital or skilled nursing facility, and/or (b) persons already in such facilities who need assistance returning to the community. Waivers include older adults, persons with disabilities, persons with intellectual disability, persons with chronic mental illness, and persons with acquired immunodeficiency syndrome (AIDS).
- ▶ Limit expenditures for nursing facility and home and community-based services for person 65 years and

older, so that they do not exceed a projected amount, determined by taking base year expenditure (the last year before the waiver), and adjusting for inflation. Also eliminates requirements that programs be statewide and be comparable for all target populations. Income rules for eligibility can also be waived.

In 1997, the federal government created the State Children's Health Insurance Program (SCHIP), a companion program for Medicaid that is designed to cover uninsured children in families with incomes at or below 200% of the federal poverty level, but above the Medicaid income eligibility level.[3]

CLINICAL PEARL

- ▶ Primary Care Case Management (PCCM). A Medicaid managed care option allowed under section 1915(b) of the Social Security Act in which each participant is assigned to a single primary care provider who must authorize most other services such as specialty physician care before they can be reimbursed by Medicaid.
- ▶ Medicaid Prudent Pharmaceutical Purchasing Act (MPPPA). Enacted as part of the Omnibus Budget Reconciliation Act of 1990, MPPPA provides that Medicaid must receive the best-discounted price of any institutional purchaser of pharmaceuticals. In doing so, drug companies provide rebates to Medicaid that are equal to the difference between the discounted price and the price at which the drug is sold. This bill has resulted in cost shifting throughout the health industry.

- ▶ *Managed care plans.* There are three major forms of managed care[2]:
  - *Fee-for-service reimbursement with utilization review.* The third-party payer (whether a private insurance company, or a government agency) has the authority to deny payment for expensive or unnecessary medical interventions.
  - *Preferred provider organizations (PPOs).* Under this form of managed care, there is a contract with a limited number of physicians and hospitals that have agreed to care for a group of patients within the PPO, usually on a discounted fee-for-service basis with utilization review.
  - *Health maintenance organizations (HMOs).* These are organizations whose patients are required (except in emergencies) to receive their care from providers within that HMO. Several types of HMOs exist.

ACCESS TO HEALTHCARE

Access to healthcare is the ability to obtain health services when needed.[5] The organizational task facing healthcare systems is one of ensuring that the right patient receives the right service at the right time in the right place, and with the right caregiver.[6,7] Health insurance coverage (see Types of Health Insurance, earlier), whether public or private, is a key factor in making healthcare accessible, and health insurance is often related to employment level. Individuals whose employers choose not to provide health insurance are technically self-employed and must find ways to obtain their own health insurance. In 2011, 48.6 million people in the United States were uninsured.[8]

CLINICAL PEARL

A number of regulations monitor the accessibility of healthcare. These include:

▶ Health Maintenance Organization Act of 1973.

▶ Anti-discriminatory restrictions (including the Rehabilitation Act of 1973, Pregnancy Discrimination Act of 1978, Americans with Disabilities Act of 1990, and Child Abuse Prevention and Treatment Act Amendments of 1984).

▶ Continuation of coverage requirements (including the Consolidated Omnibus Budget Reconciliation Act [COBRA] of 1986 and state rules).

▶ Mandated health benefits (including mandated standards of care such as bone marrow transplants. There are at present three federally mandated health insurance benefits:

  ■ The Mental Health Parity Act of 1996

  ■ Newborns' and Mothers' Protection Health Act of 1996

  ■ Women's Health and Cancer Rights Act of 1998

Despite health insurance regulation occurring at both the federal and state levels, which monitors such entities as the Blue Cross and Blue Shield carriers (which, if not for-profit, are often regulated somewhat differently than their commercial counterparts), commercial insurance companies, self-insured plans, and various types of managed care, including HMOs and PPOs, private health insurance coverage continues to decrease. The reasons for this increase in the number of people who are uninsured include[5]:

▶ The skyrocketing cost of health insurance

▶ A decrease in the number of highly paid, largely unionized, full-time manufacturing companies with employer-sponsored health insurance

▶ An increase in the overall instability and transient nature of employment, resulting in interruptions in coverage

---

CLINICAL PEARL

The uninsured suffer worse health outcomes than those with insurance, as they tend to be diagnosed at later stages, receive fewer procedures in emergency departments (EDs), and, on average, are more seriously ill when hospitalized.[9-12]

Theoretically, the uninsured population is supposed to have access to healthcare federal and state programs such as Medicaid. However, these programs have their limitations; access to care is by no means guaranteed with Medicaid coverage. One of the major reasons for this is that Medicaid pays physicians far less than does Medicare or private insurance, with the result that many physicians do not accept Medicaid patients.[5]

CLINICAL PEARL

Although the number of uninsured people is high, these people do have some access to healthcare:

▶ Hill–Burton Act: Federal legislation enacted in 1947 to support the construction and modernization of healthcare institutions. Hospitals that receive Hill–Burton funds must provide specific levels of charity care. For example, those healthcare institutions that receive tax-exemption, federal Hill–Burton grants or loans are not allowed to turn away patients because of an inability to pay. However, care is limited to emergency care only. The costs incurred by this population are covered by a surcharge on insurance payments.

▶ Individuals who cannot pay for healthcare can receive pro bono or free care through philanthropic donations and services.

Even the so-called insured patients are not guaranteed financial access to healthcare. Many people are underinsured, that is, their health insurance coverage has limitations that restrict access to needed services.[13-16] For example, many have private health insurance that leaves major expenses uncovered in the event of a serious illness.[17] Other factors that affect the insured are insurance deductibles and copayments, with many plans having high deductibles and substantial copayments.[18]

Finally, in addition to the financial barriers to healthcare, there are a number of nonfinancial barriers, including:

▶ *Gender.* In general, females have greater dissatisfaction with healthcare than males.[19,20]

▶ *Race.* Because far higher proportions of minorities than whites are uninsured, have Medicaid coverage, or are poor, access problems are amplified for these groups.[5,21]

▶ *Lack of prompt access.* Many patients resort to an ED visit because they are unable to obtain a timely appointment with their private physician.[22-24]

▶ *Shortages in qualified personnel (physicians, pharmacists, nurses).* Patients in rural areas face shortages of all types of healthcare personnel (about 20% of the U.S. population lives in areas that have a shortage of primary healthcare professionals).[25-27]

▶ *Lack of drug control.* Although drugs used in the United States must be approved for safety and efficacy, there are no constraints on either therapeutic duplication or price. Any drug that obtains approval from the U.S. Food and Drug

Administration (FDA) may be marketed in the United States, and the distributor has full discretion over the price charged.

▶ *An increasingly aging population.* The elderly often require a higher percentage of healthcare services, which can increase the burden on an already stretched healthcare system.

CLINICAL PEARL

Socioeconomic status is the dominant influence on health status and access to healthcare, although access to healthcare does not always guarantee good health.

As healthcare costs have increased, efforts to control costs by government and private entities have focused on reducing the biggest expenses to an organization—staffing—by decreasing or replacing manpower. However, decreasing or replacing manpower has the following disadvantages:

▶ The use of lower cost paraprofessionals results in an increased share of the workload being performed by aides and technicians.

▶ An increase in caseload size, resulting in less time spent with each patient.

QUALITY OF CARE REGULATORS

A number of regulations within the U.S. healthcare system attempt to ensure a high quality of care. These include:

▶ Hospital accreditation and licensure, which includes Medicare conditions of participation (COP), and the Joint Commission (formerly known as Joint Commission on Accreditation of Healthcare Organizations [JCAHO]) (see Voluntary Accreditation section)

▶ State accreditation and licensure, including the department of health (DOH)

▶ Nursing home accreditation and licensure (including the Joint Commission, COP, the Nursing Home Reform Act, part of the Omnibus Budget Reconciliation Act of 1987, and state regulations)

▶ Licensure for all other health facilities (see Voluntary Accreditation section)

▶ Peer review, encompassing Quality Improvement Organizations and the Healthcare Quality Improvement Act of 1986

▶ The Clinical Laboratory Improvement Act of 1967 as amended

▶ FDA regulation of blood banks

▶ Blood-borne pathogen requirements imposed by the Occupational Safety and Health Administration (OSHA)

▶ Health outcomes reporting systems mandated by states

CLINICAL PEARL

The goal of OSHA is to create a safe and healthy working environment for employees. Employers must provide a working environment that is free from recognized hazards and employees must adhere to health and safety standards. The National Institute for Occupational Safety and Health (NIOSH) is the research arm of OSHA. NIOSH has developed *Elements of Ergonomics Programs*, a primer based on workplace evaluations of musculoskeletal disorders that is useful in developing a program focusing on ergonomics.

Voluntary Accrediting Agencies

Accreditation of healthcare institutions is a voluntary process by which an authorized agency or organization evaluates and recognizes health services according to a set of standards describing the structures and processes that contribute to desirable patient outcomes. Outpatient centers for comprehensive rehabilitation can be accredited by the Joint Commission (JC), AC-MRDD, CORF, and/or CARF.

The Joint Commission

The Joint Commission is a private organization created in 1951 to provide voluntary accreditation to hospitals. Many states rely on JC accreditation as a substitute for their own inspection programs. The JC has high standards of quality assurance and a rigorous process of evaluation, which makes it a much-esteemed agency for accreditation. Health services certified by the JC are given "deemed status."

In the 1990s, the JC revised its standards to reflect the changing functions of hospitals, seeking to move away from departments toward the patient experience of hospital systems. In 2006, the JC changed the survey process and began unannounced surveys that focused on observations and interviews in an effort to move toward finding standards that reflect the integration of hospital services rather than examining them in isolation. Thus, surveys currently involve a "tracer methodology" whereby a survey team enters a facility, selects a number of patients, and follows those patients' treatment courses throughout the facility. Some of the JC sections that are currently surveyed are listed in Table 2-2. A series of National Patient Safety Goals (NPSGs) were introduced by the JC in 2002 (effective January 1, 2003) to help accredited organizations address specific areas of concern in regard to patient safety. The development and updating of the NPSGs is overseen by the Patient Safety Advisory Group (PSAG), a panel of widely recognized patient safety experts including nurses, physicians, pharmacists, risk managers, and clinical engineers. The NPSGs stated for 2011–12 were:

▶ Improve the accuracy of patient identification, including the use of at least two patient identifiers when providing care, treatment, and services and the elimination of transfusion errors related to patient misidentification.

▶ Improve the communication among caregivers, including the reporting of critical results of tests and diagnostic procedures on a timely basis.

TABLE 2-2	The Joint Commission Sections
Ethics, rights, responsibility, and provision of care	
Medication management	
Emergency management	
Surveillance, prevention, and control of infection	
Leadership	
Improving organizational performance	
Management of the environment of care	
Management of human resources	
Management of information	
Medical staff co-leaders	
Nursing	
National patient safety goals/sentinel events	

▶ Improve the safety of using medications, including the labeling of all medications, medication containers, and other solutions on and off the sterile field in perioperative and other procedural settings; reduce the likelihood of patient harm associated with the use of anticoagulant therapy; maintain and communicate accurate patient medication information.

▶ Reduce the risk of healthcare-associated infections, including compliance with either the current Centers for Disease Control and Prevention (CDC) hand hygiene guidelines or the current World Health Organization (WHO) hand hygiene guidelines; the implementation of evidence-based practices to prevent healthcare-associated infections due to multidrug-resistant organisms, surgical site, indwelling catheter–associated urinary tract infections (CAUTI), and central line–associated bloodstream infections in acute care hospitals.

▶ Reduce the risk of patient harm resulting from falls.

▶ Prevent healthcare-associated pressure ulcers (decubitus ulcers) by assessing and periodically reassessing each resident's risk for developing a pressure ulcer and taking action to address any identified risks.

▶ The organization is to identify safety risks inherent in certain patient populations, including those patients at risk for suicide, those at risk associated with home oxygen therapy (e.g., home fires), and to have a universal protocol for preventing Wrong Site, Wrong Procedure, and Wrong Person Surgery by conducting a pre-procedure verification process, marking the procedure site, and performing a timeout before the procedure.

CLINICAL PEARL

The JC accredits more than 80% of the nation's hospitals. It also accredits skilled nursing facilities, hospices, and other care organizations that provide home care, mental healthcare, laboratory, ambulatory care, and long-term services.

A typical accreditation process involves:

1. Organization submits an application for review.
2. A survey is conducted by the accrediting agency.

3. The organization conducts a self-study or self-assessment to examine itself based on the accrediting agency standards.

4. An individual surveyor, or a team of surveyors, visits the organization and conducts an on-site review. The whole staff of the organization is involved in the accreditation and reaccreditation process. Tasks include document preparation, hosting the site visit team, and interviews with the accreditors.

5. Accreditation surveyor or team issues a report granting or denying accreditation.

A number of disadvantages of accreditation through the JC have been listed, and include:

▶ Hospitals pay for JC surveys, and more than 70% of the JC's revenue comes directly from the organizations it is supposed to inspect.

▶ Although the JC encourages workers to speak with survey takers, most workers do not have legal protection from retaliation if they do so.

CLINICAL PEARL

The JC surveys a hospital every 3 years. Facilities must demonstrate a 12-month track record for all plans of action at the time of the survey.

Council on Quality and Leadership (CQL)

Council on Quality and Leadership (CQL) is a U.S. organization dedicated to the definition, measurement, and improvement of personal and community quality of life for people with disabilities, those with mental illness and substance abuse disorders, and older adults. CQL evolved from the work of the American Association on Mental Deficiency (AAMD; now American Association on Intellectual and Developmental Disabilities—AAIDD). During the 1980s and 1990s, the name of the organization evolved from Accreditation Council for Services for Mentally Retarded and Other Developmentally Disabled Persons (ACMRDD) to Accreditation Council on Services for People with Disabilities (ACD), and in 1997 it became the CQL. CQL provides the following services:

▶ Accreditation of organizations providing services and supports

▶ Community Life LENS—experiential community development training

▶ Certification of professionals—as personal outcome trainers, personal outcome interviewers, and certified quality analysts

▶ External independent review of public and private service systems

▶ Standards and measurement system design

Commission on Accreditation of Rehabilitation Facilities (CARF)

CARF is a nonprofit organization designed to recognize standards of excellence in rehabilitation programs across the

27

nation. CARF accreditation standards were developed with the input of consumers, rehabilitation professionals, state and national organizations, and third-party purchasers. CARF is designed to establish standards of quality for freestanding rehabilitation facilities and the rehabilitative programs of the largest hospital systems in the areas of behavioral health, employment (work hardening), and community support services and medical rehabilitation (spinal cord injury, chronic pain), and to determine how well an organization is serving its patients, consumers, and the community. Programs accredited by CARF have demonstrated that they meet the national standards for rehabilitation programs.

Comprehensive Outpatient Rehabilitation Facility (CORF)

The CORF accreditation group conducts certification surveys for compliance with federal and state regulations and investigates any complaints filed against one of these providers. Certification is achieved by adherence to federal requirements, including:

- Submission of a complete application
- Required documentation
- Successful completion of a survey

Each CORF must be surveyed for certification as directed by the CMS. An application for certification includes submission of a completed application, required documentation, and successful completion of a survey. No fees and no renewal applications are required for certification. No state licensing requirements are imposed by the agency.

Federal and State Healthcare Regulations

In the United States, healthcare regulation is undertaken to improve performance and quality through a wide variety of governmental and nongovernmental agencies. These entities have varying statutory authority, scope and remit, approaches, and outcomes, resulting in a complex, overlapping, duplicative, and sometimes contradictory regulatory environment.

Balanced Budget Act of 1997 (BBA)

This law made sweeping changes in the Medicare and Medicaid programs. Several of the significant provisions of the BBA were payment reductions to healthcare providers, new prospective payment systems for healthcare providers, and reduction of coverage of healthcare services by the Medicare and Medicaid programs.

Statutory Laws

Statutes are defined as laws that are passed by Congress and the various state legislatures. These statutes are the basis for statutory law. The legislature passes statutes that are later put into the federal code of laws or pertinent state code of laws. Statutory law consists of the acts of legislatures declaring, commanding or prohibiting something—a particular law established by the will of the legislative department of government. A number of statutory laws affect physical therapy:

- *Licensure laws.* Under the U.S. federal system of government, each state regulates the practice of all healthcare professionals by establishing licensing or regulatory agencies or boards to generate regulations. State licensing statutes establish the minimum level of education and experience required to practice, define the functions of the profession, and limit the performance of these functions to licensed persons. These laws:

  - Are designed to protect the consumer against professional incompetence and exploitation by opportunists.
  - Make a determination as to the minimal standards of education. In the case of physical therapy, the minimal standards required include:
    - Graduation from an accredited program or its equivalent in physical therapy
    - Successful completion of a national licensing examination (NPTE)
  - Licensure examination and related activities are the responsibility of the Federation of State Boards of Physical Therapy.
  - Determine the ethical and legal standards relating to the continuing practice of physical therapy.
  - Each state determines the criteria to practice and issue a license.

- *Workers' Compensation Acts.* The rules and regulations of individual state's workers' compensation systems are the primary factors influencing the provision of physical therapy services for patients with work-related injuries. Workers' compensation laws are designed to ensure that employees who are injured or disabled on the job are provided with fixed monetary awards, eliminating the need for litigation. The laws provide a no-fault system that pays all medical benefits and replaces salary (usually at 66%) until recovery occurs. In turn, employees forfeit the right to sue their employers for damages. These rules and regulations also provide benefits for dependents of workers who die as a result of a work-related accident or illness. Some of the rules and regulations also protect employers and fellow workers by limiting the amount an injured employee can recover from an employer and by eliminating the liability of co-workers in most accidents. State workers' compensation statutes establish this framework for most employment. Federal statutes are limited to federal employees or those workers employed in some significant aspect of interstate commerce. The laws vary from state to state, but most states identify four types of disability:

  - *Temporary partial*—the injured worker is able to do some work but is still recuperating from the effects of the injury and is thus temporarily limited in the amount or type of work that can be performed compared to the preinjury work.
  - *Temporary total*—the injured worker is unable to work during a period when he/she is under active medical care and has not yet reached what is called "maximum medical improvement."
  - *Permanent partial*—the injured worker is capable of employment but is not able to return to the former

job. Benefits are usually paid according to a prescribed schedule for a fixed number of weeks.

- *Permanent total*—the injured worker cannot return to any gainful employment, and lifetime benefits are provided to the employee.

Workers' compensation programs:

- Are financed by covered employers insured or self-insured under property and casualty lines and are mandatory for employers in almost all states.
- Have a limit on the number of visits in some states based on the diagnosis, and/or require a preapproval process to be followed for reimbursement. Other states require the total number of visits or total number of weeks (duration) and the number of treatments per week (frequency) to be usual, customary, and reasonable.
- Must be offered by all large employers (10 or more employees) or high-risk employers.

▶ *Malpractice laws*. Malpractice can be defined as a dereliction of professional duty, or a failure to exercise an accepted degree of professional skill or learning by one rendering professional services, which results in injury, loss, or damage. Malpractice also encompasses injurious, negligent, or improper practice. Physical therapists are personally responsible for any act of negligence or other acts that result in harm to a patient through professional-patient relationships.

- Negligence is defined as failure to do what reasonably competent practitioners would have done under similar circumstances.
- To find a practitioner negligent, harm must have occurred to the patient. Examples could include:
  - A burn caused by a hot pack
  - Using defective equipment that results in injury
  - Failing to prevent a patient from falling
  - Causing an injury to a patient through improper prescription of exercises
  - Performing any action or inaction that is inconsistent with the Code of Ethics or the Standards of Practice

CLINICAL PEARL

- ▶ Every individual (PT, PTA, student PT, or student PTA) is liable for his or her own negligence.
- ▶ Supervisors or superiors may also be found "vicariously" negligent because of the actions of their workers if they provided faulty supervision or inappropriate delegation of responsibilities.
- ▶ Institutions can be found vicariously negligent if a patient is harmed as a result of an environmental problem such as a slippery floor or a poorly lit area, or if an employee is deemed to be incompetent or not properly licensed.

THE PATIENT

The clinician must always consider a situation from the patient's perspective and understand that all patients have rights within any given healthcare system.

Patient Rights

In 1998, the U.S. Advisory Commission on Consumer Protection and Quality in the Healthcare Industry endorsed the following areas of consumer rights and responsibilities:

I. *Information disclosure.* Consumers have the right to receive accurate, easily understood information and some require assistance in making informed healthcare decisions about their health plans, professionals, and facilities.

II. *Choice of providers and plans.* Consumers have the right to a choice of healthcare providers that is sufficient to ensure access to appropriate high-quality healthcare.

III. *Access to specialists.* Consumers with complex or serious medical conditions who require frequent specialty care should have direct access to a qualified specialist of their choice within a plan's network of providers. Authorizations, when required, should be for an adequate number of direct access visits under an approved treatment plan.

IV. *Access to emergency services.* Consumers have the right to access emergency healthcare services when and where the need arises. Health plans should provide payment when a consumer presents to an emergency department with acute symptoms of sufficient severity—including severe pain—such that a "prudent layperson" could reasonably expect the absence of medical attention to result in placing that consumer's health in serious jeopardy, serious impairment to bodily functions, or serious dysfunction of any bodily organ or part.

V. *Participation in treatment decisions.* Consumers have the right and responsibility to fully participate in all decisions related to their healthcare and to expect healthcare providers to abide by the informed decisions. Consumers who are unable to fully participate in treatment decisions have the right to be represented by parents, guardians, family members, or other conservators.

VI. *Respect and nondiscrimination.* Consumers have the right to considerate, respectful care from all members of the healthcare system at all times and under all circumstances. An environment of mutual respect is essential to maintain a quality healthcare system.

VII. *Confidentiality of health information.* Consumers have the right to communicate with healthcare providers in confidence and to have the confidentiality of their individually identifiable healthcare information protected. Consumers also have the right to review and copy their own medical records and request amendments to their records.

29

VIII. Complaints and Appeals. All consumers have the right to a fair and efficient process for resolving differences with their health plans, healthcare providers, and the institutions that serve them, including a rigorous system of internal review and an independent system of external review.

IX. Consumer Responsibilities. In a healthcare system that protects consumers' rights, it is reasonable to expect and encourage consumers to assume reasonable responsibilities. Greater individual involvement by consumers in their care increases the likelihood of achieving the best outcomes and helps support a quality improvement, cost-conscious environment.

CLINICAL PEARL

A complete description of the Patient's Bill of Rights can be seen at: http://www.opm.gov/insure/archive/health/cbrr.htm

The Patient Self-Determination Act (PSDA) requires many Medicare and Medicaid providers (hospitals, nursing homes, hospice programs, HHAs, and HMOs) to give adult individuals, at the time of inpatient admission or enrollment, certain information about their rights under state laws, including:

1. The right to participate in and direct their own healthcare decisions
2. The right to accept or refuse medical or surgical treatment
3. The right to prepare an advance directive
4. Information on the provider's policies that govern the utilization of these rights

The act also prohibits institutions from discriminating against a patient who does not have an advance directive.

CLINICAL PEARL

An advance directive is a written instruction, such as a living will or a durable power of attorney for healthcare, that provides instructions for the provision of medical treatment *in anticipation* of those times when the individual executing the document no longer has decision-making capacity.

Medical Records

Medical records contain sensitive information, and increasing computerization and other policy factors have increased threats to their privacy. Besides information about physical health, these records may include information about family relationships, sexual behavior, substance abuse, and even the private thoughts and feelings that come with psychotherapy. Threats to medical record privacy include the following:

▶ *Administrative actions.* This includes errors that release, misclassify, or lose information. This includes compromised accuracy, misuse by legitimate users, and uncontrolled access.

▶ *Computerization.* Although in some situations computerization increases privacy protection (for example, by adding passwords to sensitive areas), it may also decrease privacy protection for the following reasons:

■ Computerization enables storage of large amounts of data in small spaces. Thus, when an intruder gains access, that access is not just to certain discrete amounts of data, but to larger collections, and perhaps keys to even further information.

■ Networked information is accessible from anywhere at any time, allowing a larger number of people access. This increases the possibility of mistakes or other problems such as misuse or leaks of data.

■ New databases and different types of data sets are more easily created. This both drives demand for new information and makes possible its creation.

■ Information is easily gathered, exchanged, and transmitted. Thus, potential dissemination is theoretically limitless.

■ Access by unrelated parties is possible.

▶ *Insurance companies.* Insurance companies may check records either before approving treatment or before extending coverage.

▶ *Financial institutions.* The federal Gramm-Leach-Bliley Act (GLB) allows financial companies such as banks, brokerage houses, and insurance companies to operate as a single entity.

▶ *Drug companies.* These companies may have deals with doctors and hospitals and may get access to patient lists that can be used for marketing.

▶ *Employers.* Employers could use sensitive information against employees.

▶ *Court subpoenas.* Often a patient will be unaware when his or her records have been subpoenaed. Even worse, unnecessary information is often included when the records are not adequately screened.

Current protections for medical records privacy include:

▶ Medical ethics.

▶ The privacy portion of the Hippocratic Oath: "Whatsoever I shall see or hear in the course of my intercourse with men, if it be what should not be published abroad, I will never divulge, holding such things to be holy secrets."

▶ The 1992 AMA statement that states that medical information must be kept confidential to the greatest possible degree.

▶ The Privacy Act of 1974, which states that no federal agency may disclose information without the consent of the person. Agencies must also meet certain requirements for protecting the information.

▶ *Tort law.* This may include defamation, breach of contract, and other privacy-related torts.

▶ Health Insurance and Portability and Accountability Act (HIPAA) Privacy Rule—see the next section.

▶ The U.S. Department of Health and Human Services (HHS).

Health Insurance and Portability and Accountability Act (HIPAA)

The purpose of this act was to protect the individual from excessive personal expenditures and to protect healthcare-related information. This 1996 federal legislation makes long-term care insurance premiums tax deductible if nonreimbursable medical expenses, including part or all of long-term care premiums, exceed 7.5% of an individual's gross income. HIPAA also excludes long-term care insurance benefits from taxable income. Not all long-term care insurance coverage qualifies for this benefit.

> **CLINICAL PEARL**
>
> Regulatory controls within the U.S. healthcare system include the fraud and abuse provisions included in the Health Insurance Portability and Accountability Act (HIPAA) of 1996 and the 1997 Balanced Budget Act and those listed in Table 2-3.

HIPAA also issued a Privacy Rule to implement the requirement of the HIPAA Act of 1996. The Privacy Rule standards address the use and disclosure of individuals' health information (called "protected health information" or PHI) by organizations subject to the Privacy Rule (called "covered entities"), as well as standards for individuals' privacy rights to understand and control how their health information is used. A major goal of the Privacy Rule is to ensure that individuals' health information is properly protected while allowing the flow of health information needed to provide and promote high-quality healthcare and to protect the public's health and well-being.

▶ The Privacy Rule applies to anyone who transmits health information in electronic form in connection with transactions.

▶ The Privacy Rule protects all "individually identifiable health information" (protected health information) held or transmitted by a covered entity (health plans, healthcare clearinghouses, and any healthcare provider) or its business associate (limited to legal, actuarial, accounting, consulting, data aggregation, management, administrative, accreditation, or financial services), in any form or medium, whether electronic, paper, or oral.

TABLE 2-3	Fiscal Regulations within the U.S. Healthcare System
Regulation	**Description**
False Claims Act of 1863	First signed into law in 1863. Underwent significant changes in 1986. Allows citizens to bring law suits against groups or other individuals that are defrauding the government through programs, agencies, or contracts (overbilling for services, "upcoding").
Medicare and Medicaid antifraud statutes	Stipulates that an individual who knowingly and willfully offers, pays, solicits, or receives any remuneration in exchange for referring an individual for the furnishing of any item or service (or for the purchasing, leasing, ordering, or recommending of any good, facility, item, or service) paid for in whole or in part by Medicare or a state healthcare program (i.e., Medicaid) shall be guilty of a felony. Often referred to as the "antikickback" statute.
The Civil Monetary Penalties Law (CMPL)	Authorizes the Secretary of Health and Human Services to impose civil money penalties, an assessment, and program exclusion for various forms of fraud and abuse involving the Medicare and Medicaid programs.
Federal self-referral prohibitions	Also known as Stark I and II. The first Self-Referral Prohibitions (Stark I) prohibited physicians from referring lab specimens obtained from Medicare patients to clinical laboratories with which the physician or an immediate family member of the physician had a financial relationship. In addition, any clinical laboratory that received a Medicare referral from a physician with which it had a financial relationship could not bill Medicare for the performance of that procedure. A financial relationship is defined as either an ownership/investment interest or a compensation relationship. The expanded Physician Self-Referral prohibitions (Stark II), introduced in 1995, prohibits self-referrals (Medicaid and Medicare) of not only lab services, but also many other designated health services, including physical therapy.
Pharmaceutical price regulation scheme	A scheme that ensures the national health system has access to good-quality branded medicines at reasonable prices and promotes a healthy, competitive pharmaceutical industry. Includes federal average wholesale price restrictions for Medicaid and state pharmaceutical regulations.
Certificate of Need (CON)	Intended to regulate major capital expenditures that may adversely affect the cost of health care services, to prevent the unnecessary expansion of health care facilities, and to encourage the appropriate allocation of resources for healthcare purposes. CON laws became part of almost every state by 1978 after the 1974 National Health Act was passed.

According to HIPAA's Privacy Rule, PHI includes all of the following:

▶ Demographic data, which relate to the individual's past, present, or future physical or mental health condition

▶ The provision of healthcare to the individual

▶ The past, present, or future payment for the provision of healthcare to the individual

Individually identifiable health information includes the name, address, date of birth, and Social Security number of the patient.

Further details can be found at: http://www.hhs.gov/ocr/hipaa

A covered entity must disclose protected health information in only two situations:

▶ To individuals (or their personal representatives) specifically when they request access to, or an accounting of disclosures of, their protected health information.

▶ To Health and Human services (HHS) when it is undertaking a compliance investigation or review or enforcement action.

A covered entity is permitted, but not required, to use and disclose protected health information, without an individual's authorization, for the following purposes or situations:

▶ To the individual (unless required for access or accounting of disclosures)

▶ Treatment, payment, and healthcare operations

▶ Opportunity to agree or object

▶ Incident to an otherwise permitted use and disclosure

▶ Public interest and benefit activities and Office for Civil Rights (OCR) Privacy Rule Summary

▶ Limited data set: for the purposes of research, public health, or healthcare operations

Covered entities may rely on professional ethics and best judgments in deciding which of these permitted uses and disclosures to make.

▶ *Workforce training and management.* Workforce members include employees, volunteers, trainees, and may also include other persons whose conduct is under the direct control of the entity (whether or not they are paid by the entity). A covered entity must train all workforce members on its privacy policies and procedures, as necessary and appropriate for them to carry out their functions. A covered entity must have and apply appropriate sanctions against workforce members who violate its privacy policies and procedures or the Privacy Rule.

▶ *Data safeguards.* A covered entity must maintain reasonable and appropriate administrative, technical, and physical safeguards to prevent intentional or unintentional use or disclosure of protected health information in violation of the Privacy Rule and to limit its incidental use and disclosure pursuant to otherwise permitted or required use or disclosure. For example, such safeguards might include shredding documents containing protected health information before discarding them, and securing medical records with lock and key or pass code and limiting access to keys or pass codes.

▶ *Documentation and record retention.* A covered entity must maintain, until six years after the later of the date of their creation or last effective date, its privacy policies and procedures, its privacy practices notices, disposition of complaints, and other actions, activities, and designations that the Privacy Rule requires to be documented.

▶ *Criminal penalties.* A person who knowingly obtains or discloses individually identifiable health information in violation of HIPAA faces a fine of $50,000 and up to 1 year imprisonment. The criminal penalties increase to $100,000 and up to 5 years imprisonment if the wrongful conduct involves false pretenses, and to $250,000 and up to 10 years imprisonment if the wrongful conduct involves the intent to sell, transfer, or use individually identifiable health information for commercial advantage, personal gain, or malicious harm.

Informed Consent

Informed consent is the process by which a fully informed individual can participate in choices about his or her healthcare. It originates from the legal and ethical right the patient has to direct what happens to his or her body and from the ethical duty of the physician, or healthcare provider, to involve the patient in his or her healthcare.

The most important goal of informed consent is that the patient must have an opportunity to be an informed participant in his or her healthcare decisions. Basic consent entails letting the patient know what you would like to do and asking them if they agree. The more formal process should include a discussion of the following elements:

▶ The nature of the decision/procedure

▶ Reasonable alternatives to the proposed intervention

▶ The relevant risks, benefits, and uncertainties related to each alternative

▶ Assessment of patient understanding

▶ The acceptance of the intervention by the patient

In order for the patient's consent to be valid, he/she must be considered competent to make the decision and his/her consent must be voluntary.

Emergency Medical Treatment and Labor Act (EMTALA)

The Emergency Medical Treatment and Labor Act (EMTALA), or the Patient Anti-Dumping Law, requires most hospitals to provide an examination and needed stabilizing treatment, without consideration of insurance coverage or ability to pay, when a patient presents to an emergency room for attention with an emergency medical condition.

The Patient Protection and Affordable Care Act (PPACA)

The Patient Protection and Affordable Care Act (PPACA) is a federal statute that was signed into United States law in March 2010, along with the Healthcare and Education Reconciliation Act of 2010 (also signed into law in March 2010). The law includes numerous health-related provisions to take effect over a four-year period beginning in 2010:

▶ Guaranteed issue and community rating—insurers must offer the same premium to all applicants of the same age, sex, and geographical location regardless of whether the applicant has a pre-existing condition

▶ Medicaid eligibility is expanded to include individuals and families up to 133% of poverty level.

▶ New health insurance exchanges in each state to enhance competition by offering a marketplace where individuals and small businesses can compare policy premiums on a like-for-like basis and buy insurance (with a government subsidy if eligible). Low-income persons and families above the Medicaid level and up to 400% of poverty level will receive subsidies on a sliding scale if they choose to purchase insurance via a health insurance exchange.

▶ Introduction into the tax code of a "shared responsibility payment," which is a fine paid by any large employer (with 50 or more employees) if the government has had to subsidize an employee who bought insurance in the exchange because the employer did not offer a minimum coverage plan or better. Another form of shared responsibility payment or fine is imposed on certain persons who do not have minimum essential coverage for at least one month in the year (individual mandate), though being insured is not actually mandated by law.

▶ Improved benefits for Medicare prescription drug coverage.

▶ Establishment of national voluntary insurance program for purchasing community living assistance services and support.

▶ Very small businesses to get subsidies if they purchase insurance health insurance through the exchange.

▶ Additional support provided for medical research and the National Institutes of Health (NIH).

Medical Errors

The importance of patient safety cannot be overstated, but even with the best intentions, medical/clinical errors continue to occur. The two main causes of medical error are:

▶ An intervention does not go according to plan. Examples include surgical errors and improperly functioning or poorly maintained equipment. From a rehabilitation perspective, activities that place the patient at risk, such as ambulation, aerobic exercise, and transfers, should always be performed with caution:

  ■ Diminished skin integrity can lead to skin breakdown during transfers, positioning, or exercise.

  ■ A decrease in bone density can result in a fracture during transfers, manual techniques, and ambulation.

▶ An incorrect intervention was used. Examples include errors in medication prescriptions or regimens, and laboratory report inaccuracies. An adverse drug error (ADE) is an example of a medication error. The three most common types of medication errors are failure to administer an ordered medication; a deviation in the prescribed dose, strength, or quantity of a drug; and the dispensing or administering of the incorrect drug.

CLINICAL PEARL

The six rights of the drug administration, used by nurses when administering drugs, include:

▶ Right individual
▶ Right medication
▶ Right dose
▶ Right time
▶ Right route
▶ Right documentation

The consequences of a medical error run the gamut from causing the patient no harm to causing the death of the patient. A number of agencies work cooperatively to develop strategies and standards that are designed to reduce medical errors. These agencies include:

▶ The Institute of Medicine (IOM)
▶ The Agency for Health Research and Quality (AHRQ)
▶ The Joint Commission

The focus of these agencies is to examine and analyze policies and procedures within the institution that have the potential to cause harm, including:

▶ The complexity of the healthcare delivery system. In large institutions, it is easy for a patient to become a number rather than a person.

▶ The number of caregivers involved in the patient's care. The more caregivers that are involved in a patient's care, the greater the chance of an error.

▶ Flaws in the design of systems or equipment. These flaws can be inherent in the equipment design or in the physical layout of the treatment area. One of the most common problems is overcrowding of equipment that does not permit sufficient space between items for safe negotiation. Another common problem is the physical location of one department in relation to another. Systems and departments should be designed to enhance patient flow.

TABLE 2-4	Examples of a Sentinel Event

- Any patient death, paralysis, coma, or other major permanent loss of function (e.g., loss of a limb) associated with a medication or procedural error
- Any suicide of a patient in a setting where the patient is housed around-the-clock, including suicides following elopement from such a setting
- Any elopement, that is, unauthorized departure, of a patient from an around-the-clock care setting resulting in a temporally related death (suicide or homicide) or major permanent loss of function
- Any procedure on the wrong patient, wrong side of the body, or wrong organ
- Any intrapartum (related to the birth process) maternal death
- Any perinatal death unrelated to a congenital condition in an infant having a birth weight greater than 2500 grams
- Assault, homicide, or other crime resulting in patient death or major permanent loss of function
- A patient fall that results in death or major permanent loss of function as a direct result of the injuries sustained in the fall
- Hemolytic transfusion reaction involving major blood group incompatibilities

- Improper or faulty installation and maintenance of equipment. All electrical equipment must be checked annually for safety. For example, extension cables should not be used, and neither should portable heaters.
- Incorrect design of a treatment area. In many cases areas are used for a specialty when they were designed for another specialty.

The Joint Commission categorizes a medical error as either a sentinel (adverse) event or a potential adverse event:

- Sentinel event: an unexpected occurrence that involves death or serious injury, or the risk thereof, and which may have been avoided through appropriate care or alternative interventions. Such events are called *sentinel* because they signal the need for immediate investigation and response. Examples of a sentinel event are provided in Table 2-4.
- Potential adverse event: no actual harm occurs.

CLINICAL PEARL

The terms *sentinel event* and *medical error* are not synonymous; not all sentinel events occur because of an error, and not all errors result in sentinel events.

The Joint Commission reviews organizations' activities in response to sentinel events. Healthcare providers are required to alert the Joint Commission, and often state licensing authorities, of all sentinel events, including a review of risk factors, preventative measures, and root cause analysis (RCA). The RCA is designed to determine what happened, why or how it happened, and what could be done to prevent a recurrence of the event.

Material Safety Data Sheet

The various products used by a clinical facility, especially cleaning chemicals, are one further cause of potential injury to a patient.

TABLE 2-5	Recommended Safety Precautions
Hand hygiene	This is the single most important procedure to prevent the spread of infection and cross-contamination and should be performed before and after each treatment session.
Staff competency	All personnel who provide patient care should be trained, qualified, and competent in their assigned duties.
Patient protection	As appropriate, the patient should be protected with safety straps, bed rails, and so forth according to established regulatory state and federal guidelines. Patient transfers should not be attempted unless sufficient staff is present.
Sufficient space	The clinician should always plan ahead so that sufficient space to maneuver any equipment or to perform a task is available.
Treatment area	Remove any clutter, including equipment that is not being used or is blocking a walkway, electrical cords, loose rugs/floor mats, and any water spills.
Equipment	All equipment should be regularly assessed to ensure that it functions properly.
Preparation	The clinician should obtain any equipment or supplies that are needed before a patient arrives for treatment, so that the patient will not be left unattended.

In the United States, OSHA requires that a material safety data sheet (MSDS) or safety data sheet (SDS) available to employees for potentially harmful substances handled in the workplace under the Hazard Communication regulation. The MSDS is also required to be made available to local fire departments and local and state emergency planning officials under Section 311 of the Emergency Planning and Community Right-to-Know Act. Table 2-5 lists a number of safety recommendations (see also Chapter 8).

Incident/Occurrence Reporting

The purpose of incident/occurrence reporting is to understand the underlying/contributing conditions that led to, or contributed to, the occurrence of a safety incident; identify appropriate corrective actions that must be taken to address these underlying/contributing conditions; and implement timely and effective corrective actions. An incident/occurrence report typically contains the following information:

- The name or description of the incident/occurrence. Attention should be paid to making the report simple, clear, and inclusive.
- Time and date of incident/occurrence.
- A brief description of the incident/occurrence location. A simple, chronological narrative works best.
- A brief description of the actual incident.
- First and last names and titles of persons involved, if appropriate.
- What is being done and/or will be done next.

- Other departments involved or to become involved in the incident (emergency services, physician, etc.), as appropriate.
- The name and title of the person submitting the report.

AMERICANS WITH DISABILITIES ACT

Over the years, much federal legislation has been designed to protect individuals from discrimination. These have included the Civil Rights Act of 1964, the Fair Housing and Architectural Barriers Act of 1968, Section 504 of the Rehabilitation Act of 1973, and the Education for All Handicapped Children Act of 1975. In 1990, the Americans with Disabilities Act (ADA),[28] a wide-ranging civil rights law, marked the first explicit national goal of achieving equal opportunity, independent living, and economic self-sufficiency for individuals with disabilities.[29] The original act was later amended with the ADA Amendments Act of 2008 (ADAAA), which was signed into law to give broader protections for disabled workers, with changes effective January 1, 2009. The ADA affords protections against discrimination to Americans with disabilities similar to the protections in the Civil Rights Act of 1964, which made it illegal to discriminate based on race, religion, sex, national origin, and other characteristics.

CLINICAL PEARL

The Civil Rights Act of 1991 is a federal law that capped compensatory and punitive damages under Title I of the ADA for intentional job discrimination. The law also amended the ADA's definition of an employee, adding "with respect to employment in a foreign country, such term includes an individual who is a citizen of the United States."

The ADA, which has five titles (Table 2-6), does not function in isolation but is related to other state and federal laws, such as the Family and Medical Leave Act (FMLA) and the Occupational Safety and Health Act (OSHA).

TABLE 2-6	The Five Titles of the ADA
Title	**Name and Description**
I. Employment	Prohibits employers (an employment agency, labor organization, or joint labor-management committee) from discriminating against a qualified individual with a disability with regard to job application procedures, hiring, advancement and discharge of employees, workers' compensation, job training, and other terms, conditions, and privileges of employment, on the basis of that disability alone. Examples of workplace accommodations include:
- Modification of work schedule
- Modification of job activities or requirements
- Modification to the physical plant
- The provision of assistive devices such as a telephone amplifier
- Modification of existing furniture or equipment
- Access to accessible restrooms, entrances, hallways, doorways, and parking areas.

This usually necessitates a review of the application form, process, and procedures; selection and hiring procedures; and evaluation, advancement, and training opportunities and activities. Each job description should be written in functional terms (e.g., able to lift 25 pounds, able to stand for one hour at a time). |
| II. Public services and transportation | Prohibits disability discrimination by all public entities at the local (school district, municipal, city, and county) and state level. Access includes physical access described in the ADA Standards for Accessible Design, and programmatic access that might be obstructed by discriminatory policies or procedures of the entity. Access into a facility or establishment for persons with disabilities, freedom of movement, and access to goods and services once inside the facility should be given immediate attention. |
| III. Public accommodations | No individual may be discriminated against on the basis of disability with regard to the full and equal enjoyment of the goods, services, facilities, or accommodations of any place of public accommodation by any person who owns, leases (or leases to), or operates a place of public accommodation (most places of lodging [hotel or motel], recreation, transportation, education, dining, stores, care providers, park or zoo, and places of public displays). For existing facilities and those to be constructed, structural physical barriers must be removed or not included. This title usually requires removal, modification, or alteration of structural barriers when the changes can be made reasonably and accomplished without significant difficulty or expense. Examples include the installation of ramps, the widening of doorways, the use of door hardware that is more functional than a knob, installation of support bars or rails, auxiliary services and aids for individuals with a vision or hearing impairment (telecommunication display device [TDD]), increased space in restrooms to accommodate a wheelchair, water fountains accessible from the wheelchair, and curb cutouts.

Exempted entities include private clubs and establishments that are exempt from Title II of the Civil Rights Act of 1964, religious organizations or entities controlled by religious organizations, and entities operated by governments that are exempt from Titles I and II. |
| IV. Telecommunications | Requires that all telecommunications companies in the United States take steps to ensure functionally equivalent services for consumers with disabilities, notably those who are deaf or hard of hearing and those with speech impairments. |
| V. Other provisions | Includes technical provisions such as the fact that nothing in the ADA amends, overrides, or cancels anything in Section 504, in addition to an anti-retaliation or coercion provision. |

TABLE 2-7	Major Life Activities

Social/Emotional:

▶ Interaction with others (e.g., speech difficulties such as pressured speech, lack of clarity, withdrawal or responding with difficulty or too quickly; self-absorption; inability to relate to or listen to others, including inability to relate due to paranoia, delusions, hallucinations, obsessive-compulsive ideation, negativity; inability to regulate mood and anxiety; inability to maintain appropriate distance from others)

▶ Forming and maintaining relationships with others

▶ Communication with others (e.g., answering questions, following directions, using intelligible speech, recognizing and expressing emotions appropriately, expressing needs, following a sequence)

Cognitive:

▶ Concentration—as a major life activity itself and also resulting in limitations on other major life activities, such as interaction with others, self care

▶ Making decisions

▶ Complex thinking (e.g., planning, reconciling perceptions from different senses [seeing and hearing], sorting relevant from irrelevant details, problem solving, changing from one task to another)

▶ Abstract thinking (e.g., difficulty generalizing or transferring learning from one setting to another, such as difficulty transferring the skill of cooking in one kitchen to another kitchen)

▶ Memory—long or short term

▶ Attention

▶ Perception

▶ Distinguishing real from unreal events

▶ Initiating and completing actions

▶ Processing information

Physical:

▶ Taking care of personal needs, such as eating, dressing, toileting, bathing, hygiene, household chores, managing money, following medication or treatment regimens, following safety precautions

▶ Eating (e.g., inability to regulate amounts appropriately, or to maintain appropriate diet; need for strict eating schedule)

▶ Sleeping (e.g., inability to fall asleep, obtain restful sleep, or sleep without interruption; excessive sleeping)

▶ Reproduction

▶ Sexual activity

▶ Traveling

TABLE 2-8	Glossary of ADA Terms

Term	Definition
Accessible	Refers to a site, facility, work environment, service, or program that is easy to approach, enter, operate, participate in, and/or use safely and with dignity by a person with a disability.
Affirmative-action	A set of positive steps that employers use to promote equal employment opportunity and to eliminate discrimination.
Employer	A person engaged in an industry affecting commerce that has 15 or more employees for each working day in each of 20 or more calendar weeks in the current or preceding calendar year, and any agent of such person. Exceptions: The term "employer"" does not include the United States, a corporation wholly owned by the government of the United States, or an Indian tribe; or a bona fide private membership club.
Equal Employment Opportunity Commission (EEOC)	A federal agency charged with enforcing Title I of the ADA.
Major life activity	Activities that an average person can perform with little or no difficulty. Major life activities include, but are not limited to: caring for oneself, performing manual tasks, seeing, hearing, eating, sleeping, walking, standing, sitting, reaching, lifting, bending, speaking, breathing, learning, reading, concentrating, thinking, communicating, interacting with others, and working; and the operation of a major bodily function.
Reasonable accommodation	Under Title I, a modification or adjustment to a job, the work environment, or the way things usually are done that enables a qualified individual with a disability to enjoy an equal employment opportunity. Reasonable accommodation is a key nondiscrimination requirement of the ADA.
Undue burden	With respect to complying with Title II or Title III of the ADA, significant difficulty or expense incurred by a covered entity, when considered in light of certain factors. These factors include: the nature and cost of the action; the overall financial resources of the site or sites involved; the number of persons employed at the site; the effect on expenses and resources.

To qualify as a person with a disability, the individual must have a physical or mental impairment that substantially limits the performance of one of life's major activities (Table 2-7).

To fully understand the ADA, it is important to be able to understand the terminology (Table 2-8). Working in concert with the ADA are the Americans with Disabilities Act Accessibility Guidelines (ADAAG—http://www. access-board.gov/adaag/html/adaag.htm) that detail the technical requirements to be applied during the design, construction, and alteration of buildings and facilities covered by Titles II and III of the ADA to the extent required by regulations issued by federal agencies, including the Department of Justice and the Department of Transportation (Table 2-9).

CLINICAL PEARL

Detailed information about the ADA can be found at http://www.ada.gov/cguide.htm

ASSESSING THE HOME AND WORK ENVIRONMENTS

The Guide to Physical Therapist Practice includes examination of environmental home, and work (job/school/play) barriers among the list of categories of tests and measures that may be used by physical therapists.[30] Treating

TABLE 2-9	Design Specifications for Accessibility
Ramps	Grade: not greater than 1:12 (8.3%) for new construction, with a vertical rise of not greater than 30 inches. Not greater than 1:10 (10%) for existing sites, with a vertical rise of not greater than 6 inches if space does not permit construction of a grade of 1:12 or less. Not greater than 1:8 (12.5%) for existing sites, with a vertical rise of not greater than 3 inches if space does not permit construction of a grade of 1:12 or less. Minimum width of 36 inches. Must have hand rails on both sides. 12 inches of length for each inch of vertical rise. Handrails required for a rise of 6 inches or more or for horizontal runs of 72 inches or more.
Grade of approach	Not greater than 1:20 (5%) unless requirements for a ramp are met.
Height	Not less than 80 inches vertical clearance. If vertical clearance along an accessible route is less than 80 inches, a warning barrier must be provided.
Doorways	Minimum width of 32 inches. Maximum depth of 24 inches.
Thresholds	Less than ¾ inch for sliding doors. Less than ½ inch for other doors.
Carpet	Requires ½-inch pile or less.
Hallway clearance	36-inch width.
Wheelchair turning radius (U-turn)	60-inch width. 78-inch length.
Forward reach in wheelchair	Low reach 15 inches. High reach 48 inches.
Side reach in wheelchair	Reach over obstruction to 24 inches.
Bathroom sink	Not less than 29-inch height. Not greater than 40 inches from floor to bottom of mirror or paper dispenser. 17 inches minimum depth under sink to back wall.
Bathroom toilet	17–19 inches from floor to top of toilet. Grab bars should be 1¼-1½ inches in diameter. 1-inch spacing between grab bars and wall. Grab bar placement 33 to 36 inches up from floor level.
Hotels	Approximately 2% of total rooms must be accessible.
Parking spaces	96 inches wide. 240 inches in length. Adjacent aisle must be 60 inches × 240 inches. Approximately 2% of the total spaces must be accessible.

the injured worker or person with a disability requires that the physical therapist must be knowledgeable regarding the following[31]:

▶ An understanding of all aspects of the patient's community, home, and work. This includes the physical environment in which an individual functions, including both built and natural objects. This aspect of the examination may entail the clinician visiting the patient's home or worksite. Detailed information about the patient's work history and available resources at the worksite may also be obtained from the company representative responsible for implementing change on the worker's behalf.

▶ The psychosocial issues and cultures of the patient's environment.

▶ The most appropriate avenues for minimizing loss of function while maximizing recovery for a specific patient and workplace.

▶ *Accessibility:* the degree to which an environment affords use of its resources with respect to an individual's level of function.

▶ *Universal design (life-span design):* this design concept emphasizes social inclusion by creating environments that are usable by a wide range of individuals of different ages, stature, sizes, and abilities as well as addressing the changing needs of human beings across the life span.[32]

▶ *Environmental barriers:* defined as physical impediments to prevent individuals from functioning optimally in their surroundings. Environmental barriers can be external or internal.[30,33]

■ *Exterior barriers.* External barriers include sidewalks, driveways, garage/carport accessibility, access to the grounds, and entry into the accommodation. Exterior access routes include consideration of the frequency and mode of transportation typically used to reach the destination, parking, lighting in the parking area, and safety traveling to the entrance. Outside steps should have a maximum height of 7 inches and depth of at least 11 inches and should not have tread lip projections.[32] If the patient has to use a ramp for home or work, the clinician should ensure that the patient can safely ascend and descend it and that it is soundly built. For safety and ease of use, a ramp should ideally have an incline of at least 1-foot length for each inch of rise (1:12 ratio). For example, a six-inch step leading into the home/building requires a six-foot ramp.[33] Handrails should be fitted for patients who ambulate with difficulty and for those with impaired balance, especially on any steps and ramps.

■ *Interior barriers.* Interior access routes should be checked to ensure that there is enough space for basic mobility in and out of rooms with any assistive device the patient requires. The clinician should make note of the type and resistance of any floor coverings. Doorways must be at least 32 inches wide for a standard wheelchair to pass and ideally 1 to 2 inches wider than this to account for inaccurate maneuvering and the usual oblique approach to doors.[33] The clinician should check that lighting in all areas is bright enough for safe task performance and that light switches can be reached by the patient or the lights come on automatically as the patient enters the environment.[33] In addition, it is important to assess the height of and access to electrical outlets/switches, the size and space available in each room, the location and access to communication units such as telephones and computers, the location and access to heating/cooling controls, and the location and access to safety devices (smoke/carbon monoxide detectors, circuit breaker panel, etc.).

CLINICAL PEARL

Functional range of motion, rather than individual joint motion, is generally most relevant to the examination of environmental barriers. Similarly, functional muscle testing, such as whether the individual has the strength to operate levers, lift, carry, push, and pull objects as required by the expected roles, is more useful than examination of strength by measurement of individual muscle performance with manual muscle testing or other approaches.[33]

Guidelines for wheelchair accessible home are described in Table 2-10.

CLINICAL PEARL

The Multidirectional Reach test is an effective test of functional range of motion.[34,35] Another measure of functional ROM is a map of the patient's reach zones, which look like semicircles extending in front of and to the side of the patient.[33] These items can be classified as primary, secondary, or tertiary. Objects are then placed in the zones according to frequency of use.

▶ *Primary zone:* Frequently used objects, which can be used while keeping elbows at the side of the body.

▶ *Secondary zone:* all objects that are used 4 to 10 times an hour and which can be reached without the elbow moving further forward than the anterior portion of the rib cage.

▶ *Tertiary zone:* infrequently used objects, which can be reached without exceeding full elbow extension or 90 degrees of shoulder flexion.

TABLE 2-10   Guidelines for a Wheelchair-Accessible Home

Full Access
▶ Clearance of 30" × 48" in front of and adjacent to any fixtures or workspaces, and appliance.
▶ Height of any fixture/control is not to exceed 48" above the floor.

Feedback
▶ Those with vision or hearing impairments use clicks, beeps, and lights to verify a switch is activated.

Comfort Zone
▶ The reach zone in which a person can comfortably perform a task. The standard reach zone for a standing adult is from 28" to 75". The standard reach zone for a seated adult is from 20" to 44".

Neutral Handedness
▶ Placement of fixtures, workspaces, and appliances so they can be approached from the left- and right-hand sides.

Site/Foundation
▶ Contours of the site allow all entrances to be at the same level as the driveway, for no-step entrances.

Walkways
▶ 5' wide, flat, smooth, and firm.
▶ All approaches from the street to span from the curb to the entrance.
▶ Mailboxes to be located beside walkways and within comfort zone.

Garage
▶ There should be an electric door with 9' height clearance to accommodate van.
▶ Interior measurements account for 5' clearance on each side of vehicles for chair lifts.

Entryways
▶ Walkways to extend a minimum of 25' beyond latch side of door.
▶ Thresholds are to be flush and a minimum of 3' wide.
▶ Guest entrances are to have doorbell installed 36" from the ground and have two peepholes (one at 40" one at 60").
▶ Gated entries need 36" thresholds and easy open latches.

Doors/Hardware
▶ All doors to have flush thresholds and must be 36" wide with an 18" clearance on the latch side.
▶ Doorknobs to be lever handle type.
▶ Locks must be easily operated with one hand.
▶ Knobs and locks installed below 36" and to be of the immediate feedback style if required.

Windows/Hardware
▶ Casement and vertical sliding sash windows are the preferred styles.
▶ Lock hardware should have large levers and be easy to operate.
▶ Lifts, pulls, cranks, and locks should be large and accessible.

Floors/Carpet
▶ Smooth, hard finishes (wood, linoleum) with matte surfaces are preferred.
▶ Carpet to be firm, ½ " (or less) cut pile.
▶ Tile is to have nonslip surface.

Electrical
▶ Service panels must be located in a prominent, fully accessible area.
▶ All controls to be rocker type with feedback.
▶ Thermostats, outlets, and controls are to be accessible and between 18" and 48" off the floor.
▶ Extra outlets and controls placed in bedrooms if required by buyer.

Grab Bars
▶ 1.25" to 1.5" in diameter with spacing of 1.5" between wall and bar.

Gas
▶ Meters with earthquake shutoff valves or full access to meter for emergency shutoff is a must.

Telephone
▶ Phone jacks are to be in all rooms.

Smoke and Carbon Monoxide Detectors
▶ Smoke and carbon monoxide detectors are to be placed in kitchen and in hall outside sleeping areas.

(continued)

TABLE 2-10	Guidelines for a Wheelchair-Accessible Home (continued)

Bathrooms

▶ Walls to be sheathed in ¾″ plywood to allow grab bar installation anywhere.
▶ Door is to either open outward or be pocket type (a door that slides into a hollow cavity).
▶ Clear floor space around each fixture is required for full accessibility.
▶ Outlets to have ground-fault circuit interrupters.
▶ Sinks mounted to walls or sitting vanity styles should have insulation covers on pipes or plumbing shields.
▶ Bowls with a front depth of 3″ and sloping back to 6″ are recommended.
▶ Faucets with lever handles are easiest to operate for both water and temperature control.
▶ Drain stops that are rubber plugs on a chain are preferred over plunger controls located behind the spout.
▶ Toilet is to have 18″ seat height for ease in lateral transfer and be fully accessible.
▶ Toilet paper dispenser to be installed within buyers comfort zone.
▶ Grab bars and handholds should be placed anywhere needed.
▶ Tubs to be a minimum of 30″ × 60″ × 18″ deep.
▶ Roll-in showers to be a minimum of 30″ × 60″.
▶ Showers to be a minimum of 36″ × 36″ and have built-in seats.
▶ Cabinets should be accessible, frameless, and have doors that easily open with one hand.
▶ Wet rooms need to be tiled in slip-proof tile and be sloped for drainage.
▶ Heat lamps should be included.

Kitchens

▶ Counters and workspaces are to be offered at different heights (32″-34″-36″) and various depths (16″-19″-24″).
▶ Appliances should be fully accessible. Braille and large-print dials should be offered.
▶ Cabinets should be accessible and frameless with "D" style pulls.
▶ Cook tops need smooth surfaces with staggered burners and controls that are easy to operate.
▶ Ovens that are built in with side hinges are the best design to use.
▶ Microwave ovens need to be mounted within comfort zone.
▶ Pullout shelves underneath ovens and cook tops add convenience.
▶ Sink to have a height between 32″ and 36″ and depth between 8″ and 5″ with drains and disposals in the rear. Plumbing shields installed in the knee recesses prevent burns.
▶ Faucets that control the temperature and flow of water and have retractable hose sprays should be used.
▶ Dishwasher to have push-button controls and to be located within comfort zone.
▶ Outlets for small appliances are to be located within comfort zone.
▶ Controls for disposals/fans to be located within comfort zone.

Laundry

▶ Easy access to front-loading machines.
▶ Counters, poles, and ironing areas to be accessible and within comfort zone.

Stairway

▶ Should be at least 48″ wide with handrails on both sides.
▶ The landings at both the top and bottom should be no smaller than 36″ × 36″.
▶ Chair and seat lifts can traverse curves and corners; motors can be located in remote locations (closets) or at the top or bottom of stairs.
▶ If chair and seat lifts are inadequate, elevators can be constructed. Home elevators need a floor space area of at least 4 × 6 square feet on each floor to accommodate the elevator car.

Hallways

▶ A width of 40″ is required for easy movement through halls.

Data from Lema AR: Simplified disabled housing, 2006. http://www.freepatentsonline.com/y2006/0059797.html.

REFERENCES

1. Bodenheimer TS, Grumbach K: Introduction: the paradox of excess and deprivation, in Bodenheimer TS, Grumbach K (eds): Understanding Health Policy: A Clinical Approach (ed 5). New York, McGraw-Hill, 2009, pp 1-3.
2. Bodenheimer TS, Grumbach K: Reimbursing healthcare providers, in Bodenheimer TS, Grumbach K (eds): Understanding Health Policy: A Clinical Approach (ed 5). New York, McGraw-Hill, 2009, pp 31-41.
3. Bodenheimer TS, Grumbach K: Paying for healthcare, in Bodenheimer TS, Grumbach K (eds): Understanding Health Policy: A Clinical Approach (ed 5). New York, McGraw-Hill, 2009, pp 5-16.
4. American Physical Therapy Association: Today's Physical Therapist: A Comprehensive Review of a 21st-Century Health Care Profession. Alexandria, Va, American Physical Therapy Association, 2011.
5. Bodenheimer TS, Grumbach K: Access to healthcare, in Bodenheimer TS, Grumbach K (eds): Understanding Health Policy: A Clinical Approach (ed 5). New York, McGraw-Hill, 2009, pp 17-30.
6. Rodwin VG: The Health Planning Predicament. Berkeley, Calif, University of California Press, 1984.
7. Bodenheimer TS, Grumbach K: How health care is organized, in Bodenheimer TS, Grumbach K (eds): Understanding Health Policy: A Clinical Approach (ed 5). New York, McGraw-Hill, 2009, pp 43-57.
8. U.S. Census Bureau: Overview of the Uninsured in the United States, 2011, September 2011, pp 1-5.
9. Moser JW, Applegate KE: Imaging and insurance: do the uninsured get less imaging in emergency departments? J Am Coll Radiol 9:50-57, 2012.
10. Bradley CJ, Dahman B, Shickle LM, et al: Surgery wait times and specialty services for insured and uninsured breast cancer patients: does hospital safety net status matter? Health Serv Res 47:677-697, 2012.
11. Leither MD, Ontrop ND: Improving diabetes care in the uninsured: the success of the Access To Care program in Cook County, Illinois. J Health Care Poor Underserv 23:460-473, 2012.
12. Pollack HA: High-risk pools for the sick and uninsured under health reform: too little and thus too late. J Gen Intern Med 26:91-94, 2011.

13. Young Q: Will America enact national health insurance in 2009? Medscape J Med 10:175, 2008.
14. Pol L: Health insurance in rural America. Rural Policy Brief 5:1-10, 2000.
15. Health insurer's denial of coverage upheld by Fifth Circuit. *Irion v. Prudential Insurance Company of America*. Hosp Law Newsl 10:11, 1993.
16. Wilson DL: The health insurance crisis in America. Natl J (Wash) 22:3110, 1990.
17. Seifert RW, Rukavina M: Bankruptcy is the tip of a medical-debt iceberg. Health Aff (Millwood) 25:w89-92, 2006.
18. Sipkoff M: Higher copayments and deductibles delay medical care, a common problem for Americans. Manag Care 19:46-49, 2010.
19. Henderson JT, Hudson Scholle S, Weisman CS, et al: The role of physician gender in the evaluation of the National Centers of Excellence in Women's Health: test of an alternate hypothesis. Women Health Issues 14:130-139, 2004.
20. Roter DL, Hall JA: Physician gender and patient-centered communication: a critical review of empirical research. Annu Rev Public Health 25:497-519, 2004.
21. Todd KH, Deaton C, D'Adamo AP, et al: Ethnicity and analgesic practice. Ann Emerg Med 35:11-16, 2000.
22. Eroglu SE, Toprak SN, Urgan O, et al: Evaluation of non-urgent visits to a busy urban emergency department. Saudi Med J 33:967-972, 2012.
23. Sommers AS, Boukus ER, Carrier E: Dispelling myths about emergency department use: majority of Medicaid visits are for urgent or more serious symptoms. Res Brief 1-10, 1-3, 2012.
24. Fieldston ES, Alpern ER, Nadel FM, et al: A qualitative assessment of reasons for nonurgent visits to the emergency department: parent and health professional opinions. Pediatr Emerg Care 28:220-225, 2012.
25. Garrett N, Martini EM: The boomers are coming: a total cost of care model of the impact of population aging on the cost of chronic conditions in the United States. Dis Manag 10:51-60, 2007.
26. Hootman JM, Helmick CG: Projections of U.S. prevalence of arthritis and associated activity limitations. Arthritis Rheum 54:226-229, 2006.
27. Uphold CR, Rane D, Reid K, et al: Mental health differences between rural and urban men living with HIV infection in various age groups. J Community Health 30:355-375, 2005.
28. Americans with Disabilities Act of 1989: 104 Stat 327.101-336, 42 USC 12101 s2 (a) (8), 1989.
29. Waddell G, Waddell H: A review of social influences on neck and back pain disability, in Nachemson AL, Jonsson E (eds): Neck and Back Pain: The Scientific Evidence of Causes, Diagnosis, and Treatment. Philadelphia, Lippincott Williams & Wilkins, 2000, pp 13-55.
30. American Physical Therapy Association: Guide to Physical Therapist Practice. (ed 2). Phys Ther 81:1-746, 2001.
31. Lechner D, Daly J, Maltchev K, et al: The work-injured population, in Boissonnault WG (ed): Primary Care for the Physical Therapist: Examination and Triage. St Louis, Elsevier Saunders, 2005, pp 271-287.
32. Schmitz TJ: Examination of the environment, in O'Sullivan SB, Schmitz TJ (eds): Physical Rehabilitation (ed 5). Philadelphia, FA Davis, 2007, pp 401-467.
33. Paterson M, Mets T: Environmental assessment: home, community, and work, in Cameron MH, Monroe LG (eds): Physical Rehabilitation: Evidence-Based Examination, Evaluation, and Intervention. St Louis, Saunders/Elsevier, 2007, pp 918-936.
34. Mackenzie M: A simplified measure of balance by functional reach. Physiother Res Int 4:233-236, 1999.
35. Duncan PW, Weiner DK, Chandler J, et al: Functional reach: a new clinical measure of balance. J Gerontol 45:M192-M197, 1990.

Evidence-Informed Practice

CHAPTER 3

CHAPTER OBJECTIVES

*At the completion of this chapter,
the reader will be able to:*

1. Provide a historical perspective on the evolution of evidence-informed practice (EIP)

2. Discuss the importance of EIP

3. List some of the reasons why EIP became important in healthcare

4. Describe the various research designs and their advantages and disadvantages

5. Differentiate among the experimental, quasi-experimental, and nonexperimental research designs

6. Differentiate between the form and uses of the null and research hypotheses

7. Differentiate among and discuss the roles of independent, dependent, and extraneous variables

8. Discuss the concept of research validity of a study

9. List the various threats to validity

10. Describe the different types of reliability and the roles they play in EIP

11. Discuss the various hierarchies of evidence

12. Discuss how EIP can be used in clinical decision making

OVERVIEW

An important component of the Vision 2020 statement set forth by the American Physical Therapy Association (APTA)[1] is achieving direct access through independent, self-determined, professional judgment and action.[1] With the majority of states now permitting direct access to physical therapists, many physical therapists now have the primary responsibility for being the gatekeepers of health care and for making medical referrals. In light of the APTA's movement toward realizing "Vision 2020," an operational definition of *autonomous practice* and the related term *autonomous*

physical therapist practitioner is given by the APTA's board as follows:

▶ "Autonomous physical therapist practice is practice characterized by independent, self-determined professional judgment and action."

▶ "An autonomous physical therapist practitioner within the scope of practice defined by the *Guide to Physical Therapist Practice* provides physical therapy services to patients who have direct and unrestricted access to their services, and may refer as appropriate to other healthcare providers and other professionals and for diagnostic tests."[2]

Through the history and physical examination, a physical therapist diagnoses and classifies different types of information for use in clinical reasoning and the intervention.[3] This requires that the clinician have a high level of knowledge, including an understanding of the concepts of medical screening and differential diagnosis. In addition, the clinician must be able to determine the quality of the research evidence before integrating that evidence into his or her practice.

Evidence is used comprehensively in clinical decision making within the healthcare professions. The physical therapy profession has expressed a commitment to the development and use of evidence through a variety of initiatives including the American Physical Therapy Association's introduction of a periodic feature in their journal, "Evidence in Practice," and a database of research articles, "Hooked on Evidence." Evidence-informed practice (EIP) refers to practice that is associated with epidemiological evidence and healthcare needs.[4]

CLINICAL PEARL

The production of evidence to support physical therapy services is only truly effective when practitioners integrate evidence into their practice.

The term *EIP* is used to refer to specific evidence-supported interventions—according to Sackett and colleagues,[5] EIP involves the integration of best research evidence with clinical expertise and patient values. This is in contrast to the old-fashioned reliance on knowledge gained from authority, hearsay, habit, or tradition.

The relatively recent interest in the use of EIP has resulted from a number of issues, including[6–13]:

▶ The continued increase in healthcare costs

▶ Extensive documentation of apparently unexplained practice variations in the management of a variety of conditions

▶ An increase in publicity surrounding medical errors

▶ The identification of potential or actual harm resulting from previously approved medications or techniques

▶ Recent trends in technology assessment and outcomes research

▶ The rapid evolution of Internet technology

▶ The need for proof to commercial and government insurance payers of the efficacy of a particular treatment or technique

Physical therapists are responsible for thoroughly examining each patient and then either treating the patient according to established guidelines, or referring the patient to a more appropriate healthcare provider.[14] Ultimately, given the role of physical therapists as movement specialists, task analysis should form the basis of the diagnosis.[15] A good test must differentiate the target disorder from other disorders with which it might otherwise be confused.[16] For example, when a physical therapist performs an examination and evaluation, he or she can use evidence to choose, apply, and interpret findings from a wide variety of available tests and measures, thereby enhancing the efficiency and effectiveness of service delivery.[6]

EVIDENCE-INFORMED PRACTICE

Research involves a controlled, systematic approach to obtain an answer to a question.[17] A search for relevant evidence to answer the question is then followed by critical appraisal of its qualities, applicability, and conclusions. This requires knowledge of the evidence appraisal process, access to the evidence, and the ability to discriminate between stronger and weaker evidence. Ideally, the located evidence will address specifically the test, diagnostic classification system, risk factor, treatment technique, or outcome that the physical therapist is considering relative to an individual patient/client—the research has more credibility if the subjects in the study have characteristics that are similar to the patient/client about whom the physical therapist has a clinical question.[18]

CLINICAL PEARL

EIP is best supported by research that is relevant and that advances knowledge in the professional field.[19]

In addition, there are a number of criteria that must be met, including[18]:

▶ The credibility of the research in terms of its design and execution. A number of research designs are outlined in Table 3-1. Research designs can be viewed as a continuum in terms of their usefulness.

TABLE 3-1	Research Designs
Type of Design	**Description**
Experimental	Purposeful manipulation of subjects who have been randomly assigned into two or more groups with measurement of their resulting behavior. Experimental designs are the most restrictive in terms of the amount of control imposed on study participants and conditions. The classic experimental study design is the randomized controlled trial (RCT).
Quasi-experimental	Maintains the purposeful manipulation of the experimental design but involves no randomization of subjects to groups, or may have only one subject group to evaluate. Often used when researchers have difficulty obtaining sufficient numbers of subjects, or when group membership is predetermined by a subject characteristic (whether or not the subject received a particular medical or surgical intervention). Single-system designs are a type of quasi-experimental study that can be used to investigate the usefulness of an intervention.
Nonexperimental or observational	Researchers are simply observers who collect information about the phenomenon of interest; there is no experimental manipulation of subjects. These designs have less control than quasi-experimental studies, as they have similar limitations with respect to their groupings.
Physiologic studies	Focus only on cellular, anatomical, or physiological systems and not on personal level function.
Case report	Describes what occurred with a patient/client.
Case-control studies	A retrospective approach in which subjects who are known to have the diagnosis of interest are compared to a control group known to be free of the diagnosis.
Cohort design	Refers to a group of subjects who are followed over time and who usually share a common characteristic such as gender, occupation, or diagnosis.
Narrative review	A summary of prior research on a particular topic without using a systematic search and critical appraisal process.
Systematic review	A narrative review that addresses a specific research question. Includes detailed inclusion and exclusion criteria for selection of studies to review and preestablished quality criteria with which to rate the value of the individual studies, usually applied by blinded reviewers. A meta-analysis involves additional statistical analysis using a pooling of the data from the individual studies in a systematic review.

CLINICAL PEARL

▶ Qualitative research: a research approach that assumes that truth is subjective and relative to each individual, such that multiple realities exist, the measurement of which is influenced by the interdependence of researchers and the subjects.[20] Data are provided in words rather than in numbers through interviews, surveys, or other mechanisms.

▶ Quantitative research: a research approach that assumes that an objective reality exists that can be measured through the use of standardized numerical measures that can be evaluated to determine cause-and-effect relationships by researchers who are independent of the subjects.[20]

▶ Whether or not the research article is peer reviewed.

▶ The relevance of the findings for the field and/or the specific journal. Ideally, the study should address the specific clinical question the clinician is trying to answer, and the subjects in the study should have characteristics that are similar to the patient/client in question.[18] The standard for the assessment of the efficacy and value of a test or intervention is the clinical trial, that is, a prospective study assessing the effect and value of a test or intervention against a control in human subjects.[21]

▶ The contribution to the body of knowledge about the topic.

▶ The date of the publication.

The gathering of evidence must occur in a systematic, reproducible, and unbiased manner to select and interpret diagnostic tests and to assess potential interventions.[22] The EIP process generally occurs in five steps[23]:

1. Formulating a clinical question, including details about the patient type or problem, the intervention being considered, a comparison intervention, and the outcome measure to be used.

2. Searching for the best evidence, which can include a literature search on Ovid, EMBASE, PubMed, PEDro, or other medical search engine database using the keywords from the clinical question.

3. Critical appraisal of the evidence. In general there are two types of clinical studies—those that analyze primary data and those that analyze secondary data.[24] Studies that collect and analyze primary data include case reports and series, case-control, cross-sectional, cohort (both prospective and retrospective), and randomized controlled trials (RCTs) (Table 3-2).[24] Analysis of second-rate data

TABLE 3-2	Randomized Controlled Trials, Systematic Reviews, and Clinical Practice Guidelines
Randomized controlled trials (RCTs)	Experimental designs that focus on treatment efficacy. Involve experiments on people. Less exposed to bias. Ensures comparability of groups. Typically, volunteers agreed to be randomly allocated to groups receiving one of the following: ▶ Treatment and no treatment ▶ Standard treatment and standard treatment plus a new treatment ▶ Two alternate treatments The common feature is that the experimental group receives the treatment of interest and the control group does not. At the end of the trial, outcomes of subjects in each group are determined—the difference in outcomes between groups provides an estimate of the size of the treatment effect. Best suited to answer questions about whether an experimental intervention has an effect and whether that effect is beneficial or harmful to the subjects.
Systematic reviews	Reviews of the literature conducted in a way that is designed to minimize bias. Can be used to assess the effects of health interventions, the accuracy of diagnostic tests, or the prognosis for a particular condition. Usually involve criteria to determine which studies will be considered, the search strategy used to locate studies, the methods for assessing the quality of the studies, and the process used to synthesize the findings of individual studies. Particularly useful for busy clinicians who may be unable to access all the relevant trials in an area and may otherwise need to rely on their own incomplete surveys of relevant trials.
Clinical practice guidelines	Recommendations for management of a particular clinical condition. Involve compilation of evidence concerning needs and expectations of recipients of care, the accuracy of diagnostic tests, and effects of therapy and prognosis. Usually necessitates the conduct of one or sometimes several systematic reviews. Maybe presented as clinical decision algorithms. Can provide a useful framework on which clinicians can build clinical practice.

Data from Maher CG, Herbert RD, Moseley AM, et al: Critical appraisal of randomized trials, systematic reviews of randomized trials and clinical practice guidelines, in Boyling JD, Jull GA (eds), Grieve's Modern Manual Therapy: The Vertebral Column. Philadelphia, Churchill Livingstone, 2004, pp 603-614; Petticrew M: Systematic reviews from astronomy to zoology: myths and misconceptions. BMJ 322:98-101, 2001.

occurs in systematic reviews or meta-analyses for the purpose of pooling or synthesizing data to answer a question that is perhaps not practical or answerable within an individual study.[24] Another way to broadly categorize studies is as *experimental*, where an intervention is introduced to subjects, or *observational*, in which no active treatment is introduced to the subjects.[24]

4. Applying the evidence to the patient. Once the evidence has been critically appraised, the clinician must consider the evidence in the context of his or her clinical expertise and the patient's values and preferences or goals.

5. Evaluation of the outcome. The outcome is the end product of the patient/client management process and should be distinguished from treatment effects. An outcome reflects the patient/client's goals for the physical therapy episode of care from the patient/client's point of view.

Research Article

Each research article consists of a number of elements, which include[25]:

▶ *Title*. The purpose of the title is to identify the major variables studied and to provide clues about whether the purpose of the research is description, relationship analysis, or difference analysis.

▶ *Abstract*. This element briefly summarizes the purpose of the research, the methods, and the results.

▶ *Introduction*. This element defines the broad problems that underlie the study, states the specific purposes of the study, and places the problem and purposes into the theoretical context of previous work.

▶ *Method*. This portion is usually subdivided into Subjects (the method used for their selection, inclusion and exclusion criteria, methods used to assign them to various groups, and any other significant features of the subjects including mean age and sex), Dependent Variables, Design, Instruments, Procedures, and Data Analysis sections—see later.

▶ *Results*. This element presents the results without comment on their meaning.

▶ *Discussion*. The purpose of the discussion is to present the authors' interpretation of the results, along with their assessment of study limitations and directions for future research.

▶ *Conclusions*. As its name suggests, this element concisely restates the important findings of the research and presents a conclusion for each purpose outlined in the introduction.

▶ *References*. List of references cited in the text of the article.

Hypotheses

Most research begins with a question or a purpose statement. For example, does age predict whether a patient will be discharged to home or inpatient rehabilitation following a total knee replacement? A hypothesis attempts to offer a prediction. Every hypothesis-testing situation begins with the statement of a hypothesis—a prediction about the outcome of the study.[26] In the previous example, the prediction may be "Yes, age does predict whether a patient will be discharged to home or inpatient rehabilitation following a total knee replacement."

There are two types of statistical hypothesis of each situation: the null hypothesis (H_0), and the alternative hypothesis (H_A).

▶ *Null hypothesis (H_0)*: a hypothesis that states that there will be no difference between the groups or variables.[26] The null hypothesis is also referred to as the statistical hypothesis. The premise behind this approach is that a study's results may be due to chance rather than due to the experiment or phenomenon of interest.[19]

▶ *Alternative (research) hypothesis (H_A)*: a hypothesis that there will be a difference between the groups or variables.[26] The alternative hypothesis is also referred to as the research hypothesis. The premise behind this approach is that a study's results included directional statements such as more/less than and positive/negative.[19]

Subject Selection

Whenever clinical research is performed, data are collected from people, specifically a target population based on the research question or purpose—for example, all athletes who undergo rotator cuff surgery. Unfortunately, not every member of these target populations may be accessible to the researchers, so the researchers use a collection of subjects called a *sample* that best represent the population from which they are drawn.

CLINICAL PEARL

▶ A population consists of all subjects (human or otherwise) that are being studied.

▶ A sample is a group of subjects selected from a population. One of the challenges facing researchers is to achieve an adequate sample size to avoid an incorrect conclusion.

To avoid any biasing of the collected information, samples must be collected in a systematic fashion. Sampling can occur using a probabilistic method or a nonprobabilistic method. Probabilistic methods include:

▶ *Random sampling*: all items have the same chance of selection, thereby minimizing sampling bias—for example, drawing numbers out of a hat.

▶ *Systematic sampling*: in which potential subjects are organized according to an identifier such as a birth date, Social Security number, or medical record number.

▶ *Stratified sampling*: sometimes called *proportional* or *quota* random sampling; involves dividing the population into homogeneous subgroups called strata, and then taking a simple random sample from each subgroup to highlight a specific subgroup. Thus, stratified sampling ensures that the overall population will be represented in addition to key subgroups of the population. For example, the most common strata used to formulate subgroups include age, gender, religion, educational achievement, socioeconomic status, and nationality.

▶ *Cluster sampling:* involves dividing the population into groups or clusters (such as geographic boundaries), then randomly selecting sample clusters and using all members of the selected clusters as subjects of the samples. For example, it may not be possible to list all of the patients of a chain of physical therapy clinics. However, it would be possible to randomly select a subset of clinics (stage 1 of cluster sampling) and then interview a random sample of patients who visit those clinics (stage 2 of cluster sampling).

Nonprobabilistic methods include[27]:

▶ *Convenience sampling:* in which researchers recruit easily available individuals who meet the criteria for the study—for example, requesting students to volunteer.

▶ *Snowball sampling:* in which the researchers start with a few subjects and then recruit more via word of mouth from the original participants.

▶ *Purposive sampling:* in which the researchers make specific choices about who will serve as subjects in this study by handpicking individuals with certain characteristics.

Variables

Studies about a diagnostic test require information about the specific test performed and the diagnoses obtained, whereas studies about an intervention require information about the interventions provided and their effects.[28] The tests, diagnoses, interventions, and effects are referred to generically as variables.[28]

> ### CLINICAL PEARL
>
> A variable is a measurement of phenomena that can assume more than one value or more than one category.[17] The two traits of a variable that should always be achieved include:
>
> ▶ Each variable should be *exhaustive*: it should include all possible answerable responses.
>
> ▶ Each variable should be *mutually exclusive*: no respondent should be able to have two attributes simultaneously.

Dependency refers to the "role" of the variable in the experiment or study. Different study designs require different types of variables. Two common types of variables include the independent variable and dependent variable:

▶ *Independent variable:* one that is purposely manipulated by the researcher; independent variables are controlled or fixed in order to observe their effect on dependent variables. An example of an independent variable would be the treatment received by a subject.

▶ *Dependent variable:* the variable that is the outcome of interest in a study. Using pain as an example, if a study examines the effects of iontophoresis on pain levels, the iontophoresis is the independent variable and the measurement of pain levels is the dependent variable.

> ### CLINICAL PEARL
>
> An extraneous variable is a factor other than the independent variable that is set to influence, or confound, the dependent variable.[29] Examples of extraneous variables include subjects, equipment, and environmental conditions.

Measurement of Variables

Variables can be classified by how they are categorized, counted, or measured. This type of classification uses measurement scales. The four classic scales (or levels) of measurement include[30]:

▶ *Nominal (classificatory; categorical):* classifies data into mutually exclusive, exhausting categories in which no order or ranking can be imposed. Examples include arbitrary labels, such as zip codes, religion, and marital status.

▶ *Ordinal (ranking):* classifies data into categories that can be ranked, although precise differences between the ranks do not exist. Examples include letter grades (A, B, C, etc.) and body builds (small, medium, large).

▶ *Interval:* ranks data where precise differences between units of measure do exist, although there is no meaningful zero. Examples include temperature (degrees Celsius, degrees Fahrenheit), IQ, calendar dates.

▶ *Ratio:* possesses all the characteristics of interval measurement, and there exists a true zero. Examples include height, weight, age, and salary.

Validity

After determining the question being asked in a study, and having an overview of the types of studies used in clinical research, the next step is to look at data analysis, which validates the answer to the question. Research or test validity is defined as the degree to which a test measures what it purports to be measuring, and how well it correctly classifies individuals with or without a particular condition.[31–33]

> ### CLINICAL PEARL
>
> A test is considered to have diagnostic accuracy if it has the ability to discriminate between patients with and without a specific disorder.[34]

There are a number of forms of measurement validity that may be evaluated to determine the potential validity of a study:

▶ *Construct validity.* Construct validity refers to the ability of a test to represent the underlying construct (the theory developed to organize and explain some aspects of existing knowledge and observations). Construct validity refers to overall validity.

▶ *Face validity.* Face validity refers to the degree to which the questions or procedures incorporated within a test make sense to the users. The assessment of face validity is generally informal and nonquantitative and is the lowest standard of assessing validity—it is based on the notion that the finding is valid "on the face of it." For example, if a weighing scale indicates that a normal-sized person weighs 2000 pounds, that scale does not have face validity.

▶ *Content validity.* Content validity refers to the assessment by experts that the content of the measure is consistent with what is to be measured. Content validity is concerned with sample-population representativeness—that is, the knowledge and skills covered by the test items should be representative of the larger domain of knowledge and skills. In many instances, it is difficult, if not impossible, to administer a test covering all aspects of knowledge or skills. Therefore, only several tasks are sampled from the population of knowledge or skills. In these circumstances, the proportion of the score attributable to a particular component should be proportional to the importance of that component to total performance. In content validity, evidence is obtained by looking for agreement in judgments by judges. In short, one person can determine face validity, but a panel should confirm content validity.

▶ *Convergent validity.* A method with which to evaluate the construct validity of an instrument by assessing the relationship between scores on the instrument of interest, and scores on another instrument that is said to measure the same concept or constructs.

▶ *Discriminant validity.* Discriminant validity is the ability of a test to distinguish between two different constructs and is evidenced by a low correlation between the results of the test and those of tests of a different construct.

▶ *Criterion validity.* Criterion validity is determined by comparing the results of a test to those of a test that is accepted as a "gold standard" test (a test that is accepted as being close to 100% valid).[35]

▶ *Concurrent validity.* The degree to which the measurement being validated agrees with an established measurement standard administered at approximately the same time. Concurrent validity is a form of criterion validity.

▶ *Predictive validity.* Predictive validity is the extent to which test scores are associated with future behavior or performance.

CLINICAL PEARL

It is important to remember that there are no perfect studies because of the reciprocal nature of many of the threats to validity.

A number of factors can threaten the validity of a research project. The most common threats to validity include:

▶ *Ambiguity*—when correlation is taken for causation.

▶ *Subject assignment*—subject age, gender, ethnic and racial background, educational level, and presence of comorbidities can all threaten the validity unless randomization is used.

▶ *Errors of measurement*—random errors or systematic errors.

▶ *History*—when some critical event occurs between the pretest and posttest results.

▶ *Instrumentation*—when the researcher changes the measuring device.

▶ *Maturation*—when people change or mature physically, psychologically, emotionally, or spiritually over the research period.

▶ *Attrition*—when people die or drop out of the research project.

▶ *Testing*—subjects may appear to demonstrate improvement based on their growing familiarity with the testing procedure, or based on different instructions and cues provided by the person administering the test.

▶ *The John Henry Effect*—when groups compete to score well.

▶ *The Hawthorne Effect*—A tendency of research subjects to act atypically as a result of their awareness of being studied.

▶ *Statistical regression to the mean*—when a nonrandomized sample is selected, the average of that sample tends to regress towards the mean. For example, if a group of students is given a test (pretest) and the researchers select the group that lies at the bottom 5% of the total test takers, in the next test (posttest), the same group will often have a higher score than their pretest values. In a similar manner, if the researchers take the top 5% students on the pretest, they will probably perform more poorly in the posttest compared to the pretest when considered as a group.

Validity is directly related to the notion of sensitivity and specificity. The sensitivity and specificity of any physical test to discriminate relevant dysfunction must be appreciated to make meaningful decisions.[36] Sensitivity is the ability of the test to pick up what it is testing for, and specificity is the ability of the test to reject what it is not testing for.

▶ Sensitivity represents the proportion of patients with a disorder who test positive. A test that can correctly identify every person who has the disorder has a sensitivity of 1.0. *SnNout* is an acronym for when *sen*sitivity of a symptom or sign is high, a *n*egative response rules *out* the target disorder. Thus, a so-called highly sensitive test helps rule out a disorder. The positive predictive value is the proportion of patients with positive test results who are correctly diagnosed.

▶ Specificity is the proportion of the study population without the disorder that test negative.[35] A test that can correctly identify every person who does not have the target disorder has a specificity of 1.0. *SpPin* is an acronym for when *sp*ecificity is extremely high, a *p*ositive test result rules *in* the target disorder. Thus, a so-called highly specific test helps rule in a disorder or condition.

Reliability

Numerous physical therapy tests exist that are designed to help the clinician rule out some of the many possible diagnoses. Regardless of which test is chosen, the test must be performed reliably by the clinician in order for the test to be a valuable guide. Reliability describes the extent to which test or measurement is free from error. A test is considered reliable if it produces precise, accurate, and reproducible information.[38] Two types of reliability are often described:

▶ *Interrater*. This type of reliability determines whether two or more examiners can repeat a test consistently.

▶ *Intrarater*. This type of reliability determines whether the same single examiner can repeat the test consistently.

Reliability is quantitatively expressed by way of an index of agreement, with the simplest index being the percentage agreement value. The statistical coefficients most commonly used to characterize the reliability of the tests and measures are the intraclass correlation coefficient (ICC) and the kappa statistic (κ), both of which are based on statistical models[39]:

▶ The ICC is a reliability coefficient calculated with variance estimates obtained through an *analysis of variance* (Table 3-3).[40] The advantages of the ICC over correlation coefficients are that it does not require the same number of raters per subject, and it can be used for two or more raters or ratings.[40]

▶ The kappa statistic (κ) is a chance-corrected index of agreement that overcomes the problem of chance agreement when used with nominal and ordinal data.[41] With nominal data, the kappa statistic is applied after the percentage agreement between testers has been determined. However, with higher scale data, it tends to underestimate reliability.[42] Theoretically, κ can be negative if agreement is worse than chance. Practically, in clinical reliability studies, κ usually varies between 0.00

TABLE 3-3	Intraclass Correlation Coefficient Benchmark Values	
Value	**Description**	
<0.75	Poor-to-moderate agreement	
>0.75	Good agreement	
>90	Reasonable agreement for clinical measurements	

Data from Portney L, Watkins MP: Foundations of Clinical Research: Applications to Practice. Norwalk, Conn, Appleton & Lange, 1993.

and 1.00.[42] The κ statistic does not differentiate among disagreements; it assumes that all disagreements are of equal significance.[42]

▶ Standard error of measurement (SEM). The SEM reflects the reliability of the response when the test is performed many times and is an indication of how much change there might be when the test is repeated.[42] If the SEM is small, then the test is stable, with minimal variability between tests.[42]

Once the specificity and sensitivity of the test is established (see Validity), the predictive value of a positive test versus a negative test can be determined if the prevalence of the disease/dysfunction is known. For example, when the prevalence of the disease increases, a patient with a positive test is more likely to have the disease (a false negative is less likely). A negative result of a highly sensitive test will probably rule out a common disease, whereas if the disease is rare, the test must be much more specific for it to be clinically useful.

The likelihood ratio (LR) is the index measurement that combines sensitivity and specificity values and can be used to gauge the performance of a diagnostic test, as it indicates how much a given diagnostic test result will lower or raise the pretest probability of the target disorder.[16,35]

Four measures contribute to sensitivity and specificity (Table 3-4):

▶ *True positive*. The test indicates that the patient has the disease or dysfunction, and this is confirmed by the gold standard test.

▶ *False positive*. The clinical test indicates that the disease or dysfunction is present, but this is not confirmed by the gold standard test.

▶ *False negative*. The clinical test indicates absence of the disorder, but the gold standard test shows that the disease or dysfunction is present.

TABLE 3-4	2 × 2 Table			
			Disease/Outcome	
			Present	**Absent**
Test	Positive (+ve)		a (true +ve)	b (false +ve)
	Negative (−ve)		c (false −ve)	d (true −ve)

TABLE 3-5   Definition and Calculation of Statistical Measures

Statistical Measure	Definition	Calculation
Accuracy	The proportion of people who were correctly identified as either having or not having the disease or dysfunction	$(TP + TN)/(TP + FP + FN + TN)$
Sensitivity	A pre-test probability to determine the proportion of people with the disease or dysfunction who will have a positive test result	$TP/(TP + FN)$
Specificity	A pre-test probability to determine the proportion of people without the disease or dysfunction who will have a negative test result	$TN/(FP + TN)$
Positive predictive value	A post-test probability to determine the proportion of people who truly have the disease or dysfunction when the test is positive	$TP/(TP + FP)$
Negative predictive value	A post-test probability to determine the proportion of people who truly do not have the disease or dysfunction when the test is negative	$TN/(FN + TN)$
Positive likelihood ratio	How likely a positive test result is in people who have the disease or dysfunction as compared to how likely it is in those who do not have the disease or dysfunction	Sensitivity$/(1 -$ specificity$)$
Negative likelihood ratio	How likely a negative test result is in people who have the disease or dysfunction as compared to how likely it is in those who do not have the disease or dysfunction	$(1 -$ sensitivity$)/$specificity

TP, true positive; TN, true negative; FP, false positive; FN, false negative.

Data from Fritz JM, Wainner RS: Examining diagnostic tests: an evidence-based perspective. Phys Ther 81:1546-1564, 2001; Powell JW, Huijbregts PA: Concurrent criterion-related validity of acromioclavicular joint physical examination tests: a systematic review. J Man Manip Ther 14:E19-E29, 2006.

▶ *True negative.* The clinical and the gold standard test agree that the disease or dysfunction is absent.

These values are used to calculate the statistical measures of accuracy, sensitivity, specificity, negative and positive predictive values, and negative and positive likelihood ratios (LRs), as indicated in Table 3-5. Another way to summarize diagnostic test performance is to use Table 3-4 through the diagnostic odds ratio (DOR): DOR = true/false = $(a \times d)/(b \times c)$. The DOR of a test is the ratio of the odds of positivity in disease relative to the odds of positivity in the nondiseased. The value of a DOR ranges from 0 to infinity, with higher values indicating better discriminatory test performance. A score of 1 means a test does not discriminate between patients with the disorder and those without.

CLINICAL PEARL

The DOR value rises steeply when sensitivity or specificity becomes near perfect.

The quality assessment of studies of diagnostic accuracy (QUADAS)[45] is an evidence-based quality assessment tool currently recommended for use in systematic reviews of diagnostic accuracy studies. The aim of a diagnostic accuracy study (DAS) is to determine how good a particular test is at detecting the target condition. DAS allow the calculation of various statistics that provide an indication of "test performance"—how good the index test is at detecting the target condition. These statistics include sensitivity, specificity, positive and negative predictive values, positive and negative likelihood ratios, and diagnostics odds ratios. The QUADAS

tool is a list of 14 questions that should each be answered "yes," "no," or "unclear" (Table 3-6). A score of 10 or more "yes" answers is indicative of a higher quality study, whereas a score of fewer than 10 "yes" answers suggests a poorly designed study.

USING EVIDENCE IN CLINICAL DECISION MAKING

Decision making encompasses the selection of tests in the examination process, interpretation of data from the detailed history and examination, establishment of the diagnosis, estimation of the prognosis, determination of intervention strategies, sequence of therapeutic procedures, and establishment of discharge criteria.[2] Ideally, the evidence located will address specifically the test, classification system, risk factors, treatment technique, or outcome that the clinician is considering relative to an individual patient/client.[18] The methodologic hierarchy or rating of scientific studies is well documented in the literature (Table 3-7). Clinicians must constantly remind themselves that without information gathered from controlled clinical trials, they have limited scientific basis for their tests or interventions.[46]

In order to evaluate the literature, the following six-step generic sequence is recommended[25]:

1. *Classify the research and variables.* For example, if the reader determines that the research is experimental, the authors are likely to make causal statements about their results; if the reader determines that the research is nonexperimental, the expectation about causal statements should change. If the dependent variables of interest are such things as range of motion measures, the reader should expect clean, easily understood results, as

TABLE 3-6	The QUADAS Tool			
Item		**Yes**	**No**	**Unclear**
1.	Was the spectrum of patients representative of the patients who will receive the test in practice?	( )	( )	( )
2.	Were selection criteria clearly described?	( )	( )	( )
3.	Is the reference standard likely to correctly classify the target condition?	( )	( )	( )
4.	Is the time period between reference standard and index test short enough to be reasonably sure that the target condition did not change between the two tests?	( )	( )	( )
5.	Did the whole sample, or a random selection of the sample, receive verification using a reference standard of diagnosis?	( )	( )	( )
6.	Did patients receive the same reference standard regardless of the index test result?	( )	( )	( )
7.	Was the reference standard independent of the index test (i.e., the index test did not form part of the reference standard)?	( )	( )	( )
8.	Was the execution of the index test described in sufficient detail to permit replication of the test?	( )	( )	( )
9.	Was the execution of the reference standard described in sufficient detail to permit its replication?	( )	( )	( )
10.	Were the index test results interpreted without knowledge of the results of the reference standard?	( )	( )	( )
11.	Were the reference standard results interpreted without knowledge of the results of the index test?	( )	( )	( )
12.	Were the same clinical data available when test results were interpreted as would be available when the test is used in practice?	( )	( )	( )
13.	Were uninterpretable/intermediate test results reported?	( )	( )	( )
14.	Were withdrawals from the study explained?	( )	( )	( )

Data from Whiting P, Rutjes AW, Reitsma JB, et al: The development of QUADAS: a tool for the quality assessment of studies of diagnostic accuracy included in systematic reviews. BMC Med Res Methodol 3:25, 2003.

opposed to the results found when measuring patterns of interaction between a patient and a clinician.

2. *Compare purposes and conclusions.* This comparison serves two purposes: it indicates whether or not the study is internally consistent and also provides guidance for the critique of the methods, results, and discussion.

3. *Describe design and control elements.* The reader must determine both the design of the study and the level of control the researchers exerted over implementation of the independent variable, selection and assignment of participants, extraneous variables related to the setting or participants, measurement, and information.

4. *Identify threats to research validity.* As previously mentioned, the threats to research validity can be divided into construct, internal, and external validity.

5. *Place the study in the context of other research.* The reader must determine how much new information the study adds to what is already known about a topic.

6. *Evaluate the personal utility of the study.* During this step, the reader determines whether the study has meaning for his or her own practice.

When integrating evidence into clinical decision making, an understanding of how to appraise the quality of the evidence offered by clinical studies is important. One of the major problems in evaluating studies is that the volume of literature makes it difficult for the busy clinician to obtain and analyze all of the evidence necessary to guide the clinical decision-making process.[38] The other problem involves deciding whether the results from the literature are definite enough to indicate an effect other than chance. Judging the strength of the evidence becomes an important part of the decision-making process.

CLINICAL PEARL

Clinical prediction rules (CPRs) are tools designed to assist clinicians in decision making when caring for patients. However, although there is a growing trend toward designing a number of CPRs for physical therapy, few presently exist.

The best evidence for making decisions about interventions comes from randomized controlled trials, systematic reviews,

TABLE 3-7 A Hierarchy of Evidence Grading

	Level of Evidence Grading = 1a	Level of Evidence Grading = 1b	Level of Evidence Grading = 1c	Level of Evidence Grading = 2a	Level of Evidence Grading = 2b	Level of Evidence Grading = 2c	Level of Evidence Grading = 3a	Level of Evidence Grading = 3b	Level of Evidence Grading = 4	Level of Evidence Grading = 5
Type of Study	Systematic review of randomized clinical trials that do not have statistically significant variation in the direction or degrees of results	Individual randomized clinical trial with narrow confidence interval	All-or-none study (a study in which some or all patients died before treatment became available, and then none die after the treatment)	Systematic review of cohort studies that do not have statistically significant variation in the direction or degrees of results	Individual cohort study (including low-quality randomized clinical trial)	Outcomes research nonexperimental research that evaluates outcomes of care in *real-world* clinical conditions	Nonrandomized trial with concurrent or historical controls Study of sensitivity and specificity of a diagnostic test Population-based descriptive study	Individual case-control study	Cross sectional study Case series study-Case report	Expert consensus Clinical experience

Data from Sackett DL: Rules of evidence and clinical recommendations on the use of antithrombotic agents. Chest 89:2S-3S, 1986; and the Oxford Center for Evidence-based Medicine (www.cebm.net).

and evidence-based clinical practice guidelines.[47] At the other end of the continuum is the unsystematic collection of patient/client data. In between the two ends of the evidence continuum are the study designs outlined in Table 3-1, with quasi-experimental designs being the strongest and narrative reviews being the weakest. Proponents of evidence-informed medicine have attempted to make the study selection process easier by developing hierarchies, or levels of evidence (see Table 3-7).

It may also be possible to discriminate between high- and low-quality trials by asking three simple questions[47]:

1. Were subjects randomly allocated to conditions? Random allocation implies that a nonsystematic, unpredictable procedure was used to allocate subjects to conditions.

2. Was there blinding of assessors and patients? Blinding of assessors and patients minimizes the risk of the placebo effect and the "Hawthorne effect."[48]

3. Was there adequate follow-up? Ideally, all subjects who enter the trial should subsequently be followed up to avoid bias. In practice this rarely happens. As a general rule, losses to follow-up of less than 10% avoid serious bias, but losses to follow-up of more than 20% cause potential for serious bias.

Patients may be referred to physical therapy with a nonspecific diagnosis, an incorrect diagnosis, or no diagnosis at all.[49] A diagnosis can only be made when all potential causes for the signs and symptoms have been ruled out. The best indicator for the correctness of a diagnosis is the quality of the hypothesis considered, because if the appropriate diagnosis is not considered from the start, any subsequent inquiries will be misdirected.[50] Once impairments have been highlighted, a determination can be made as to the reason for those impairments and the relationship between the impairments and the patient's functional limitations or disabilities.

The decision-making process is a multifaceted fluid process that combines tacit knowledge with accumulated clinical experience.[51] The experienced clinician is able to recognize patterns and extrapolate information from them using forward reasoning, to develop an accurate working hypothesis.[52] This is accomplished through an estimate of the proportional contribution of tissue pathology and *impairment clusters* to the patient's functional limitations.[53] Using this information, the clinician puts a value on examination findings, considering relevant environmental, social, cultural, psychological, medical, and physical findings, and clusters the information into recognizable, understandable, or identifiable diagnoses, dysfunctions, or classification syndromes.[53] According to Kahney,[54] the expert seems to do less problem solving than the novice, because the former has already stored solutions to many of the clinical problems previously encountered.[55]

One of the problems for the clinician is how to attach relevance to all the information gleaned from the examination. This judgment process can be viewed as a continuum. At one end of the continuum is the novice who uses very clear-cut signposts; at the other end there is the experienced clinician who has a vast bank of clinical experiences from which to draw.[55] Experts are able to see meaningful relationships, possess enhanced memory, are skilled in qualitative analysis, and have well-developed reflection skills.[51] This combination

of skills allows the expert to systematically organize the information to make efficient and effective clinical decisions.

What differentiates diagnosis by the physical therapist from diagnosis by the physician is not the process itself but the phenomena being observed and clarified.[56] Sackett and colleagues[22] proposed three strategies of clinical diagnosis:

▶ *Pattern recognition.* This is characterized by the clinician's instantaneous realization that the patient conforms to a previously learned pattern of disease.

▶ *History and physical examination.* This method requires the clinician to consider all hypotheses of the potential etiology.

▶ *Hypothetico-deductive method.* In this method, the clinician identifies early clues and formulates a short list of potential diagnoses/working hypotheses.

The clinician's knowledge base is critical in the evaluation process.[50] Experienced clinicians appear to have a superior organization of knowledge, and they use a combination of hypothetico-deductive reasoning and pattern recognition to derive the correct diagnosis or working hypothesis.[50]

A number of frameworks have been applied to clinical practice for guiding clinical decision making and providing structure to the healthcare process.[57-63] Whereas the early frameworks were based on disablement models, the more recent models have focused on enablement perspectives using algorithms. An algorithm is a systematic process involving a finite number of steps that produces the solution to a problem. Algorithms used in healthcare allow for clinical decisions and adjustments to be made during the clinical reasoning and decision-making process because they are not prescriptive or protocol driven.[51] The most commonly used algorithm in physical therapy is the *hypothesis-oriented algorithm for clinicians* (HOAC) designed by Rothstein and Echternach.[60] The HOAC is designed to guide the clinician from evaluation to intervention planning with a logical sequence of activities. It also requires the clinician to generate working hypotheses early in the examination process, which is a strategy often used by expert clinicians.

REFERENCES

1. American Physical Therapy Association House of Delegates: Vision 2020, HOD 06-00-24-35. Alexandria, Va, American Physical Therapy Association, 2000.
2. Guide to Physical Therapist Practice. Second Edition. American Physical Therapy Association. Phys Ther 81:9-746, 2001.
3. DuVall RE, Godges J: Introduction to physical therapy differential diagnosis: the clinical utility of subjective examination, in Wilmarth MA (ed): Medical Screening for the Physical Therapist. Orthopaedic Section Independent Study Course–14.1.1, La Crosse, Wisconsin, Orthopaedic Section, APTA, Inc, 2003, pp 1-44.
4. Dean E: Physical therapy in the 21st century (Part I): toward practice informed by epidemiology and the crisis of lifestyle conditions. Physiother Theory Pract 25:330-353, 2009.
5. Sackett DL, Strauss SE, Richardson WS, et al: Evidence Based Medicine: How to Practice and Teach EBM (ed 2). Edinburgh, Scotland, Churchill Livingstone, 2000.
6. Jewell DV: Introduction, Guide to Evidence-Based Physical Therapy Practice. Sudbury, Mass, Jones & Bartlett, 2008, pp 5-18.
7. Sheth SA, Kwon CS, Barker FG 2nd: The art of management decision making: from intuition to evidence-based medicine. Otolaryngol Clin North Am 45:333-351, viii, 2012.

8. Saitz, R: "Evidence-based design: part of evidence-based medicine?" Evid Based Med 18: 1, 2013.

9. Rosner AL: Evidence-based medicine: revisiting the pyramid of priorities. J Bodyw Mov Ther 16:42-49, 2012.

10. Rhee JS, Daramola OO: No need to fear evidence-based medicine. Arch Facial Plast Surg 14:89-92, 2012.

11. Matthews DR: Wisdom-based and evidence-based medicine. Diabetes Obes Metab 14 Suppl 1:1-2, 2012.

12. Mansi IA, Banks DE: Evidence-based medicine for clinicians. South Med J 105:109, 2012.

13. Mansi IA, Banks DE: The challenge of evidence-based medicine. South Med J 105:110-113, 2012.

14. Leerar PJ: Differential diagnosis of tarsal coalition versus cuboid syndrome in an adolescent athlete. J Orthop Sports Phys Ther 31:702-707, 2001.

15. Schenkman M, Deutsch JE, Gill-Body KM: An integrated framework for decision making in neurologic physical therapist practice. Phys Ther 86:1681-1702, 2006.

16. Jaeschke R, Guyatt G, Sackett DL: Users guides to the medical literature. III. How to use an article about a diagnostic test. B. What are the results and will they help me in caring for my patients? JAMA 27:703-707, 1994.

17. Underwood FB: Clinical research and data analysis, in Placzek JD, Boyce DA (eds): Orthopaedic Physical Therapy Secrets. Philadelphia, Hanley & Belfus, 2001, pp 130-139.

18. Jewell DV: General characteristics of desirable evidence, in Guide to Evidence-Based Physical Therapy Practice. Sudbury, Mass, Jones & Bartlett, 2008, pp 19-34.

19. Jewell DV: Questions, theories, and hypotheses, in Guide to Evidence-Based Physical Therapy Practice. Sudbury, Mass, Jones & Bartlett, 2008, pp 81-95.

20. Domholdt E, Carter R, Lubinsky J: Qualitative research, Rehabilitation Research: Principles and Applications. St. Louis, Mo, Elsevier Saunders, 2010, pp 157-173.

21. Friedman LM, Furberg CD, DeMets DL: Fundamentals of Clinical Trials (ed 2). Chicago, Mosby-Year Book, 1985, pp 2, 51, 71.

22. Sackett DL, Haynes RB, Tugwell P: Clinical Epidemiology: A Basic Science for Clinical Medicine. Boston, Mass, Little, Brown, 1985.

23. Straus SE, Richardson WS, Glasziou P, et al: Evidence-Based Medicine, University Health Network, http://www.cebm.utoronto.ca, 2006.

24. Fisher C, Dvorak M: Orthopaedic research: What an orthopaedic surgeon needs to know, Orthopaedic Knowledge Update: Home Study Syllabus. Rosemont, Ill, American Academy of Orthopaedic Surgeons, 2005, pp 3-13.

25. Carter RE, Lubinsky J, Domholdt E: Evaluating evidence one article at the time, in Carter RE, Lubinsky J (eds): Rehabilitation Research: Principles and Applications (ed 4), Elsevier Saunders, 2011, pp 341-358.

26. Bluman AG: Hypothesis testing, in Bluman AG (ed): Elementary Statistics: A Step by Step Approach (ed 4). New York, McGraw-Hill, 2008, pp 387-455.

27. Jewell DV: Research subjects, in Guide to Evidence-Based Physical Therapy Practice. Sudbury, Mass, Jones & Bartlett, 2008, pp 127-143.

28. Jewell DV: Variables and their measurement, in Guide to Evidence-Based Physical Therapy Practice. Sudbury, Mass, Jones & Bartlett, 2008, pp 145-167.

29. Domholdt E, Carter R, Lubinsky J: Variables, Rehabilitation Research: Principles and Applications. St. Louis, Mo, Elsevier Saunders, 2010, pp 67-74.

30. Bluman AG: The nature of probability and statistics, in Bluman AG (ed): Elementary Statistics: A Step by Step Approach (ed 4). New York, McGraw-Hill, 2008, pp 1-32.

31. Feinstein AR: Clinimetrics. Westford, Mass, Murray, 1987.

32. Marx RG, Bombardier C, Wright JG: What we know about the reliability and validity of physical examination tests used to examine the upper extremity. J Hand Surg 24A:185-193, 1999.

33. Roach KE, Brown MD, Albin RD, et al: The sensitivity and specificity of pain response to activity and position in categorizing patients with low back pain. Phys Ther 77:730-738, 1997.

34. Schwartz JS: Evaluating diagnostic tests: what is done—what needs to be done. J Gen Intern Med 1:266-267, 1986.

35. Van der Wurff P, Meyne W, Hagmeijer RHM: Clinical tests of the sacroiliac joint, a systematic methodological review. Part 2: validity. Man Ther 5:89-96, 2000.

36. Jull GA: Physiotherapy management of neck pain of mechanical origin, in Giles LGF, Singer KP (eds): Clinical Anatomy and Management of Cervical Spine Pain. The Clinical Anatomy of Back Pain. London, England, Butterworth-Heinemann, 1998, pp 168-191.

37. Davidson M: The interpretation of diagnostic tests: A primer for physiotherapists. Aust J Physiother 48:227-233, 2002.

38. Cleland J: Introduction, in Orthopedic Clinical Examination: An Evidence-Based Approach for Physical Therapists. Carlstadt, NJ, Icon Learning Systems, 2005, pp 2-23.

39. Wainner RS: Reliability of the clinical examination: how close is "close enough"? J Orthop Sports Phys Ther 33:488-491, 2003.

40. Huijbregts PA: Spinal motion palpation: A review of reliability studies. J Man Manip Ther 10:24-39, 2002.

41. Laslett M, Williams M: The reliability of selected pain provocation tests for sacroiliac joint pathology. Spine 19:1243-1249, 1994.

42. Portney L, Watkins MP: Foundations of Clinical Research: Applications to Practice. Norwalk, Conn, Appleton & Lange, 1993.

43. Feinstein AR: Clinical biostatistics XXXI: on the sensitivity, specificity & discrimination of diagnostic tests. Clin Pharmacol Ther 17:104-116, 1975.

44. Anderson MA, Foreman TL: Return to competition: functional rehabilitation, in Zachazewski JE, Magee DJ, Quillen WS (eds): Athletic Injuries and Rehabilitation. Philadelphia, WB Saunders, 1996, pp 229-261.

45. Whiting P, Rutjes AW, Reitsma JB, et al: The development of QUADAS: a tool for the quality assessment of studies of diagnostic accuracy included in systematic reviews. BMC Med Res Methodol 3:25, 2003.

46. Schiffman EL: The role of the randomized clinical trial in evaluating management strategies for temporomandibular disorders, in Fricton JR, Dubner R (eds): Orofacial Pain and Temporomandibular Disorders (Advances in Pain Research and Therapy, Vol 21). New York, Raven Press, 1995, pp 415-463.

47. Maher CG, Herbert RD, Moseley AM, et al: Critical appraisal of randomized trials, systematic reviews of radomized trials and clinical practice guidelines, in Boyling JD, Jull GA (eds): Grieve's Modern Manual Therapy: The Vertebral Column. Philadelphia, Churchill Livingstone, 2004, pp 603-614.

48. Wickstrom G, Bendix T: The "Hawthorne effect"—what did the original Hawthorne studies actually show? Scand J Work Environ Health 26:363-367, 2000.

49. Clawson AL, Domholdt E: Content of physician referrals to physical therapists at clinical education sites in Indiana. Phys Ther 74:356-360, 1994.

50. Jones MA: Clinical reasoning in manual therapy. Phys Ther 72:875-884, 1992.

51. Hoogenboom BJ, Voight ML: Clinical reasoning: An algorithm-based approach to musculoskeletal rehabilitation, in Voight ML, Hoogenboom BJ, Prentice WE (eds): Musculoskeletal Interventions: Techniques for Therapeutic Exercise. New York, McGraw-Hill, 2007, pp 81-95.

52. Brooks LR, Norman GR, Allen SW: The role of specific similarity in a medical diagnostic task. J Exp Psychol Gen 120:278-287, 1991.

53. Sullivan PE, Puniello MS, Pardasaney PK: Rehabilitation program development: clinical decision-making, prioritization, and program integration, in Magee D, Zachazewski JE, Quillen WS (eds): Scientific Foundations and Principles of Practice in Musculoskeletal Rehabilitation. St Louis, Mo, Saunders, 2007, pp 314-327.

54. Kahney H: Problem Solving: Current Issues. Buckingham, England, Open University Press, 1993.

55. Coutts F: Changes in the musculoskeletal system, in Atkinson K, Coutts F, Hassenkamp A (eds): Physiotherapy in Orthopedics. London, Churchill Livingstone, 1999, pp 19-43.

56. Jette AM: Diagnosis and classification by physical therapists: A special communication. Phys Ther 69:967, 1989.

57. Higgs J, Jones M: Clinical Reasoning in the Health Professions (ed 2). London, Butterworth-Heinemann, 2000, pp 118-127.

58. Rothstein JM, Echternach JL, Riddle DL: The Hypothesis-Oriented Algorithm for Clinicians II (HOAC II): a guide for patient management. Phys Ther 83:455-470, 2003.

59. Echternach JL, Rothstein JM: Hypothesis-oriented algorithms. Phys Ther 69:559-564, 1989.

60. Rothstein JM, Echternach JL: Hypothesis-oriented algorithm for clinicians. A method for evaluation and treatment planning. Phys Ther 66:1388-1394, 1986.

61. Schenkman M, Butler RB: A model for multisystem evaluation, interpretation, and treatment of individuals with neurologic dysfunction. Phys Ther 69:538-547, 1989.

62. Schenkman M, Butler RB: A model for multisystem evaluation treatment of individuals with Parkinson's disease. Phys Ther 69:932-943, 1989.

63. Schenkman M, Donovan J, Tsubota J, et al: Management of individuals with Parkinson's disease: rationale and case studies. Phys Ther 69:944-955, 1989.

Foundations of Movement

CHAPTER 4

CHAPTER OBJECTIVES

*At the completion of this chapter,
the reader will be able to:*

1. Discuss the various periods of normal prenatal development

2. Describe the normal sequence in which nervous tissue, connective tissue, and skeletal muscle develop

3. Describe how the motor unit works

4. List the different kinds of feedback receptors

5. Describe the various physiologic processes by which the body produces energy

6. Discuss the external and internal forces of the body that are either generated or resisted during the course of daily activities

7. Describe the various types of levers and give real-life examples of each

8. Describe the various components of the stresses and strains that occur with connective tissues

9. List the various planes and axes of the body

10. Explain the concept of degrees of freedom and give examples of each

11. Explain the difference between osteokinematic motion and arthrokinematic motion

12. Discuss the difference between open and closed kinetic chains

13. Describe the various theories of motor development, motor control, and motor learning

14. List the different kinds of motor tasks and describe the differences

15. Describe how early motion develops in terms of stability and mobility

16. Discuss the various methods of skill acquisition

17. Describe the factors that affect normal development and the impact that physical therapy can have

OVERVIEW

Normal movement, which is an amalgamation of strength, endurance, speed, and accuracy, is essential to normal functioning. In turn, normal functioning is dependent on normal development. A physical therapist can be viewed as an expert on movement, both normal and abnormal, through an acquired knowledge of neuromusculoskeletal development. This working knowledge is applied to make a number of decisions about the overall clinical program of a patient (see Chapter 7).

HUMAN DEVELOPMENT

Human development is a continuum, starting with fertilization, prenatal development, birth, and ending with growth up to adulthood. Embryology is the study of prenatal development. Prenatal development, or fetal development, is the term given to the process of gestation (pregnancy) that an embryo undergoes. Human gestation lasts an average of 266 days (38 weeks) from conception (fertilization) to parturition (childbirth).

CLINICAL PEARL

Because the date of conception is seldom known with certainty, the gestational calendar is usually measured from the day a woman's last menstrual period began, and birth is predicted to occur about 280 days (40 weeks) thereafter.[1]

From a clinical perspective, the course of pregnancy is divided into three-month intervals called trimesters:

▶ First trimester (first 12 weeks)

▶ Second trimester (weeks 13 to 24)

▶ Third trimester (week 25 to birth)

From a biological perspective, human development occurs in three main stages. The first two weeks (approximately 16 days) after conception are known as the pre-embryonic period; day 17 through the eighth week are known as the embryonic period; and the time from the beginning of the ninth week until birth is known as the fetal period.

The internal physiologic changes that occur in all body systems throughout these developmental periods provide a substrate for movement. In particular, maturation of the nervous system occurs in the presence of a continually changing musculoskeletal system. Movement itself influences the quality of muscle contractions, shapes the body's joints, and prepares body parts for stabilizing or mobilizing functions.

Pre-embryonic Period

The early embryonic events, such as body axis formation, gastrulation, and neurulation, are crucial for normal embryogenesis and greatly influence both the formation of the basic body plan. This two-week period involves three main processes:

▶ Cleavage (cell division) (Figure 4-1)

▶ Implantation, in which the egg becomes embedded in the mucosal lining of the uterus (see Figure 4-1)

▶ Embryogenesis, in which the embryonic cells migrate and differentiate into three tissue layers called the ectoderm, mesoderm, and endoderm

CLINICAL PEARL

A gamete is a cell that fuses with another cell during fertilization (conception). The female gamete is an ovum, whereas the male gamete is the sperm. Human cells normally have 46 chromosomes each. To combine the cells from two parents, a process called meiosis (reduction division) reduces the chromosome number by half as the gamete's are formed, so that gamete's have only 23 chromosomes—half as many as other cells of the body. They are called haploid for this reason, whereas the other cells in the body are diploid.

The human ovary usually releases one egg (oocyte) per month around day 14 of a typical 28-day ovarian cycle. In order for normal fertilization to occur, a number of conditions need to be met:

▶ An egg must be present in the uterine (fallopian) tube. The egg is swept into the fallopian tube by the beating of cilia on the tube's epithelial cells. The egg is surrounded by a thin layer of protein and polysaccharides, called the zona pellucida (see Figure 4-1), and a layer of granulocytic cells, called the corona radiata, both of which provide a protective shield around the egg as it enters the uterine tube during its three-day journey. If the egg is not fertilized, it dies within 24 hours and gets no more than one third of the way to the uterus.[1]

▶ Large numbers of spermatozoa must be ejaculated. Only about 100 of the spermatozoa survive to encounter the ovum in the uterine tube. The anterior tip of the sperm contains a specialized lysosome called an *acrosome*, a packet of enzymes used to penetrate the egg and certain barriers around it.

The main function of fertilization is to combine the haploid sets of chromosomes from two individuals into a single

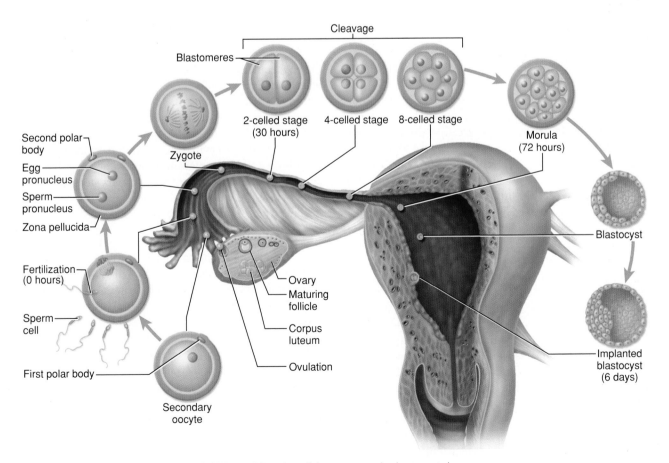

FIGURE 4-1 Migration of the oocyte and subsequent cleavage

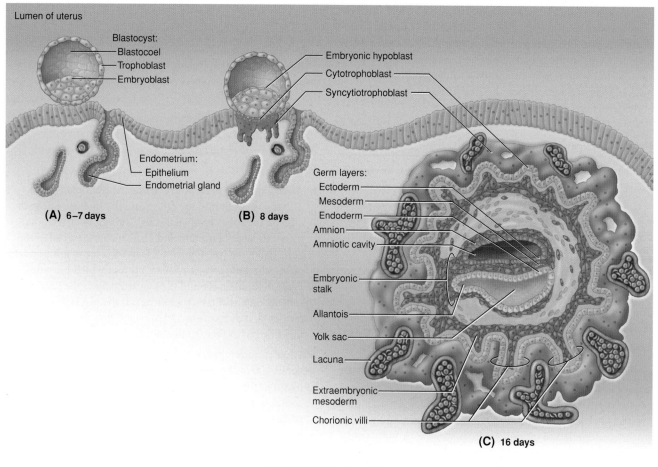

Lumen of uterus

Blastocyst:
 Blastocoel
 Trophoblast
 Embryoblast

Embryonic hypoblast
Cytotrophoblast
Syncytiotrophoblast

Endometrium:
 Epithelium
 Endometrial gland

(A) 6–7 days

(B) 8 days

Germ layers:
 Ectoderm
 Mesoderm
 Endoderm
 Amnion
 Amniotic cavity

Embryonic
stalk

Allantois

Yolk sac

Lacuna

Extraembryonic
mesoderm

Chorionic villi

(C) 16 days

FIGURE 4-2 Implantation

diploid complement of chromosomes—the zygote (fertilized ovum).

After fertilization, the embryogenesis starts. Within 30 hours following fertilization, the zygote undergoes a mitotic division called cleavage, progressing through 2-cell, 4-cell, 8-cell, and 16-cell stages (morula) (see Figure 4-1). The morula floats within the uterine cavity for approximately three days, as it gradually fills with fluid and forms two distinct groups of cells. At this time, the structure becomes known as a blastocyst (see Figure 4-1), and its fluid-filled sac is called a blastocyst cavity (Figure 4-2). The outer layer of cells of the blastocyst is referred to as the trophoblast, whereas the inner layer is called the embryoblast. The trophoblast cells eventually contribute to fetal membrane systems; the inner cell mass plays a large role in the formation of the embryo and fetus. The developmental characteristics of the embryo and fetus according to gestational age are outlined in Table 4-1. The termination of the cleavage stage of development terminates with the formation of the blastocyst. The process of implantation occurs as the blastocyst embeds itself into the endometrium of the uterine wall and prevents itself from being aborted by secreting a hormone that indirectly prevents menstruation.

During the second week of development, the embryoblast becomes completely embedded within the endometrium surface and undergoes marked differentiation, with the appearance of a slit-like space called the amniotic cavity between the embryoblast and the invading trophoblast. The embryoblast flattens into the embryonic disk, which consists of two germ layers: an upper ectoderm, which is closer to the amniotic cavity, and a lower endoderm, which borders the blastocyst cavity (Figure 4-3). A short time later, a third layer called the mesoderm forms between the endoderm and ectoderm. These three primary germ layers give rise to all of the specific tissues and organs in the developing embryo:

▶ *Ectoderm:* gives rise to the outer layer of the skin (epidermis) including hair, nails, skin glands, and portions of the sensory organs, as well as the neural crest, and other tissues that eventually form the nervous system. Neurulation, the formation of a neural plate, a thickening of the ectoderm, occurs around week 3. An invagination of the neural plate produces a longitudinal neural grooves, and closure of this groove results in the formation of a neural tube and neural crest:

 ■ *Neural tube:* gives rise to the brain and spinal cord (central nervous system). By approximately the fourth week, the cranial end of the neural tube expand into three primary brain vesicles (prosencephalon, mesencephalon, and rhombencephalon), which in turn subdivide to form five secondary brain vesicles

TABLE 4-1	Developmental Characteristics of the Embryo and Fetus According to Gestational Age
Gestational Age	**Developmental Characteristics**
2.5 weeks	Neural plate formation; shape and length begin to be determined.
Three weeks	Cell differentiation occurs—formation of ectoderm (nervous system, sensory systems and many other tissues), mesoderm (muscles, skeleton, and other tissues), endoderm (respiratory system, digestive system, and other tissues). Early in the third week, a thick linear band called the *primitive streak* appears along the posterior midline of the embryonic disk. Derived from mesodermal cells, the primitive streak establishes a structural foundation for embryonic morphogenesis along a longitudinal axis. As the primitive streak elongates, a prominent thickening called the *primitive node* appears at its cranial end, which later gives rise to the mesodermal structures of the head and to a rod of mesodermal cells called the notochord. It is the notochord that forms a midline axis that is the basis for the embryonic skeleton.
Four weeks	The embryo increases about 4 mm (0.16 inches), reaching a length of 0.75 to 1 cm and weighing 400 mg. A *connecting stalk*, which is later involved in the formation of the umbilical cord, is established from the body of the embryo to the developing placenta. By this time, a rudimentary heart is already pumping blood with a regular rhythm to all parts of the embryo, the head and jaw are apparent, and the primordial tissue that will form the eyes, brain, spinal cord, lungs, and digestive organs has developed.
	Lateral wings bend forward, meeting at the center, and will eventually form the body.
	Head tilts forward and makes up about one-third of the entire structure.
	The superior and inferior limb buds have the appearance of small swellings on the lateral body walls.
Fifth week	The head enlarges, and the developing eyes, ears, and nasal pit become obvious.
	The embryo reaches a length of 2.5 cm (1 in) and weighs 20 g.
	The heart has a definite septum and valves.
	The appendages have formed from the limb buds, and paddle-shaped hand and foot plates develop.
	External genitalia are evident, but gender is not obvious.
Sixth week	The embryo reaches a length of 16–24 mm (0.64–0.96 inches).
	The head is larger than the trunk, and the brain has undergone marked differentiation.
	The limbs lengthen and are slightly flexed.
	Considered as the most critical time for the development for many organs.
Seventh and eighth weeks	The embryo reaches a length of 28–40 mm (1.12–1.6 inches).
	The body organs are formed, and the nervous system starts to coordinate body activity.
	The body systems are developed by the end of the eighth week, and from this time on the embryo is called a fetus.
9 to 12 weeks	By the beginning of the ninth week, the head of the fetus is as large as the rest of the body.
	Head growth slows during the next three weeks, while lengthening of the body accelerates.
	Ossification centers appear in most bones during the ninth week.
	By the end of the 12th week the fetus is 87 mm (3.5 inches) long and weighs about 45 g (1.6 ounces).
	The nervous system and muscle coordination are developed so that the fetus will withdraw its leg if tickled. Some movement is occurring, but it is usually too faint for the mother to feel.
	The fetal heart can be heard with an electronic device called a Doppler.
13 to 16 weeks	The facial features of the fetus are well formed.
	Epidermal structure such as eyelashes, eyebrows, hair on the head, fingernails, and nipples begin to develop.
	Liver and pancreatic secretions are present.
	Fetus starts to make sucking motions with the mouth.
	The fetal heartbeat can be detected using a stethoscope.
	By the end of the 16th week, the fetus reaches a length of 140 mm (5.5 inches) and weighs 200 g (7 ounces).
17 to 20 weeks	The mother starts to feel fetal movement (quickening).
	Development of the fetal position, with the head flexed down and in contact with the flexed knees.
	A 20-week-old fetus is about 119 mm (7.5 inches) long and weighs about 460 g (16 ounces).
21 to 25 weeks	The fetus increases weight substantially to about 900 g (32 ounces).
	Pupils are reactive to light.
	Surfactant, a phospholipid substance essential to lung function, is formed and excreted by cells in the alveoli.

(continued)

TABLE 4-1	Developmental Characteristics of the Embryo and Fetus According to Gestational Age (continued)
Gestational Age	**Developmental Characteristics**
26 to 29 weeks	Toward the end of this stage, the fetus reaches a length of 275 mm (11 inches) and weighs approximately 1300 g (46 ounces). Fetus could possibly be viable if born now and cared for in a neonatal intensive care unit, but the mortality rate is high. Testes begin descent into the scrotal sac from the lower abdominal cavity if the fetus is male. The brain is rapidly developing. Eyelids, which fused in the 12th week, start to open. The fetus rotates to a vertical position in which the head is directed toward the cervix.
30 to 38 weeks	At the end of 38 weeks, the fetus is considered full term. The fetus reaches a length of 360 mm (14 inches) and weighs about 3400 g (7.5 pounds). Fetus hears sounds and responds with movement. Soles of the feet have only one or two creases. The central nervous system has greater control over body functions. Iron stores begin to develop.

Data from Van de Graaff KM, Fox SI: Developmental anatomy and inheritance, in Van de Graaff KM, Fox SI (eds): Concepts of Human Anatomy and Physiology. New York, WCB/McGraw-Hill, 1999, pp 954-984.

(telencephalon, diencephalon, mesencephalon, metencephalon, and myelencephalon) (Table 4-2).

- *Neural crest:* this is sometimes referred to as the fourth germ layer because of its importance. It gives rise to the neurons and glial cells of the sensory, sympathetic, and parasympathetic nervous systems (peripheral nervous system).

CLINICAL PEARL

Pharyngeal (branchial) pouches, five pairs of pockets that form in the walls of the future throat of the embryo at around 4 to 5 weeks' gestation, are separated by pharyngeal arches (Figure 4-4). Pharyngeal pouches give rise to the middle ear cavity, palanquin tonsil, thymus, parathyroid glands, and part of the thyroid gland.[1]

▶ Mesoderm, which eventually forms the skeleton, muscles, blood, reproductive organs, dermis of the skin, and connective tissue. Formation of the notochord from mesoderm during gastrulation results in delineation of the primitive axis of the embryo. The mesoderm on either side of the notochord subdivides into paraxial, intermediate, and lateral columns.

- *Paraxial.* Further subdivision of the paraxial mesoderm gives rise to somites, from which are formed the bones of the appendicular skeleton as well as the muscles, bones, and connective tissue of the axial skeleton (excluding the skull). Typical somites further differentiate into three components: a superficial posterolateral mass, the dermatome; a deeper posterolateral mass, the myotome; and an anteromedial mass, the sclerotome.[2] The dermatomes extend the nisi overlying ectoderm and are destined to become the dermis and hypodermis. Striated, voluntary, skeletal muscle originates from several sources. The axial muscles (the muscles that attach to the head, neck, vertebral column, thorax, abdomen, and pelvis) develop from myotomal mesoderm of the somites. The appendicular muscles (the muscles of the upper and

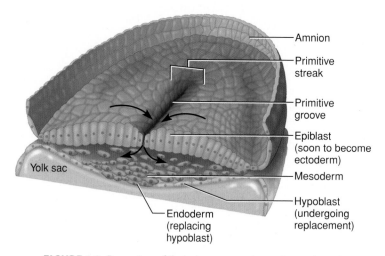

FIGURE 4-3 Formation of the primary germ layers (gastrulation)

	Region	Structure	Description/Function
TABLE 4-2	**Derivation and Functions of the Major Brain Structures**		
Prosencephalon (forebrain)	Telencephalon	Cerebrum	Consists of six paired lobes within two convoluted hemispheres. The outer part of the cerebral hemispheres is called the cerebral cortex. The elevated folds of the convolutions (crests) are called the cerebral gyri, and the depressed grooves (fissures) are the cerebral sulci.
		Limbic system	Phylogenetically, the oldest part of the brain. Controls most sensory and motor activities; reasoning, memory, intelligence, etc. Instinctual and limbic functions include basic emotional behavior, such as anger, fear, sex, and hunger.
	Diencephalon	Thalamus	The principal function of the thalamus is to act as a relay center for all sensory impulses, except smell, to the cerebral cortex and subcortical regions. Also performs initial autonomic response to pain and crude awareness.
		Hypothalamus	Regulation of food and water intake, body temperature, heartbeat, etc.; control of secretory activity in the anterior pituitary; instinctual and limbic functions.
		Epithalamus	Production of cerebrospinal fluid by the choroid plexus. Influence of the circadian rhythm through the release of hormones from the pineal gland. Integration of olfactory, visceral, and somatic afferent pathways via the habenular nuclei.
		Pituitary gland	Regulation of various endocrine functions.
Mesencephalon (midbrain)	Mesencephalon	Corpora quadrigemina	Consists of the superior colliculi (visual reflexes, hand-eye coordination) and the inferior colliculi (auditory reflexes).
		Cerebral peduncles	Cylindrical structures composed of ascending and descending projection fiber tracts that support and connect the cerebrum to other regions of the brain to allow reflex coordination.
		The mesencephalic aqueduct (Sylvius)	Connects the third and fourth ventricle.
		Red nucleus	Functions in reflexes concerned with motor coordination and maintenance of posture.
		Substantia nigra	Functions to inhibit involuntary movements. It is a major element of the basal ganglia. Degeneration of pigmented neurons in the substantia nigra region is the principal pathology that underlies Parkinson's disease.
Rhombencephalon (hindbrain)	Metencephalon	Pons	Balance and motor coordination. The nuclei of the pons serve a number of important functions: ▶ Some of the nuclei function with nuclei of the medulla oblongata to regulate the rate and depth of breathing. ▶ Several nuclei (tegmentum) within the pons are associated with specific cranial nerves (trigeminal [V], abducens [VI], facial [VII], and vestibulocochlear [VIII]). ▶ The surface fibers extend transversely to connect with the cerebellum through the middle cerebellar peduncles. ▶ Raphe nuclei are involved with pain modulation and the control of arousal.
		Cerebellum	The principal functions of the cerebellum include: ▶ Coordination of skeletal muscle contractions by recruiting precise motor units within the muscles, such as accurate force, direction, and extent of movement, and sequencing of movements (neocerebellum). ▶ Equilibrium, and regulation of muscle tone via the flocculonodular lobe and proprioceptive input. ▶ Modification of muscle tone and synergistic actions of muscles.
	Myelencephalon	Medulla oblongata	Relay center that connects the spinal cord with the pons; contains many nuclei; visceral autonomic center (e.g., respiration, heart rate, vasoconstriction). ▶ Composed of vital nuclei and white matter that form all of the descending and ascending tracks communicating between the spinal cord and various parts of the brain. ▶ Most of the fibers within these tracks cross over (decussate) to the opposite side through the pyramidal region of the medulla oblongata permitting one side of the brain to receive information from, and send information to, the opposite side of the body.

Data from Van de Graaff KM, Fox SI: Central nervous system, in Van de Graaff KM, Fox SI (eds): Concepts of Human Anatomy and Physiology. New York, WCB/McGraw-Hill, 1999, pp 407-446.

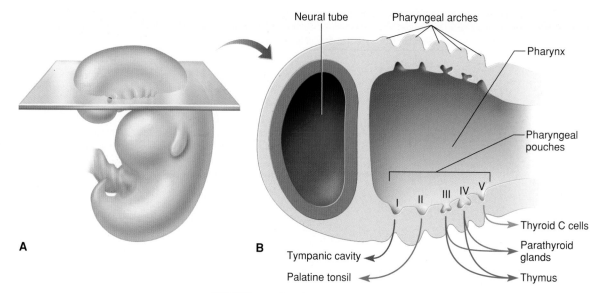

A   **B**

Neural tube

Pharyngeal arches

Pharynx

Pharyngeal pouches

Thyroid C cells

Parathyroid glands

Thymus

Tympanic cavity

Palatine tonsil

I II III IV V

FIGURE 4-4 The pharyngeal pouches

lower extremities) develop from mesenchyme of the limb buds. The mesenchymal cells differentiate into myoblasts, which further develop into muscle fibers and myofilaments.

- *Intermediate.* This is located between the paraxial mesoderm and the lateral plate and develops into the part of the urogenital system (kidneys and gonads), as well as the reproductive system.

- *The lateral plate.* This separates into posterior (somatic) and anterior (visceral) layers. Cells from the lateral plate mesoderm and the myotome migrate to the limb field and proliferate to create the limb bud.

▶ Endoderm, which gives rise to the epithelium lining of the digestive system, the respiratory system, the urinary bladder and urethra, and organs associated with the digestive system, including the liver and pancreas.

CLINICAL PEARL

Bone formation occurs by two different methods:

▶ *Intramembranous ossification.* The bones develop directly from mesenchymal cells.

▶ *Endochondral ossification.* Involves replacement of a pre-existing cartilaginous model by bone.

CLINICAL PEARL

The 206 bones of the fully formed body are divided into:

▶ *Axial skeleton*: 80 bones including the human skull, the ossicles of the middle ear, the hyoid bone, the rib cage, sternum and the vertebral column

▶ *Appendicular skeleton*: 126 bones including the clavicles, scapulae, and the bones of the upper and lower extremities

Embryonic Period

During this stage of development, which begins around day 16 and extends to the end of week 8, the placenta and other accessory structures develop, and all of the organ systems begin to develop from the three germ layers. The formation of organs and organ systems during this time, which is called organogenesis, requires a precise integration of many developmental processes that involve the coordination of complex genetic and developmental networks, including the provision of:

▶ Nutrients and oxygen through the formation of a vascular connection between the uterus of the mother and the embryo (the placenta and umbilical cord). The blood vessel that will become the heart starts to pulse.

▶ Internal and external structural support for the embryo. In weeks 3 to 4, the embryo grows rapidly and folds around the yolk sac, converting the flat embryonic disk into a somewhat cylindrical form. As the superior and inferior ends curve around the ends of the yolk sac, the embryo becomes T-shaped, with the head and tail almost touching (Figure 4-5). Around the fourth week, the head begins to form, quickly followed by the eyes, nose, ears, and mouth.

▶ A protective environment around the embryo (the amniotic sac).

▶ A structural foundation along a longitudinal axis to allow for morphogenesis—the embryo begins to fold on itself in both the sagittal and transverse planes, producing a posterior convexity and an anterior concavity. By about the fifth week, the limb buds begin to direct themselves anteriorly; in addition, the upper limbs externally rotate 90° and the lower limbs internally rotate 90° so that the elbows are directed posteriorly and the knees are projected anteriorly.[2]

At approximately the 10th week of development, the embryo has all of the basic organs and parts except those of the sex organs.

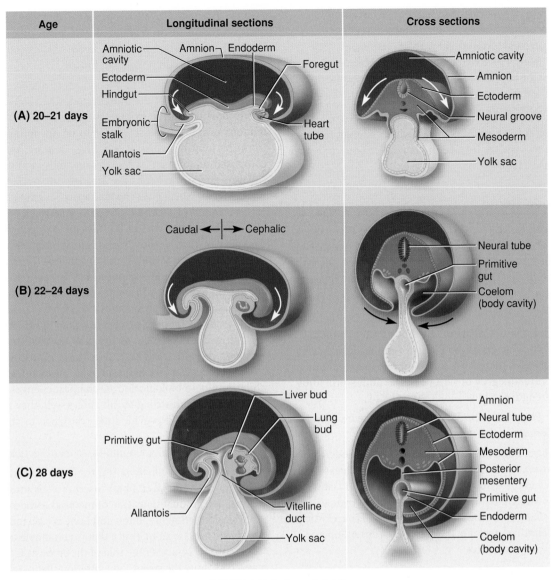

FIGURE 4-5 Embryonic folding

Fetal Period

Once cell differentiation is mostly complete, the embryo becomes known as a fetus. The primary changes in the fetal period are that the organ systems become functional and the fetus rapidly gains weight and becomes more human looking.[1] The early body systems and structures established in the embryonic stage continue to develop, with the limbs growing more rapidly than the trunk. The neural tube develops into the brain and spinal cord, and neurons form. Sex organs begin to appear during the third month of gestation. The heart, which has been beating since the fourth week, now circulates blood and grows stronger. Fingernails, hair, eyelashes, and toenails form.

CLINICAL PEARL

A birth defect, or congenital anomaly, is the abnormal structure or position of an organ at birth, resulting from a defect in prenatal development.[1] Although there are known causes of congenital anomalies, in 50% to 60% of cases the cause is unknown.

NORMAL DEVELOPMENT OF MOVEMENT COMPONENTS

Throughout the human body, there are four major types of tissues:

► *Epithelial.* Covers all internal and external body surfaces and include structures such as the skin and the inner lining of the blood vessels.

► *Connective.* Connective tissue (CT) is the most abundant, widely distributed, and histologically variable of the primary tissues,[3] and one of its variants, fibrous connective tissue, includes bone, cartilage, tendons, ligaments, and blood tissue. CT provides protection, movement, and structural and metabolic support for other tissues and organs of the body.

► *Nervous.* Nervous tissue provides communication between the central nervous system (the brain and spinal cord), the peripheral nervous system, muscles, organs, and various other systems.

▸ *Muscle.* Muscles are classified functionally as either voluntary or involuntary, and structurally as either smooth, striated (skeletal). or cardiac. There are approximately 430 skeletal muscles in the body, each of which can be considered anatomically as a separate organ. Of these 430 muscles, about 75 pairs provide the majority of body movements and postures.[4]

Neuromusculoskeletal structures, which interact together to produce movement, include the nervous, connective, and skeletal muscle tissues.

Connective Tissue

Connective tissue (CT) is divided into subtypes according to the matrix that binds the cells. CT proper has a loose flexible matrix, called *ground substance*. The most common cell within CT proper is the fibroblast. Three types of protein fibers are found in fibrous connective tissue: collagenous, reticular, and elastic fibers.

▸ *Collagenous fibers.* Collagen is the body's most abundant protein.[3] The collagens are a family of extracellular matrix (ECM) proteins that play a dominant role in maintaining the structural integrity of various tissues and in providing tensile strength to tissues.

▸ *Reticular fibers.* These fibers form a spongelike framework for such organs as the spleen and lymph nodes.[3]

▸ *Elastic fibers.* Elastic fibers are composed of a protein called *elastin*. As its name suggests, elastin provides elastic properties to the tissues in which it is situated.[5] Elastin fibers can stretch, but they normally return to their original shape when the tension is released. Thus, elastic fibers of elastin determine the patterns of distention and recoil in most structures.

Fibrous connective tissue is divided into two broad categories according to the relative abundance of fiber: loose and dense CT. The various anatomic and functional characteristics of loose and dense collagen are summarized in Table 4-3. Collagenous and elastic fibers are sparse and irregularly arranged in loose CT but are tightly packed in dense CT.[6] Bundles of collagen and elastin combine to form a matrix of CT fascicles. This matrix is organized within the primary collagen bundles as well as between the bundles that surround them.[7]

The various types of fibrous CT as relates to the musculoskeletal system are described as follows.

Fascia. Fascia is viewed as a loose CT that provides support and protection to the joint, and acts as an interconnection between tendons, aponeuroses, ligaments, capsules, nerves, and the intrinsic components of muscle.[8,9]

Tendons. The function of a tendon is to attach a muscle to a bone at each end of the muscle, and, when stretched, store elastic energy that contribute to movement.[10] In addition, tendons enable the muscle belly to be an optimal distance from the joint on which it is acting. Tendons are primarily composed of collagen, proteoglycans, cells, and water.[10] The collagen fibers of tendons are arranged in a quarter-stagger arrangement, which gives the tendon a characteristic banding pattern and provides high strength and stability.[11] A loose CT matrix surrounds the bundles of collagen fibrils. The thickness of each tendon varies and is proportional to the size of the muscle from which it originates. Tendons display viscoelastic mechanical properties that confer time- and rate-dependent effects on the tissue. Specifically, tendons are more elastic at lower strain rates and stiffer at higher rates of tensile loading. Tendons deform less than ligaments under an applied load and are able to transmit the load from muscle to bone.[7] As with all CT, tendons have a positive adaptive response to repeated physiologic mechanical loading, which results in biologic and mechanical changes. Although tendons withstand strong tensile forces well, they resist shear forces less well and provide little resistance to compression force.[7]

A tendon can be divided into three main sections[10]:

▸ *The bone-tendon junction.* At most bone-tendon interfaces, the collagen fibers insert directly into the bone, in a gradual transition of material composition. The physical junction of tendon and bone is referred to as an enthesis[12] and is an interface that is vulnerable to acute and chronic injury.[13] One role of the enthesis is to absorb and distribute the stress concentration that occurs at the junction over a broader area.

▸ *The tendon midsubstance.* Overuse tendon injuries can occur in the midsubstance of the tendon, but not as frequently as at the enthesis.

▸ *The musculotendinous junction (MTJ).* The MTJ is the site where the muscle and tendon meet. The MTJ comprises numerous interdigitations between muscle cells and tendon tissue, resembling interlocked fingers. Despite its viscoelastic mechanical characteristics, the MTJ is very vulnerable to tensile failure.[14,15]

TABLE 4-3	Loose and Dense Collagen		
Joint Type	**Anatomic Location**	**Fibers**	**Mechanical Specialization**
Dense irregular connective tissue (CT)	Composes the external fibrous layer of the joint capsule; forms ligaments, bone, aponeuroses, and tendons	Parallel, tightly aligned fibers	Ligament: binds bones together and restrains unwanted movement at the joints; resists tension in several directions. Tendon: attaches muscle to bone
Loose irregular connective tissue	Found in capsules, muscles, nerves, fascia, and skin	Random fiber orientation	Provides structural support

CLINICAL PEARL

The MTJ is the location of most common muscle strains caused by tensile forces in a normal muscle-tendon unit.[7,16] In particular, a predilection for a tear near the MTJ has been reported in the biceps and triceps brachii, rotator cuff muscles, flexor pollicis longus, fibularis (peroneus) longus, medial head of the gastrocnemius, rectus femoris, adductor longus, iliopsoas, pectoralis major, semimembranosus, and the entire hamstring group.[17-19]

Ligaments. Skeletal ligaments are fibrous bands of dense CT that connect bones across joints. Ligaments can be named for the bones into which they insert (coracohumeral), their shape (deltoid), or their relationships to each other (cruciate).[20] The gross structure of a ligament varies according to location (e.g., intra-articular or extra-articular, or capsular) and function.[21] The collagen in ligaments has a less unidirectional organization than it does in tendons, but its structural framework still provides stiffness (resistance to deformation).[22] Small amounts of elastin are present in ligaments, with the exception of the ligamentum flavum and the nuchal ligament of the spine, which contain more. The cellular organization of ligaments makes them ideal for sustaining tensile load, with many containing functional subunits that are capable of tightening or loosening in different joint positions.[23] At the microscopic level, closely spaced collagen fibers (fascicles) are aligned along the long axis of the ligament and are arranged into a series of bundles.[20] Ligaments contribute to the stability of joint function by preventing excessive motion,[24] acting as guides or checkreins to direct motion, and providing proprioceptive information for joint function through sensory nerve endings and the attachments of the ligament to the joint capsule.[25-27] Many ligaments share functions. For example, although the anterior cruciate ligament of the knee is considered the primary restraint to anterior translation of the tibia relative to the femur, the medial and lateral collateral ligaments together with the posterior capsule of the knee also help in this function.[20] The vascular and nerve distribution to ligaments is not homogenous. For example, the middle of the ligament is typically avascular, whereas the proximal and distal ends enjoy a rich blood supply. Similarly, the insertional ends of the ligaments are more highly innervated than the midsubstance.

Cartilage. Cartilage is a relatively stiff CT with a semisolid, flexible. Cartilage tissue exists in three forms: hyaline, elastic, and fibrocartilage.

▶ Hyaline cartilage, also referred to as articular cartilage, covers the ends of long bones and permits almost frictionless motion to occur between the articular surfaces of a synovial joint.[28] The various types of joints, and their classifications, are outlined in Table 4-4. Articular cartilage is a highly organized viscoelastic material composed of cartilage cells called *chondrocytes*, water, and an ECM. Articular cartilage, the most abundant cartilage within the body, is devoid of any blood vessels, lymphatics, and nerves.[29,30] Most of the bones of the body form first as hyaline cartilage, and later become proper bone in a process called *endochondral ossification* (see Bone). The normal thickness of articular cartilage is determined by the contact pressures across the joint—the higher the peak pressures, the thicker the cartilage.[21] Articular cartilage functions to distribute the joint forces

TABLE 4-4	The Classification of Joints		
Major Type of Joint	**Other Name(s)**	**Description**	**Example**
Bony	Synostosis	An immobile joint formed when the gap between two bones ossifies and they become, in effect, a single bone. A bony joint can form by ossification of either fibrous or cartilaginous joints.	The attachment of the first rib to the sternum, and the epiphysis and diaphysis of long bones with maturation
Fibrous	Synarthrosis	A point at which adjacent bones are bound by collagen fibers that emerge from the matrix of one bone, cross the space between them, and penetrate into the matrix of the other. Three types are recognized: sutures, gomphosis, and syndesmosis.	Suture: bind the bones of the skull to each other Gomphosis: a tooth socket Syndesmosis: the interosseous membrane between the radius and ulna
Cartilaginous	Amphiarthrosis	Occur when two bones are linked by either hyaline cartilage (synchondroses) or fibrocartilage (symphyses).	Synchondroses: the epiphyseal plate of a long bone in a child Symphysis: the pubic symphysis
Synovial	Diarthrosis	The facing surfaces of two bones are covered with articular cartilage and are lubricated by synovial fluid. Synovial joints can be classified as ball and socket, condylar, saddle, plane, hinge, or pivot.	Ball and socket: shoulder, hip Condylar: radiocarpal Saddle: trapeziometacarpal joint Plane: carpal bones of the wrist Hinge: elbow, knee, and interphalangeal joints Pivot: Atlantoaxial joint

Data from Saladin, KS: Joints, in Human Anatomy. New York, McGraw-Hill, 2012, pp 204-234.

over a large contact area, dissipating the forces associated with the load. This distribution of forces allows the articular cartilage to remain healthy and fully functional throughout decades of life. The patella has the thickest articular cartilage in the body.

CLINICAL PEARL

Chondrocytes are specialized cells that are responsible for the development of cartilage and the maintenance of the extracellular matrix.[31] Chondrocytes produce aggrecan, link protein, and hyaluronan, all of which are extruded into the extracellular matrix, where they aggregate spontaneously.[32] The aggrecans form a strong, porous-permeable, fiber-reinforced composite material with collagen. The chondrocytes sense mechanical changes in their surrounding matrix through intracytoplasmic filaments and short cilia on the surface of the cells.[21]

Articular cartilage may be grossly subdivided into four distinct zones with differing cellular morphology, biomechanical composition, collagen orientations, and structural properties, as follows:

■ *The superficial zone.* The superficial zone, which lies adjacent to the joint cavity, comprises approximately 10 to 20% of the articular cartilage thickness and functions to protect deeper layers from shear stresses. The collagen fibers within this zone are packed tightly and aligned parallel to the articular surface. This zone is in contact with synovial fluid and is responsible for most of the tensile properties of cartilage.

■ *The middle (transitional) zone.* In the middle zone, which provides an anatomic and functional bridge between the superficial and deep zones, the collagen fibril orientation is obliquely organized. This zone comprises 50% of the total cartilage volume. Functionally, the middle zone is the first line of resistance to compressive forces.

■ *The deep or radial layer.* The deep layer comprises 30% of the matrix volume. It is characterized by radially aligned collagen fibers that are perpendicular to the surface of the joint and which have a high proteoglycan content. Functionally, the deep zone is responsible for providing the greatest resistance to compressive forces.

■ *The tidemark.* The tidemark distinguishes the deep zone from the calcified cartilage, the area that prevents the diffusion of nutrients from the bone tissue into the cartilage.

▶ Elastic cartilage is a very specialized CT, primarily found in locations such as the outer ear and portions of the larynx.

▶ Fibrocartilage functions as a shock absorber in both weight-bearing and non–weight-bearing joints. Its large fiber content, reinforced with numerous collagen fibers, makes it ideal for bearing large stresses in all directions. Fibrocartilage is an avascular, alymphatic, and aneural tissue and derives its nutrition by a double-diffusion system.[33] Examples of fibrocartilage include the symphysis pubis, the intervertebral disks, and the menisci of the knee.

Bone. The function of bone is to provide support, enhance leverage, protect vital structures, provide attachments for both tendons and ligaments, and store minerals, particularly calcium. Bones also may serve as useful landmarks during the palpation phase of the examination. Bone is a highly vascular form of CT, composed of collagen, calcium phosphate, water, amorphous proteins, and cells. It is the most rigid of the CTs because of its calcified matrix. Despite its rigidity, bone is a dynamic tissue that undergoes constant metabolism and remodeling. Normal, healthy bone will deform under moderate load, returning to the original position once the loads have been removed. It is the different physical characteristics of bone, as well as variables related to the type of imposed loads, that determine a bone's exact response to loading. The collagen of bone is produced in the same manner as that of ligament and tendon, but by a different cell, the osteoblast.[6] At the gross anatomic level, each bone has a distinct morphology comprising both cortical bone and cancellous bone.

▶ Cortical bone is found in the outer shell.

▶ Cancellous bone is found within the epiphyseal and metaphyseal regions of long bones as well as throughout the interior of short bones.[14]

The development of bone occurs in one of two ways:

▶ *Intramembranous ossification.* Mesenchymal stem cells within mesenchyme or the medullary cavity of a bone initiate the process of intramembranous ossification. This type of ossification occurs in the flat bones of the cranium and facial bones and, in part, in the ribs, clavicle, and mandible.

▶ *Endochondral ossification.* The first site of ossification occurs in the primary center of ossification, which is in the middle of the diaphysis (shaft). About the time of birth, a secondary ossification center appears in each epiphysis (end) of long bones. Between the bone formed by the primary and secondary ossification centers, cartilage persists as the epiphyseal (growth) plate between the diaphysis and the epiphysis of a long bone. This type of ossification occurs in the long and short bones of the appendicular and axial bones.

The periosteum is formed when the perichondrium that surrounds the cartilage develops into the periosteum. Chondrocytes in the primary center of ossification begin to grow (hypertrophy) and begin secreting alkaline phosphatase, an enzyme essential for mineral deposition. Calcification of the matrix follows, and apoptosis of the hypertrophic chondrocytes occurs. This creates cavities within the bone. The exact mechanism of chondrocyte hypertrophy and apoptosis is currently unknown. The hypertrophic chondrocytes (before apoptosis) also secrete a substance called *vascular endothelial cell growth factor* that induces the sprouting of blood vessels from the perichondrium. Blood vessels forming the periosteal bud invade the cavity left by the chondrocytes and branch in opposite directions along the length of the shaft. The blood vessels carry osteoprogenitor cells and hematopoietic cells inside the cavity, the latter of which later form the bone marrow. Osteoblasts, differentiated from the osteoprogenitor cells that enter the cavity via the periosteal bud, use the calcified matrix as a scaffold and begin to secrete osteoid, which forms the bone trabecula. Osteoclasts, formed from macrophages, break down the spongy bone to form the medullary cavity (bone marrow). The strength of a bone is related directly to its density. Of importance to the clinician, is the difference between maturing bone and mature bone. The epiphyseal plate or growth plate of a maturing bone can be divided into four distinct zones[34]:

▶ *Reserve zone:* produces and stores matrix.

▶ *Proliferative zone:* produces matrix and is the site for longitudinal bone cell growth.

▶ *Hypertrophic zone:* subdivided into the maturation zone, degenerative zone, and zone of provisional calcification. It is within the hypertrophic zone that the matrix is prepared for calcification, and is here that the matrix is ultimately calcified. The hypertrophic zone is the most susceptible of the zones to injury because of the low volume of bone matrix and the high amounts of developing immature cells in this region.[35]

▶ *Bone metaphysis:* the part of the bone that grows during childhood.

Nervous Tissue

The development and maturation of the nervous system have the most significant impact on the development of movement. The greatest rate of growth of the brain occurs at birth, and rapid growth occurs during the first six months of life. In utero movements begin as stereotypical movements involving simple flexion-extension motions, which then become goal-directed during the first 6 to 10 months of life. When movements become goal directed, it is critical that a normal sensorimotor system be in place so that these movements can become refined.

The nerve cell, or neuron, which serves to store and process information, is the functional unit of the nervous system. The other cellular constituent is the neuroglial cell, or glia, which function to provide structural and metabolic support for the neurons.[36]

Although neurons come in a variety of sizes and shapes, there are four functional parts to each nerve fiber (Figure 4-6):

▶ *Dendrite.* Dendrites serve a receptive function and receive information from other nerve cells or the environment.

▶ *Axon.* The axon cylinder, in which there is a bi-directional flow of axoplasm, conducts information and nutrition to other nerve cells and the tissues that the nerve innervates. Many axons are covered by myelin, a lipid-rich membrane. In myelinated fibers, there is a direct proportional relationship between fiber diameter and conduction velocity.[37] This membrane is divided into segments about 1 mm long by small gaps, called nodes of Ranvier, where the myelin is absent.[38] Myelin has a high electrical resistance and low capacitance and serves to increase the nerve conduction velocity of

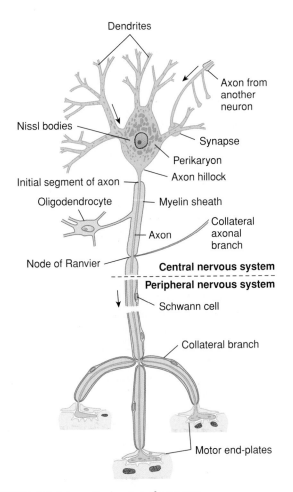

FIGURE 4-6 Schematic drawing of a neuron

neural transmissions through a process called *salutatory conduction.*

▶ *Cell body.* The cell body contains the nucleus of the cell and has important integrative functions.

▶ *Axon terminal.* The axon terminal is the transmission site for action potentials, the messengers of the nerve cell.

The communication of information from one nerve cell to another occurs at junctions called synapses, where a chemical is released in the form of a neurotransmitter. A difference in concentration of potassium, sodium, and chloride ions exists across the cell membrane. These ions can selectively permeate ion channels in the membrane so that an unequal distribution of net charge occurs. The resting membrane potential results from an internal negativity resulting from the active transport of sodium from inside to outside the cell, and potassium from outside to inside the cell.[37]

The central nervous system (CNS) consists of the brain and an elongated spinal cord. The spinal cord participates directly in the control of body movements, the processing and transmission of sensory information from the trunk and limbs, and the regulation of visceral functions.[39] The spinal cord also provides a conduit for the two-way transmission of messages between the brain and the body. These messages travel along pathways, or tracts, that are fiber bundles of similar groups of neurons. Tracts may descend or ascend.

The spinal cord has an external segmental organization. Each of the 31 pairs of spinal nerves that arise from the spinal cord has an anterior (ventral) root and a posterior (dorsal) root, with each root made up of one to eight rootlets and consisting of bundles of nerve fibers.[38] In the posterior (dorsal) root of a typical spinal nerve lies a spinal (sensory) ganglion (posterior [dorsal] root ganglion), a swelling that contains nerve cell bodies.

Three membranes, or meninges, envelop the structures of the CNS: dura mater, arachnoid, and pia mater. The meninges and related spaces are important to both the nutrition and the protection of the spinal cord. The cerebrospinal fluid that flows through the meningeal spaces, and within the ventricles of the brain, provides a cushion for the spinal cord. The meninges also form barriers that resist the entrance of a variety of noxious organisms.

The peripheral nervous system consists of the cranial nerves (with the exception of cranial nerve II—the optic nerve) and the spinal nerves. Cranial nerves (CNs), of which there are traditionally 12 pairs, emerge directly from the brain, whereas spinal nerves emerge from segments of the spinal cord. As a simplistic description, cranial nerves bring information from the sense organs to the brain, control some muscles, or help control the function of glands or internal organs such as the heart and lungs. The term *spinal nerve* generally refers to a mixed spinal nerve, which carries motor, sensory, and autonomic signals between the spinal cord and the body. Each spinal nerve is formed by the combination of nerve fibers from the anterior and posterior roots of the spinal cord. The anterior roots carry efferent motor axons, whereas the posterior roots carry afferent sensory axons.

Feedback Receptors

All synovial joints of the body are provided with an array of receptor endings (nociceptors, thermoreceptors, and mechanoreceptors) embedded in articular, muscular, and cutaneous structures with varying characteristic behaviors and distributions (Table 4-5). These receptors provide information for the somatosensory system, which mediates signals related to multiple sensory modalities (pain, temperature, and proprioception). The nociceptors provide information with regard to pain, whereas the thermoreceptors provide feedback related to temperature. The mechanoreceptors, which are stimulated by mechanical forces (soft-tissue elongation, relaxation, compression, and fluid tension), are usually classified into three groups based on receptor type: joint, muscle, or cutaneous. There are four primary types of joint receptors that include Pacinian corpuscles, Ruffini endings, Golgi tendon organ (GTO)-like endings, and bare nerve endings.[40-42]

CLINICAL PEARL

The term *musculotendinous kinesthesia* refers to the capacity for musculotendinous structures to contribute proprioception information. Two types of muscle receptors are commonly described: muscle spindles and GTO (Box 4-1). It is most likely that the muscle and joint receptors work in a complementary fashion to one another in this complex afferent system, with each modifying the function of the other.[43] The muscle spindle functions as a stretch receptor, whereas the GTO functions as a monitor for the degree of tension within a muscle and tendon. Based on extensive work of Voss,[44] Peck et al[45] proposed that in the extremities, smaller muscles with high muscle spindle concentrations, arranged in parallel with larger, less spindle-dense muscles, function primarily as kinesthetic monitors.[46]

TABLE 4-5	Classification of Afferent, Cutaneous, and Efferents	
Type	Conduction Velocity (m/s)	Function
Afferents		
I	70–120	Provide input from muscle and tendon receptors
II	36–72	Afferents from muscle spindles
III	27–68	Pressure/nociceptive afferents from joints and aponeuroses
IV	1–4	Pain
Cutaneous		
Aα, β	30–70	Tactile receptors
Aδ	12–30	Cold; fast nociception
C	0.5–1.0	Warmth; tissue damage nociception
Efferents		
α	60–100	Extrafusal muscle fibers
γ	10–30	Intrafusal muscle fibers
B	3–30	Preganglionic autonomic
C	0.5–2.0	Postganglionic autonomic

Box 4-1 Muscle Spindle and Golgi Tendon Organ

Muscle Spindle

Muscle spindles are encapsulated spindle-shaped structures lying in parallel with skeletal muscle fibers in the muscle belly. Essentially, the purpose of the muscle spindle is to compare the length of the spindle with the length of the muscle that surrounds the spindle. Spindles have three main components[1]:

▶ *Intrafusal muscle fibers.* 2–12 long, slender, and specialized skeletal muscle fibers. The central portion of the intrafusal fiber is devoid of actin or myosin and thus is incapable of contracting. As a result, these fibers are capable of putting tension on the spindle only. These intrafusal fibers are of two types: nuclear bag fibers and nuclear chain fibers. Nuclear bag fibers primarily serve as sensitivity meters for the changing lengths of the muscle.[2,3] Nuclear chain fibers each contain a single row or chain of nuclei and are attached at their ends to the bag fibers.

▶ *Sensory neuron endings that wrap around the intrafusal fibers.* The sensory neurons are afferent structures (groups Ia and II afferents) that send information regarding static muscle length and changes in muscle length to the posterior root ganglia of the spinal cord. The group Ia afferents relay information regarding rates of change, whereas the group II afferents relay information regarding steady-state muscle length.

▶ *Motor axons.* Whereas muscles are innervated by alpha motor neurons, muscle spindles have their own motor supply, namely gamma motor neurons.

The muscle spindle can be stimulated in two different ways:

▶ By stretching the whole muscle, which stretches the mid portion of the spindle and depolarizes the Ia afferents. Ia afferents depolarization can trigger two separate responses[1]:

1. A monosynaptic or disynaptic spinal reflex

2. A long loop transcortical reflex

▶ By contracting only the end portion of the intrafusal fibers, exciting the receptor (even if muscle length does not change).

If the length of the muscles surrounding the spindle is less than that of the spindle, a decrease in intrafusal fiber afferent activity occurs. For example, a quick stretch applied to a muscle reflexively produces a quick contraction of the agonistic and synergistic muscle (extrafusal) fibers. This has the effect of producing a smooth contraction and relaxation of muscle and eliminating any jerkiness during movement. The firing of the type Ia phasic nerve fibers is influenced by the rate of stretch: the faster and greater the stimulus, the greater the effect of the associated extrafusal fibers.[3,4]

Golgi Tendon Organs

Golgi tendon organs (GTOs) are small, encapsulated structures spaced in series along the musculotendinous junction that become activated by stretch.[1] In contrast to the muscle spindle, GTOs function to protect muscle attachments from strain or avulsion, by using a postsynaptic inhibitory synapse of the muscle in which they are located.[5] The signals from the GTO may go both to local areas within the spinal cord and through the spinocerebellar tracts to the cerebellum.[6] The local signals result in excitation of interneurons, which in turn inhibit the anterior α motor neurons of the GTO's own muscle and synergist, while facilitating the antagonists.[6] This is theorized to prevent overcontraction, or stretch, of a muscle.[5]

1. Rose J: Dynamic lower extremity stability, in Hughes C (ed): Movement disorders and neuromuscular interventions for the trunk and extremities—Independent Study Course 18.2.5. La Crosse, WI, Orthopaedic Section, APTA, 2008, pp 1-34.
2. Grigg P: Peripheral neural mechanisms in proprioception. J Sport Rehabil 3:1-17, 1994.
3. Swash M, Fox K: Muscle spindle innervation in man. J Anat 112:61-80, 1972.
4. Wilk KE, Voight ML, Keirns MA, et al: Stretch-shortening drills for the upper extremities: theory and clinical application. J Orthop Sports Phys Ther 17:225-239, 1993.
5. de Jarnette B: Sacro-occipital technique. Nebraska City, Major Bertrand de Jarnette, DC, 1972.
6. Pollard H, Ward G: A study of two stretching techniques for improving hip flexion range of motion. J Man Physiol Ther 20:443–447, 1997.

▶ *Ruffini endings.* These slow-adapting, low-threshold stretch receptors are important postural mediators, signaling actual joint position or changes in joint positions.[47] They are primarily located on the *flexion* side (detect the stretch with extension of the joint) of the joint capsule, but are also found in ligaments, primarily near the origin and insertion.[48,49] These slowly adapting receptors continue to discharge while the stimulus is present and contribute to reflex regulation of postural tone, to coordination of muscle activity, and to a perceptional awareness of joint position. An increase in joint capsule tension by active or passive motion, posture, mobilization, or manipulation causes these receptors to discharge at a higher frequency.[42,50]

▶ *Pacinian corpuscles.* These rapidly adapting, low-threshold receptors function primarily in sensing joint compression and increased hydrostatic pressure in the joint.[51] They are primarily located in the subcapsular fibroadipose tissue, the cruciate ligaments, the annulus fibrosis, and the fibrous capsule. These receptors are entirely inactive in immobile joints but become active for brief periods at the onset of movement and during rapid changes in tension. They also fire during active or passive motion of a joint, or with the application of traction. This behavior suggests their role as a control mechanism to regulate motor unit activity of the prime movers of the joint.

▶ *Golgi tendon organ–like receptors.* These receptors, also referred to as Golgi ligament organs (Box 4-1), are found in the joint capsule, ligaments, and menisci.[52] These slow-adapting and high-threshold receptors function to detect large amounts of tension. They only become active in the extremes of motion such as when strong manual techniques are applied to the joint. Their function is protective—to prevent further motion that would over displace the joint (a joint protective reflex)—and their firing is inhibitory to those muscles that would contribute to excessive forces.

▶ *Bare nerve endings.* These high-threshold, nonadapting, free nerve ending receptors are inactive in normal circumstances but become active with marked mechanical deformation or tension.[53,54] They may also become active in response to direct mechanical or chemical irritation, and their sensitivity usually increases when joints are inflamed or swollen.[55]

Structurally, the CNS is organized in a hierarchical and parallel fashion, with the most complex processing located in the cortical centers of the brain and the most basic processing located in the spinal cord.[48] At the upper end of the hierarchy, the motor cortex has a motor program, defined as an abstract plan of movement that, when initiated, results in the production of a coordinated movement sequence.[56,57] At the lower end of the hierarchy, specific motor units must contract to accomplish the movement. Rapid motor responses to somatosensory feedback mediated in the spinal cord are referred to as spinal reflexes.[48] These reflex actions include preparatory postural adjustments[58] and reaction movements. Although the hierarchy is well established, research suggests that these components also work in parallel so that any of the components may predominate in controlling some aspects of movement; the system is built for efficiency and redundancy (see normal Development of Motor Control and Motor Learning).[56]

Skeletal Muscle

The microstructure and composition of skeletal muscle have been studied extensively. The class of tissue labeled *skeletal muscle* consists of individual muscle cells or fibers that work together to produce the movement of bony levers. A single muscle cell is called a *muscle fiber* or *myofiber*. Individual muscle fibers are wrapped in a CT envelope called *endomysium*. Bundles of myofibers, which form a whole muscle (fasciculus), are encased in the perimysium. The perimysium is continuous with the deep fascia. Groups of fasciculi are surrounded by a connective sheath called the epimysium. Under an electron microscope, it can be seen that each of the myofibers consists of thousands of *myofibrils*, which extend throughout its length. Myofibrils are composed of sarcomeres arranged in series.[59] All skeletal muscles exhibit four characteristics[60]:

1. Excitability, the ability to respond to stimulation from the nervous system

2. Elasticity, the ability to change in length or stretch

3. Extensibility, the ability to shorten and return to normal length

4. Contractility, the ability to shorten and contract in response to some neural command. The tension developed in skeletal muscle can occur passively (stretch) or actively (contraction). When an activated muscle develops tension, the amount of tension present is constant throughout the length of the muscle, in the tendons, and at the sites of the musculotendinous attachments to bone.[1] The tensile force produced by the muscle pulls on the attached bones and creates torque at the joints crossed by the muscle. The magnitude of the tensile force is dependent on a number of factors.

One of the most important roles of fibrous CT is to mechanically transmit the forces generated by the skeletal muscle cells to provide movement. Each of the myofibrils contains many fibers called *myofilaments*, which run parallel to the myofibril axis. The myofilaments are made up of two different proteins: actin (thin myofilaments) and myosin (thick myofilaments), which give skeletal muscle fibers their striated (striped) appearance.[59]

CLINICAL PEARL

The sarcomere is the contractile machinery of the muscle. The graded contractions of a whole muscle occur because the number of fibers participating in the contraction varies. Increasing the force of movement is achieved by recruiting more cells into cooperative action.

The striations are produced by alternating dark (A) and light (I) bands that appear to span the width of the muscle fiber. The A bands are composed of myosin filaments, whereas the I bands are composed of actin filaments. The actin filaments of the I band overlap into the A band, giving the edges of the A band a darker appearance than the central region (H band), which contains only myosin. At the center of each I band is a thin, dark Z line. A *sarcomere* represents the distance between each Z line. Each muscle fiber is limited by a cell membrane called a *sarcolemma*. The protein *dystrophin* plays an essential role in the mechanical strength and stability of the sarcolemma.[61] Dystrophin is lacking in patients with Duchenne muscular dystrophy.

CLINICAL PEARL

The sarcoplasm is the specialized cytoplasm of a muscle cell that contains the usual subcellular elements along with the Golgi apparatus, abundant myofibrils, a modified endoplasmic reticulum known as the sarcoplasmic reticulum (SR), myoglobin, and mitochondria. Transverse tubules (T-tubules) invaginate the sarcolemma, allowing impulses to penetrate the cell and activate the SR.

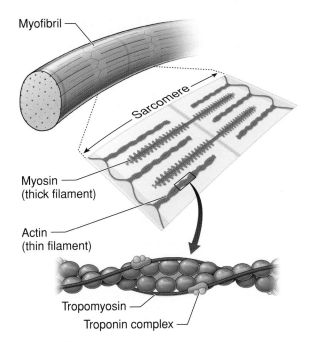

Myofibril

Sarcomere

Myosin
(thick filament)

Actin
(thin filament)

Tropomyosin

Troponin complex

FIGURE 4-7 Troponin and tropomyosin

Structures called *cross-bridges* serve to connect the actin and myosin filaments. The myosin filaments contain two flexible, hinge-like regions, which allow the cross-bridges to attach and detach from the actin filament. During contraction, the cross-bridges attach and undergo power strokes, which provide the contractile force. During relaxation, the cross-bridges detach. This attaching and detaching is asynchronous, so that some are attaching while others are detaching. Thus, at each moment, some of the cross-bridges are pulling, while others are releasing.

The regulation of cross-bridge attachment and detachment is a function of two proteins found in the actin filaments: tropomyosin and troponin (Figure 4-7). Tropomyosin attaches directly to the actin filament, whereas troponin is attached to the tropomyosin rather than directly to the actin filament.

The Motor Unit. Each muscle fiber is innervated by a somatic motor neuron. One neuron and the muscle fibers it innervates constitute a motor unit, or functional unit of the muscle. Each motor neuron branches as it enters the muscle to innervate a number of muscle fibers.

The release of a chemical called acetylcholine from the axon terminals at the neuromuscular junction (NMJ) causes electrical activation of the skeletal muscle fibers. When an action potential propagates into the transverse tubule system (narrow membranous tunnels formed from and continuous with the sarcolemma), the voltage sensors on the transverse tubule membrane signal the release of Ca^{2+} from the terminal cisternae portion of the sarcoplasmic reticulum (SR; a series of interconnected sacs and tubes that surround each myofibril).[62] The released Ca^{2+} then diffuses into the sarcomeres and binds to troponin, displacing the tropomyosin, and allowing the actin to bind with the myosin cross-bridges (see Figure 4-7). Whenever a somatic motor neuron is activated, all of the muscle fibers that it innervates are stimulated and contract with *all-or-none* twitches. Although the muscle fibers produce all-or-none contractions, muscles are capable of a wide variety of responses, ranging from activities requiring a high level of precision, to activities requiring high tension.

At the end of the contraction (the neural activity and action potentials cease), the SR actively accumulates Ca^{2+} and muscle relaxation occurs. The return of Ca^{2+} to the SR involves active transport, requiring the degradation of adenosine triphosphate (ATP) to adenosine diphosphate. (ADP*).[62] Because SR function is closely associated with both contraction and relaxation, changes in its ability to release or sequester Ca^{2+} markedly affect both the time course and magnitude of force output by the muscle fiber.[63]

Muscle Fibers

On the basis of their contractile properties, two major types of muscle fiber have been recognized within skeletal muscle: type I (slow-twitch fibers), and type II (fast-twitch fibers) (Table 4-6).[64] Slow-twitch fibers are richly endowed with mitochondria and have a high capacity for oxygen uptake. They are, therefore, suitable for activities of long duration or endurance, including the maintenance of posture. In contrast, fast-twitch fibers are suited to quick, explosive actions, including such activities as sprinting. A number of muscle subtypes

---

*The most readily available energy for skeletal muscle cells is stored in the form of ATP and phosphocreatine (PCr). Through the activity of the enzyme ATPase, ATP promptly releases energy when required by the cell to perform any type of work, whether it is electrical, chemical, or mechanical.

TABLE 4-6	Comparison of Muscle Fiber Types			
Characteristics	**Type I**	**Type IIA**	**Type IIAB**	**Type IIB**
Size (diameter)	Small	Intermediate	Large	Very large
Resistance to fatigue	High	Fairly high	Intermediate	Low
Glycogen content	Low	Intermediate	High	High
Twitch rate	Slow	Fast	Fast	Fast
Myosin ATPase content	Low	High	High	High
Major storage fuel	Triglycerides	Creatine phosphate Glycogen	Creatine phosphate Glycogen	Creatine phosphate Glycogen

ATP, Adenosine triphosphate.

have been recognized based on their qualities and aerobic to anaerobic capabilities.

▸ *Type A:* possess good aerobic and anaerobic characteristics

▸ *Type B:* possess fair aerobic and poor anaerobic characteristics

▸ *Type AB:* possess aerobic and anaerobic characteristics somewhere between types A and B

Based on the above, four fiber types can be distinguished: I, IIA, IIB, and IIAB.[65] The type II (fast-twitch) fibers are separated based on mitochondria content into those that have a high complement of mitochondria (type IIA) and those that are mitochondria poor (type IIB). Type IIAB fibers exhibit structural features of both red and white fibers and thus have fast contraction times and good fatigue resistance. Within this list, there appears to be a consistent order of recruitment based on fiber size: type I fibers first, followed by IIA, IIAB, and, finally, IIB fibers.[65] The smaller type I fibers are the easiest to stimulate as they have the smaller motor units.

CLINICAL PEARL

In fast-twitch fibers, the sarcoplasmic reticulum embraces every individual myofibril. In slow-twitch fibers, it may contain multiple myofibrils.[66]

Theory dictates that a muscle with a large percentage of the total cross-sectional area occupied by slow-twitch type I fibers should be more fatigue resistant than one in which the fast-twitch type II fibers predominate.

Different activities place differing demands on a muscle (Table 4-7).[66] For example, movement activities involve a predominance of fast-twitch fiber recruitment, whereas postural activities and those activities requiring stabilization entail more involvement of the slow-twitch fibers. In humans, most limb muscles contain a relatively equal distribution of each muscle fiber type, whereas the back and trunk demonstrate a predominance of slow-twitch fibers. Although it would seem possible that physical training may cause fibers to convert from slow twitch to fast twitch or the reverse, this has not

been shown to be the case.[67] However, fiber conversion from type IIB to type IIAB and IIA, and vice versa, has been found to occur with training.[68]

The effectiveness of a muscle in producing movement depends on a number of factors. These include the location and orientation of the muscle attachment relative to the joint, the tightness or laxity present in the musculotendinous unit, the type of contraction, the point of application, and the actions of other muscles that cross the joint.[4]

TABLE 4-7	Functional Division of Muscle Groups
Movement Group	**Stabilization Group**
Primarily type IIA	Primarily type I
Prone to develop tightness	Prone to develop weakness
Prone to develop hypertonicity	Prone to muscle inhibition
Dominate in fatigue and new movement situations	Fatigue easily
Generally cross two joints	Primarily cross one joint
Examples	**Examples**
Gastrocnemius/Soleus	Peronei
Tibialis posterior	Tibialis anterior
Short hip adductors	Vastus medialis and lateralis
Hamstrings	Gluteus maximus, medius, and minimus
Rectus femoris	Serratus anterior
Tensor fascia lata	Rhomboids
Erector spinae	Lower portion of trapezius
Quadratus lumborum	Short/deep cervical flexors
Pectoralis major	Upper limb extensors
Upper portion of trapezius	Rectus abdominis
Levator scapulae	
Sternocleidomastoid	
Scalenes	
Upper limb flexors	

Data from Jull GA, Janda V: Muscle and motor control in low back pain, in Twomey LT, Taylor JR (eds), Physical Therapy of the Low Back: Clinics in Physical Therapy. New York, Churchill Livingstone, 1987, p 258.

CLINICAL PEARL

Following the stimulation of a muscle, a brief period elapses before the muscle begins to develop tension. This period is referred to as the *electromechanical delay* (EMD). The length of the EMD varies considerably among muscles. Fast-twitch fibers have shorter periods of EMD when compared with slow-twitch fibers.[69] It has been suggested that injury increases the EMD and, therefore, increases the susceptibility to injury.[70] One of the purposes of neuromuscular reeducation through physical therapy is to return the EMD to a normal level.[71]

Types of Muscle Contractions

As previously mentioned, depending on the type of muscular contraction, the length of a muscle can remain the same (isometric), shorten (concentric), or lengthen (eccentric). The rate of muscle shortening or lengthening substantially affects the force that a muscle can develop during contraction.

▶ *Shortening contractions.* As the speed of a muscle shortening increases, the force it is capable of producing decreases.[72,73] The slower rate of shortening is thought to produce greater forces than can be produced by increasing the number of cross-bridges formed. This relationship can be viewed as a continuum, with the optimum velocity for the muscle somewhere between the slowest and fastest rates. At very slow speeds, the force that a muscle can resist or overcome rises rapidly up to 50% greater than the maximum isometric contraction.[72,73]

▶ *Lengthening contractions.* The following changes in force production occur during an eccentric contraction:

- Rapid lengthening contractions generate more force than do slow ones (slower lengthening contractions).
- During slow lengthening muscle actions, the work produced approximates that of an isometric contraction.[72,73]

CLINICAL PEARL

The number of cross-bridges that can be formed is dependent on the extent of the overlap between the actin and myosin filaments.[74] Thus, the force a muscle is capable of exerting depends on its length. For each muscle cell, there is an optimum length, or range of lengths, at which the contractile force is strongest. At the optimum length of the muscle, there is near-optimal overlap of actin and myosin, allowing for the generation of maximum tension at this length.

▶ If the muscle is in a shortened position, the overlap of actin and myosin reduces the number of sites available for cross-bridge formation. *Active insufficiency*

of a muscle occurs when the muscle is incapable of shortening to the extent required to produce full range of motion at all joints crossed simultaneously.[4,75–77] For example, the finger flexors cannot produce a tight fist when the wrist is fully flexed, as they can when it is in neutral position.

▶ If the muscle is in a lengthened position compared with the optimum length, the actin filaments are pulled away from the myosin heads such that they cannot create as many cross-bridges.[78] *Passive insufficiency* of the muscle occurs when the two-joint muscle cannot stretch to the extent required for full range of motion in the opposite direction at all joints crossed.[4,75–77] For example, a larger range of hyperextension is possible at the wrist when the fingers are not fully extended.

The force and speed of a muscle contraction are based on the requirements of an activity and are dependent on the ability of the central nervous system to control the recruitment of motor units.[4] The motor units of slow-twitch fibers generally have lower thresholds and are relatively easier to activate than those of the fast-twitch motor units. Consequently, the slow-twitch fibers are the first to be recruited, even when the resulting limb movement is rapid.[79]

As the force requirement, speed requirement, or duration of an activity increases, motor units with higher thresholds are recruited. Type IIA units are recruited before type IIB.[80]

CLINICAL PEARL

The term *temporal summation* refers to the summation of individual contractile units. The summation can increase the muscular force by increasing the muscle activation frequency.[81]

Force Production

Although each muscle contains the contractile machinery to produce the forces for movement, it is the tendon that transmits these forces to the bones in order to achieve movement or stability of the body in space.[7] The angle of insertion the tendon makes with a bone determines the line of pull, whereas the tension generated by a muscle is a function of its angle of insertion. A muscle generates the greatest amount of torque when its line of pull is oriented at a 90-degree angle to the bone, and it is attached anatomically as far from the joint center as possible.[4]

Just as there are optimal speeds of length change, and optimal muscle lengths, there are optimal insertion angles for each of the muscles. The angle of insertion of a muscle, and therefore its line of pull, can change during dynamic movements.[78] The *angle of pennation* is the angle created between the fiber direction and the line of pull. When the fibers of a muscle lie parallel to the long axis of the muscle, there is no angle of pennation. The number of fibers within a fixed volume of muscle increases with the angle of pennation.[78] Although maximum tension can be improved with pennation, the range of shortening of the muscle is reduced. Muscle fibers can contract to about 60% of their resting length. Because the muscle fibers in pennate muscles are shorter than the nonpennate equivalent, the amount of contraction is similarly reduced. Muscles that need to have large changes in length without the need for very high tension, such as the sartorius, do not have pennate muscle fibers.[78] In contrast, pennate muscle fibers are found in those muscles in which the emphasis is on a high capacity for tension generation rather than range of motion (e.g., gluteus maximus).

INTRODUCTION TO PHYSICAL THERAPY AND PATIENT SKILLS

CLINICAL PEARL

Skeletal muscle blood flow increases 20-fold during muscle contractions.[82] The muscle blood flow generally increases in proportion to the metabolic demands of the tissue, a relationship reflected by positive correlations between muscle blood flow and exercise. As body temperature rises, the speeds of nerve and muscle functions increase, resulting in a higher value of maximum isometric tension and a higher maximum velocity of shortening possible with fewer motor units at any given load.[83] Muscle function is most efficient at 38.5°C (101°F).[84]

Cardiovascular System

The heart is a hollow, muscular organ that functions to pump blood around the body through the blood vessels using repeated, rhythmic contractions. The human heart (Latin *cor*) is derived embryologically from mesoderm that forms the heart tube. The muscle tissue of the heart is composed of muscle fibers called myocardium.

CLINICAL PEARL

The cardiovascular system functions to provide the fuel for movement. The newborn has a cardiac output and metabolic rate twice that of an adult.

Cardiac muscle fibers have numerous mitochondria, exhibit rhythmicity of contraction, and can work continuously without fatigue.

CLINICAL PEARL

Cardiac muscle has a myogenic origin (an inherent source of contraction), whereas skeletal (striated) muscle has a neurogenic source for contraction (its motor nerve supply).

The heart consists of four chambers, the two upper atria (singular: atrium) and the two lower ventricles. Blood is pumped through the heart chambers aided by four heart valves.

CLINICAL PEARL

Valves are flap-like structures that allow blood to flow in one direction. The heart has two kinds of valves, atrioventricular and semilunar valves.

Right Atrium

The right atrium (RA) receives blood from the systemic circulation via the superior vena cava, which drains the upper part of the body, and the inferior vena cava, which drains the lower part of the body. The coronary sinus is an additional venous return into the right atrium, receiving blood from the heart itself. Blood passes from the right atrium into the right ventricle via the right atrioventricular (AV) valve (also known as the tricuspid valve, because it is formed of three triangular leaflets or cusps).

CLINICAL PEARL

The AV valves are held in position by chordae tendineae, which in turn are secured to the ventricular wall by the papillary muscles.

► The papillary muscles serve to maintain approximation of the valve leaflets during contraction of the ventricles.

► The chordae tendineae prevent the valves from everting when the ventricles contract, thereby stopping any back flow of blood.

Right Ventricle

The right ventricle (RV) receives blood from the RA. The ventricular contraction causes the right AV valve to close and the oxygen-depleted blood to leave the RV via the pulmonary trunk to the lungs. The blood then enters the capillaries of the right and left pulmonary arteries, where gaseous exchange takes place and the blood releases carbon dioxide into the lung cavity and picks up oxygen. The oxygenated blood then flows through pulmonary veins to the left atrium.

CLINICAL PEARL

► The blood that is pumped to the pulmonary trunk passes through the pulmonary valve (also called the pulmonary semilunar valve), which lies at the base of the pulmonary trunk and serves to prevent blood from leaking back into the right ventricle.

► Semilunar valves are half-moon–shaped flaps of endocardium and connective tissue reinforced by fibers, which prevent the valves from turning inside out. Their main function is to prevent the back flow of blood from the aorta and pulmonary arteries into the ventricles when the heart relaxes between beats. They comprise the pulmonary valve and the aortic valve (see Left Ventricle).

Left Atrium

The left atrium (LA) receives the oxygenated blood from the lungs via four pulmonary veins (two left and two right pulmonary veins). From the LA the blood passes through the mitral (bicuspid) valve to enter the left ventricle.

Left Ventricle

The left ventricle (LV), which forms most of the diaphragmatic side of the heart, receives blood from the LA. The left ventricle is longer and more conical in shape than the right.

The LV is much more muscular (1.3 to 1.5 cm thick) than the RV (0.3 to 0.5 cm thick) because it has to pump blood around the entire body, which involves exerting a considerable force to overcome the vascular pressure (because the RV only needs to pump blood to the lungs, it requires less muscle). The aortic valve allows blood to flow from the LV into the aorta, and then closes to prevent blood from leaking back into the LV.

A septum (also known as the fiber skeleton of the heart) divides the right atrium and ventricle from the left atrium and ventricle, preventing blood from passing between them. Even though the ventricles lie below the atria, the two vessels through which the blood exits the heart (the pulmonary artery and the aorta) leave the heart at its top side.

The function of the right side of the heart is to collect deoxygenated blood from the body and pump it into the lungs so that carbon dioxide can be dropped off and oxygen picked up. This happens through a process called diffusion. The left side collects oxygenated blood from the lungs and pumps it out to the body.

Respiratory System

The pulmonary or respiratory system is contained within the sternum, 12 pairs of ribs, the clavicle, and the vertebrae of the thoracic spine, which together form the thoracic cage.

The primary function of the respiratory system is to exchange gases (oxygen and carbon dioxide) between tissue, the blood, and the environment so that arterial blood oxygen, carbon dioxide, and pH levels remain within specific limits throughout many different physiologic limits.[86] The pulmonary system also plays a number of other roles, including contributing to temperature homeostasis via evaporative heat loss from the lungs, and filtering, humidifying, and warming or cooling the air to body temperature.[86] These processes protect the remainder of the respiratory system from damage caused by dry gases or harmful debris.[86]

The respiratory system is arranged basically as an upside-down tree, which can be divided into two main portions:[86]

▶ The conducting portion includes the upper airways, the lower airway (trachea, bronchi, and bronchioles). Within this portion, air moves by bulk flow under the pressure gradients created by the respiratory muscles and the elastic recoil of the lungs. The left main bronchus branches at a more acute angle and is longer than the right main bronchus, which is more directly in line with the trachea.[86] This relationship predisposes to aspiration of material into the right rather than the left lung.[86] Two body defense mechanisms are located within the walls of the trachea and bronchi:

■ *Cilia and goblet cells.* These function to eliminate inhaled minute particulate matter.

■ *Irritant receptors.* These receptors, which are located in the larynx, trachea, bronchi, pleura, and diaphragm, are responsible for the cough reflex.

▶ The respiratory portion includes the terminal portion of the bronchial tree and alveoli, the site of gas exchange.[87] The total cross-sectional area rapidly increases at the respiratory zone. Forward velocity of air flow therefore decreases, and the gases readily move by diffusion through the alveoli into the pulmonary capillaries.

CLINICAL PEARL

The transitional zone, consisting of the respiratory bronchioles, separates the conducting and respiratory portions.

The diaphragm, innervated by the phrenic nerve, is the primary muscle of inspiration, contributing two thirds of the airflow in the sitting or standing position, and three quarters of the airflow in the supine position. The diaphragm, which forms a partition between the thoracic and the abdominal cavities, is made up of two hemidiaphragms, each with a central tendon. When the diaphragm is at rest, the hemidiaphragms are arched high into the thorax. When the diaphragm contracts, it descends over the abdominal contents, flattening the dome, which causes the lower ribs, which serve as levers, to move outward, resulting in protrusion of the abdominal wall. In addition, the contracting diaphragm causes a decrease in intrathoracic pressure, which pulls air into the lungs.[88] The other muscles of respiration include the external intercostal muscles, which are active on inspiration, and the internal intercostals, which are active during forced expiration. A number of accessory inspiratory muscles are recognized and include the scalenus and sternocleidomastoid. The abdominal muscles can be used for forceful exhalation.

Respiratory muscle activity involves multiple components of the neural, mechanical, and chemical control and is closely integrated with the cardiovascular system.[89] The spontaneous neuronal activity that produces cyclic breathing originates in the respiratory centers in the posterior region of the medulla, which is influenced by two control centers in the pons[86]:

▶ *Apneustic:* appears to promote inspiration by stimulating neurons in the medulla.

▶ *Pneumotaxic:* seems to antagonize the apneustic center and inhibit inspiration.

In addition to the neural and mechanical influences, the automatic control of breathing is also influenced by chemoreceptors.[86] Chemoreceptor input to the brainstem maintains the rate and depth of breathing at an efficient level. Of the two respiratory gases, carbon dioxide is the most tightly controlled.[86]

CLINICAL PEARL

Three chemical levels in particular play a critical role in controlling respiration: the blood acid-base balance (pH—a measure of the concentration of free-floating hydrogen ions within the body), the partial pressure of carbon dioxide within the arterial blood bicarbonate ($PaCO_2$), and the amount of bicarbonate ions within the arterial blood (HCO_3^-).

The central chemoreceptors monitor the carbon dioxide levels of both the arterial blood and cerebrospinal fluid.[86] A second group of chemoreceptors, the peripheral chemoreceptors, are located in the carotid and aortic bodies[86]:

▶ The carotid chemoreceptors are stimulated by low arterial oxygen tensions, high arterial carbon dioxide tensions, and acidosis (arterial pH below 7.35).

▶ The aortic chemoreceptors are not involved in ventilation, but produce reflex cardiovascular responses (i.e., stimulation increases the heart rate and raises the blood pressure). In addition to responding to the same stimuli as the carotid chemoreceptors, they are also stimulated by a low oxygen content of the arterial blood.

CLINICAL PEARL

▶ The normal range for arterial pH is 7.36–7.44. Acidosis refers to an arterial pH below 7.35, and alkalosis refers to an arterial pH above 7.5.

▶ The normal range of PCO_2 is 40 mm Hg. A rise in PCO_2, called hypercapnia, is caused by hypoventilation. Conversely, hyperventilation results in a fall in PCO_2, hypocapnia.

The Energy for Movement

Movement requires muscular and neural activity. The energy required to power muscular activity is derived from the hydrolysis of ATP to ADP and inorganic phosphate (P_i). Despite the large fluctuations in energy demand just mentioned, muscle ATP remains practically constant and demonstrates a remarkable precision of the system in adjusting the rate of the ATP-generating processes to the demand.[90] There are three energy systems that contribute to the resynthesis of ATP via ADP rephosphorylation. These energy systems are as follows:

▶ *Phosphagen system.* The phosphagen system is an anaerobic process—it can proceed without oxygen (O_2). Within the skeletal muscle cell at the onset of muscular contraction, phosphocreatine (PCr) represents the most immediate reserve for the rephosphorylation of ATP. The phosphagen system provides ATP primarily for short-term, high-intensity activities (i.e., sprinting) and is active at the start of all exercises regardless of intensity.[91] One disadvantage of the phosphagen system is that because of its significant contribution to the energy yield at the onset of near-maximal exercise, the concentration of PCr can be reduced to less than 40% of resting levels within 10 seconds of the start of intense exercise.[92]

▶ *Glycolysis system.* The glycolysis system is an anaerobic process that involves the breakdown of carbohydrates—either glycogen stored in the muscle or glucose delivered in the blood—into pyruvate to produce ATP. Pyruvate is then transformed into lactic acid. Because this system relies on a series of nine different chemical reactions, it is slower to become fully active. However, glycogenolysis has a greater capacity to provide energy than does PCr, and therefore it supplements PCr during maximal exercise and continues to rephosphorylate ADP during maximal exercise after PCr reserves have become essentially depleted.[91] The process of glycolysis can go one of two ways, termed fast glycolysis and slow glycolysis, depending on the energy demands within the cell. If energy must be supplied at a high rate, fast glycolysis is used primarily. If the energy demand is not as high, slow glycolysis is activated. The main disadvantage of the fast glycolysis system is that during very high-intensity exercise, hydrogen ions dissociate from the glycogenolytic end product of lactic acid.[90] The accumulation of lactic acid in the contracting muscle is recognized in sports and resistance training circles. An increase in hydrogen ion concentration is believed to inhibit glycotic reactions and directly interfere with muscle excitation–contraction and coupling, which can potentially impair contractile force during exercise.[91] This inhibition occurs once the muscle pH drops below a certain level, prompting the appearance of phosphofructokinase (PFK), resulting in local energy production ceasing until replenished by oxygen stores.

▶ *Oxidative system.* As its name suggests, the oxidative system requires O_2 and is consequently termed the "aerobic" system. The oxidative system is the primary source of ATP at rest and during low-intensity activities. It is worth noting that at no time during either rest or exercise does any single energy system provide the complete supply of energy. Although it is unable to produce ATP at an equivalent rate to that produced by PCr breakdown and glycogenolysis, the oxidative system is capable of sustaining low-intensity exercise for several hours.[91] However, because of its greater complexity, the time between the onset of exercise and when this system is operating at its full potential is around 45 seconds.[93] A phenomenon, called *steady state*, occurs after some 5 to 6 minutes of exercise at a constant intensity level.[94] During steady state, the rate of mitochondrial ATP production is closely matched to the rate of ATP hydrolysis and demonstrates the existence of efficient cellular mechanisms to control mitochondrial ATP synthesis in a wide dynamic range.[95]

The relative contribution of these energy systems to ATP resynthesis has been shown to depend on the intensity and duration of exercise, with the primary system used being based on the duration of the event[96]:

▶ 0–10 seconds: ATP-PCr
▶ 10–30 seconds: ATP-PCr plus anaerobic glycolysis
▶ 30 seconds-2 minutes: anaerobic glycolysis
▶ 2–3 minutes: anaerobic glycolysis plus oxidative system
▶ >3 minutes and rest: oxidative system

Recovery

The performance of any activity requires a certain rate of oxygen consumption, so that an individual's ability to perform an activity is limited by the maximal amount of oxygen the person is capable of delivering into the lungs.[97] Fatigue and recovery from fatigue are complex processes that depend on physiologic and psychological factors. The physiologic factors include the adequacy of the blood supply to the working muscle and the maintenance of a viable chemical environment, whereas the psychological factors include motivation and incentive.[98] After an intense exercise session, anaerobic energy sources must be replenished before they can be called on again to provide energy for muscular contraction. The anaerobic energy sources of ATP-PCr and lactic acid are ultimately replenished by the oxidative energy system. The extra oxygen that is taken in to replenish the anaerobic energy sources after cessation of the exercise effort was previously referred to as the *oxygen debt*, but is now more accurately referred to as *excess postexercise oxygen consumption* (EPOC).

Muscle Performance

Movement of the body, or any of its parts, involves considerable muscular activity from those muscles directly responsible for the movement. Muscle is the only biological tissue capable of actively generating tension. This characteristic enables human skeletal muscle to perform important functions including the maintenance of an upright body posture, the movement of body parts, and the absorption of the various forces that act on the body. The ability of a muscle to carry out its various roles is a measure of muscle performance. Muscle performance can be measured using a number of parameters. These include strength, endurance, and power.

▶ *Strength.* Strength may be defined as the amount of force that may be exerted by an individual in a single maximum muscular contraction against a specific resistance, or the ability to produce torque at a joint. Three types of contraction are commonly recognized: isometric, concentric, and eccentric.[99]

■ *Isometric contraction.* Isometric contractions do not produce any appreciable change in muscle length.

■ *Concentric contraction.* A concentric contraction produces a shortening of the muscle length. When a muscle contracts concentrically, the distance between the Z lines decreases, the I band and H bands disappear, but the width of the A band remains unchanged.[62] This shortening of the sarcomeres is not produced by a shortening of the actin and myosin filaments, but by a sliding of actin filaments over the myosin filaments, which pulls the Z lines together (sliding filament theory).

■ *Eccentric contraction.* An eccentric contraction produces a "lengthening" of the muscle length. In reality, the muscle does not actually lengthen, it merely returns from its shortened position to its normal resting length.

▶ *Endurance.* Muscular endurance is the ability of a muscle, or group of muscles, to continue to perform without fatigue. The nature of muscular endurance encourages the body to work aerobically—*steady state*. Endurance exercise training produces an increase in mitochondrial volume density in all three muscle fiber types[100] and thus muscle aerobic power. With a higher mitochondrial density in trained muscle, the rate of substrate flux per individual mitochondrion will be less at any given rate of ATP hydrolysis.[95] Therefore, the required activation of mitochondrial respiration by adenosine diphosphate (ADP) to achieve a given rate of ATP formation will be less, resulting in increased ADP sensitivity of muscle oxidative phosphorylation.[95]

▸ *Power.* Mechanical power is the product of force and velocity. *Muscular power*, the maximum amount of work an individual can perform in a given unit of time, is the product of muscular force and velocity of muscle shortening. Muscular power is an important contributor to activities requiring both strength and speed. Maximum power occurs at approximately one-third of maximum velocity.[101] Muscles with a predominance of fast-twitch fibers generate more power at a given load than those with a high composition of slow-twitch fibers.[102] The ratio for mean peak power production by type IIB, type IIA, and type I fibers in skeletal tissue is 10:5:1.[67]

These three components of muscle performance are important in functional activities as they can allow a patient to interact with the environment in a more efficient and pain-free way through increased movement control and capacity.

CLINICAL PEARL

The ultimate source of energy for muscular contraction is the adenosine triphosphate (ATP) molecule. The catabolic breakdown of the chemical bonds of the ATP molecule provides the energy necessary to allow myosin cross-bridges to pull the actin filaments across the myosin filaments, which results in muscle contraction.

To assess muscle performance, strength values using manual muscle testing (MMT) (see Chapter 12) have traditionally been used between similar muscle groups on opposite extremities, or antagonistic ratios. Strength measures the ability with which musculotendinous units act across a bone-joint lever-arm system to actively generate motion, or passively resist movement against gravity and variable resistance.[103]

Range of Motion and Flexibility

The terms *range of motion* and *flexibility* are often used synonymously by clinicians, yet they are not the same.

▸ Range of motion refers to the distance and direction a joint can move. Each specific joint has a normal range of motion that is expressed in degrees. Within the field of physical therapy, goniometry is commonly used to measure the total amount of available motion at a specific joint (see Chapter 11). Range of motion of a joint may be limited by the shape of the articulating surfaces and by capsular and ligamentous structures surrounding that joint.

▸ Flexibility refers to the ability to move a joint or series of joints through a full, nonrestricted, injury- and pain-free range of motion. Flexibility is dependent on a combination of joint range of motion, muscle flexibility, and neuromuscular control. When injury occurs, there is almost always some associated loss of the ability to move normally due to the pain, swelling, muscle guarding or spasm. The subsequent inactivity results in a shortening of connective tissue and muscle, loss of neuromuscular control, or a combination of these factors.[104]

When referring to range of motion, three major movements are recognized[104]:

▸ *Passive range of motion (PROM).* PROM, refers to the degree to which a joint can be passively moved to the endpoint in the range of motion. PROM is indicated when the patient's own muscle force is inadequate to produce sufficient motion at a joint, when active contraction of the muscle would be harmful, or as a means of educating a patient about a particular movement. PROM does not prevent muscle atrophy, increase strength or endurance, or assist circulation to the same extent that active, voluntary muscle contraction does. PROM is contraindicated during stages of tissue healing in which motion could prevent or inhibit tissue repair, in the presence of muscle guarding, or in the presence of increasing pain.

▸ *Active range of motion (AROM).* AROM refers to the degree to which a joint can be moved by a single muscle contraction, usually through the mid-range of movement. AROM is indicated when the patient is able to perform a movement safely, effectively, and with minimum pain. AROM does not maintain or increase strength, or develop skill or coordination except in the movement patterns used. AROM is contraindicated in the acute stage of healing (12–48 hours after the trauma) or in the presence of any adverse response to the motion (pain that persists more than two hours after the activity, an undesired cardiopulmonary response, or an increase in effusion/inflammation).

▸ *Active assisted range of motion (AAROM).* AAROM is active range of motion where the effect of gravity has been removed or when manual assistance is necessary to complete the motion. For example, performing shoulder abduction while lying supine removes the effect of gravity.

CLINICAL PEARL

In the early stages of the rehabilitation process, range of motion exercises are performed in the following sequence: Passive ROM → Active assisted ROM → Active ROM. When making the transition from PROM to AAROM or AROM, it is important to remember that gravity has a significant impact, especially in individuals with weak musculature. These individuals may require assistance when the segment moves up against gravity or moves downward with gravity. Once AROM can be performed without pain or substitution, the next progression is to introduce resistance.

When referring to flexibility, two types are recognized, static and dynamic.

▶ *Static flexibility*. Static flexibility is defined as the passive range of motion available to a joint or series of joints.[105,106] Increased static flexibility should not be confused with joint hypermobility, or laxity, which is a function of the joint capsule and ligaments. Decreased static flexibility indicates a loss of motion. The end-feel encountered may help the clinician differentiate the cause among adaptive shortening of the muscle (muscle stretch), a tight joint capsule (capsular), and an arthritic joint (hard). Static flexibility can be measured by a goniometer or by a number of tests, such as the toe touch and the sit and reach, all of which have been found to be valid and reliable.[107,108]

▶ *Dynamic flexibility*. Dynamic flexibility refers to the ease of movement within the obtainable range of motion. Dynamic flexibility is measured actively. The important measurement in dynamic flexibility is *stiffness*, a mechanical term defined as the resistance of a structure to deformation.[109,110] An increase in range of motion around a joint does not necessarily equate to a decrease in the passive stiffness of a muscle.[111–113] However, strength training, immobilization, and aging have been shown to increase stiffness.[114–117] The converse of stiffness is pliability. When a soft tissue demonstrates a decrease in pliability, it has usually undergone an adaptive shortening, or an increase in tone, termed *hypertonus*. There is a growing research to suggest that the limiting factors to preventing increases in range of motion are not only the connective tissues but are also the result of neurophysiologic phenomena controlled by the higher centers of the CNS.[118]

NORMAL DEVELOPMENT OF FUNCTIONAL MOVEMENT

In addition to the normal development of the neuromusculoskeletal structures as previously described, the normal development of functional movement depends on many fundamental factors, including an efficient production of energy and the ability to produce and overcome forces. The physical therapist needs an appreciation of these underlying factors as well as a working knowledge of the biomechanics of movement.

▶ Kinesiology is the study of movement.

▶ Kinetics is the term applied to the forces acting on an individual segment (e.g., hand) or combined segment (e.g., upper extremity) of the body.

▶ Kinematics is the branch of classical mechanics that describes the motion of points, objects, and groups of objects without consideration of the causes of the motion.

Although a deeper study of biomechanics will be provided to the reader as part of the physical therapy curriculum, this section provides a basic outline to form a foundation for an understanding of the fundamental principles. A working knowl-

TABLE 4-8	Potential Forces That Can Be Applied to the Body
Type of Force	**Definition**
Tension	A force that pulls on each end of a surface or attempts to stretch or lengthen a tissue.
Distraction	A pulling force that tries to separate two surfaces from each other.
Compression	A force that pushes two surfaces together. Axial compression is a compressive force that is directed along the long axis of a structure.
Pressure	The amount of force across a given area. A force over a small area increases pressure, whereas applying the same amount of force over a large area decreases pressure.
Shear	Two forces acting in opposite directions that are parallel to the contact surface.
Bending	A combination of tension and compression that bends a structure around a pivot point.
Torsion	A twisting force that occurs about a structure's long axis.

edge of the mechanics behind each movement enables the clinician to both diagnose and treat a movement dysfunction. This knowledge also helps the clinician in decision making during such activities as dependent patient transfers and mobility tasks.

Kinetics

Posture and movement are both governed by the control of forces. The same forces that move and stabilize the body also have the potential to deform and injure the body.[119] Broadly speaking, *force* can be defined as a *push* or *pull* that can produce, halt, or modify movement. A combination of push and pull forces produce rotations. Forces can be further differentiated as external or internal. A wide range of external and internal forces are either generated or resisted by the human body during the course of daily activities (Table 4-8). Examples of these external forces include ground reaction force, gravity, and applied force through contact. Examples of internal forces include muscle contraction, joint contact, and joint shear forces (Figure 4-8). Whether the body is able to respond to these stresses depends on the extent of the stress and the health of the tissues sustaining the stress. It is important to remember that too little stress, such as occurs with immobilization or decreased activity levels, can be as detrimental as too much stress. The former can result in muscle atrophy, bone loss, and weakening of ligaments and tendons, whereas the latter can lead to tissue damage.

CLINICAL PEARL

▶ *Force*: a force can act on an object in a linear (in a line), rotational (in a circle), or angular (at an angle) manner. Most movements involve a combination of linear and angular forces. Forces can be further differentiated as external (e.g., gravity) or internal (e.g., joint reaction forces). Forces are often depicted graphically as vectors using arrows. Forces

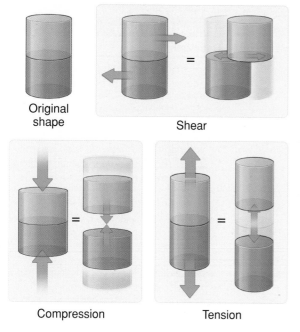

FIGURE 4-8 Internal forces acting on the body

act on a line of action, which represents the orientation and direction of the force. For example, the line of action of a muscle is parallel to the muscle fibers.

▶ *Mass:* the amount of matter of which an object, segment, or body is composed, which remains the same regardless of the situation in which the mass exists.

▶ *Center of mass:* for every individual segment (arm, hand, leg, and foot), combined segment of the body (upper extremity, lower extremity, and trunk), or the entire body, there is a balance point at which no movement occurs and which is called the center of mass (COM) of that object. The COM is often referred to as the center of gravity (COG). The COM of the human body in a standing position is located just anterior to the S2 vertebral segment within the pelvis, but as the positions of the body segments change, the COM may even be located outside the body. Factors affecting the COM include the size of the base of support (BOS), the relation of the line of gravity to the BOS, and the height of the COM.

▶ *Base of support:* The region bounded by an object or body parts in contact with a support surface or surfaces. A smaller BOS provides less stability than a larger BOS. Consider the stability of a unicycle versus a tricycle.

A number of forces can act on the body. These include compression, tension, shear, and torsion (see Figure 4-8).

▶ *Compression.* Compression can be viewed as a squeezing force that pushes two surfaces together. Pressure is defined as the amount of force acting over a given area.

▶ *Axial compression.* Axial compression occurs when a compressive force is directed along the long axis of a

structure. Axial compression occurs throughout the spine in weight bearing, whether in standing or sitting.

▶ *Tension.* Tensile force is the opposite of a compressive force and can be viewed as a pulling or stretching force.

▶ *Distraction.* A distraction force is one that attempts to separate two surfaces from each other.

▶ *Shear.* Shear forces tend to cause one portion of an object to slide or displace with respect to another portion of the object. Whereas compressive and tensile forces act along the longitudinal axis of a structure to which they are applied, shear forces act parallel or tangent to a surface. For example, when bending forward at the waist, shear forces are produced between the lumbar vertebral bodies and their respective intervertebral disks.

▶ *Torsion.* Torsional forces (torque) occur when a structure is made to twist about its longitudinal axis, typically when one end of the structure is fixed. For example, torsional forces occur in the lower extremity if a directional change is attempted while the sole of the foot is planted firmly on the ground.

CLINICAL PEARL

A bending force creates a combination of both tension and compression. The tension force is created on the opposite side of the direction of the bend, while the compression force is created on the same side of the direction of the bend.

One of these responses to resist internal and/or external forces is the maintenance of balance as the body's center of mass (COM) shifts as the segments of the body change position, or if weight is added to or removed from the body. For example, if a weight is added to a body segment, the COM moves toward the added weight, whereas if a weight is removed, the COM moves away from the removed weight.

Newton's laws of motion help to explain the relationship between forces and their impact on body segments, as well as on total body motion (Table 4-9).

CLINICAL PEARL

Two of the most common forces that the body must resist during functional activities are:

▶ *Gravity:* a natural phenomenon by which physical bodies attract with a force proportional to their mass. Under normal circumstances, the effects of gravity go unnoticed. However, in a weakened individual, gravity provides an additional challenge when moving against it.

▶ *Friction:* a force that acts between two contacting surfaces in an opposite direction to the desired movement. Generally speaking, functional movements can be made easier by decreasing friction. However, too little friction can result in slips and falls.

TABLE 4-9   Newton's Laws of Motion

	Definition	Description	Real-life Example	Clinical Example
First law (inertia)	An object continues to move in a state of constant velocity unless acted on by an external net force or resultant force. Directly connects inertia with the concept of relative velocities.	Describes the reluctance of an object that is in a state of equilibrium to change its movement pattern. The larger the mass or inertia of an object, the more difficult it is to alter its motion.	While traveling in a moving vehicle at a constant velocity, a person can throw a ball straight up in the air and catch it without worrying about applying a force in the direction the vehicle is moving.	It is easier to start and stop an empty wheelchair than it is to start or stop a wheelchair in which a patient is seated.
Second law (force = mass × acceleration)	Motion is inversely related to mass. An unbalanced force acting on an object will result in the object's momentum changing over time. The relationship between an object's mass m, its acceleration a, and the applied force F is $F = ma$.	Can be used to determine how velocities change when forces are applied—a measurement of the strength of forces. More force is required to change the speed of a heavy object than a lighter one.	Landing from a jump with the knees extended is much harder than bending the hips and knees when landing.	The patient who is having difficulty overcoming inertia in order to come from a sitting position to a standing position will often roll forward and backward to gain momentum.
Third law (action-reaction)	For every action there is an equal and opposite reaction.	All forces are *interactions* between different bodies.	During gait, when the foot strikes the ground, the ground applies a force in the opposite direction (ground reaction force) depending on the firmness of the surface.	Using the hands to push up from a stable surface during a sit-to-stand transfer.

Levers

Biomechanical levers can be defined as rotations of a rigid surface about a pivot point or axis. The majority of body movements involve the use of levers. For simplicity's sake, biomechanical levers are usually described using a straight bar, which is the lever, and the fulcrum, which is the point on which the bar is resting. Two sources of effort are required: a load and an effort. A load is typically an external force placed on an object or structure (see Table 4-8). The effort forces attempt to cause movement of the load. That part of the lever between the fulcrum and the load is the load arm. There are three types of levers (Figure 4-9):

► *First-class:* occurs when two forces are applied on either side of an axis and the fulcrum lies between the effort and

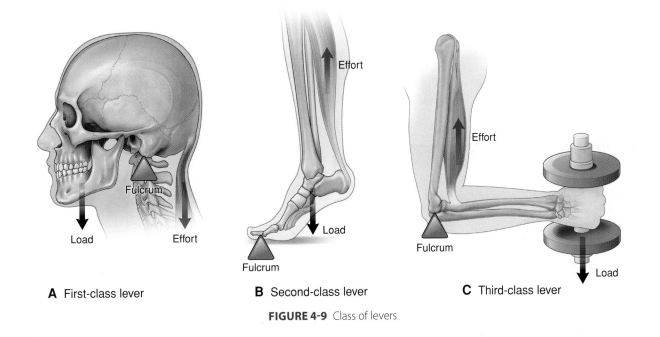

A First-class lever   **B** Second-class lever   **C** Third-class lever

FIGURE 4-9 Class of levers

the load (see Figure 4-9), like a seesaw. Examples in the human body include the contraction of the triceps at the elbow joint, or tipping of the head forward and backward.

▶ *Second-class:* occurs when the load (resistance) is applied between the fulcrum and the point where the effort is exerted (see Figure 4-9). This has the advantage of magnifying the effects of the effort so that it takes less force to move the resistance. Examples of second-class levers in everyday life include the nutcracker, and the wheelbarrow—with the wheel acting as the fulcrum. Examples of second-class levers in the human body include weight-bearing plantarflexion (rising up on the toes) (see Figure 4-9). Another would be an isolated contraction of the brachioradialis to flex the elbow, which could not occur without the other elbow flexors being paralyzed.

▶ *Third class:* occurs when the load is located at the end of the lever (see Figure 4-9) and the effort lies between the fulcrum and the load (resistance), like a drawbridge or a crane. The effort is exerted between the load and the fulcrum. The effort expended is greater than the load, but the load is moved a greater distance. Most movable joints in the human body function as third-class levers—an example is flexion at the elbow.

Moments

A moment (sometimes erroneously referred to as torque) is a mathematical value defined as the product of the force and the moment arm, with the moment arm defined as the distance from the linear force to the axis—the perpendicular distance from the point of rotation. In practice, the terms *torque* and *moment* are not interchangeable:

▶ *Torque:* the rate of change of angular momentum of an object such that one or both of the angular velocity or the moment of inertia of an object are changing. Inertia is the property of any physical object to resist a change in its state of motion or rest, or the inclination of an object to resist any change in its motion.

▶ *Moment:* the tendency of one or more applied forces to rotate an object about an axis, but not necessarily to change the angular momentum of the object.

Although muscles produce linear forces, motions at joints are all rotary. The rotary force is the product of the linear force and the moment arm (mechanical advantage) of the muscle about the joint's center of rotation.

CLINICAL PEARL

The principle of moments occurs if an object is balanced so that the sum of the clockwise moments about a pivot is equal to the sum of the anticlockwise moments about the same pivot.

To understand the concept of a moment arm, an understanding of the anatomy and movement (kinematics) of the joint of interest is necessary. For example, some joints can be considered to rotate about a fixed point. A good example of

such a joint is the elbow. At the elbow joint, where the humerus and ulna articulate, the resulting rotation occurs primarily about a fixed point, referred to as the center of rotation (COR). In the case of the elbow joint, this COR is relatively constant throughout the joint range of motion. However, in other joints (for example, the knee) the COR moves in space as the knee joint rotates because the articulating surfaces are not perfect circles. In the case of the knee, it is not appropriate to discuss a single COR—rather, we must speak of a COR corresponding to a particular joint angle, or, using the terminology of joint kinematics, we must speak of the instant center of rotation (ICR), that is, the COR at any "instant" in time or space. Thus, the moment arm is defined as the perpendicular distance from the line of force application to the axis of rotation.

Force Couples

A special case of moments is a force couple. A force couple consists of two parallel forces that are equal in magnitude, opposite in direction, and do not share a line of action. A force couple does not produce any translation, only rotation about a pivot point. For example, a force couple is involved when two hands work together to turn a steering wheel. A number of force couples exist throughout the body, particularly at the shoulder, where various muscles work together to help the scapula rotate during arm elevation. Force couples can also be used in a number of functional movements. For example, scooting forward in a chair rotates the pelvis around a pivot point.

Mechanical Advantage

When a machine puts out more force than is put in, the machine is said to have mechanical advantage (MA). Moments and moment arms can be internal or external. The MA of the musculoskeletal lever is defined as the ratio of the internal moment arm to the external moment arm. Depending on the location of the axis of rotation, the first-class lever can have an MA equal to, less than, or greater than 1.[119] Second-class levers always have an MA greater than 1. Third-class levers always have an MA less than 1. The majority of muscles throughout the musculoskeletal system function with an MA of much less than 1. Therefore, the muscles and underlying joints must "pay the price" by generating and dispersing relative large forces, respectively, even for seemingly low-load activities.[119]

Stress and Strain

During activities of daily living, the body is subject to a number of forces, including gravity. The terms *stress* and *strain*, which are commonly used to describe some of these forces, have specific mechanical meanings.

▶ *Stress.* Stress or load is given in units of force per area and is used to describe the type of force applied. Stress is independent of the amount of a material, but is directly related to the magnitude of force and inversely related to the unit area.[120]

▶ *Strain.* Strain is defined as the change in length of a material due to an imposed load divided by the original length.[120] The two basic types of strain are linear strain, which causes a change in the length of a structure, and shear strain, which causes a change in the angular relationships within a structure. It is the concentration of proteoglycans in solution that is responsible for influencing the mechanical properties of the tissue, including compressive stiffness, shear stiffness, osmotic pressure, and regulation of hydration.[121]

The inherent ability of a tissue to tolerate stress or strain can be observed experimentally in graphic form.

▶ Linear forces (line of action) are depicted as straight arrows in which the arrowhead points in the direction of the force being exerted. When a force is acting at an angle to a surface, the components of the force can be divided into those forces acting perpendicular to the surface and those forces acting in parallel to the surface.

▶ Gravity is represented as a vertical force pointing downward.

When any stress is plotted on a graph against the resulting strain for a given material, the shape of the resulting load-deformation curve depends on the kind of material involved. The load-deformation curve, or stress-strain curve, of a structure (Figure 4-10) depicts the relationship between the amount of force applied to a structure and the structure's response in terms of deformation or acceleration. The horizontal axis (deformation or strain) represents the ratio of the tissue's deformed length to its original length. The vertical axis of the graph (load or stress) denotes the internal resistance generated as a tissue resists its deformation, divided by its cross-sectional area. The load-deformation curve can be divided into four regions, each region representing a biomechanical property of the tissue (see Figure 4-10):

▶ *Toe region.* Collagen fibers have a wavy, or folded, appearance at rest. When a force that lengthens the collagen fibers is initially applied to connective tissue, these folds are affected first. As the fibers unfold, the slack is taken up (see Crimp later). The toe region is an artifact caused by this take-up of slack, alignment, and/or seating of the test specimen. The length of the toe region depends on the type of material and the waviness of the collagen pattern.

▶ *Elastic deformation region.* Within the elastic deformation region the structure imitates a spring—the geometric deformation in the structure increases linearly with increasing load, and after the load is released, the structure returns to its original shape. The slope of the elastic region of the load-deformation curve from one point in the curve to another is called the modulus of elasticity, or Young's modulus, and represents the extrinsic stiffness or rigidity of the structure—the stiffer the tissue, the steeper the slope. Young's modulus is a numerical description of the relationship between the amount of stress a tissue undergoes and the deformation that results. The ratio of stress to strain in an elastic material is a measure of its stiffness. Mathematically, the value for stiffness is found by dividing the load by the deformation at any point in the selected range. All normal tissues within the musculoskeletal system exhibit some degree of stiffness. Young's modulus is independent of specimen size and is therefore a measure of the intrinsic stiffness of the material. The greater the Young's modulus for a material, the better it can withstand greater forces. Larger structures will have greater rigidity than smaller structures of similar composition.

▶ *Plastic deformation region.* The end of the elastic range and the beginning of the plastic range represents the point

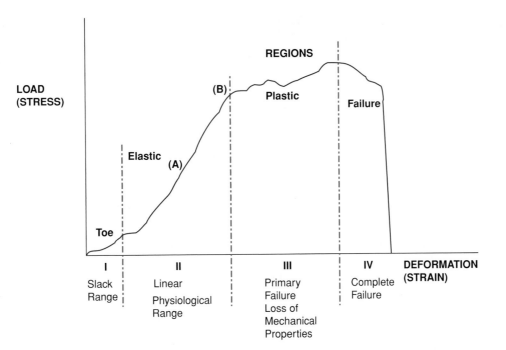

FIGURE 4-10 The stress–strain curve

where an increasing level of stress on the tissue results in progressive failure and microscopic tearing of the collagen fibers. Further increases in strain result in microscopic damage and in permanent deformation. The permanent change results from the breaking of bonds and their subsequent inability to contribute to the recovery of the tissue. Unlike the elastic region, removal of the load in this region will not result in a return of the tissue to its original length.

▶ *Failure region.* Deformations exceeding the ultimate failure point (see Figure 4-10) produce mechanical failure of the structure, which in the human body may be represented by the fracturing of bone or the rupturing of soft tissues.

CLINICAL PEARL

Stiffness = force/deformation. The gradient in the linear portion of the load-deformation graph immediately after the toe region of the load displacement curve represents the stiffness value. The load-deformation curve does not indicate the variable of time.

Elastic modulus = stress/strain. The larger the Young's modulus for a material, the greater stress needed for a given strain.

Biological tissues are anisotropic, which means they can demonstrate differing mechanical behavior as a function of test direction. The properties of extensibility and elasticity are common to many biologic tissues. Extensibility is the ability to be stretched, and elasticity is the ability to return to normal length after extension or contraction.[122]

A number of protective mechanisms exist in connective tissue to help respond to stress and strain, including crimp, viscoelasticity, creep and stress relaxation, plastic deformation, and stress response.

CLINICAL PEARL

Protective tissue mechanisms include:

▶ Crimp
▶ Viscoelasticity
▶ Creep and stress relaxation
▶ Plastic deformation
▶ Stress response

Crimp

The crimp of collagen is one of the major factors behind the viscoelastic properties of connective tissue. Crimp, a collagen tissue's first line of response to stress, is different for each type of connective tissue, providing each with different viscoelastic properties. Collagen fibers are wavy in appearance and are oriented obliquely when relaxed. However, when a load is applied, the fibers line up in the direction of the applied force as they uncrimp. Crimping is seen primarily in ligaments, tendons, and joint capsules and occurs in the toe phase of the stress-strain curve (see Figure 4-10).

CLINICAL PEARL

If a load is applied to connective tissue and then removed immediately, the material recoils to its original size. If, however, the load is allowed to remain, the material continues to stretch. After a period of sustained stretch, the stretching tends to reach a steady-state value. Realignment of the collagen fibers in the direction of the stress occurs, and water and proteoglycans are displaced from between the fibers.

Viscoelasticity

Viscoelasticity is the time-dependent mechanical property of a material to stretch or shorten over time and to return to its original shape when a force is removed. The mechanical qualities of a tissue can be separated into categories based on whether the tissue acts primarily like a solid, a fluid, or a mixture of the two. Solids are described according to their elasticity, strength, hardness, and stiffness. Bone, ligaments, tendons, and skeletal muscle are all examples of elastic solids. Biological tissues that demonstrate attributes of both solids and fluids are viscoelastic. The viscoelastic properties of a structure determine its response to loading. For example, a ligament demonstrates more viscous behavior at lower loads, whereas at higher loads, elastic behaviors dominate.[20]

Creep and Stress Relaxation

Creep and stress relaxation are two characteristics of viscoelastic materials that are used to document their behavior quantitatively.[122]

Creep is the gradual rearrangement or deformation of collagen fibers, proteoglycans, and water that occurs because of a constantly applied force after the initial lengthening caused by crimp has ceased. Creep is a time-dependent and transient biomechanical phenomenon. Short-duration stresses (less than 15 minutes) do not have sufficient time to produce this displacement; however, longer times can produce it. Once creep occurs, the tissue has difficulty returning to its initial length (see later discussion).

Stress relaxation is a phenomenon in which stress or force in a deformed structure decreases with time, while the deformation is held constant.[122] Unlike creep, stress relaxation responds with a high initial stress that decreases over time until equilibrium is reached and the stress equals zero; hence the label *relaxation*. As a result, no change in length is produced.

Thus, stress to connective tissues can result in no change, a semipermanent change, or a permanent change to the microstructure of the collagenous tissue. The semipermanent or permanent changes may result in either *microfailure* or *macrofailure*.

Plastic Deformation

Plastic deformation of connective tissue occurs when a tissue remains deformed and does not recover its pre-stress length. Once all of the possible realignment has occurred, any further loading breaks the restraining bonds, resulting in microfailure. On average, collagen fibers are able to sustain a 3% increase in elongation (strain) before microscopic damage occurs.[123] Following a brief stretch, providing the chemical bonds remain intact, the collagen and proteoglycans gradually recover their original alignment. The recovery process occurs at a slower rate and often to a lesser extent. The loss of energy that occurs between the lengthening force and the recovery activity is referred to as *hysteresis*. The more chemical bonds that are broken with applied stress, the greater the hysteresis. If the stretch is of sufficient force and duration and a sufficient number of chemical bonds are broken, the tissue is unable to return to its original length until the bonds are re-formed. Instead, it returns to a new length and to a new level of strain resistance. Increased tissue excursion is now needed before tension develops in the structure. In essence, this has the effect of decreasing the stabilizing capabilities of the connective tissue.

Stress Response

Exercises may be used to change the physical properties of both tendons and ligaments, as both have demonstrated adaptability to external loads with an increase in strength: weight ratios.[124–126] The improved strength results from an increase in the proteoglycan content and collagen cross-links.[124–126]

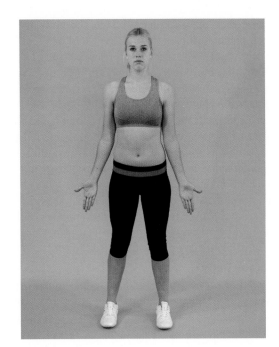

FIGURE 4-11 The anatomic reference position

CLINICAL PEARL

Three biomechanical attributes of connective tissue can have a clinical significance:

▶ Structural behavior

▶ Material behavior

▶ Viscoelastic behavior

Movements of the Body Segments

When describing movements, it is necessary to have a starting position as the reference position. This starting position is referred to as the *anatomic reference position*. The anatomic reference position for the human body is described as the erect standing position with the feet just slightly separated and the arms hanging by the side, the elbows straight, and the palms of the hand facing forward (Figure 4-11).

In general, there are two types of motions: translation, which occurs in either a straight or curved line, and rotation, which involves a circular motion around a pivot point. Movements of the body segments occur in three dimensions along imaginary *planes* and around various *axes* of the body.

Planes of the Body

There are three traditional planes of the body corresponding to the three dimensions of space: sagittal, frontal, and transverse[127] (Figure 4-12).

▶ *Sagittal.* The sagittal plane, also known as the *anterior-posterior or median plane,* divides the body vertically into left and right halves of equal size.

▶ *Frontal.* The frontal plane, also known as the *lateral* or *coronal plane,* divides the body equally into front and back halves.

▶ *Transverse.* The transverse plane, also known as the *horizontal plane,* divides the body equally into top and bottom halves.

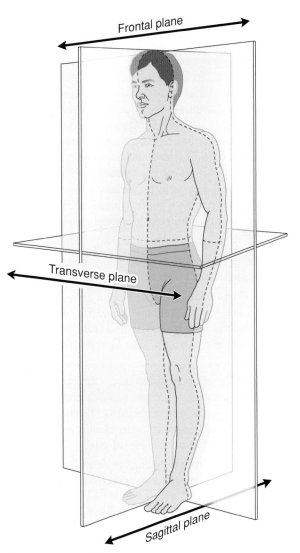

FIGURE 4-12 Planes of the body

Because each of these planes bisects the body, it follows that each plane must pass through the COM or COG.* If the movement described occurs in a plane that passes through the COM, that movement is deemed to have occurred in a *cardinal* plane. An *arc of motion* represents the total number of degrees traced between the two extreme positions of movement in a specific plane of motion.[103] If a joint has more than one plane of motion, each type of motion is referred to as a *unit of motion*. For example, the wrist has two units of motion: flexion-extension (anterior-posterior plane), and ulnar-radial deviation (lateral plane).[103]

Few movements involved with functional activities occur in the cardinal planes. Instead, most movements occur in an infinite number of vertical and horizontal planes parallel to the cardinal planes (see discussion that follows).

Axes of the Body

Three reference axes are used to describe human motion: frontal, sagittal, and longitudinal (Figure 4-13). The axis around which the movement takes place is always perpendicular to the plane in which it occurs.

- *Frontal.* The frontal axis, also known as the *M-L axis,* is perpendicular to the sagittal plane.
- *Sagittal.* The sagittal axis, also known as the *A-P axis*, is perpendicular to the frontal plane.
- *Longitudinal.* The longitudinal axis, also known as the *vertical axis,* is perpendicular to the transverse plane.

Most movements occur *in* planes and *around* axes that are somewhere in between the traditional planes and axes. However, nominal identification of every plane and axis of movement is impractical. The structure of the joint determines the possible axes of motion that are available. For example, a hinge joint has only one axis. Condyloid (ovoid) joints have two axes. Ball-and-socket joints have three axes. The axis of rotation remains stationary only if the convex member of a joint is a perfect sphere and articulates with a perfect reciprocally shaped concave member. The planes and axes for the more common planar movements (Figure 4-14) are as follows:

- Flexion, extension, hyperextension, dorsiflexion, and plantarflexion occur in the sagittal plane around a M-L axis.
- Abduction and adduction, side flexion of the trunk, elevation and depression of the shoulder girdle, radial and ulnar deviation of the wrist, and eversion and inversion of the foot occur in the frontal plane around a sagittal axis.
- Rotation of the head, neck, and trunk; internal rotation and external rotation of the arm or leg; horizontal adduction and abduction of the arm or thigh; and pronation and supination of the forearm occur in the transverse plane around the vertical axis.
- Arm circling and trunk circling are examples of *circumduction*. Circumduction involves an orderly

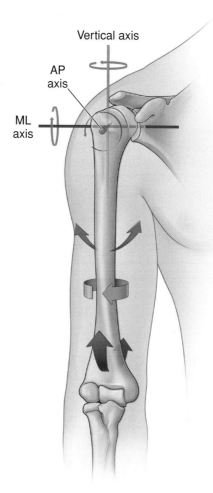

FIGURE 4-13 Axes of the body
A-P - Anterior-posterior
M-L - Medial-lateral

sequence of circular movements that occur in the sagittal, frontal, and intermediate oblique planes, so that the segment as a whole incorporates a combination of flexion, extension, abduction, and adduction. Circumduction movements can occur at biaxial and triaxial joints. Examples of these joints include the tibiofemoral, radiohumeral, hip, glenohumeral, and spinal joints.

Both the configuration of a joint and the line of pull of the muscle acting at a joint determine the motion that occurs at a joint:

- A muscle that has a line of pull that is lateral to the joint is a potential abductor.
- A muscle that has a line of pull that is medial to the joint is a potential adductor.
- A muscle that has a line of pull that is anterior to a joint has the potential to extend or flex the joint. At the knee, an anterior line of pull may cause the knee to extend, whereas at the elbow joint, an anterior line of pull may cause flexion of the elbow.
- A muscle that has a line of pull that is posterior to the joint has the potential to extend or flex a joint (refer to preceding example).

---

*The center of mass may be defined as the point at which the three planes of the body intersect each other. The line of gravity is defined as the vertical line at which the two vertical planes intersect each other.

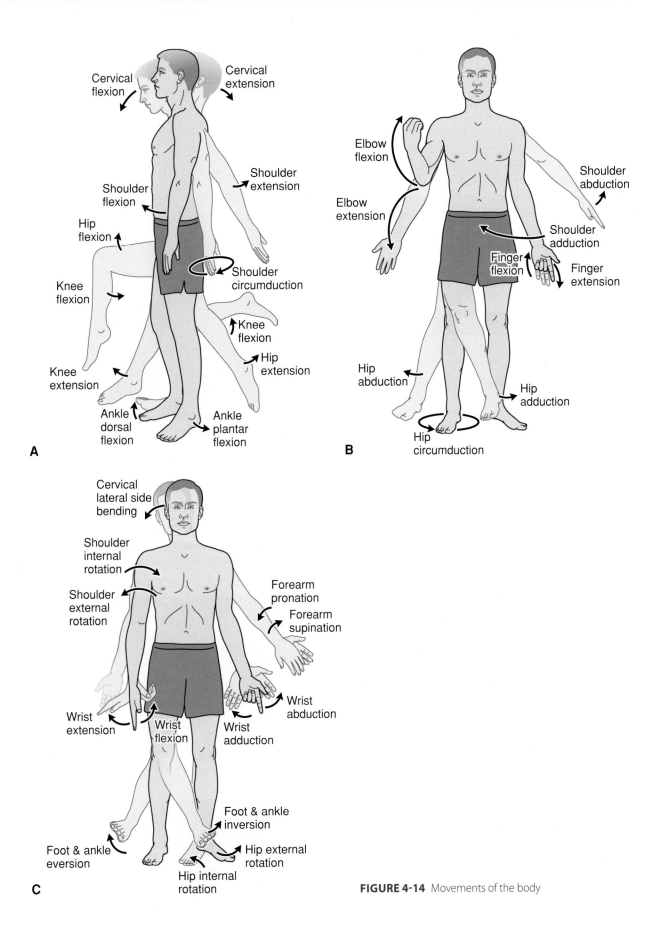

A

B

C

FIGURE 4-14 Movements of the body

Degrees of Freedom

The number of independent modes of motion at a joint is called the *degrees of freedom (DOF)*. A joint can have up to 3 degrees of angular freedom, corresponding to the three dimensions of space.[119] If a joint can swing in one direction or can only spin, it is said to have 1 DOF.[128–131] The proximal interphalangeal joint is an example of a joint with 1 DOF. If a joint can spin and swing in one way only *or* it can swing in two completely distinct ways, but not spin, it is said to have 2 DOF.[128–131] The tibiofemoral joint, temporomandibular joint, proximal and distal radioulnar joints, subtalar joint, and talocalcaneal joint are examples of joints with 2 DOF. If the bone can spin and also swing in two distinct directions, then it is said to have 3 DOF.[128–131] Ball-and-socket joints such as the shoulder and hip have 3 DOF.

> ### CLINICAL PEARL
>
> Joint motion that occurs only in one plane is designated as one degree of freedom; in two planes, two degrees of freedom; and in three planes, three degrees of freedom.

Because of the arrangement of the articulating surfaces—the surrounding ligaments and joint capsules—most motions around a joint do not occur in straight planes or along straight lines. Instead, the bones at any joint move through space in curved paths. This can best be illustrated using *Codman's paradox.*

1. Stand with your arms by your side, palms facing inward, thumb extended. Notice that the thumb is pointing forward (Figure 4-15).

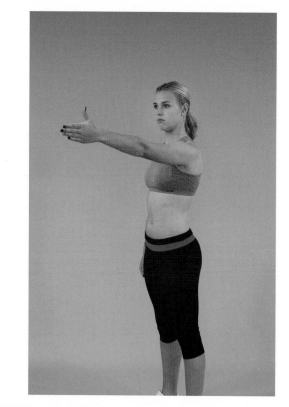

FIGURE 4-16 Codman's paradox: 90° of glenohumeral flexion

2. Flex one arm to 90 degrees at the shoulder so that the thumb is pointing up (Figure 4-16).

3. From this position, horizontally extend your arm so that the thumb remains pointing up but your arm is in a position of 90 degrees of glenohumeral abduction (Figure 4-17).

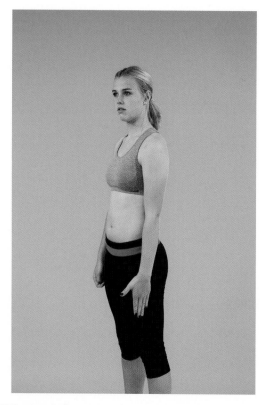

FIGURE 4-15 Codman's paradox: start position

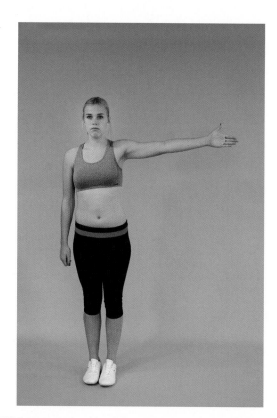

FIGURE 4-17 Codman's paradox: 90° of glenohumeral abduction

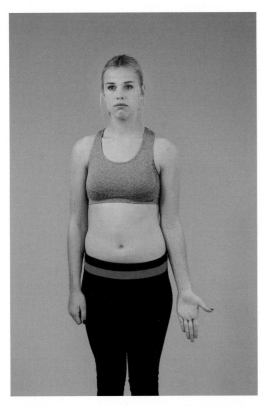

FIGURE 4-18 Codman's paradox: end position Codman's paradox: end position

4. From this position, without rotating your arm, return the arm to your side and note that your thumb is now pointing away from your thigh (Figure 4-18).

Referring to the start position, and using the thumb as the reference, it can be seen that the arm has undergone an external rotation of 90 degrees. But where and when did the rotation take place? Undoubtedly, it occurred during the three separate, straight-plane motions or *swings* that etched a triangle in space. What you have just witnessed is an example of a conjunct rotation—a rotation that occurs as a result of joint surface shapes—and the effect of inert tissues rather than contractile tissues. Conjunct rotations can only occur in joints that can rotate internally or externally. Although not always apparent, most joints can so rotate. Consider the motions of elbow flexion and extension. While fully flexing and extending your elbow a number of times, watch the pisiform bone and forearm. If you watch carefully you should notice that the pisiform and the forearm move in a direction of supination during flexion and pronation during extension of the elbow. The pronation and supination motions are examples of conjunct rotations.

Most habitual movements, or those movements that occur most frequently at a joint, involve a conjunct rotation. However, the conjunct rotations are not always under volitional control. In fact, the conjunct rotation is only under volitional control in joints with 3 DOF (glenohumeral and hip joints). In joints with fewer than 3 DOF (hinge joints, such as the tibiofemoral and ulnohumeral joints), the conjunct rotation occurs as part of the movement but is not under voluntary control. The implications become important when attempting to restore motion at these joints: the mobilizing techniques must take into consideration both the relative shapes of the articulating surfaces and the conjunct rotation that is associated with a particular motion.

Kinematics

In studying kinematics, two major types of motion are involved: (1) osteokinematic and (2) arthrokinematic.

Osteokinematic Motion

Osteokinematic motion occurs when any object forms the radius of an imaginary circle about a fixed point. The axis of rotation for osteokinematic motions is oriented perpendicular to the plane in which the rotation occurs.[127] The distance traveled by the motion may be a small arc or a complete circle and is measured as an angle, in degrees. All human body segment motions involve osteokinematic motions. Examples of osteokinematic motion include abduction or adduction of the arm, flexion of the hip or knee, and side bending of the trunk.

Arthrokinematic Motion

The motions occurring at the joint surfaces are termed *arthrokinematic* movements (Figure 4-19). At each synovial articulation, the articulating surface of each bone moves relative to the shape of the other articulating surface. A normal joint has an available range of active, or physiologic, motion, which is limited by a physiologic barrier as tension develops within the surrounding tissues, such as the joint capsule, ligaments, and CT. At the physiologic barrier, there is an additional amount of passive, or accessory, range of motion. The small motion, which is available at the joint surfaces, is referred to as *accessory* motion, or *joint-play* motion. This motion can only occur when resistance to active motion is applied, or when the patient's muscles are completely relaxed.[132]

Beyond the available passive range of motion, the anatomic barrier is found (Figure 4-20). This barrier cannot be exceeded without disruption to the integrity of the joint.

Both the physiologic (osteokinematic) and accessory (arthrokinematic) motions occur simultaneously during movement and are directly proportional to each other, with a small increment of accessory motion resulting in a larger increment of osteokinematic motion. Normal arthrokinematic motions must occur for full-range physiologic motion to take place. Mennell[133,134] introduced the concept that full, painless, active range of motion is not possible without these motions and that a restriction of arthrokinematic motion results in a decrease in osteokinematic motion.

Kinematic Chains

When a body moves, it will do so in accordance with its kinematics, which in the human body takes place through arthrokinematic and osteokinematic movements. The expression *kinematic chain* is used in rehabilitation to describe the function or activity of an extremity or trunk in terms of a series of linked chains. A kinematic chain refers to a series of articulated segmented links, such as the connected pelvis, thigh, leg, and foot of the lower extremity.[119]

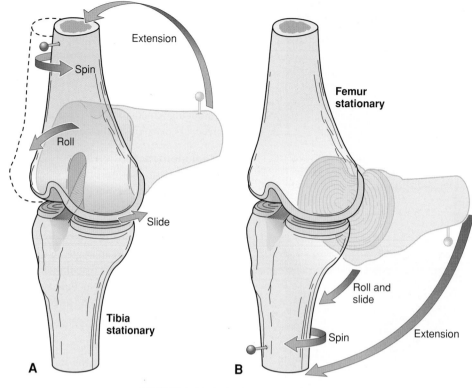

FIGURE 4-19 Arthrokinematics of motion

CLINICAL PEARL

When muscle force is diminished throughout a kinetic chain, momentum is sometimes used to compensate. For example, a patient with trunk and lower extremity weakness will lower the legs off the edge of the bed while moving from supine to sitting to use the weight of the lower extremities as momentum.

According to kinematic chain theory, each of the joint segments of the body involved in a particular movement constitutes a link along the kinematic chain. Because each motion of a joint is often a function of other joint motions, the efficiency of an activity can be dependent on how well these chain links work together.[135]

CLINICAL PEARL

The number of links within a particular kinematic chain varies, depending on the activity. In general, the longer kinematic chains are involved with the more strenuous activities.

Two types of kinematic chain systems are recognized: *closed kinematic chain* (CKC) systems and the *open kinematic chain* (OKC) system (Table 4-10).[136]

Examples of closed kinematic chain exercises (CKCEs) involving the lower extremities include the squat and the leg press. The activities of walking, running, jumping, climbing, and rising from the floor all incorporate closed kinematic chain components. An example of a CKCE for the upper extremities is the push-up (Figure 4-21), or when using the arms to rise out of a chair.

CLINICAL PEARL

In most activities of daily living, the activation sequence of the links involves a closed chain whereby the activity is initiated from a firm base of support and transferred to a more mobile distal segment.

Open kinematic chain exercises (OKCEs) involving the lower extremity include the seated knee extension and prone knee flexion. Example OKCEs of the upper extremity include hitting

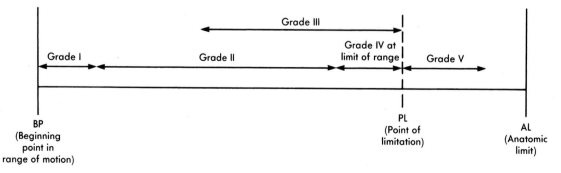

FIGURE 4-20 Various ranges of motion

TABLE 4-10	Differential Features of OKC and CKC Exercises		
Exercise Mode	**Characteristics**	**Advantages**	**Disadvantages**
Open kinematic chain	1. Single muscle group 2. Single axis and plane 3. Emphasizes concentric contraction 4. Non–weight-bearing	1. Isolated recruitment 2. Simple movement pattern 3. Isolated recruitment 4. Minimal joint compression	1. Limited function 2. Limited complexity 3. Limited eccentrics 4. Less proprioception and joint stability with increased joint shear forces
Closed kinematic chain	1. Multiple muscle groups 2. Multiple axes and planes 3. Balance of concentric and eccentric contractions 4. Weight-bearing exercise	1. Functional recruitment 2. Functional movement patterns 3. Functional contractions 4. Increase proprioception and joint stability	1. Difficult to isolate 2. More complex 3. Loss of control of target joint 4. Compressive forces on articular surfaces

Data from Greenfield BH, Tovin BJ: The application of open and closed kinematic chain exercises in rehabilitation of the lower extremity. J Back Musculoskel Rehabil 2:38-51, 1992.

a ball (Figure 4-22), the biceps curl, and the military press, using very light weights.

Once significant resistance is applied to the end of an extremity, there is some debate as to whether the activity or exercise changes from an OKCE to a CKCE. For example, many activities that include a load on the end segment, such as swimming and cycling, have been traditionally viewed as OKC activities even though the end segment is not "fixed" and restricted from movement. This ambiguity of definitions for CKC and OKC activities has allowed some activities to be classified in opposing categories.[137] Thus, there has been a growing need for clarification of OKC and CKC terminology, especially when related to functional activities.

Motor Progression

Motor progression refers to the complex processes of change in motor behavior that start in utero and continue over the life span. These changes in human motor behavior are influenced by psychomotor, physiologic, biochemical, biomechanical, psychosocial, and even gender considerations.[138,139] The study of motor progression helps with the early detection of problems in individuals who do not develop normally by using references that are developmentally appropriate. Two such references are:

▶ *Age-appropriate.* This refers to individuals who pass through the predictable sequences of growth and development through which most children pass. An understanding of these sequences provides a basis from which to provide the best rehabilitation approach.

▶ *Individual-appropriate.* This refers to individuals who do not pass through the sequences in the same manner or within the same period, but is based more on the stage of a specific individual's development.

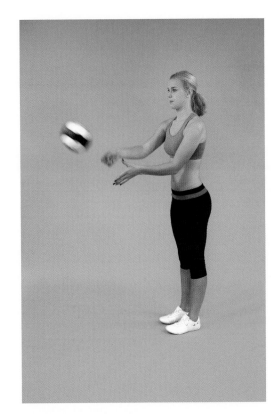

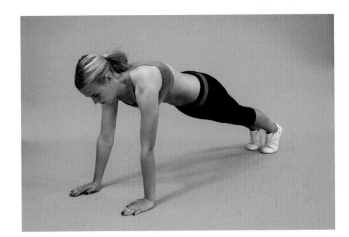

FIGURE 4-21 Upper extremity closed kinetic chain exercise

FIGURE 4-22 Upper extremity open kinetic chain activity

CLINICAL PEARL

Developmental change can occur in a number of different ways:

► Qualitative, in which the components of a skill change as does the product outcome (learning to jump farther)

► Cumulative, in which motor behavior is aggregated (progressing from assisted to unassisted standing)

► Sequential, in which there are identifiable sequences of progression (prone crawling to crawling on all fours)

► Directional, in which skill can either progress or regress because of such things as aging or disease.

► Structural, in which development occurs because of growth (height and weight)

► Functional, in which development occurs because of maturation (brain changes result in cognitive development)

There are many theories as to how motor progression occurs. These include:

► *Cephalocaudal:* progression occurs from the top of the body (head) to the tail (feet).

► *Proximodistal:* progression occurs from points close to the center of the body to points close to the periphery.

► *Differentiation:* progression occurs from gross, immature movement to precise, well-controlled, intended movement.

► *Integration:* progression occurs from the integration of the various systems, particularly the neuromuscular system, to produce a well-controlled, intended movement.

There are two main schools of thought with regard to how best enhance motor progression:

► *Product approach.* This is a task-oriented approach that measures the development of a skill based on the end results or outcome.

TABLE 4-11	Major Milestones
Milestone	Approximate Age (in months) Able to Perform
Roll	3–4
Sit independently	5–6
Belly crawl	7–8
Creep (quadruped)	8–9
Pull to stand	9–10
Cruise	11
Walk	12

Data from van Blankenstein M, Welbergen UR, de Haas JH: Le Developpement du Nourrisson: Sa Premiere Annee en 130 Photographies. Paris, Presses Universitaires de France, 1962.

► *Process approach.* This is a process-oriented approach that emphasizes the movement itself with little attention to the outcome.

The Development of Early Movement

A milestone is a significant point in development or a significant functional ability achieved during the developmental process. The various developmental milestones for both sensory and motor development are depicted in Tables 4-11, 4-12, and 4-13. An analysis of the progressions involved in the developmental milestones reveals the following progressive sequence:

► Prone
► Prone on elbows
► Rolling, sidelying
► Supine
► Sitting
► Quadruped
► Kneeling
► Half kneeling
► Standing

TABLE 4-12	Gross Motor Checklist	
Month/Year	Position/Activity	Milestone
One month	Prone	Lifts head and turns to side
Two months	Vertical Prone Supported sitting	Rights head Recurrently lifts head to 45° Head erect and bobbing
Three months	Prone	Lifts head to 45° (sustained) Recurrently lifts head to 90° Supports self on forearms Rolls to side
Four months	Prone Supine Supported sitting	List head to 90° (sustained) Rolls to supine Rolls to prone Assists with head when pulled to sit Head steady, set forward

TABLE 4-12	Gross Motor Checklist (continued)	
Month/Year	**Position/Activity**	**Milestone**
Five months	Prone	Supports self on extended arms
		Rolls to supine segmentally
	Supine	Lifts head when pulled to sitting.
		Rolls to prone segmentally
	Supported sitting	Head erect and steady
	Standing	Takes weight on lower extremities
Six months	Prone	Can lift one arm and weight bear on the other
		Pivots in a circle
	Sitting	Erect for one minute with hands propped forward
		Protective extension sideways
Seven months	Prone	Up on all fours
		Progress is forward in any manner
	Sitting	Erect without support but unsteady
		Protective extension forward
Eight months	Prone	Crawls in any manner
	Sitting	Erect without support
	Standing	Pulls to stand
Nine months	Prone/supine	Rotates to sitting
	Sitting	Goes to prone
		Protective extension backwards
	Standing	Pulls to standing with rotation and support
10 months	Sitting	Pivots
	Locomotion	Cruises
12 months	Locomotion	Stands up without support
		Walks with high guard
15 months	Kneeling	Kneels without support
	Locomotion	Walks with medium guard
		Can stop, start, and change directions without falling
18 months	Locomotion	Walks with no guard carrying object
		Walks fast with feet flat
		Squats to play
		Goes up/down stairs on all fours
Two years	Locomotion	Walks up/down stairs one at the time holding rail
		Walks with heel-total gait
		Runs forward well
Three years	Locomotion/Skills	Jumps forward on both feet
		Alternates feet going upstairs
		Walks backward easily
		Hops up to six times
Four years	Locomotion/Skills	Walks downstairs with alternating feet, holding rail
		Skips on one foot
		Throws overhand
		Moves backward and forward with equal agility
Five years	Locomotion/Skill	Pedals and steers tricycle well
		Able to walk long distances on toes
		Gallops
		Hops up to nine times on one foot
		Smooth reciprocal movements in walking and running
Six years	Skill	Throws a small ball at a target and hits the target
		Broad jumps up to three feet

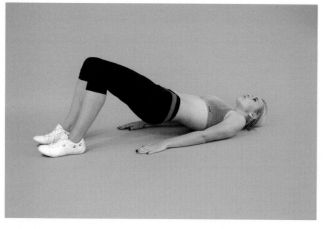

FIGURE 4-23 Bridging

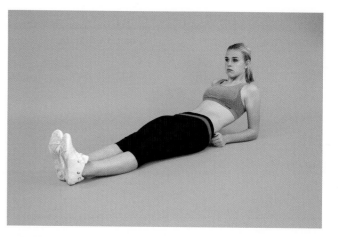

FIGURE 4-24 Supine on elbows

CLINICAL PEARL

The basic components of movement that allow an individual to produce head control, trunk control, and trunk rotation are typically developed by six months of age. The degree to which these basic components are involved in a particular activity is related to the patient position:

▸ Supine—bilateral symmetrical flexion against gravity with concurrent elongation of the antagonist extensors

▸ Prone—bilateral symmetrical extension against gravity with concurrent elongation of the antagonist flexors

▸ Sidelying—unilateral symmetrical contraction of trunk flexors and extensors on one side with the concurrent elongation of the antagonist trunk flexors and extensors.

Although this progressive sequence appears to be somewhat arbitrary, it is the same sequence that is used to progress a patient who has undergone a compromise to the neuromotor system with such tasks as bed mobility training and balance retraining. Other components worth mentioning because of their importance in neuromuscular rehabilitation but which may not appear in the foregoing developmental sequence of milestones are bridging, supine on elbows, and hooklying.

▸ *Bridging.* This involves the lifting of the hips and lower back while in the supine position (Figure 4-23). To avoid putting too much stress on the cervical spine while achieving trunk extension, the patient can use the upper arms to push down into the bed. In addition, assistance can be provided by stabilizing the patient's feet or by having the patient wear shoes to increase the grip. From a functional perspective, acquisition of this skill allows items such as bedpans to be placed underneath the patient, provides pressure relief, and serves as a precursor to scooting in supine.

▸ *Supine on elbows* (Figure 4-24). This position involves the raising of the trunk and head off the bed and both elbows placed on the bed to support the position. From a functional perspective, this position is a precursor

for scooting in supine in a variety of directions, which is particularly important for bed mobility training (see Chapter 10).

▸ *Hooklying* (Figure 4-25). This position involves flexion of both hips and knees in the supine position. From a functional perspective, it is the precursor for bridging, scooting, and rolling (see Chapter 10).

NORMAL DEVELOPMENT OF MOTOR CONTROL AND MOTOR LEARNING

The term *motor control* refers to processes of the brain and spinal cord that govern the mechanisms essential to regulate or direct posture and movement using perception and cognition.[138] The hallmarks of cognition are observable: selection, sequence generation, and working memory.

Motor learning is a complex set of internal processes that involve the relatively permanent acquisition and retention of a skill or task through practice or the reacquisition of skills that are difficult to perform or cannot be performed because of injury or disease.[140–142]

The traditional study of motor control and development was characterized by detailed observations of progressive

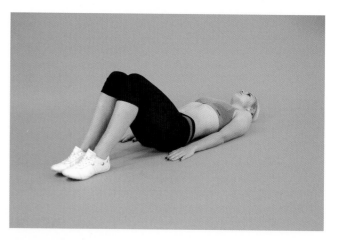

FIGURE 4-25 Hooklying

TABLE 4-13   Development Milestones According to Position

Age	Prone	Supine	Sitting	Standing	Comments
Neonate: 0 to 14 days	Physiologic flexor activity in the ankles, knees, hips, and elbows.		Lack of trunk muscular control—the back is round and the head flops forward.	Demonstrates the remarkable capabilities of primary standing—automatic walking when supported.	Grasp is a reflex in which the hand automatically closes on objects the baby touches because of tactile stimulation of the palm of the hand. The hands will randomly swing out wide (neonatal reaching). No organized response to postural perturbations.
Newborn (0–1 month)	Arms and hands tucked in close to the body, rounded shoulders, elbows flexed. Hands are closed loosely and positioned close to mouth.	No control of neck flexion in supine is present, so the baby cannot maintain the head in midline, but keeps it rotated to one side.	Sacral sitting if supported.		Period dominated by physiological flexion. Poor head control. Very active when awake. Random wide-ranging movements primarily in supine. Soft tissue tightness holds the hips in flexion/abduction/external rotation. The baby touches and feels, and is soon sucking and learning about the hands. Vision limited to 8–9 feet. Skeletal characteristics include coxa valgus, genu varum, tibial varum and torsion, calcaneal varus, and occasionally, metatarsus adductus.
1 month	Head lifting in prone may appear to be improved. Increased cervical rotation mobility. Elbows moving forward, arms away from body.	Head to one side resulting in lateral vision becoming dominant, and eye-hand regard and uncontrolled swiping at toys at the baby's side is frequently observed. Wider ranges of movement. Heels hit surface.		Positive support and primary walking reflexes in supported standing.	Decreasing physiologic flexion (less "recoil"). Increasing level of arousal. Neonatal reaching. Able to visually track a moving object horizontally.
2 months	Able to hold the head steady in all positions and to raise it about 45° because of increased activity of active shoulder abduction. The arms and hands begin to work to support the actions of the head and trunk. Hand movements more goal directed.	Increased asymmetry with more visual interaction.	Head lag occurs with pull to sit. Begins to develop head and trunk control and more attempts at sustained extension. Head bobs in supported sitting.	May not accept weight on lower extremities (astasia-abasia). No more neonatal stepping.	Increasing asymmetry/decreased tone. Increased head and trunk control lets the baby use the arms for reaching and playing rather than for support. Holds objects placed in the hand.

(continued)

TABLE 4-13   Development Milestones According to Position (continued)

Age	Prone	Supine	Sitting	Standing	Comments
3 months	Change occurs in the general position of the arms, from a position where the arms are tucked in close to the body with the elbows near the ribs, to one in which the elbows are almost in line with the shoulders, which allows for forearm weight-bearing. Legs abducted and externally rotated. Face can be raised 45–90° when prone.	Beginning of symmetry is evident—the head is in midline with chin tucking and the hands are in midline on the chest/to mouth.	Attempts pull to sit but falls forward.	Minimal weight through extended legs.	Period of controlled symmetry. The grasp becomes more controlled and voluntary, and the hands can adjust to the shape of objects. Symmetry is very obvious in the lower extremities as they assume their "frog legged" position of hip abduction, external rotation and flexion, and knee flexion. The feet come together and the baby is able to take some weight with toes curled in supported standing.
4 months	Able to prop up on the forearms and look around. The head and chest are lifted and maintained in midline. Prone pivots.	Can roll from prone to side and from supine to side, although these are usually accidental occurrences. Able to bring the hands together in the space above the body due to increased shoulder girdle control. Hands to knees. Active anterior and posterior pelvic tilt.	Assists in pull to sit by flexing elbows. Very minimal head bobbing—stabilized through shoulder elevation. Tends to sit in a slumped position. Protective reactions develop, first laterally, then forward, and then backward.	Because of the increased head-neck-trunk control, the baby is able to take more of his/her weight when placed in standing and can now be held by the hands instead of at the chest. Legs are extended and the toes are clawed.	Ulnar palmar grasp develops. Able to perform bilateral reaching with the forearm pronated when the trunk is supported. Side lying. Starts hand-to-mouth activities. Emerging righting and equilibrium reactions. Findings of concern include poor midline orientation (persistent ATNR), imbalance between flexors and extensors, poor visual attention/tracking, persistent wide base of support in standing, and poor antigravity strength.
5 months	Equilibrium reactions begin in prone position. Can roll from prone to supine. Able to assume and maintain a position of extended arm weight bearing in prone and can weight shift from one forearm to the other end to reach out to with one arm.	Chin tuck, downward gaze. Feet to mouth. Anterior and posterior pelvic tilt more active. Active role to sideline. Manipulation and transfer of toys.	There is no head lag when the baby is pulled from supine to sit. Assists during pull to sit with chin tuck and head lift. Able to control head in supported sitting, although still leans forward from the hips.	Tends to be able to bear almost all weight.	Finding of concern include: ▲ Poor antigravity flexion. ▲ Poor tolerance for prone/inability to bear weight to extended arms/poor weight shifting.
6 months	Completes turning and can roll from prone to supine. Can lie prone on hands with the elbows extended and is able to weight shift on extended arms from hand to hand and to reach forward because of sufficient shoulder girdle control.	Active hip extension. Transfers toys. Flexes head independently.	Can sit independently, although initially uses the arms and hands for support.	In standing, is able to bear weight on both legs and bounce and can independently hold onto the support of a person because of sufficient trunk and hip control.	Uses rolling for locomotion. Findings of concern include: ▲ Poor tolerance for prone position. ▲ Paucity of movement patterns. ▲ Inability to sit independently. ▲ Inability to roll or rolling with neck hyperextension.

Age	Prone	Supine	Sitting	Standing	Hand function / Findings of concern
7 months	Trunk and arms free Able to achieve and maintain the quadruped position, although the prone is usually the preferred position. Can pivot on belly, often moving body in a circle.	Tends to avoid except for playing.	Protective reactions more consistent. Able to perform trunk rotation in sitting. Can assume the sitting position from the quadruped position.	Can often pull to stand from the quadruped position. Able to actively flex and extend both legs simultaneously while standing and supporting standing independently.	Very active with large variety of movements and positions available. May show fear of strangers. Findings of concern include: ▲ Lack of weight shifting in prone. ▲ Reliance on more primitive movement patterns as compensations in order to explore. ▲ Inability to assume or maintain quadruped. ▲ Poor weight-bearing in supported stance.
8 months	Minimal time spent in prone.		Full equilibrium reactions in sitting, and the beginning of equilibrium reactions in quadruped. Able to side-sit and is also able to go from sitting to quadruped. May also kneel.	Can stand by leaning on supporting surfaces. Able to pull to stand. Early walking, cruising.	Can reach out for objects and reach across the midline of the body without losing balance. The thumb can wrap around objects—now the baby can hold two small objects, such as cubes, in one hand. Findings of concern include: ▲ Poor sitting ability. ▲ Unable to use hand for play. ▲ Overall reliance on upper extremities.
9 months	Able to creep/crawl in the quadruped position as the primary means of locomotion.		Large variety of sitting positions and movement. Pivoting/long sitting. Sitting often used as a transitional position.	Uses arms, hands, and body together while pulling up to standing through half-kneel position (nine months). Immature stepping. The sequence in rising to standing is kneeling, half kneeling, weight shift forward, squat, then upright.	The index finger starts to move separately from the rest of the hand when poking at objects. This leads to the pincer grasp, with the tips of the thumb and index finer meeting in a precise pattern. The baby's ability to let go of an object smoothly has also improved. Findings of concern include: ▲ Poor standing control. ▲ Poor/inadequate sitting. ▲ Inability to assume quadruped.
10 months			Arms reach above shoulders. Active site sitting. Rarely stationary.	Creeping/climbing. Legs very active. "High guard" Cruising with wide base of support.	
11 months			Able to play and move hands across midline.	Mostly using legs. Very symmetrical standing with a wide base of support.	
12 to 15 months				Many babies are walking unassisted.	Able to self feed.
Two years				Runs well. Goes upstairs using reciprocal pattern (reciprocal stair climbing).	Can build a tower of two cubes.

Data from van Blankenstein M, Welbergen UR, de Haas JH: Le Developpement du Nourrisson: Sa Premiere Annee en 130 Photographies. Paris, Presses Universitaires de France, 1962. ATNR - Asymmetrical tonic neck reflex

changes of different kinds of motor sequences, including actions such as grasping, rolling, crawling, and walking (see Motor Progression). Until fairly recently, many of the theoretical concepts used in physical therapy evaluation and therapeutic intervention were based on the theoretical constructs developed in the 1930s and 1940s. Specifically much credence was given to the neuromaturational theory of development, in which structure preceded function such that changes in motor development were thought to be the results of maturation of the CNS. With development of the CNS, higher centers inhibited lower centers, thereby eliciting voluntary movements through a process of hierarchical control. Since the late 1980s, the CNS has been hypothesized to be multilevel and multisystem rather than hierarchical.

Motor Control

The field of motor control is directed at understanding the control of those movements already acquired and how the neuromuscular system functions to activate and coordinate the muscles and limbs involved in the performance of a motor skill.[143] It is thought that infants attain gross and fine motor control along a predetermined and sequential path. Factors that affect motor control include the task, the environment, and the neuromotor capabilities of the individual. Over the years, many theories concerning motor control have evolved in an attempt to describe how movement is controlled. A description of the various theories of motor control follows.

Reflex Theory. In this theory, a stimulus triggers a combined action of individual reflex circuits that create a complex response, such that the performer is a passive recipient responding to the stimuli present in the environment and with which he or she is confronted. The problem with this theory is that not all movement is spontaneous, or activated by an environmental agent. In addition, there is no room for goal-oriented or goal-directed behavior within such a theory.

Hierarchical Theory. The hierarchical theory of motor control describes how motor programs begin with a definition of a fixed set of commands that can be structured before movement initiation. These motor patterns emerge in orderly predetermined genetic sequences and are based on a number of parameters that specify how a particular movement pattern is to be expressed in terms of the overall duration of a movement, the overall force needed to accomplish the movement, the temporal phasing of the movement pattern, and the spatial and temporal order in which the components of the movement are to be executed. Hierarchical theorists consider that basic motor skills, such as standing and walking, are not learned by experience but are the result of cerebral maturation. More recently, this theory has been modified to recognize the fact that each level of the nervous system can act on other levels (higher and lower) depending on the task and that reflexes are not considered the sole determinant of motor control, but as one of the many processes important to the generation and control of movement.[144]

CLINICAL PEARL

A number of physical therapy approaches initially developed according to the hierarchical model:

▶ Pediatric physical therapy with its emphasis on the assessment of reflex development and motor milestones as reflections of increasingly higher levels of neural maturation.[145] The intervention for children with CNS dysfunction, particularly cerebral palsy, was based around methods to inhibit the primitive reflexes and emphasize the facilitation of the righting and equilibrium reactions.[146]

▶ *Stroke rehabilitation.* Signe Brunnstrom used a reflex hierarchical theory to describe disordered movement following a motor cortex lesion.

Motor Programming Theory. Although reflex theories are useful in explaining certain stereotyped patterns of movement, they cannot be used to explain all types of movement. It is currently believed that there are certain motor program generators for movement patterns that are inherent in the CNS, and that these naturally develop during the maturation process of the CNS. For example, gait on a level surface is controlled by a set of neural circuits known as a central pattern generator (CPG). CPGs are neural networks that can endogenously (i.e., without rhythmic sensory or central input) produce rhythmic patterned outputs; these networks underlie the production of most rhythmic motor patterns, such as the gait cycle.[57,147–149]

Once this pattern is formed, the individual no longer has to concentrate on performing the activity, but can do so with very little cortical involvement. The motor program for each of these activities is saved in an *engram* (a hypothetical means by which a patterned response has been stabilized at the level of unconscious competence) within the cerebral cortex.[150–152] Thousands of repetitions (practice) are required to begin the engram formation, and millions are needed to perfect it.[152] Skilled performance is developed in proportion to the number of repetitions of an engram practiced just below the maximal level of ability to perform.[153,154]

CLINICAL PEARL

▶ A motor plan is defined as an idea or plan for purposeful movement that is made up of component motor programs.[147]

▶ A motor program is defined as an abstract representation that, when initiated, results in the production of a coordinated movement sequence.[57] Motor programs are codes within the nervous system that when initiated, produce coordinated movement sequences.[57] These programs are usually under central control. Sensory input is used extensively in selecting the appropriate motor program, in monitoring whether or not movement is consistent with expectations, and in reflexively modulating the movement so that it is specific to environmental variables.[48,57]

- Reflexes are evoked responses and depend on a stimulus to be initiated. They are involuntary, stereotyped, and graded responses to sensory input, and they have no threshold except that the stimulus must be great enough to activate the relevant sensory input pathway.

- Fixed action patterns (sneezing, orgasm) are involuntary and stereotyped, but typically have a stimulus threshold that must be reached before they are triggered and are less graded and more complex than reflexes.

- Directed movements (reaching) are voluntary and complex, but are generally neither stereotyped nor repetitive.

- Rhythmic motor patterns (walking, scratching, breathing) are complex (unlike reflexes), stereotyped (unlike directed movements), and, by definition, repetitive (unlike fixed action patterns), but are subject to continuous voluntary control.

Many different mechanisms seem to be involved in controlling the timing of movements, from CPGs, to cerebellar estimators, to cortical mechanisms.[155] In much the same way as there is a CPG for locomotion, the nervous system has a number of built-in corrections that can occur rapidly and automatically to counteract perturbations and continually adjust its position in space. As the infant learns to move against gravity, a number of reactions occur in response to sensory input. These include righting, protective, and equilibrium reactions.

- *Righting.* Righting reactions function to keep the correct orientation of the head and the body in relation to the ground.

- *Protective.* Protective reactions are extremity responses to rapid displacement of the body by horizontal or diagonal forces.

- *Equilibrium.* Equilibrium reactions occur when the center of gravity is changed either by movement of the supporting surface or of the body. The three most common equilibrium reactions include:

  - Trunk rotation away from the weight shift

  - Lateral head and trunk righting away from the weight shift

  - Abduction of the arm and leg away from the weight shift

Anticipatory postural adjustments occur in response to internal perturbations such as voluntary movements of the body by activating muscle synergies in advance of the actual perturbation. Research has shown that anticipatory postural adjustments are highly adaptable and vary according to the task demands.[156–158] For example, postural muscles in standing humans are activated before (and during) voluntary movement of an upper limb and are specific to this movement. Anticipatory postural adjustments have also been studied during leg movements,[159,160] trunk movements,[161,162] and arm movements in standing subjects,[156,163] and during load release from extended arms.[164–166]

Whereas anticipatory reactions are initiated by the subject, compensatory reactions, which occur later, are initiated by sensory feedback triggering signals. With anticipatory reactions, the CNS tries to predict postural perturbations associated with a planned movement and minimize them with anticipatory corrections in a feedforward manner. Compensatory reactions deal with actual perturbations of balance that occur because of the suboptimal efficacy of the anticipatory components. Another motor program that is particularly important is the one responsible for postural stability—the ability to maintain stable upright stance against internal and external perturbations. Postural balance results from an integration of three components[167]:

- The nervous system, which provides sensory processing for perception of body orientation in space provided mainly by the visual, vestibular, and somatosensory systems. The sensory motor integration provides motor strategies for the planning, programming, and execution of balance responses.[168]

- Musculoskeletal contributions including postural alignment, flexibility, joint integrity, muscle performance, and mechanoreceptor sensation.

- Contextual effects that interact with the nervous and musculoskeletal systems. These effects include whether the environment is closed (predictable) or open (unpredictable), the support surface, the amount of lighting, the effects of gravity and inertial forces on the body, and the characteristics of the task (new versus well learned, predictable versus unpredictable, single versus multiple).

The Equilibrium Point (EP).[169] The EP theory was first described in the 1960s and 1970s. Over the past 50 years, it has been revised and refined to a theory addressing the production of complex movements, such as multijoint movement and locomotion, while uniting the processes underlying movement production and perception. Fundamental to the EP theory is the concept that *threshold position control* triggers intentional motor actions such that electrochemical influences descending from the brain in the presence of proprioceptive feedback to the motoneurons are transformed into modifications in the threshold muscle lengths or joint angles at which these motoneurons begin to be recruited, thus setting the spatial activation range in reference to the body geometry. This allows control levels of the CNS to specify *where*, in spatial coordinates, muscles are activated without being concerned about the exact details on *when* and *how* they are activated.

Motor Learning

Certain assumptions are made with regard to motor learning[170]:

- The nervous system has the ability to modify neural connections to perform more efficiently, known as neural plasticity.

- Short-term, or working, memory is necessary for learning new movements.

- Long-term memory, the ability to save and retrieve, is necessary for lasting change.

- Motor learning occurs naturally during task performance.

Learning, unlike performance, is not something that can be directly measured. Rather, we measure behavior and infer learning when a set of processes associated with practice or experience results in a change in behavior that seems relatively permanent.[171]

CLINICAL PEARL

Learning can be measured indirectly using retention tests or transfer tests:

- *Retention test:* involves allowing sufficient time between practice and testing to assess whether a relatively permanent change has occurred.

- *Transfer tests:* involves the ability to transfer a skill used in one task to other situations.

Learning involves both acquisition and retention of a skill. Two main types of learning are recognized[171]:

1. Declarative or explicit—the learning of factual knowledge that can be consciously recalled and thus requires processes such as awareness, attention, and reflection. Examples include buttoning a shirt and tying a shoelace.

2. Nondeclarative or implicit—learning that is dependent on practice, association (associating a particular stimulus with another stimulus, or a certain stimulus with a certain response, or a certain response with a certain result), adaptation (making adjustments based on previous results), habituation (filtering out irrelevant stimuli), and sensitization (integration of relevant stimuli). Procedural learning, another type of nondeclarative learning, refers to the learning of a task that can be performed automatically without attention or conscious thought, like a habit.[143]

The most commonly recognized motor learning theories associated with complex skills are discussed next.

Adams' Closed-loop Theory.[172] In a closed-loop process, sensory feedback is used for the ongoing production of skilled movement. The closed-loop theory of motor learning also proposes that two distinct types of memory are important in this process:

- *Memory trace:* used in the selection and initiation of the movement

- *Perceptual trace:* built up over a period of practice and becomes the internal reference of correctness

This theory proposes that when learning a new movement skill, movement is selected and initiated by a memory trace, which is modified by a perceptual trace with repeated practice, and that the more an individual practices the specific movement, the stronger the perceptual trace becomes. Theoretically, the more time spent in practicing the movement as accurately as possible, the better the learning. However, Adams' theory has been refuted by studies involving animals and humans that have demonstrated that motor learning can occur without sensory feedback, and studies that have indicated that variability in practice may be superior in promoting motor learning than errorless practice.

Schmidt's Schema Theory.[172,173] This theory emphasizes open-loop control processes and the generalized motor program (GMP) concept—a set of general rules that can be applied to a variety of contexts. The schema is a generalized motor program that consists of four parts:

- Initial situation (start of the movement)

- Response specifications (the parameters used in the execution of the movement, e.g., speed)

- Sensory consequence (how the movement feels)

- Response outcome (knowledge of result)

These four parts are stored in the memory following the movement as a GMP. A GMP is created from every past movement, and these GMPs are recalled from memory to influence the motor performance of a new task. As a movement is repeated, the GMP becomes stronger. The GMP is considered to contain the rules for creating the spatial and temporal patterns of muscle activity needed to carry out a given movement. A *recall schema* initiates the GMP that closely resembles the desired movement, and the *recognition schema* evaluates the last executed movement attempt based on the initial conditions, past actual outcomes, and past sensory information.[174] The recall schema is then modified by the movement experience. For example, with every attempt, the recall schema updates the instruction to the muscles based on the recognition schema (it continually revises the initial conditions, past outcomes, and past sensory consequences), which eventually leads to a more accurate response. A major limitation of the original schema theory is that it did not explain how GMPs are initially formed. However, Schmidt's theory has evolved over time and has provided the important motor learning notions of knowledge of results (KR) and variability of practice (see Chapter 7).[173]

Ecological Theory. This theory, which clarifies the role of perception in motor learning, is based on the concept of search strategies—during practice there is a search for optimal strategies to solve the task, based on the task constraints. The hypothesis behind this theory is that constraints in the sensory system and biases in the motor system may have an important adaptive role in ontogeny.

CLINICAL PEARL

According to ecological theory, certain boundaries limit the movement capabilities of the individual, including[175]:

- *Structural or functional:* body shape, weight, height, emotional, cognitive, etc.

- *Environmental:* gravity, temperature, light, wind, etc. Wind affects the force and direction of throwing a discus.

- *Task constraints:* rules of the game, goal of the task, and the implement used (i.e., size, shape, and weight).

Critical to the search for optimal strategies is the exploration of the perceptual-motor workspace, or environment, which requires exploring all possible perceptual cues to identify those that are most relevant to the performance of a specific task. Actions require perceptual information that is specific to a desired goal-directed action performed within a specific environment such that the organization of action is specific to the task and the environment in which the task is being performed.[144]

Dynamic Systems Theory (DST).[176-178] One of the most currently accepted approaches to motor and skill learning appears to be Thelen's[176-178] dynamical functional perspective. DST places less emphasis on the nervous system by viewing movement as emerging from the interaction of three general systems: the person, the task, and the environment.

<table>
<tr><td>
CLINICAL PEARL

Systems, dynamic, dynamic action, and dynamic action systems are all terms that are often used interchangeably, although there are subtle differences.[144]
</td></tr>
</table>

<table>
<tr><td>
CLINICAL PEARL

Thelen's dynamic systems theory (DST)[176,179]:

▶ Emphasizes process rather than product or hierarchically structured plans (see Motor Development)

▶ Places neural maturation on an equal plane with other structures and processes that interact to promote motor learning

▶ Emphasizes that the environment is as important as the organism, and change is seen not as a series of discrete stages, but as a series of states of stability, instability, and phase shifts in which new states becomes stable aspects of behavior
</td></tr>
</table>

In contrast to the hierarchical concept of the nervous system, no subsystem has higher control than another, and development is a nonlinear process. Instead, movement is produced from the interaction of multiple subsystems within the framework of degrees of freedom and within the context of a specific task within the context of self-organization. According to the DST, cooperating systems, which include musculoskeletal components, sensory systems, central sensorimotor integrated mechanisms, and arousal and motivation, spontaneously self-organize, or come together and interact in a specific way, to produce the most efficient movement solution for each specific task to gradually optimize skilled function.[179,180] Thus, movements can emerge as a result of interacting elements that interact with one another to either support or constrain movement without the need for specific commands or motor programs within the nervous system. A small but critical change in one subsystem can cause the whole system to shift, resulting in a new motor behavior.

<table>
<tr><td>
CLINICAL PEARL

Movement emerges from the interaction of three factors[144]:

1. The individual, which is a factor of the health condition, dysfunction or damage, age, gender, etc., of the individual and involves the cooperative efforts of the nervous and musculoskeletal systems. This includes control of the muscles and joints, the control of perception, and the control of attention, motivation, and emotional aspects. Cognitive development normally occurs in a sequential manner (Table 4-14).

2. The task, which can be defined as a continuum from the most difficult task to the easiest task, but also includes how meaningful or preferred a task is.

3. The environment, which includes all relevant contexts including such things as the type of walking surface; the size, shape, and weight of an object to be picked up; and the presence of visual or auditory distractions.
</td></tr>
</table>

According to this theory, the number of biomechanical degrees of freedom of the motor system is dramatically reduced through the development of coordinative structures or temporary accumulations of muscle complexes.[181] Degrees of freedom refer to the gradual increase in smoothness

TABLE 4-14	Cognitive Development
Age Group	**Cognitive Development**
Preschool (3–6 years)	Can remember basic information and recall that information on demand Can answer simple who and what questions Tend to learn from trial and error Have short attention spans (5–15 minutes) and selective attention Can identify the missing parts of familiar objects Can follow simple rules but need visual cues and frequent reminders
Middle childhood (6–11 years)	See things as here and now, right or wrong, and black or white Engage in magical thinking and may believe they have unique powers Can understand the intent of instructions given and can follow directions Can apply factual knowledge to familiar situations Can recognize differences between personal performance and the performance or skill of others

of performance of a skilled movement. DST theory suggests that when a novice or an infant is first learning a new skill, the degrees of freedom available in the body are constrained as they perform the task. Descriptive evidence has highlighted that in some tasks the number of degrees of freedom is initially reduced and subsequently increased.[182] Although an individual can reasonably perform the task in the early stages of learning, the movement is not efficient and the individual is not able to adapt to environmental changes. Starting with fewer degrees of freedom has been shown to enable a more efficient exploration of the sensorimotor space, and although this does not necessarily lead to optimal task performance, it guides the coordination of additional degrees of freedom.[183] Bernstein[182] showed that this release of additional degrees of freedom allows for optimal task performance and more tolerance and adaptation to environmental interaction. Several other studies have reported a freezing of joint segments in the initial stage of learning a motor task, including adults learning to write a signature with the nondominant hand[184] and to perform tasks while using a ski simulator.[185] Based on these observations, three stages of motor learning have been described[185-187]:

▶ *Novice.* During this stage, the learner simplifies the movement in order to reduce the number of individual elements (degrees of freedom) that must be controlled—he or she freezes the degrees of freedom. Examples of freezing the degrees of freedom include blocking some joints within limbs so that the limb moves as a single unit rather than as a multijoint system.

▶ *Advanced.* During the advanced stage, the learner begins to free up movement possibilities so that the previously frozen joints are incorporated into larger and more sophisticated units of action (synergies) over the course of practice.

▶ *Expert.* The expert stage is one in which the individual has learned to release all the degrees of freedom necessary to perform the task and has learned to take advantage of the mechanics of the musculoskeletal system and of the environment to optimize the efficiency of the movement. Thus, the learner learns to exploit the internal and external forces to achieve the most energetically efficient movement patterns.

The reduced complexity of the motor system theorized in DST encourages the development of functionally preferred or "attractor" states to support goal-directed actions. Within each of these attractor regions, the system dynamics are highly ordered and stable, leading to a consistent movement pattern for a specific task. A highly illustrative example of this arises from a series of studies[188,189] focusing on the orientation behaviors of the common house fly. Detailed analysis revealed that, as flies orient toward moving objects as part of their mating behavior, the circuitry underlying this behavior forms a motion detection system fed by luminance changes on the fly's facet eye, which in turn drives the flight motor, generating a sufficient amount of torque that is a function of where the motion was detected on the sensory surface. For example, if the speck of motion is detected on the right, a torque to the right is generated and vice versa. This meaningful

behavior emerges as a stable state, an attractor, from the neural circuitry that links the sensory surface to the flight motor which, together with the physics of flight, establishes a dynamical system. The research also found that the fly's simple nervous system was able to compute an expected visual motion from its own motor commands and treat the detected visual motion that matched the predicted motion differently than extraneous motion signals related to movement of an object relative to the fly. So even this very simple control system provides hints that uncovering the dynamics from which behavior emerges requires more than a simple input–output analysis.

CLINICAL PEARL

▶ Attractor states: An important concept in describing movement from a DST perspective is that of attractor states. Attractor states may be considered efficient patterns of movement that develop with practice and experience and that are preferred to accomplish common activities of daily life. Practice and experience alter the formation of movement patterns through interaction with the environment and the demands of the task.

▶ Control parameters: Subsystems that have the potential to change. These may be the target of therapeutic intervention to improve motor learning.

DST has emerged as a viable framework for rehabilitation. Patterns of movement are flexible, adaptable, and dynamic, yet have "preferred" paths. However, flexible and adaptive motor system behavior results from variations between these multiple attractor regions, which encourage the exploration of performance contexts by an individual. Stable movement patterns are those movement patterns that are difficult to change, whereas unstable movement patterns are those that are relatively easy to change. How people switch intentionally from one pattern of movement to another is constrained by stability.[190] Only when states are released from stability does behavioral flexibility arise. This release from stability takes the form of instabilities created when the restoring forces around an attractor become too weak to resist change. It would appear that movement coordination emerges as a stable state from a nonlinear, potentially multistable dynamics, realized by neural networks coupled to the body in a structured environment. Movement plans evolve continuously in time[191] and are updated at any time during movement preparation when sensory information changes.[192] This paradoxical relationship between the stability inherent in simple tasks and the variability in more complex tasks explains why skilled athletes are capable of persistent changes in motor output during high-level sports performance. Eventually, the explored task and environmental constraints become stable motor solutions over time, thereby enhancing the coordination of body segments to optimize energy and momentum transfer.

To help organize functional behavior, the DST approach emphasizes the use of functional tasks that promote an interaction between the individual and their environment, combined with the utilization of motor experiences using different strategies, which all help the individual determine the most optimal (effective and efficient) patterns or solutions for any given motor problem. The resultant behavioral changes, which are the individual's attempts to compensate to achieve task performance, vary from individual to individual because of the uniqueness of the patient factors and the environmental contexts.[193,194]

Task-oriented Approach.[144] This approach is based on DST in addition to the newest theories and concepts that are emerging from research in the fields of motor control, motor learning, and rehabilitation science. Similar to DST, this theory assumes that normal movement emerges as an interaction among many different systems, each contributing different aspects of control.[144] In addition, it is theorized that movement is organized around a behavioral goal that is controlled by the environment, so that the role of sensation in normal movement is not limited to a stimulus/response reflex mode, but is crucial to predictive and adaptive control of movement as well. Under this theory, impairments within one or more of the systems controlling movement will result in abnormal motor control such that abnormal movement occurs because of a combination of the lesion itself and the efforts of the remaining systems to compensate for the loss while still being functional.[144]

From a rehabilitation standpoint, it is important that the clinician select functional tasks that are contextually suitable for the specific patient, rather than movement patterns for movement's sake alone, so that the patient learns by actively attempting to solve the problems inherent in a functional task rather than repetitively practicing normal patterns of movement.[144] Clinical practice strategies must emphasize

functional, age-appropriate tasks incorporated into naturally occurring activities during the day coupled with maximizing practice time (see Chapter 7).

Skilled Movement: Stability and Mobility

Motor function is the ability to demonstrate the skillful and efficient assumption, maintenance, modification, and control of voluntary postures and movement patterns.[195] Multiple variables contribute to the initiation and execution of a functional movement (Table 4-15). The criteria for simple motor patterns are that the movement[196,197]:

► Is performed exactly in the desired direction
► Is smooth and of a constant speed
► Follows the shortest and most efficient path
► Is performed in its full range

The necessary motor responses for functional movements rely on processing and planning at different levels: spinal cord, the brainstem and cerebellum, and the cerebral cortex. The complexity of the processing affects the speed of motor responses, with spinal reflexes representing the shortest neuronal pathway and consequently the most rapid response to afferent stimuli. The criteria for complex motor patterns are as follows[196]:

► Synchronization between the primary movers in the distal regions with those more proximal
► Smooth propagation of motion from one region of the body to another
► Absence of inefficient movement patterns or muscle recruitment
► Optimal relationship between the speed of motion initiated in one region and the speed of motion in other regions

For purposeful and skilled motions to take place, the muscles producing movement must have a stable base from

TABLE 4-15	Motor Control Variables
Variable	**Description**
Sensorimotor	Those physiologic mechanisms or processes that reside within the nervous system, e.g., central pattern generators (CPGs). Movement synergies and neural mechanisms that alter or regulate them.
Mechanical	Changes in total body mass and relative distribution of mass during development are accompanied by changes in length and center of mass of the body segment, which in turn alter inertial forces due to gravity and during movement. The viscoelastic properties of musculoskeletal tissues.
Cognitive	May include variables that are dependent on conscious and subconscious processes such as reasoning, memory, or judgment to optimize performance (arousal, motivation, anticipatory or feedforward strategies, a selective use of feedback, practice, and memory).
Task requirements	May include any variable that can contribute to or in some way alter movement, including biomechanical requirements, meaningfulness, predictability, or any other variable associated with a given movement context.

Data from Bradley NS, Westcott SL: Motor control: Developmental aspects of motor control in skill acquisition, in Campbell SK, Vander Linden DW, Palisano RJ (eds): Physical Therapy for Children (ed 3). St Louis, Saunders, 2006, pp 77-130.

which to work. Thus, integral to the performance of functional movements is the ability to produce a delicate balance between stability and mobility. Stability, the ability of something to remain in place, can be either static or dynamic. Mobility, which refers to the ease at which something can be moved, can be either controlled or uncontrolled. Both stability and mobility are related to the BOS and the COM.

CLINICAL PEARL

Stability is enhanced when:

▶ The BOS covers a large area.

▶ The COM is low and closer to the BOS.

▶ The line of action produced by gravity that acts on the COM is at or near the center of the BOS.

▶ The distance between the COM and the BOS is minimized.

▶ *Static stability:* the ability to maintain the COM within the BOS so that the body's orientation in space is controlled without movement. For example, an individual who is able to sit upright while maintaining his or her arms down by the sides demonstrates static stability.

▶ *Dynamic stability:* the ability to maintain and control the body's orientation in space (the COM within the BOS) during movement. For example, the ability to sit upright while the upper extremities perform reaching activities requires dynamic stability.

▶ *Controlled mobility:* occurs when the COM can be moved beyond and then back within the BOS. The fall that occurs at the initiation of gait so that an individual must take the first step is controlled by the central nervous system.

▶ *Uncontrolled mobility:* occurs when the COM moves outside the BOS to a point that it cannot be moved back within the BOS. Such an occurrence results in either a stumble or a fall.

CLINICAL PEARL

Whereas the objective in standing is to maintain a static equilibrium of forces, the objective with mobility is to create and control dynamic, unbalanced forces to produce movement.[56] Mobility is enhanced when:

▶ The BOS covers a small area.

▶ The COM is high and further away from the BOS.

▶ The line of action produced by gravity that acts on the COM moves beyond the center of the BOS.

▶ The distance between the COM and the BOS is maximized.

In both the spine and the extremities, certain muscles work as either mobilizers or stabilizers. The peripheral stabilizers rely on stabilization of the two primary dynamic bases or core structures—the pelvis and the scapula. The pelvis acts as a base for the whole body, especially for the spine and the lower limbs, whereas the scapula acts as a base for its respective upper limb.[81] During peripheral joint movement, the peripheral stabilizer muscles normally contract first to stabilize the core structures from which the mobilizers work.[81,198] The mobilizers then contract, resulting in a controlled movement pattern. For example, during upper extremity activity, the scapular stabilizers contract first to stabilize the scapula before the other shoulder muscles move the upper extremity into a functional position. However, with injury, a pathologic process, or other abnormality, an abnormal stabilizer recruitment pattern can develop, resulting in a dominance of the mobilizer muscles and eventual weakening of the local stabilizers.[81,198] The clinician must therefore ensure that a stable base is present from which the mobilizers can act. The body has several natural stabilization methods including muscle contraction, muscle spasm, osteophyte formation, scar tissue formation, and adaptive shortening of inert tissue or muscle.[81] Although the clinician cannot affect some of these natural stabilization methods such as osteophyte and scar tissue formation, the clinician can use muscle contraction and adaptive shortening to the patient's advantage. Factors that the clinician can control include the COM of an object and the BOS (see Kinetics earlier).

CLINICAL PEARL

Mobility and stability often demonstrate an inverse relationship. Increasing mobility often decreases stability and vice versa. Consider a patient using a walker versus a cane—the walker increases the patient's stability but slows down the gait speed, whereas the cane allows for a faster gait at the expense of decreased stability.

Gravity also has an impact on stability. When the line of gravity intersects the BOS in such a way that it provides for the greatest range of movement within the base, stability is enhanced. To promote stability, the clinician must minimize the distance between the COM and the BOS (crouching, kneeling, or sitting lower the COM and increase stability) and ensure that the force of gravity on the COM is acting at or near the center of the BOS. In contrast, to promote mobility, the clinician should reduce the BOS, allow the force of gravity to act beyond the center of the BOS, and increase the distance between the COM and the BOS.

CLINICAL PEARL

▶ The greater the mass, the greater the stability.

▶ The greater the friction, the greater the stability.

▶ The larger the BOS, the greater the stability.

▶ The lower the COM, the greater the stability.

▶ The more the BOS is widened in the direction of the line of force, the greater the stability.

The various applications of these principles are described throughout a number of chapters in the second half of this book.

REFERENCES

1. Saladin KS: Human development, in Human Anatomy (ed 3). New York, McGraw-Hill, 2011, pp 82-105.

2. Christian EL: Embryology and the evolution of movement and function, in Scully RM, Barnes MR (eds): Physical Therapy (ed 1). Philadelphia, JB Lippincott, 1989, pp 48-62.

3. Saladin KS: Histology—The study of tissues, in Human Anatomy (ed 3). New York, McGraw-Hill, 2011, pp 52-81.

4. Hall SJ: The biomechanics of human skeletal muscle, in Hall SJ (ed): Basic Biomechanics. New York, McGraw-Hill, 1999, pp 146-185.

5. Starcher BC: Lung elastin and matrix. Chest 117(5 Suppl):229S-34S, 2000.

6. Engles M: Tissue response, in Donatelli R, Wooden MJ (eds): Orthopaedic Physical Therapy (ed 3). Philadelphia, Churchill Livingstone, 2001, pp 1-24.

7. Teitz CC, Garrett WE Jr, Miniaci A, et al: Tendon problems in athletic individuals. J Bone Joint Surg 79A:138-152, 1997.

8. Barnes J: Myofascial Release: A Comprehensive Evaluatory and Treatment Approach. Paoli, PA, MFR Seminars, 1990.

9. Smolders JJ: Myofascial pain and dysfunction syndromes, in Hammer WI (ed): Functional Soft Tissue Examination and Treatment by Manual Methods—The Extremities. Gaithersburg, MD, Aspen, 1991, pp 215-234.

10. Curwin SL: Tendon pathology and injuries: Pathophysiology, healing, and treatment considerations, in Magee D, Zachazewski JE, Quillen WS (eds): Scientific foundations and principles of practice in musculoskeletal rehabilitation. St Louis, Mo, WB Saunders, 2007, pp 47-78.

11. Amiel D, Woo SL-Y, Harwood FL: The effect of immobilization on collagen turnover in connective tissue: A biochemical–biomechanical correlation. Acta Orthop Scand 53:325-332, 1982.

12. Benjamin M, Toumi H, Ralphs JR, et al: Where tendons and ligaments meet bone: attachment sites ("entheses") in relation to exercise and/or mechanical load. J Anat 208:471-490, 2006.

13. Maganaris CN, Narici MV, Almekinders LC, et al: Biomechanics and pathophysiology of overuse tendon injuries: ideas on insertional tendinopathy. Sports Med 34:1005-1017, 2004.

14. Reid DC: Sports Injury Assessment and Rehabilitation. New York, Churchill Livingstone, 1992.

15. Garrett W, Tidball J: Myotendinous junction: Structure, function, and failure, in Woo SL-Y, Buckwalter JA (eds): Injury and Repair of the Musculoskeletal Soft Tissues. Rosemont, Ill, AAOS, 1988.

16. Garrett WE Jr: Muscle strain injuries: clinical and basic aspects. Med Sci Sports Exerc 22:436-443, 1990.

17. Garrett WE: Muscle strain injuries. Am J Sports Med 24:S2-S8, 1996.

18. Safran MR, Seaber AV, Garrett WE: Warm-up and muscular injury prevention: An update. Sports Med 8:239-249, 1989.

19. Huijbregts PA: Muscle injury, regeneration, and repair. J Man Manip Ther 9:9-16, 2001.

20. Hildebrand KA, Hart DA, Rattner JB, et al: Ligament injuries: pathophysiology, healing, and treatment considerations, in Magee D, Zachazewski JE, Quillen WS (eds): Scientific Foundations and Principles of Practice in Musculoskeletal Rehabilitation. St Louis, Mo, WB Saunders, 2007, pp 23-46.

21. Vereeke West R, Fu F: Soft tissue physiology and repair, Orthopaedic Knowledge Update 8: Home Study Syllabus. Rosemont, Ill, American Academy of Orthopaedic Surgeons, 2005, pp 15-27.

22. Amiel D, Kleiner JB: Biochemistry of tendon and ligament, in Nimni ME (ed): Collagen. Boca Raton, FL, CRC Press, 1988, pp 223-251.

23. Woo SL-Y, An K-N, Arnoczky SP, et al: Anatomy, biology, and biomechanics of tendon, ligament, and meniscus, in Simon S (ed): Orthopaedic Basic Science. Rosemont, Ill, American Academy of Orthopaedic Surgeons, 1994, pp 45-87.

24. Safran MR, Benedetti RS, Bartolozzi AR, III et al: Lateral ankle sprains: a comprehensive review: part 1: etiology, pathoanatomy, histopathogenesis, and diagnosis. Med Sci Sports Exerc 31:S429-S437, 1999.

25. Smith RL, Brunolli J: Shoulder kinesthesia after anterior glenohumeral dislocation. Phys Ther 69:106-112, 1989.

26. McGaw WT: The effect of tension on collagen remodelling by fibroblasts: a stereological ultrastructural study. Connect Tissue Res 14:229, 1986.

27. Inman VT: Sprains of the ankle, in Chapman MW (ed): AAOS Instructional Course Lectures, 1975, pp 294-308.

28. Cohen NP, Foster RJ, Mow VC: Composition and dynamics of articular cartilage: structure, function, and maintaining healthy state. J Orthop Sports Phys Ther 28:203-15, 1998.

29. Junqueira LC, Carneciro J, Kelley RO: Basic Histology. Norwalk, Conn, Appleton and Lange, 1995.

30. Lundon K, Bolton K: Structure and function of the lumbar intervertebral disk in health, aging, and pathological conditions. J Orthop Sports Phys Ther 31:291-306, 2001.

31. Mankin HJ, Mow VC, Buckwalter JA, et al: Form and function of articular cartilage, in Simon SR (ed): Orthopaedic Basic Science. Rosemont, IL, American Academy of Orthopaedic Surgeons, 1994, pp 1-44.

32. Muir H: Proteoglycans as organizers of the extracellular matrix. Biochem Soc Trans 11:613-622, 1983.

33. Buchbinder D, Kaplan AS: Biology, in Kaplan AS, Assael LA (eds): Temporomandibular disorders diagnosis and treatment. Philadelphia, WB Saunders, 1991, pp 11-23.

34. Tippett SR: Considerations for the pediatric patient, in Voight ML, Hoogenboom BJ, Prentice WE (eds): Musculoskeletal Interventions: Techniques for Therapeutic Exercise. New York, McGraw-Hill, 2007, pp 803-820.

35. Iannotti JP, Goldstein S, Kuhn J, et al: The formation and growth of skeletal tissues, in Buckwalter JA, Einhorn TA, Simon SR (eds): Orthopedic Basic Science. Rosemont, Ill, American Academy of Orthopedic Surgeons, 2000, pp 77-109.

36. Waxman SG: Correlative Neuroanatomy (ed 24). New York, McGraw-Hill, 1996.

37. Butler DS, Tomberlin JP: Peripheral nerve: structure, function, and physiology, in Magee D, Zachazewski JE, Quillen WS (eds): Scientific foundations and principles of practice in musculoskeletal rehabilitation. St Louis, Mo, WB Saunders, 2007, pp 175-189.

38. Pratt N: Anatomy of the Cervical Spine. La Crosse, Wisc, Orthopaedic Section, APTA, 1996.

39. Martin J: Introduction to the central nervous system, in Martin J (ed): Neuroanatomy: Text and Atlas (ed 2). New York, McGraw-Hill, 1996, pp 1-32.

40. Chusid JG: Correlative Neuroanatomy & Functional Neurology (ed 19). Norwalk, Conn, Appleton-Century-Crofts, 1985, pp 144-148.

41. Freeman MAR, Wyke BD: An experimental study of articular neurology. J Bone Joint Surg 49B:185, 1967.

42. Wyke BD: The neurology of joints: a review of general principles. Clin Rheum Dis 7:223-239, 1981.

43. Voight ML, Cook G: Impaired neuromuscular control: Reactive neuromuscular training, in Voight ML, Hoogenboom BJ, Prentice WE (eds): Musculoskeletal Interventions: Techniques for Therapeutic Exercise. New York, McGraw-Hill, 2007, pp 181-212.

44. Voss H: [Tabulation of the absolute and relative muscular spindle numbers in human skeletal musculature]. Anat Anz 129:562-72, 1971.

45. Peck D, Buxton DF, Nitz A: A comparison of spindle concentrations in large and small muscles acting in parallel combinations. J Morphol 180:243-252, 1984.

46. Nyland J, Lachman N, Kocabey Y, et al: Anatomy, function, and rehabilitation of the popliteus musculotendinous complex. J Orthop Sports Phys Ther 35:165-179, 2005.

47. Grigg P, Hoffmann AH: Properties of Ruffini afferents revealed by stress analysis of isolated sections of cat knee capsule. J Neurophysiol 47:41-54, 1982.

48. Williams GN, Krishnan C: Articular neurophysiology and sensorimotor control, in Magee D, Zachazewski JE, Quillen WS (eds): Scientific foundations and principles of practice in musculoskeletal rehabilitation. St Louis, Mo, WB Saunders, 2007, pp 190-216.

49. Zimny ML: Mechanoreceptors in articular tissues. Am J Anat 182:16-32, 1988.

50. Wyke BD: Articular neurology and manipulative therapy, in Glasgow EF, Twomey LT, Scull ER, et al (eds): Aspects of Manipulative Therapy (ed 2). New York, Churchill Livingstone, 1985, pp 72-77.

51. Grigg A, Hoffman AH, Fogarty KE: Properties of Golgi–Mazzoni afferents in cat knee joint capsule, as revealed by mechanical studies of isolated joint capsule. J Neurophysiol 47:31-40, 1982.

52. Schutte MJ, Happel RT: Joint innervation in joint injury. Clin Sports Med 9:511-517, 1990.

53. Milne RJ, Foreman RD, Giesler GJ, et al: Convergence of cutaneous and pelvic visceral nociceptive inputs onto primate spinothalamic neurons. Pain 11:163-183, 1981.

54. Vierck CJ, Greenspan JD, Ritz LA: Long-term changes in purposive and reflexive responses to nociceptive stimulation following anterior–lateral chordotomy. J Neurosci 10:2077-2095, 1990.

55. Schaible HG, Schmidt RF: Discharge characteristics of receptors with fine afferents from normal and inflamed joints: influence of analgesics and prostaglandins. Agents Actions Suppl 19:99-117, 1986.

56. Rose J: Dynamic lower extremity stability, in Hughes C (ed): Movement Disorders and Neuromuscular Interventions for the Trunk and Extremities—Independent Study Course 18.2.5. La Crosse, Wisc, Orthopaedic Section, APTA, Inc, 2008, pp 1-34.

57. Schmidt R, Lee T: Motor control and learning (ed 4). Champaign, Ill, Human Kinetics, 2005.

58. Lee WA: Anticipatory control of postural and task muscles during rapid arm flexion. J Mot Behav 12:185-196, 1980.

59. Jones D, Round D: Skeletal muscle in health and disease. Manchester, UK, Manchester University Press, 1990.

60. Loitz-Ramage B, Zernicke R: Bone biology and mechanics, in Zachazewski J, Magee D, Quillen W (eds): Athletic Injuries and Rehabilitation. Philadelphia, WB Saunders, 1996.

61. Armstrong RB, Warren GL, Warren JA: Mechanisms of exercise-induced muscle fibre injury. Med Sci Sports Exerc 24:436-443, 1990.

62. Van de Graaff KM, Fox SI: Muscle tissue and muscle physiology, in Van de Graaff KM, Fox SI (eds): Concepts of Human Anatomy and Physiology. New York, WCB/McGraw-Hill, 1999, pp 280-305.

63. Williams JH, Klug GA: Calcium exchange hypothesis of skeletal muscle fatigue. A brief review. Muscle Nerve 18:421, 1995.

64. Brooke MH, Kaiser KK: The use and abuse of muscle histochemistry. Ann N Y Acad Sci 228:121, 1974.

65. Staron RS, Hikida RS: Histochemical, biochemical, and ultrastructural analyses of single human muscle fibers, with special reference to the C-fiber population. J Histochem Cytochem 40:563-568, 1992.

66. Jull GA, Janda V: Muscle and motor control in low back pain, in Twomey LT, Taylor JR (eds): Physical Therapy of the Low Back: Clinics in Physical Therapy. New York, Churchill Livingstone, 1987, pp 258-278.

67. Fitts RH, Widrick JJ: Muscle mechanics; adaptations with exercise training. Exerc Sport Sci Rev 24:427-473, 1996.

68. Allemeier CA, Fry AC, Johnson P, et al: Effects of spring cycle training on human skeletal muscle. J Appl Physiol 77:2385, 1994.

69. Nilsson J, Tesch PA, Thorstensson A: Fatigue and EMG of repeated fast and voluntary contractions in man. Acta Physiol Scand 101:194, 1977.

70. Sell S, Zacher J, Lack S: Disorders of proprioception of arthrotic knee joint. Z Rheumatol 52:150-155, 1993.

71. Mattacola CG, Lloyd JW: Effects of a 6 week strength and proprioception training program on measures of dynamic balance: a single case design. J Athl Training 32:127-135, 1997.

72. McArdle W, Katch FI, Katch VL: Exercise Physiology: Energy, Nutrition, and Human Performance. Philadelphia, Lea and Febiger, 1991.

73. Astrand PO, Rodahl K: The Muscle and its Contraction: Textbook of Work Physiology. New York, McGraw-Hill, 1986.

74. Edman KAP RC: The sarcomere length–tension relation determined in short segments of intact muscle fibres of the frog. J Physiol 385:729-732, 1987.

75. Boeckmann RR, Ellenbecker TS: Biomechanics, in Ellenbecker TS (ed): Knee Ligament Rehabilitation. Philadelphia, Churchill Livingstone, 2000, pp 16-23.

76. Brownstein B, Noyes FR, Mangine RE, et al: Anatomy and biomechanics, in Mangine RE (ed): Physical Therapy of the Knee. New York, Churchill Livingstone, 1988, pp 1-30.

77. Deudsinger RH: Biomechanics in clinical practice. Phys Ther 64:1860-1868, 1984.

78. Lakomy HKA: The biomechanics of human movement, in Maughan RJ (ed): Basic and Applied Sciences for Sports Medicine. Woburn, Mass, Butterworth-Heinemann, 1999, pp 124-125.

79. Desmendt JE, Godaux E: Fast motor units are not preferentially activated in rapid voluntary contractions in man. Nature 267:717, 1977.

80. Gans C: Fiber architecture and muscle function. Exerc Sport Sci Rev 10:160, 1982.

81. Magee DJ, Zachazewski JE: Principles of stabilization training, in Magee D, Zachazewski JE, Quillen WS (eds): Scientific foundations and principles of practice in musculoskeletal rehabilitation. St Louis, Mo, WB Saunders, 2007, pp 388-413.

82. Lash JM: Regulation of skeletal muscle blood flow during contractions. Proc Soc Exp Biol Med 211:218-235, 1996.

83. Rosenbaum D, Henning EM: The influence of stretching and warm-up exercises on Achilles tendon reflex activity. J Sports Sci 13:481, 1995.

84. Astrand PO, Rodahl K: Physical Training: Textbook of Work Physiology. New York, McGraw-Hill, 1986.

85. Grimes K: Heart disease, in O'Sullivan SB, Schmitz TJ (eds): Physical Rehabilitation (ed 5). Philadelphia, FA Davis, 2007, pp 589-641.

86. Shaffer TH, Wolfson MR, Gault JH: Respiratory Physiology, in Irwin S, Tecklin JS (eds): Cardiopulmonary Physical Therapy (ed 2). St Louis, Mosby, 1990, pp 217-244.

87. Van de Graaff KM, Fox SI: Respiratory system, in Van de Graaff KM, Fox SI (eds): Concepts of Human Anatomy and Physiology. New York, WCB/McGraw-Hill, 1999, pp 728-777.

88. Collins SM, Cocanour B: Anatomy of the cardiopulmonary system, in DeTurk WE, Cahalin LP (eds): Cardiovascular and Pulmonary Physical Therapy: an Evidence-Based Approach. New York, McGraw-Hill, 2004, pp 73-94.

89. Schmitz TJ: Vital signs, in O'Sullivan SB, Schmitz TJ (eds): Physical Rehabilitation (ed 5). Philadelphia, FA Davis, 2007, pp 81-120.

90. Sahlin K, Tonkonogi M, Soderlund K: Energy supply and muscle fatigue in humans. Acta Physiol Scand 162:261-266, 1998.

91. McMahon S, Jenkins D: Factors affecting the rate of phosphocreatine resynthesis following intense exercise. Sports Med 32:761-784, 2002.

92. Walter G, Vandenborne K, McCully KK, et al: Noninvasive measurement of phosphocreatine recovery kinetics in single human muscles. Am J Physiol 272:C525-C534, 1997.

93. Bangsbo J: Muscle oxygen uptake in humans at onset and during intense exercise. Acta Physiol Scand 168:457-464, 2000.

94. Hoppeler H, Fluck M: Plasticity of skeletal muscle mitochondria: structure and function. Med Sci Sports Exerc 35:95-104, 2003.

95. Tonkonogi M, Sahlin K: Physical exercise and mitochondrial function in human skeletal muscle. Exerc Sport Sci Rev 30:129-137, 2002.

96. Sahlin K, Ren JM: Relationship of contraction capacity to metabolic changes during recovery from a fatiguing contraction. J Appl Physiol 67:648-54, 1989.

97. Sells P, Prentice WE: Impaired endurance: Maintaining aerobic capacity and endurance, in Voight ML, Hoogenboom BJ, Prentice WE (eds): Musculoskeletal Interventions: Techniques for Therapeutic Exercise. New York, McGraw-Hill, 2007, pp 153-164.

98. Kiser DM: Physiological and biomechanical factors for understanding repetitive motion injuries. Semin Occup Med 2:11-17, 1987.

99. Luttgens K, Hamilton K: The musculoskeletal system: The musculature, in Luttgens K, Hamilton K (eds): Kinesiology: Scientific Basis of Human Motion (ed 9). Dubuque, Iowa, McGraw-Hill, 1997, pp 49-75.

100. Howald H, Hoppeler H, Claassen H, et al: Influences of endurance training on the ultrastructural composition of the different muscle fiber types in humans. Pflugers Arch 403:369-376, 1985.

101. Hill AV: The heat and shortening and the dynamic constants of muscle. Proc R Soc Lond B126:136-195, 1938.

102. Tihanyi J, Apor P, Fekete GY: Force–velocity–power characteristics and fiber composition in human knee extensor muscles. Eur J Appl Physiol 48:331-343, 1982.

103. American Medical Association: Guides to the Evaluation of Permanent Impairment (ed 5). Chicago, American Medical Association, 2001.

104. Prentice WE: Impaired mobility: Restoring range of motion and improving flexibility, in Voight ML, Hoogenboom BJ, Prentice WE (eds): Musculoskeletal Interventions: Techniques for Therapeutic Exercise. New York, McGraw-Hill, 2007, pp 165-180.

105. The American Orthopaedic Society for Sports Medicine: Flexibility. Chicago, The American Orthopaedic Society for Sports Medicine, 1988.

106. Gleim GW, McHugh MP: Flexibility and its effects on sports injury and performance. Sports Med 24:289-299, 1997.

107. Kippers V, Parker AW: Toe-touch test: a measure of validity. Phys Ther 67:1680-1684, 1987.

108. Jackson AW, Baker AA: The relationship of the sit and reach test to criterion measures of hamstring and back flexibility in young females. Res Q Exerc Sport 57:183-186, 1986.

109. Litsky AS, Spector M: Biomaterials, in Simon SR (ed): Orthopaedic Basic Science. Chicago, The American Orthopaedic Society for Sports Medicine, 1994, pp 447-486.

110. Johns R, Wright V: Relative importance of various tissues in joint stiffness. J Appl Physiol 17:824-830, 1962.

111. Toft E, Espersen GT, Kalund S, et al: Passive tension of the ankle before and after stretching. Am J Sports Med 17:489-494, 1989.

112. Halbertsma JPK, Goeken LNH: Stretching exercises: effect of passive extensibility and stiffness in short hamstrings of healthy subjects. Arch Phys Med Rehab 75:976-981, 1994.

113. Magnusson SP, Simonsen EB, Aagaard P, et al: A mechanism for altered flexibility in human skeletal muscle. J Physiol 497:291-298, 1996.

114. Klinge K, Magnusson SP, Simonsen EB, et al: The effect of strength and flexibility on skeletal muscle EMG activity, stiffness and viscoelastic stress relaxation response. Am J Sports Med 25:710-6, 1997.

115. Lapier TK, Burton HW, Almon RF: Alterations in intramuscular connective tissue after limb casting affect contraction-induced muscle injury. J Appl Physiol 78:1065-1069, 1995.

116. McNair PJ, Wood GA, Marshall RN: Stiffness of the hamstring muscles and its relationship to function in ACL deficient individuals. Clin Biomech 7:131-137, 1992.

117. McHugh MP, Magnusson SP, Gleim GW, et al: A cross-sectional study of age-related musculoskeletal and physiological changes in soccer players. Med Exerc Nutr Health 2:261-268, 1993.

118. Hutton RS: Neuromuscular basis of stretching exercise, in Komi PV (ed): Strength and Power in Sports. Oxford, Blackwell Science, 1993, pp 29-38.

119. Neumann DA: Getting started, in Neumann DA (ed): Kinesiology of the Musculoskeletal System: Foundations for Physical Rehabilitation. St Louis, Mo, Mosby, 2002, pp 3-24.

120. Topoleski LD: Mechanical properties of materials, in Oatis CA (ed): Kinesiology: The Mechanics and Pathomechanics of Human Movement. Philadelphia, Lippincott Williams & Wilkins, 2004, pp 21-35.

121. Woo SL-Y, Buckwalter JA: Injury and Repair of the Musculoskeletal Tissue. Park Ridge, IL, American Academy of Orthopaedic Surgeons, 1988.

122. Goel VK, Khandha A, Vadapalli S: Musculoskeletal Biomechanics, Orthopaedic Knowledge Update 8: Home Study Syllabus. Rosemont, Ill, American Academy of Orthopaedic Surgeons, 2005, pp 39-56.

123. Noyes FR, Butler DL, Paulos LE, et al: Intra-articular cruciate reconstruction. I: Perspectives on graft strength, vascularization and immediate motion after replacement. Clin Orthop 172:71-77, 1983.

124. Laros GS, Tipton CM, Cooper R: Influence of physical activity on ligament insertions in the knees of dogs. J Bone Joint Surg 53B:275-286, 1971.

125. Nimni ME: Collagen: structure function and metabolism in normal and fibrotic tissue. Semin Arthritis Rheum 13:1-86, 1983.

126. Noyes FR, Torvik PJ, Hyde WB, et al: Biomechanics of ligament failure: II. An analysis of immobilization, exercise, and reconditioning effects in primates. J Bone Joint Surg 56A:1406-1418, 1974.

127. Hall SJ: Kinematic concepts for analyzing human motion, in Hall SJ (ed): Basic Biomechanics. New York, McGraw-Hill, 1999, pp 28-89.

128. Lehmkuhl LD, Smith LK: Brunnstrom's Clinical Kinesiology. Philadelphia, FA Davis, 1983, pp 361-390.

129. MacConnail MA, Basmajian JV: Muscles and Movements: A Basis for Human Kinesiology. New York, Robert Krieger, 1977.

130. Rasch PJ, Burke RK: Kinesiology and Applied Anatomy. Philadelphia, Lea and Febiger, 1971.

131. Steindler A: Kinesiology of the Human Body under Normal and Pathological Conditions. Springfield, Ill, Charles C Thomas, 1955.

132. Williams PL, Warwick R, Dyson M, et al: Gray's Anatomy (ed 37). London, Churchill Livingstone, 1989.

133. Mennell JB: The Science and Art of Joint Manipulation. London, J & A Churchill, 1949.

134. Mennell JM: Back Pain. Diagnosis and Treatment Using Manipulative Techniques. Boston, Mass, Little, Brown, 1960.

135. Marino M: Current concepts of rehabilitation in sports medicine, in Nicholas JA, Herschman EB (eds): The Lower Extremity and Spine in Sports Medicine. St Louis, Mo, Mosby, 1986, pp 117-195.

136. Blackard DO, Jensen RL, Ebben WP: Use of EMG analysis in challenging kinetic chain terminology. Med Sci Sports Exerc 31:443-448, 1999.

137. Dillman CJ, Murray TA, Hintermeister RA: Biomechanical differences of open and closed chain exercises with respect to the shoulder. J Sport Rehabil 3:228-238, 1994.

138. Van Sant AF: Concepts of neural organization and movement, in Connolly BH, Montgomery PC (eds): Therapeutic Exercise in Developmental Disabilities (ed 2). Thorofare, NJ, Slack, Inc, 2001, pp 1-12.

139. Lewis C: Physiological response to exercise in the child: considerations for the typically and atypically developing youngster, Proceedings from the American Physical Therapy Association combined sections meeting. San Antonio, Texas, 2001.

140. Winstein CJ, Knecht HG: Movement science and its relevance to physical therapy. Phys Ther 70:759-762, 1990.

141. Winstein CJ: Knowledge of results and motor learning—implications for physical therapy. Phys Ther 71:140-149, 1991.

142. Winstein CJ: Motor learning considerations in stroke rehabilitation, in Duncan PW, Badke MB (eds): Stroke Rehabilitation: The Recovery of Motor Control. Chicago, Yearbook Medical Publishers, 1987, pp 109-134.

143. Shumway-Cook A, Woollacott MH: Motor learning and recovery of function, in Shumway-Cook A, Woollacott MH (eds): Motor Control—Translating Research into Clinical Practice. Philadelphia, Lippincott Williams & Wilkins, 2007, pp 21-45.

144. Shumway-Cook A, Woollacott MH: Motor control: issues and theories, in Shumway-Cook A, Woollacott MH (eds): Motor Control—Translating Research into Clinical Practice. Philadelphia, Lippincott Williams & Wilkins, 2007, pp 3-20.

145. Horak FB: Assumptions underlying motor control for neurologic rehabilitation, in Lister MJ (ed): Contemporary Management of Motor Control Problems: Proceedings of the II STEP Conference. Alexandria, VA, Foundation for Physical Therapy, 1991, pp 11-27.

146. Campbell SK: The child's development of functional movement, in Campbell SK, Vander Linden DW, Palisano RJ (eds): Physical Therapy for Children. St Louis, Mo, Saunders, 2006, pp 33-76.

147. O'Sullivan SB: Strategies to improve motor function, in O'Sullivan SB, Schmitz TJ (eds): Physical Rehabilitation (ed 5). Philadelphia, FA Davis, 2007, pp 471-522.

148. Thompson S, Watson WH 3rd: Central pattern generator for swimming in Melibe. J Exp Biol 208:1347-1361, 2005.

149. Yamaguchi T: The central pattern generator for forelimb locomotion in the cat. Prog Brain Res 143:115-122, 2004.

150. Agnati LF, Franzen O, Ferre S, et al: Possible role of intramembrane receptor-receptor interactions in memory and learning via formation of long-lived heteromeric complexes: focus on motor learning in the basal ganglia. J Neural Transm Suppl 65:1-28, 2003.

151. Agnati LF, Fuxe K, Ferri M, et al: A new hypothesis on memory—a possible role of local circuits in the formation of the memory trace. Med Biol 59:224-229, 1981.

152. Morris C, Chaitow L, Janda V: Functional examination for low back syndromes, in Morris C (ed): Low back syndromes: Integrated clinical management. New York, McGraw-Hill, 2006, pp 333-416.

153. Kottke FJ: From reflex to skill: the training of coordination. Arch Phys Med Rehabil 61:551-561, 1980.

154. Kottke FJ, Halpern D, Easton JK, et al: The training of coordination. Arch Phys Med Rehabil 59:567-572, 1978.

155. Ivry RB, Diedrichsen J, Spencer R, et al: A cognitive neuroscience perspective on bimanual coordination and interference, in Swinnen SP, Duysens J (eds): Neuro-Behavioral Determinants of Interlimb Coordination—An Interdisciplinary Approach. Dordrecht, The Netherlands, Kluwer Academic, 2004, pp 259-295.

156. Cordo PJ, Nashner LM: Properties of postural adjustments associated with rapid arm movements. J Neurophysiol 47:287-302, 1982.

157. Nashner LM, Forssberg H: Phase-dependent organization of postural adjustments associated with arm movements while walking. J Neurophysiol 55:1382-1394, 1986.

158. Krishnamoorthy V, Latash ML: Reversals of anticipatory postural adjustments during voluntary sway in humans. J Physiol 565:675-684, 2005.

159. Rogers MW, Pai YC: Dynamic transitions in stance support accompanying leg flexion movements in man. Exp Brain Res 81:398-402, 1990.

160. Mouchnino L, Aurenty R, Massion J, et al: Coordination between equilibrium and head-trunk orientation during leg movement: a new strategy build up by training. J Neurophysiol 67:1587-1598, 1992.

161. Oddsson L, Thorstensson A: Fast voluntary trunk flexion movements in standing: motor patterns. Acta Physiol Scand 129:93-106, 1987.

162. Pedotti A, Crenna P, Deat A, et al: Postural synergies in axial movements: short and long-term adaptation. Exp Brain Res 74:3-10, 1989.

163. Friedli WG, Hallett M, Simon SR: Postural adjustments associated with rapid voluntary arm movements 1. Electromyographic data. J Neurol Neurosurg Psychiatry 47:611-622, 1984.

164. Aruin AS, Latash ML: The role of motor action in anticipatory postural adjustments studied with self-induced and externally triggered perturbations. Exp Brain Res 106:291-300, 1995.

165. De Wolf S, Slijper H, Latash ML: Anticipatory postural adjustments during self-paced and reaction-time movements. Exp Brain Res 121:7-19, 1998.

166. Benvenuti F, Stanhope SJ, Thomas SL, et al: Flexibility of anticipatory postural adjustments revealed by self-paced and reaction-time arm movements. Brain Res 761:59-70, 1997.

167. Kloos A: Mechanics and control of posture and balance, in Hughes C (ed): Movement Disorders and Neuromuscular Interventions for the Trunk and Extremities—Independent Study Course 18.2.2. La Crosse, Wisc, Orthopaedic Section, APTA, Inc, 2008, pp 1-26.

168. Horak FB: Postural orientation and equilibrium: what do we need to know about neural control of balance to prevent falls? Age Ageing 35 Suppl 2:ii7-ii11, 2006.

169. Latash ML, Levin MF, Scholz JP, et al: Motor control theories and their applications. Medicina (Kaunas) 46:382-392, 2010.

170. Cole M: Applied theories in occupational therapy: a practical approach. Thorofare, NJ, Slack Inc, 2007.

171. Buford JA: Neuroscience of motor control and learning, in Hughes C (ed): Movement Disorders and Neuromuscular Interventions for the Trunk and Extremities—Independent Study Course 18.2.1. La Crosse, Wisc, Orthopaedic Section, APTA, Inc, 2008, pp 1-23.

172. Shumway-Cook A, Woollacott MH: Motor learning and recovery of function, in Shumway-Cook A, Woollacott MH (eds): Motor Control: Theory and Practical Applications (ed 2). Philadelphia, Lippincott Williams & Wilkins, 2001, pp 26-49.

173. Schmidt RA: Motor schema theory after 27 years: reflections and implications for a new theory. Res Q Exerc Sport 74:366-375, 2003.

174. Zwicker JG, Harris SR: A reflection on motor learning theory in pediatric occupational therapy practice. Can J Occup Ther 76:29-37, 2009.

175. Newell KM: Constraints on the development of coordination, in Wade MG, Whiting HTA (eds): Motor Development in Children: aspect of Coordination and Control. Boston, Martinus Nijhoff, 1985, pp 341-360.

176. Thelen E: Motor development. A new synthesis. Am Psychol 50:79-95, 1995.

177. Thelen E, Corbetta D: Exploration and selection in the early acquisition of skill. Int Rev Neurobiol 37:75-102, 1994.

178. Thelen E, Ulrich BD: Hidden skills: a dynamic systems analysis of treadmill stepping during the first year. Monogr Soc Res Child Dev 56:1-98, 1991.

179. Palisano RJ, Campbell SK, Harris SR: Evidence-based decision-making in pediatric physical therapy, in Campbell SK, Vander Linden DW, Palisano RJ (eds): Physical Therapy for Children. St Louis, Mo, Saunders, 2006, pp 3-32.

180. Shumway-Cook A, Woollacott MH: The growth of stability: postural control from a development perspective. J Mot Behav 17:131-47, 1985.

181. Turvey MT: Coordination. Am Psychol 45:938-953, 1990.

182. Bernstein N: The Coordination and Regulation of Movement. London, Pergamon, 1967.

183. Shemmell J, Riek S, Tresilian JR, et al: The role of the primary motor cortex during skill acquisition on a two-degrees-of-freedom movement task. J Mot Behav 39:29-39, 2007.

184. Newell K, van Emmerik R: The acquisition of coordination: Preliminary analysis of learning to write. Hum Mov Sci 8:17-32, 1989.

185. Vereijken B, van Emmerik R, Whiting H, et al: Freezing degrees of freedom in skill acquisition. J Mot Behav 24:133-142, 1992.

186. Konczak J, Vander Velden H, Jaeger L: Learning to play the violin: motor control by freezing, not freeing degrees of freedom. J Mot Behav 41:243-252, 2009.

187. Newell KM, Broderick MP, Deutsch KM, et al: Task goals and change in dynamical degrees of freedom with motor learning. J Exp Psychol Hum Percept Perform 29:379-387, 2003.

188. Poggio T, Reichardt W: Visual control of orientation behaviour in the fly. Part II. Towards the underlying neural interactions. Q Rev Biophys 9:377-438, 1976.

189. Reichardt W, Poggio T: Visual control of orientation behaviour in the fly. Part I. A quantitative analysis. Q Rev Biophys 9:311-375, 428-38, 1976.

190. Scholz JP, Kelso JAS, Schöner G: Dynamics governs switching among patterns of coordination in biological movement. Phys Lett A134:8-12, 1988.

191. Ghez C, Favilla M, Ghilardi MF, et al: Discrete and continuous planning of hand movements and isometric force trajectories. Exp Brain Res 115:217-233, 1997.

192. Goodale MA, Pelisson D, Prablanc C: Large adjustments in visually guided reaching do not depend on vision of the hand or perception of target displacement. Nature 320:748-750, 1986.

193. Mathiowetz V, Bass-Haugen J: Assessing abilities and capacities: Motor behavior, in Radomski MV, Trombly-Latham CA (eds): Occupational Therapy for Physical Dysfunction (ed 6). Baltimore, Williams & Wilkins, 2008, pp 186-211.

194. Mathiowetz V: Task-oriented approach to stroke rehabilitation, in Gillen G (ed): Stroke Rehabilitation: A Function-Based Approach (ed 3). St Louis, Mo, Mosby, 2011, pp 80-99.

195. Guide to physical therapist practice. Phys Ther 81:S13-S95, 2001.

196. Vasilyeva LF, Lewit K: Diagnosis of muscular dysfunction by inspection, in Liebenson C (ed): Rehabilitation of the Spine: A Practitioner's Manual. Baltimore, Lippincott Williams & Wilkins, 1996, pp 113-142.

197. Janda V: Muscle Function Testing. London, Butterworths, 1983.

198. Comerford MJ, Mottram SL: Movement and stability dysfunction—contemporary developments. Man Ther 6:15-26, 2001.

CHAPTER 5

Patient/Client Management

CHAPTER OBJECTIVES

*At the completion of this chapter,
the reader will be able to:*

1. Describe the various models of disablement and their similarities and differences

2. List the components of the examination process

3. Conduct a thorough history

4. Understand the importance of the systems review

5. Describe the various components of the tests and measures portion of the examination

6. Discuss the importance of the physical therapy evaluation

7. Describe the purposes of documentation and the different types of documentation

8. Have an understanding of the common medical abbreviations used in healthcare

9. Describe the difference between short-term and long-term goals

10. Describe the components and importance of patient/ family/client-related instruction

11. Discuss various strategies to improve patient adherence and compliance

12. Understand the importance of the physical therapist's role in the promotion of health, wellness, and physical fitness

OVERVIEW

A profession's scope of practice is directly dependent on the education and skill of the provider, the established history of the practice scope within the profession, supporting evidence, and the regulatory environment.[1] For the physical therapist, the profession has outlined the following six steps involved in the management of a typical patient/client[2]: (1) examination of the patient; (2) evaluation of the data and identification of problems; (3) determination of the diagnosis; (4) determination of the prognosis and plan of care (POC); (5) implementation of the POC; and (6) reexamination of the patient and evaluation of treatment outcomes (Figure 5-1). Through accomplishment of this process, the physical therapist determines whether physical therapy services are needed and develops the plan of care in collaboration with the patient/client/caregiver.

MODELS OF DISABLEMENT

The Guide to Physical Therapist Practice, 2nd Edition (The Guide), promotes the practice of physical therapy based on a disablement model. A number of theoretical frameworks, or disablement models, have been proposed to describe the path from disease to disability (Table 5-1).[3-9] A disablement model is designed to detail the functional consequences and relationships of disease, impairment, and functional limitations. The Guide[10] employs an expanded version of the terminology from the Nagi disablement model (see Table 5-1),[6] but also uses components from other disablement models.[11] For example, The National Center for Medical Rehabilitation Research (NCMRR) devised a modification to Nagi's model by adding a fifth concept, that of societal limitation (see Table 5-1). In 1980 the Executive Board of the World Health Organization published a document for trial purposes, the International Classification of Functioning, Disability and Health (ICFDH-I or ICF) (see Table 5-1). In 2001, a revised edition was published (ICFDH-II) that emphasized "components of health" rather than "consequences of disease" (i.e., participation rather than disability) and environmental and personal factors as important determinants of health (see Table 5-1).[12]

Nagi's model depicts the relationship between the following series of linked events[6,13]: *pathology/pathophysiology* (the presence of disease), which may lead to *impairments* (anatomic and structural abnormalities), which may in turn lead to *functional limitations* (restrictions in basic physical and mental actions), which may then lead to *disability* (difficulty doing activities of daily life) (Table 5-2). In addition, the model focuses on persons with health, prevention, and wellness needs.

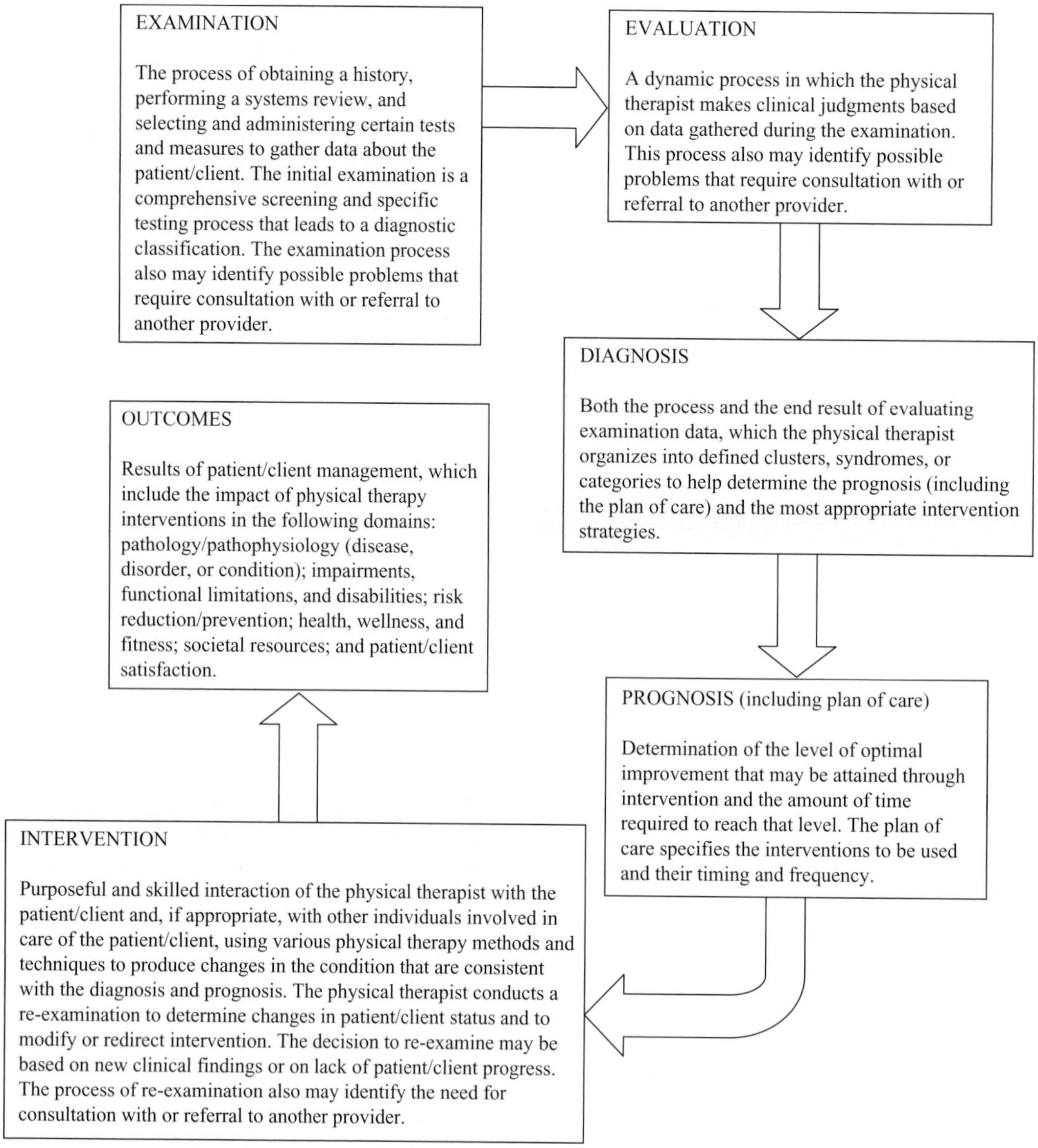

EXAMINATION

The process of obtaining a history, performing a systems review, and selecting and administering certain tests and measures to gather about the patient/client. The initial examination is a comprehensive screening and specific testing process that leads to a diagnostic classification. The examination process also may identify possible problems that require consultation with or referral to another provider.

EVALUATION

A dynamic process in which the physical therapist makes clinical judgments based on data gathered during the examination. This process also may identify possible problems that require consultation with or referral to another provider.

DIAGNOSIS

Both the process and the end result of evaluating examination data, which the physical therapist organizes into defined clusters, syndromes, or categories to help determine the prognosis (including the plan of care) and the most appropriate intervention strategies.

OUTCOMES

Results of patient/client management, which include the impact of physical therapy interventions in the following domains: pathology/pathophysiology (disease, disorder, or condition); impairments, functional limitations, and disabilities; risk reduction/prevention; health, wellness, and fitness; societal resources; and patient/client satisfaction.

PROGNOSIS (including plan of care)

Determination of the level of optimal improvement that may be attained through intervention and the amount of time required to reach that level. The plan of care specifies the interventions to be used and their timing and frequency.

INTERVENTION

Purposeful and skilled interaction of the physical therapist with the patient/client and, if appropriate, with other individuals involved in care of the patient/client, using various physical therapy methods and techniques to produce changes in the condition that are consistent with the diagnosis and prognosis. The physical therapist conducts a re-examination to determine changes in patient/client status and to modify or redirect intervention. The decision to re-examine may be based on new clinical findings or on lack of patient/client progress. The process of re-examination also may identify the need for consultation with or referral to another provider.

FIGURE 5-1 Elements of patient management leading to optimal outcomes

CLINICAL PEARL

Impairment—loss or abnormality of anatomic, physiologic, or psychological structure or function. Not all impairments are modified by physical therapy, and not all impairments cause activity limitations and participation restrictions.[14]

Primary Impairment—an impairment that can result from active pathology or disease. An example is a hip fracture with subsequent loss of ambulation and strength. Primary impairment can create secondary impairments and can lead to secondary pathology.

Secondary Impairment—an impairment that originates from primary impairment and pathology.[14] Using the hip fracture example, a secondary impairment could be the development of decubiti secondary to immobility.

Functional Limitation—a restriction of the ability to perform, at the level of the whole person, a physical action, activity, or task in an efficient, typically expected, or competent manner.[14]

Pathology and Pathophysiology

The term *pathology* is perhaps self-explanatory. It refers to any diagnosed disease, injury, disorder, or abnormal condition that is (1) characterized by a particular cluster of signs and symptoms and (2) recognized by either the patient or clinician as abnormal.[15–17]

Pathology may result in a change that manifests itself as a health condition producing an alteration in, or characteristic of, an individual's health status. Pathology is primarily identified at the cellular level and usually is determined by the physician's medical diagnosis.[16,17] The presence of pathology may lead to distress or interference with functional status. The severity of the pathology, and thus the impact that it has on a patient's functional status, depends on several factors. These factors include, but are not limited to:

► Comorbidity (the degree and location of edema, the quality of the vascular supply, the presence of infection, and the degree of atrophy)

TABLE 5-1	Disablement Model Comparisons			
WHO (ICIDH)	**NAGI Scheme**	**National Center for Medical Rehabilitation Research (NCMRR)**	**WHO (ICIDH)-2 (2001)**	**Health Related Quality of Life (HRQL)**
Disease The intrinsic pathology or disorder	**Pathology/ Pathophysiology** Interruption or interference with normal processes and efforts of an organism to regain normal state	**Pathophysiology** Interruption with normal physiologic developmental processes or structures	**Condition**	**Pathophysiology**
Impairment Loss or abnormality of psychological, physiologic, or anatomic structure or function	**Impairment** Anatomic, physiologic, mental or emotional abnormalities or loss	**Impairment** Loss of cognitive, emotional physiologic or anatomic structure or function	**Body Functions and Structure**	**Impairment**
Disability Restriction or lack of ability to perform an activity in a normal manner	**Functional limitation** Limitation in performance at the level of the whole organism or person	**Functional Limitation** Abnormality of or restriction or lack of ability to perform an action in the manner or range consistent with the purpose of an organ or organ system	**Activities** Activity limitations can cause secondary impairments	**Functional Limitation** ▶ Physical Function Component, which includes Basic Activities of Daily Living (BADLs) and Instrumental Activities of Daily Living (IADLs) ▶ Psychological Component, which includes the *various cognitive, perceptual, and personality traits of a person* ▶ Social Component, which involves the interaction of the person *within a larger social context or structure*
Handicap Disadvantage or disability that limits or prevents fulfillment of a normal role (depends on age, sex, sociocultural factors for the person)	**Disability** Limitation in performance of socially defined roles and tasks within a sociocultural and physical environment	**Disability** Limitation or inability in performing tasks, activities, and roles to levels expected within physical and social contexts	**Participation** Is context dependent (environmental and personal factors) Is one aspect of health-related quality of life	**Disability**
		Societal Limitation Restriction attributed to social policy or barriers that limit fulfillment of roles Examples include lack of accessibility and funding	**Contextual, environmental personal factors**	

ICIDH, International Classification of Impairments, Disabilities and Handicaps; WHO, World Health Organization.

▶ The patient's general physical health

▶ The age of the patient

▶ The patient's nutritional status

Patients generally are referred to physical therapy services with a medical diagnosis that is based on pathology (e.g., osteoarthritis of the hip). Although knowledge of pathology and pathophysiology can help the clinician predict the range, severity, and prognosis of a particular condition, a medical diagnosis does not tell the clinician how to manage the patient. A physical therapy diagnosis, on the other hand, is a diagnostic label that identifies the impact of a condition on function. When a patient is referred from a physician with a medical diagnosis, there may be four possible scenarios following the physical therapy examination[16]:

TABLE 5-2	Disablement Terminology
Term	**Definition**
Disease	A pathological condition of the body or abnormal entity with a characteristic group of signs and symptoms that affect the body
Signs	Directly observable or measurable evidence of physical abnormality
Symptoms	Subjective reactions to a physical abnormality
Impairments	Direct (primary): the results of pathology or disease states which can include any loss or abnormality of physiologic, anatomic, or psychologic structure or function Indirect (secondary): the sequelae or complications that originate from other systems which can result from preexisting impairments or the expanding multisystem dysfunction that occurs with prolonged inactivity, lack of adherence to suggested strategy/interventions, and ineffective plan of care, or lack of a rehabilitation intervention
Functional limitation	The restriction of the ability to perform, at the level of the whole person, a physical action, task, or activity, in an efficient, typically expected, or competent manner
Disability	An inability to perform or limitation in the performance of actions, tasks, and activities usually expected in specific social roles that are customary for the individual or expected for the person's status or role in a specific sociocultural context and physical environment (self-care, home management, work, and community/leisure)
Disablement risk factors	Behaviors (negative affect, psychosocial instability), attributes (disengaged lifestyle, limited education), or environmental influences (inadequate family support, limited financial/health resources) that increase the chances of developing impairments, functional limitations, or disability when an individual demonstrates an active pathology

Data from Guide to Physical Therapist Practice. Second Edition. American Physical Therapy Association. Phys Ther 81:9-746, 2001; O'Sullivan SB: Clinical decision-making, in O'Sullivan SB, Schmitz TJ (eds): Physical Rehabilitation (ed 5). Philadelphia, FA Davis, 2007, pp 3-24; Jette AM: Physical disablement concepts for physical therapy research and practice. Phys Ther 74:375-382, 1994.

1. The clinical findings are consistent with the physician's medical diagnosis. This scenario permits the physical therapist to proceed with interventions that are justified by changes in the patient's functional status.

2. The clinical findings suggest a pathologic or pathophysiologic condition that is inconsistent with the referring physician's diagnosis and is out of the scope of the practice of physical therapy. This scenario requires the physical therapist to either return the patient to the referring physician or make a referral to another practitioner.

3. The clinical findings suggest the presence of an additional pathologic or pathophysiologic condition that was not previously identified. If the newly identified pathophysiologic condition is within the scope of physical therapy practice, the physical therapist can continue to treat the patient. If, however, the newly identified pathophysiologic condition is not within the scope of physical therapy practice, the physical therapist is required to return the patient to the referring physician or to make a referral to another practitioner (e.g., speech therapist).

4. The clinical findings fail to identify the underlying cause. With this scenario, the physical therapist continues to test the signs and symptoms while providing interventions that are justified by changes in the patient's functional status.

If a physical therapy intervention is warranted, the goal of the intervention is to restore function, with the focus of the intervention on reducing and preventing risk factors and decreasing the impact of impairments, functional limitations, and disabilities.[16]

Impairments

The Guide defines *impairment* as any loss or abnormality of anatomic, physiologic, mental, or psychological structure or function that both (1) results from underlying changes in the normal state and (2) contributes to illness.[16] Thus, impairments can be viewed as abnormalities of structure or function as indicated by signs and symptoms. Verbrugge and Jette[3] suggest that disease symptoms are essentially impairments, and thus downstream from the pathologic process of the disease.

Impairments have the potential to create pain and subtle alterations in the normal functions of the involved joint and surrounding tissues. Impairments can be manifested objectively, for example, by reduced range of motion, articular deformity, abnormal gait, and the loss of strength, power, endurance, or proprioception. Impairments also can be manifested subjectively, for example, through pain (see later), tenderness, morning stiffness, or fatigue.

The definition of *impairment* refers to some form of loss. *Loss* or *loss of use* refers to a change from the normal or preexisting state. The term *normal* refers to a range representing healthy functioning, which can vary with age, gender, and other factors such as environmental conditions. For example, normal range of motion for knee flexion is deemed to be 150°.[17] Although a loss of more than 70° of knee flexion may prevent a patient from performing such activities as getting in and out of a bathtub and walking up and down steps, the patient may still be able to ambulate around the house.

It is important to note that physical impairment and physical functioning appear to be separate constructs that do not necessarily have a clear linear relationship. Furthermore, some measures of impairment are not correlated with patient function, bringing into question their meaningfulness as measurement tools.

One of the goals of the examination process is to determine which impairments are related to the patient's functional limitations. Once these have been identified, the clinician must then determine which impairments may be remedied by physical therapy intervention.

CLINICAL PEARL

It is worth noting that various definitions of impairment exist outside the realm of physical therapy. For example, the American Medical Association's (AMA) *Guide to the Evaluation of Permanent Impairment*[17] rate impairment using a whole person (WP) rating scale. Within this scale, a percentage score is assigned to an individual, depending on the amount of impairment. A WP rating of 0% is given to an individual with impairment if the impairment has no significant organ or body system functional consequences and does not limit the performance of common activities of daily living (ADLs). A 90% to 100% WP impairment indicates a very severe organ or body system impairment requiring the individual to be fully dependent on others for self-care, and approaching death.

Functional Limitations

A functional limitation is defined by The Guide as a restriction of the ability to perform a fundamental physical action, task, or activity in an efficient, typically expected, or competent manner.[16] In other words, functional limitations are restrictions in performing expected basic physical and mental actions. Examples of such functional limitations include difficulty with walking and an inability to put on shoes. The vast majority of the traditional tests used in physical therapy clinics, such as range of motion and strength, are measures of impairments, not function. Measurements of functional limitations include sensorimotor performance testing during such activities as walking, climbing, bending, transferring, lifting, and carrying.[16] It is important that these measurements assess the patient's ability to perform tasks that the patient feels are important (Table 5-3).

The process of identifying meaningful, achievable functional goals should be a collaborative effort between the clinician and the patient, the patient's family, or the patient's significant other.[16] To identify functional goals, Randall and McEwen[18] recommend the following steps:

1. Determine the patient's desired outcome for the intervention.
2. Develop an understanding of the patient's self-care, work, and leisure activities and the environments in which these activities occur.
3. Establish goals with the patient that relate to the desired outcomes (see Table 5-3).[18]

TABLE 5-3	Questions to Determine Desired Outcomes

1. If you were to concentrate your energies on one thing for yourself, what would it be?
2. What activities do you need help with that you would rather perform yourself?
3. What are your concerns about returning to work, home, school, or leisure activities?
4. What about your current situation would you like to be different in about 6 months? What would you like to be the same?

Data from Randall KE, McEwen IR: Writing patient-centered goals. Phys Ther 80:1197-1203, 2000; Winton PJ, Bailey DB: Communicating with families: examining practices and facilitating change, in Simeonsson JP, Simeonsson RJ (eds): Children with special needs: Family, culture, and society. Orlando, FL, Harcourt Brace Jovanovich, 1993, pp 69-89.

Once the goals have been agreed on, the clinician must write the goals so that they contain the following elements[18,19]:

▶ Who (the patient)
▶ Will do what (activities)
▶ Under what conditions (the home or work environment)
▶ How well (the amount of assistance, or number of attempts required for successful completion)
▶ By when (target date)

Thus, the functional examination creates a functional diagnosis, with functional goals. Once these functional goals are established, the clinician can grade them according to difficulty. Functional tasks can reproduce the whole task in its entirety or can break down the task to its required fundamental components and the physical demands necessary to perform each task. Regaining the smaller requirements may constitute the short-term goals, whereas completion of the whole task may become the long-term goal. For example, exercises to improve sit-to-stand transfers could be initiated by having the patient perform triceps push-ups on the chair handle, perform bilateral mini-squats, or exercise on the leg press, before progressing to the functional activity.

Disability

Disability may be defined as difficulty in the performance of social roles and tasks within a sociocultural and physical environment (from hygiene to hobbies, errands, to sleep), as a result of a health or physical problem.[6,7,9,20–23] Disability, which may be temporary or permanent, is the gap between what a person can do and what the person needs or wants to do. The Americans with Disabilities Act (ADA) of 1989[24] marked the first explicit national goal of achieving equal opportunity, independent living, and economic self-sufficiency for individuals with disabilities.[25] Disability is a problem that encompasses a wide range of issues, from very specific topics to the basic question of what it means to be human.

Three main models are generally used to describe disability: the moral, medical, and social models.[26] Table 5-4 compares these three models along seven dimensions: the

TABLE 5-4	Comparison of the Moral, Medical, and Social Models of Disability		
Measure	**Moral**	**Medical**	**Social**
Meaning of disability	A defect caused by moral lapse or sins, failure of faith, evil; test of faith	A defect in or failure of a bodily system that is inherently abnormal and pathological	A social construct; problems reside in the environment that fails to accommodate people with disability
Moral implications	Brings shame to the person with the disability and his or her family	A medical abnormality due to genetics, bad health habits, person's behavior	Society has failed a segment of its citizens and oppresses them
Sample ideas	"God gives us only what we can bear" or "There's a reason I was chosen to have this disability"	Clinical descriptions of "patient" in medical terminology; isolation of body parts	"Nothing about us without us" or "Civil rights, not charity"
Origins	Oldest model and still most prevalent worldwide	Mid-19th century; most common model in the United States; entrenched in most rehabilitation clinics and journals	1975, following demonstrations by people with disabilities in support of the yet-unsigned Rehabilitation Act
Goals of intervention	Spiritual or divine, acceptance	"Cure" or amelioration of the disability to the greatest extent possible	Political, economic, social, and policy systems, increased access and inclusion
Benefits of model	An acceptance of being selected; a special relationship with God; a sense of greater purpose to the disability	A lessened sense of shame and stigma; faith in medical intervention; spurs medical and technologic advances	Promotes integration of the disability into their self; a sense of community and pride; depathologizing of disability
Negative effects	Shame; ostracization; need to conceal the disability or person with the disability	Paternalistic; promotes benevolence and charity; services for but not by people with disabilities	Powerlessness in the face of necessary broad social and political changes; challenges to prevailing ideas

Data from Olkin R: Could you hold the door for me? Including disability in diversity. Cultur Divers Ethnic Minor Psychol 8:130-137, 2002.

meaning of disabilities, moral implications of disability, sample ideas, origins, goals of intervention, and benefits and negative effects of the model.[26] The moral and medical models share in common the perspective that disability resides within the individual and carries with it a degree of stigma or pathology.[26] In contrast, the social model locates the disablement in the environment and in society, which fail to appropriately accommodate and include people with disabilities.[26]

Disability is not necessarily related to any health impairment or medical condition, although a medical condition or impairment may cause or contribute to disability. For example, associations between pathology and disability have been found for several health conditions. These include diabetes,[27-29] cardiovascular diseases,[30,31] musculoskeletal diseases,[22,32,33] and vision-related diseases.[34] The rating of perceived difficulty in performing various activities can be considered the primary assessment of disability, whereas the rating of actual dependence on assistance is an assessment of the consequence of disability.[35]

For any given level of health or specific diagnosis, some people will be disabled and others will not. Thus, impairments and functional limitations are not related to disability in a linear fashion. It is even possible for two patients who have the same disease and similar impairments and functional limitations to have two different levels of disability. For example, degenerative joint disease of the spine that prevents heavy lifting likely has a greater impact on a construction worker than it does on a bank president.

CLINICAL PEARL

While many functional limitations can be categorized using the various disablement models, difficulty arises when trying to categorize such limitations as poor postural control, dysfunctional gait, and poor balance. This is because these limitations are controlled by multiple systems, making it difficult to categorize them as impairments or functional limitations.

Although a degree of inevitability is implied in many of the disablement models, many factors can have an impact on the pathology–disability pathway or disablement process. Some of these factors are modifiable; some are not. Characteristics of an illness that are not amenable to modification may be termed *contextual variables*. These innate characteristics of a person include age, sex, ethnic background, and socioeconomic status. In contrast, modifiable factors are characteristics that an individual can control or adjust. The impact that the modifiable factors have on the pathology–disability pathway or disablement process can depend on both the capacities of the individual and the expectations that are imposed on the individual by those in the immediate social and occupational environment.[25] Escalante and del Rincon[36] use the term *external modifiers* to describe those secondary conditions that may influence the level of disability but are not directly related to the disease process itself. These external modifiers can include the presence of depression or comorbidity (e.g., pressure sores, contractures, urinary tract infections). Broader definitions for these conditions include self-concept, work and social participation, health-related economic consequences for the individual or family, and other family members.[9,37] Specific examples of modifiable patient factors include:

▶ *Level of activity.* A number of studies have made associations between physical activity levels and the onset of disability.[27,28,38–47]

▶ *Reaction to the illness.* Different cultural backgrounds are associated with different beliefs about pain, coping strategies, expressions of pain, and response to healthcare.[48,49] The term *sick role* has been used to define a status accorded to the individual by himself or herself and other members of society that may be variably associated with a medical condition.[25] An individual's sick role reflects not only his or her primary condition but also any additional or secondary conditions.[4,50]

▶ *Educational background.* Patients with less formal education tend to have an increased frequency of disability.[51,52]

▶ *Compensatory and coping strategies.* Some people simply do not have the emotional and social resources to deal with life, particularly in times of adversity.[53]

▶ *Pain tolerance and motivation.* Various studies[49,54] have revealed ethnic and gender differences in responses to both clinical and experimental pain. Specifically, investigators have recently indicated that African Americans report greater levels of pain than whites for such conditions as glaucoma, acquired immunodeficiency syndrome, migraine headache, jaw pain, postoperative pain, myofascial pain, angina pectoris, joint pain, nonspecific daily pain, and arthritis.[55] Interpretations of such findings remain difficult, however, because of potential group differences in disease severity and physician management.[55] There are also disparate reports about gender differences in sensitivity to pain in humans and in animals, indicating that women have a lower tolerance of pain than men.[56–58] Whether women are more willing to report pain than men are, or experience pain differently than men do, is unclear. Whatever the reasons for the differences in pain tolerance and motivation, there is perhaps reason to suppose that improved pain tolerance and motivation might be instrumental in reducing impairment and disability. The chronic pain-adaptation model of Lund and colleagues[32] describes a decreased activation of the muscles during movements in which they act as agonists and an increased activation during movements that require that they adopt the role of antagonists. These changes in muscle activation, characteristic of several types of chronic musculoskeletal pain, are described as a normal protective adaptation to avoid further pain and possible damage.[32]

▶ *Personal and health habits.* The link between disability and a health behavior, such as excessive alcohol use, is subtle because there are many potential pathways. The link between body weight and both morbidity and mortality has been examined extensively, but relatively little research has investigated the relation between body weight and disability. Among the studies that have investigated this relation, the findings are inconsistent.[59–62]

▶ *Level of social support.* The *family* is the primary unit of society and the one in which the earliest and most powerful social learning occurs.[25] The literature on the role of the family in the development and maintenance of chronic pain and disability is extensive. Dysfunctional family systems may promote, permit, and maintain chronic pain and disability.[25]

▶ *Marital status.* Considerable research shows that the spouse's reaction can modify behavior of patients with chronic pain and disability.[25]

▶ *Extent to which involved in litigation and compensation.* Few issues around disability have given rise to more controversy than the question of litigation, compensation, and secondary gain. Anecdotal clinical and legal experience shows general agreement that some claimants magnify or exaggerate their symptoms and disability to varying degrees during medical examination carried out specifically for legal proceedings.[25]

EXAMINATION

An *examination* refers to the gathering of information from the chart, other caregivers, the patient, the patient's family, caretakers, and friends in order to identify and define the patient's problem(s) and to design an intervention plan.[16] The examination process involves a complex relationship between the clinician and the patient. Given the melting-pot society that we now live in, patients are likely to come from diverse cultural and ethnic backgrounds, which are influenced by individual factors related to the psychological and socioeconomic conditions that affect health, behavioral practices, and access to care. Although most patients are amenable to a therapeutic interaction because they realize the benefits, some patients can be difficult to deal with. Groves[63] identified four types of difficult patients (Table 5-5). Every attempt should be made by the clinician to make each patient interaction a positive one. There is plenty of high-quality research pointing to the benefits of good communication between the clinician and patient, including improved diagnosis and outcomes, treatment adherence, patient satisfaction, and reduced litigation.

CLINICAL PEARL

The goal of the examination is to analyze and identify any causal relationships between the impairments, functional limitations, and disabilities. For example, an impairment such as an articular deformity may cause functional limitations that in turn can lead to disability. It is also important to remember that the absence of impairments or disease does not necessarily correlate with good health. Good health must be viewed as a combination of mental, social, and physical well-being.

TABLE 5-5	Difficult Patient Types
Type	**Description**
Dependent clingers	This type can escalate from mild requests for reassurance to repeated overt demands for explanations and affection. Unfortunately, this type may have no discernible medical illness, or they may have severe, chronic, or life-threatening disorders, which makes them difficult to treat. The high level of dependency that they display may eventually lead to aversion toward the patient. Early signs of this type are demonstrations of genuine but extreme gratitude. The clinger must be told as early as possible, and as tactfully and firmly as possible, that the clinician has limitations to time and stamina.
Entitled demanders	This type resembles dependent clingers in the profundity of their neediness, but they use intimidation, devaluation, and guilt induction, which results from a deep-seated fear of abandonment. The patient may try to control the clinician by withholding payment or threatening litigation. "Entitlement" serves for some persons the functions that faith and hope serve in better adjusted ones. Ideally, the clinician should avoid getting entangled in complicated logical (or illogical) debates with this type of patient.
Manipulative help rejecters	This type of patient appears to feel that no type of intervention will help, and following every attempt they return again and again to the clinic to report that, once again, the regimen did not work. In an attempt to maintain their relationship with the clinician, when one of their symptoms is relieved, another mysteriously appears in its place.
Self-destructive deniers	This type of patient demonstrates self-destructiveness and seem to glory in his or her own self-destruction. Although the temptation on the part of the clinician is to wash their hands of the patient, the clinician should try to work with diligence and compassion to preserve the denier as long as possible, just as one does with any other patient with a terminal illness.

Data from Groves JE: Taking care of the hateful patient. N Engl J Med 298(16):883-887, 1978.

The aims of the examination process are to provide an efficient and effective exchange and to develop a rapport between the clinician and the patient. The success of this interaction involves a myriad of factors. The primary responsibility of a clinician is to make decisions in the best interest of the patient. Although the approach to the examination should vary with each patient, and from condition to condition, there are several fundamental components to the examination process. Successful clinicians are those who demonstrate effective communication, sound clinical reasoning, critical judgment, creative decision making, and competence. To successfully perform an examination, the clinician must choose, apply, and interpret findings from a wide variety of tests and measures.

CLINICAL PEARL

From the patient's point of view, there is no substitute for interest, acceptance, and especially empathy on the part of the clinician.[64]

Much about becoming a clinician relates to an ability to communicate with the patient, the patient's family, and the other members of the healthcare team. Communication between the clinician and the patient, which involves interacting with the patient using terms he or she can understand (see Chapter 8), begins when the clinician first meets the patient and continues throughout any future sessions. The introduction to the patient should be handled in a professional yet empathetic tone. Special attention needs to be paid to cultural diversity (Table 5-6) and the avoidance of preconceived notions about a particular culture or ethnicity (Table 5-7). The nonverbal cues, such as voice volume, postures, gestures, and eye contact, are especially important, because they often are performed subconsciously and can be misinterpreted. The appearance of the clinician is also important, if a professional image is to be projected.

The examination is an ongoing process that begins with the patient referral or initial entry and continues throughout the course of rehabilitation. During the examination phase, the clinician hypothesizes the clinical problem, then chooses and implements measures to test the hypotheses. The examination must be performed with a scientific rigor that follows a predictable and strictly ordered thought process. The purpose of the examination is to obtain information that identifies and measures a change from normal. This is determined using information related by the patient, in conjunction with clinical signs, symptoms, and findings.

CLINICAL PEARL

▶ A sign is an observable, objective measure that can often be quantified by using valid and reliable measurement instruments.

▶ A symptom is a subjective report from a patient that accompanies a pathology or dysfunction.

TABLE 5-6	Culture and Ethnicity
Culture	The integration of learned, not inherited, behaviors that are characteristic to a society. These behavioral standards include fundamental values, beliefs, and customs.
Ethnicity	An affiliation with a group of people who share a common racial, national, religious, linguistic, or cultural background.

TABLE 5-7	Interacting with Culturally Diverse Patient Populations

▶ Avoid using stereotypes. Although an individual may share characteristics with others of the same culture, each individual will also have unique differences.

▶ Respect cultural and religious differences.

▶ Avoid interpreting ethical cultural preferences based on dress, manner, and physical appearance.

Data from Metzgar ED: The health history, in Morton PG (ed): Health Assessment (ed 2). Philadelphia, FA Davis, 1995, pp 1-32.

The examination should not be viewed as an algorithm. Rather, it is a framework that has specific points that can be applied to a variety of situations. The strength of an examination relies on the accuracy of the findings of the testing procedures. Diagnostic tests are divided into two main categories[65]:

1. Tests that result in a discrete outcome—they permit interpretations from the test as present/absent, disease/not disease, mild/moderate/severe.

2. Tests that result in a continuous outcome—they provide data on an interval or scale of measurement such as degrees of range of motion.

For the clinician to formulate an appropriate interpretation and accurate final diagnosis, the tests chosen must be useful. Examination tools can be divided into two categories[66]:

▶ *Performance-based or self-report measures.* Performance-based measures involve the clinician's performance of the test or observation of patient performance. Examples include assessment of joint mobility, muscle strength, or balance. Self-report measures involve the patient rating his or her performance during activities such as walking, stair climbing, or sporting activity based on the ability to perform a task, difficulty with the task, help needed for the task, and pain during performance of the task. The perception of pain is highly specific, and different individuals may be impaired by pain to differing degrees. Although absolute quantification of pain is not possible, its severity may be estimated using a visual analogue scale or a numeric scale. More complex scales exist including the Pain Disability Index (PDI)[67-69] (Table 5-8) and the McGill Pain Questionnaire (MPQ) (Table 5-9).[70-72]

The PDI is a self-report instrument that has been used to assess the degree to which chronic pain interferes with various daily activities. The PDI consists of a series of 0-to-10 scales on which an individual rates pain-related interference. The seven categories that make up the scale are family/home responsibilities, recreation, social activity, occupation, sexual behavior, self-care, and life-support activities (e.g., eating, sleeping, and breathing). An initial study[69] found the PDI to be effective in discriminating patients immediately post-surgery (high impairment) from patients several months removed from surgery (low impairment).[69] A subsequent study[68] showed the PDI to be sensitive to differences between outpatients (low impairment) and inpatients (high impairment) with chronic pain.[67]

The MPQ contains a list of words chosen to reflect the sensory, affective, and evaluative components of the pain experience.

▶ *Generic or disease-specific measures.* A number of generic or disease-specific measures currently exist that examine the performance of functional activities. Disease-specific measures are questionnaires that concentrate on a region of primary interest that is generally relevant to the patient and clinician.[73] As a result of this focus on a regional disease state, the likelihood of increased responsiveness is higher. Some examples of the primary focus of these instruments include populations (rheumatoid arthritis), symptoms (back pain), and function (activities of daily living).[73] The disadvantage of a disease-specific outcome is that general information is lost, and therefore, it is generally recommended that when assessing patient outcomes, both a disease-specific and a generic outcome measure should be used.[73]

CLINICAL PEARL

The clinician must always remember that measurements may appear to be objective but that the interpretation of any measurement is always subjective.[74]

Patient discomfort should always be kept to a minimum. It is important that examination procedures only be performed to the point at which symptoms are provoked or begin to increase, if they are not present at rest.

The examination consists of three components of equal importance: (1) patient history, (2) systems review, and (3) tests and measures.[16] These three components are closely related, in that they often occur concurrently. One further element, observation, occurs throughout.

History

One of the purposes of the history is to focus the examination. The history usually precedes the systems review and the tests and measures components of the examination, but it may also occur concurrently. Whenever it occurs, it should always be used in conjunction with the findings from the system review and the tests and measures rather than performed in a vacuum. Information about the patient's history and current health status is obtained from interviews and review of the medical record. In general, the history can help the clinician to:

▶ Develop a working relationship with the patient and establish lines of communication with the patient. To help establish a rapport with the patient, the clinician should discuss the information provided on the medical history form with the patient at either the initial or subsequent visits.

▶ Determine the chief complaint, its mechanism of injury, its severity, and its impact on the patient's function. It is worth remembering that a patient's chief complaint can sometimes differ from the chief concern, but both should be addressed.

TABLE 5-8	The Pain Disability Index

The rating scales below are designed to measure the degree to which several aspects of your life are presently disrupted by chronic pain. In other words, we would like to know how much your pain is preventing you from doing what you would normally do, or from doing it as well as you normally would. Respond to each category by indicating the *overall* impact of pain in your life, not just the pain at its worst.

For each of the 7 categories of life activity listed, please circle the number on the scale that describes the level of disability you typically experience. A score of 0 means no disability at all, and a score of 10 signifies that all of the activities in which you would normally be involved have been totally disrupted or prevented by your pain.

(1) FAMILY/HOME RESPONSIBILITIES

This category refers to activities related to the home or family. It includes chores or duties performed around the house (e.g., yard work) and errands or favors for other family members (e.g., driving children from school).

0	1	2	3	4	5	6	7	8	9	10
No disability										Total disability

(2) RECREATION

This category includes hobbies, sports, and other similar leisure-time activities.

0	1	2	3	4	5	6	7	8	9	10
No disability										Total disability

(3) SOCIAL ACTIVITY

This category refers to activities that involve participation with friends and acquaintances other than family members. It includes parties, theater, concerts, dining out, and other social functions.

0	1	2	3	4	5	6	7	8	9	10
No disability										Total disability

(4) OCCUPATION

This category refers to activities that are a part of or directly related to one's job. This includes nonpaying jobs as well, such as that of a housewife or volunteer worker.

0	1	2	3	4	5	6	7	8	9	10
No disability										Total disability

(5) SEXUAL BEHAVIOR

This category refers to the frequency and quality of one's sex life.

0	1	2	3	4	5	6	7	8	9	10
No disability										Total disability

(6) SELF-CARE

This category includes activities that involve personal maintenance and independent daily living (e.g., taking a shower, driving, getting dressed, etc.).

0	1	2	3	4	5	6	7	8	9	10
No disability										Total disability

(7) LIFE-SUPPORT ACTIVITY

This category refers to basic life-supporting behaviors such as eating, sleeping, and breathing.

0	1	2	3	4	5	6	7	8	9	10
No disability										Total disability

Data from Pollard CA: Preliminary validity study of Pain Disability Index. Percep Motor Skills 59:974, 1984.

- ▶ Ascertain the specific location and nature of the symptoms.
- ▶ Determine the irritability of the symptoms.
- ▶ Establish a baseline of measurements.
- ▶ Ascertain which medications the patient is currently taking and whether they are prescribed or over-the-counter.
- ▶ Elicit information about the history of the current condition.

- ▶ Confirm that the patient does not have any physiologic changes that could adversely affect tolerance and ability to perform various tasks or activities. This is particularly important in the elderly population where changes in vision, auditory acuity, mental capacity, and tactile sense may be diminished.
- ▶ Determine the goals and expectations of the patient from the physical therapy intervention. It is important that

TABLE 5-9	Modified McGill Pain Questionnaire

Patient's Name _____ Date _____

Directions: Many words can describe pain. Some of these words are listed below. If you are experiencing any pain, check (√) every word that describes your pain.

A. Flickering
   Quivering
   Pulsing
   Throbbing
   Beating
   Pounding

B. Jumping
   Flashing
   Shooting

C. Pricking
   Boring
   Drilling
   Stabbing

D. Sharp
   Cutting
   Lacerating

E. Pinching
   Pressing
   Gnawing
   Cramping
   Crushing

F. Tugging
   Pulling
   Wrenching

G. Hot
   Burning
   Scalding
   Searing

H. Tingling
   Itchy
   Smarting
   Stinging

I. Dull
   Sore
   Hurting
   Aching
   Heavy

J. Tender
   Taut
   Rasping
   Splitting

K. Tiring
   Exhausting

L. Sickening
   Suffocating

M. Fearful
   Frightful
   Terrifying

N. Punishing
   Grueling
   Cruel
   Vicious
   Killing

O. Wretched
   Blinding

P. Annoying
   Troublesome
   Intense
   Unbearable

Q. Spreading
   Radiating
   Penetrating
   Piercing

R. Tight
   Numb
   Drawing
   Squeezing
   Tearing

S. Cool
   Cold
   Freezing

T. Nagging
   Nauseating
   Agonizing
   Dreadful
   Torturing

KEY TO PAIN QUESTIONNAIRE
Group A: Suggests vascular disorder
Groups B–H: Suggests neurogenic disorder
Group I: Suggests musculoskeletal disorder
Groups J–T: Suggests emotional disorder

SCORING GUIDE: ADD UP TOTAL NUMBER OF CHECKS (√):
Total: 4–8 = NORMAL
   8–10 = Focusing too much on pain
   10–16 = May be helped more by a clinical psychologist than by a physical therapist
   >16 = Unlikely to respond to therapy procedures

the clinician and patient discuss and determine mutually agreed-on anticipated goals and expected outcomes. The discussion can help the clinician determine whether the patient has realistic expectations or will need further patient education concerning his or her condition and typical recovery time frames.

▶ Elicit reports of potentially life-threatening symptoms, or *red flags*, that require an immediate medical referral.

CLINICAL PEARL

It is important to remember that symptoms can be experienced without the presence of recognized clinical signs, and that signs can be present in the absence of symptoms.

Pain. Pain, felt by everyone at some point or other, is considered an emotional experience and is the most common determinant for a patient to seek intervention. It is, therefore, often the patient's chief complaint. Pain perception and the response to a painful experience can be influenced by a variety of cognitive processes, including anxiety, tension, depression, past pain experiences, and cultural influences.[75] Pain is a broad and significant symptom that can be described using many descriptors. Perhaps the simplest descriptors for pain are acute and chronic.

Acute pain can be defined as "the normal, predicted physiological response to an adverse chemical, thermal, or mechanical stimulus . . . associated with surgery, trauma, and acute illness."[76] This type of pain usually precipitates a visit to a physician, because it has one or more of the following characteristics[77]:

117

▶ It is new and has not been experienced before.

▶ It is severe and disabling.

▶ It is continuous, lasting for more than several minutes, or recurs very frequently.

▶ The site of the pain may cause alarm (e.g., chest or eye).

▶ In addition to the sensory and affective components, acute pain is typically characterized by anxiety. This may produce a fight-or-flight autonomic response, which is normally used for survival needs. This autonomic reaction is also associated with an increase in systolic and diastolic blood pressure, a decrease in gut motility and salivatory flow, increased muscle tension, and papillary distention.[78,79]

CLINICAL PEARL

▶ Hyperalgesia is an increased response to noxious stimulus. Primary hyperalgesia occurs at the site of injury, whereas secondary hyperalgesia occurs outside the site of injury.

▶ Allodynia is defined as pain in response to a previously innocuous stimulus.

▶ Referred pain is a site adjacent to or at a distance from the site of an injury's origin. Referred pain can occur from muscle, joint, and viscera. For example, the pain felt during a myocardial infarction is often felt in the neck, shoulders, and back rather than in the chest, the site of the injury.

Acute pain following trauma, or the insidious onset of a musculoskeletal condition, is typically chemical in nature. Although motions aggravate the pain, they cannot be used to alleviate the symptoms. In contrast, cessation of movement (absolute rest) tends to alleviate the pain, although not necessarily immediately. The structures most sensitive to chemical irritation in order of sensitivity are:

▶ The periosteum and joint capsule

▶ Subchondral bone, tendon and ligament

▶ Muscle and cortical bone layer

▶ The synovium and articular cartilage

CLINICAL PEARL

The aching type of pain, associated with degenerative arthritis and muscle disorders, is often accentuated by activity and lessened by rest. Pain that is not alleviated by rest, and that is not associated with acute trauma, may indicate the presence of a serious disorder such as a tumor or aneurysm. This pain is often described as deep, constant, and boring and is apt to be more noticeable and more intense at night.[80]

Chronic pain is typically more aggravating than worrying, last for more than six months, and has the following characteristics[77]:

▶ It has been experienced before and has remitted spontaneously, or after simple measures.

▶ It is usually mild to moderate in intensity.

▶ It is usually of limited duration, although it can persist for long periods (persistent pain).

▶ The pain site does not cause alarm (e.g., knee and ankle).

▶ There are no alarming associated symptoms. However, patients with chronic pain may be more prone to depression and disrupted interpersonal relationships.[70,81–83]

The symptoms of chronic pain typically behave in a mechanical fashion, in that they are provoked by activity or repeated movements and reduced with rest or a movement in the opposite direction.

CLINICAL PEARL

Referred pain, which can be either acute or chronic, is pain perceived to be in an area that seems to have little or no relation to the existing pathology.

The production of pain typically occurs in one of four ways[84]:

1. Mechanical deformation resulting in the application of sufficient mechanical forces to stress, deform, or damage a structure.

2. Excessive heat or cold.

3. The presence of chemical irritants in sufficient quantities or concentrations. Key mediators that have been identified include bradykinin, serotonin, histamine, potassium ions, adenosine triphosphate, protons, prostaglandins, nitric oxide, leukotrienes, cytokines, and growth factors.[76]

4. Ischemia restriction of blood to a structure e.g., myocardial infarction

CLINICAL PEARL

Chemical, or inflammatory, pain is more constant and is less affected by movements or positions than mechanical pain. Thus, specific movements or positions should influence pain of a mechanical nature.

Over the past decade, researchers have begun to investigate the influence of pain on patterns of neuromuscular activation and control.[85] It has been suggested that the presence of pain leads to inhibition or delayed activation of muscles or muscle groups that perform key synergistic functions to limit unwanted motion.[86] This inhibition usually occurs in deep muscles, local to the involved joint, that perform a synergistic function in order to control joint stability.[87–89] It is now also becoming apparent that in addition to being influenced by pain, motor activity and emotional states can, in turn, influence pain perception.[85,90]

Pain may be variable, constant, or intermittent.

▶ *Variable.* This is pain that is perpetual, but that varies in intensity. Variable pain usually indicates the involvement of both a chemical and a mechanical source.

▶ *Constant.* The mechanical cause of constant pain is less understood but is thought to be the result of the deformation of collagen, which compresses or stretches the nociceptive free nerve endings, with the excessive forces being perceived as pain.[84]

CLINICAL PEARL

It is important to assume that all reports of pain by the patient are serious until proven otherwise with a thorough examination.[91]

▶ *Intermittent.* This type of pain is unlikely to be caused by a chemical irritant. Usually, this type of pain is caused by prolonged postures, a loose intra-articular body, or impingement of a musculoskeletal structure.

CLINICAL PEARL

Constant pain following an injury continues until the healing process has sufficiently reduced the concentration of noxious irritants.

Unfortunately, the source of the pain is not always easy to identify, because most patients present with both mechanical and chemical pain.

When examining a patient with complaints of pain, the clinician must determine the following details about the pain:

▶ *Location.* The location of the pain can indicate which areas need to be included in the physical examination. Information about how the location of the pain has

changed since the onset can indicate whether a condition is worsening or improving. In general, as a condition worsens, the pain distribution becomes more widespread and distal (peripheralizes). As the condition improves, the symptoms tend to become more localized (centralized). A body chart may be used to record the location of symptoms (Figure 5-2). Some of the more common causes of localized pain are depicted in Figures 5-3 through 5-6.

CLINICAL PEARL

Symptoms that are distal and superficial are easier for the patient to specifically localize than those that are proximal and deep.

It must be remembered that the location of pain for many musculoskeletal conditions is quite separate from the source, especially in those peripheral joints that are more proximal, such as the shoulder and the hip. For example, a cervical radiculopathy can produce pain throughout the upper extremity. The term *referred pain* is used to describe symptoms that have their origin at a site other than where the patient feels the pain. For example, pain due to osteoarthritis of the hip is often felt in the anterior groin and thigh along with the sclerotomes or dermatomes for L2 and L3. The concept of referred

---

Name: _____

Date: _____ **Signature:** _____

Please use the diagram below to indicate where you feel symptoms right now. Use the following key to indicate different types of symptoms.

KEY: Pins and Needles = 000000   Stabbing = ///////   Burning = XXXXX   Deep Ache = ZZZZZZ

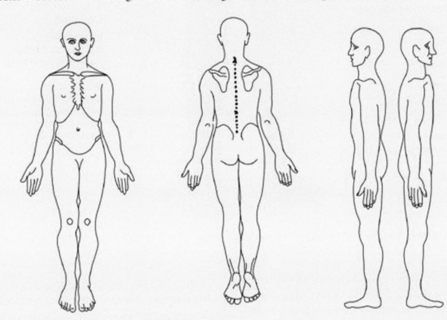

Please use the three scales below to rate your pain over the past 24 hours. Use the upper line to describe your pain level right now. Use the other scales to rate your pain at its worst and best over the past 24 hours.

RATE YOUR PAIN: 0 = NO PAIN, 10 = EXTREMELY INTENSE

1.	Right now	0	1	2	3	4	5	6	7	8	9	10
2.	At its worst	0	1	2	3	4	5	6	7	8	9	10
3.	At its best	0	1	2	3	4	5	6	7	8	9	10

FIGURE 5-2 Body chart

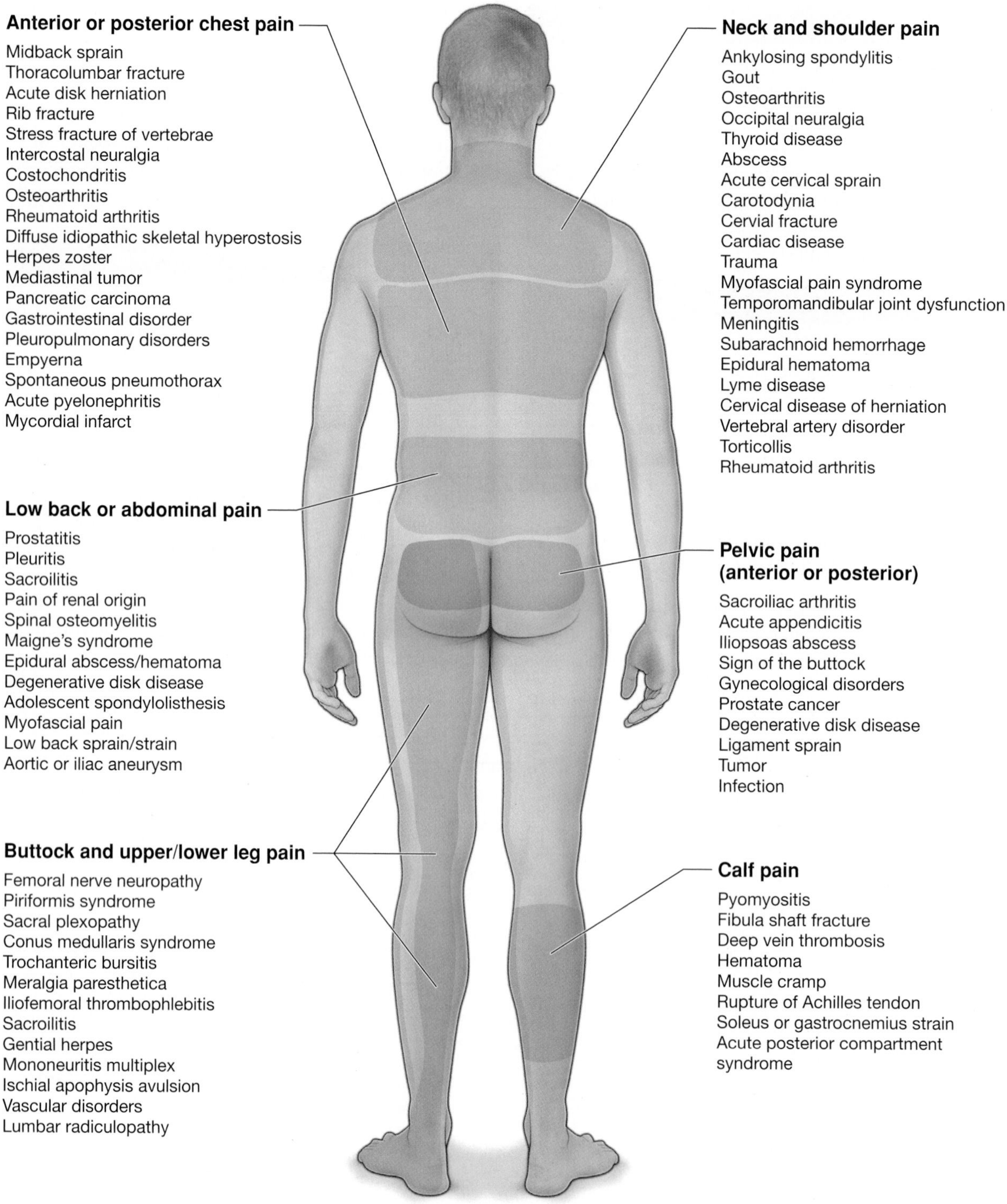

Anterior or posterior chest pain

Midback sprain
Thoracolumbar fracture
Acute disk herniation
Rib fracture
Stress fracture of vertebrae
Intercostal neuralgia
Costochondritis
Osteoarthritis
Rheumatoid arthritis
Diffuse idiopathic skeletal hyperostosis
Herpes zoster
Mediastinal tumor
Pancreatic carcinoma
Gastrointestinal disorder
Pleuropulmonary disorders
Empyerna
Spontaneous pneumothorax
Acute pyelonephritis
Mycordial infarct

Low back or abdominal pain

Prostatitis
Pleuritis
Sacroilitis
Pain of renal origin
Spinal osteomyelitis
Maigne's syndrome
Epidural abscess/hematoma
Degenerative disk disease
Adolescent spondylolisthesis
Myofascial pain
Low back sprain/strain
Aortic or iliac aneurysm

Buttock and upper/lower leg pain

Femoral nerve neuropathy
Piriformis syndrome
Sacral plexopathy
Conus medullaris syndrome
Trochanteric bursitis
Meralgia paresthetica
Iliofemoral thrombophlebitis
Sacroilitis
Gential herpes
Mononeuritis multiplex
Ischial apophysis avulsion
Vascular disorders
Lumbar radiculopathy

Neck and shoulder pain

Ankylosing spondylitis
Gout
Osteoarthritis
Occipital neuralgia
Thyroid disease
Abscess
Acute cervical sprain
Carotodynia
Cervial fracture
Cardiac disease
Trauma
Myofascial pain syndrome
Temporomandibular joint dysfunction
Meningitis
Subarachnoid hemorrhage
Epidural hematoma
Lyme disease
Cervical disease of herniation
Vertebral artery disorder
Torticollis
Rheumatoid arthritis

Pelvic pain (anterior or posterior)

Sacroiliac arthritis
Acute appendicitis
Iliopsoas abscess
Sign of the buttock
Gynecological disorders
Prostate cancer
Degenerative disk disease
Ligament sprain
Tumor
Infection

Calf pain

Pyomyositis
Fibula shaft fracture
Deep vein thrombosis
Hematoma
Muscle cramp
Rupture of Achilles tendon
Soleus or gastrocnemius strain
Acute posterior compartment syndrome

FIGURE 5-3 Potential causes of cervical, thoracic, lumbar, pelvic, and posterior lower extremity pain

pain is often difficult for patients to understand. An explanation of referred pain enables the patient to better understand and answer questions about symptoms they might otherwise have felt irrelevant. If the extremity appears to be the source of the pain, the clinician should attempt to reproduce the pain by loading the peripheral tissues. If this proves unsuccessful, a full investigation of the spinal structures must ensue.

► *Behavior of symptoms.* The presence of pain should not always be viewed negatively by the clinician. After all, its presence helps to determine the location of the injury, and its behavior aids the clinician in determining the stage of

healing and the impact it has on the patient's function. For example, whether the pain is worsening, improving, or unchanging provides information on the effectiveness of an intervention. In addition, a gradual increase in the intensity of the symptoms over time may indicate to the clinician that the condition is worsening or that the condition is nonmusculoskeletal in nature.[92,93] Maitland[94] introduced the concept of the *degree of irritability*. An irritable structure has the following characteristics:

■ *A progressive increase in the severity of the pain with movement or a specific posture.* An ability to reproduce

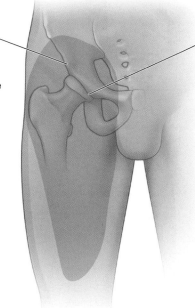

Dislocation and fracture of the hip
Hip or pelvis fracture
Pubic fracture
Femoral neck stress fracture
Osteoarthritis of the hip
Septic arthritis of the hip
Osteoid osteoma
Reiter's syndrome
Synovitis of the hip in children or adolescents
Avascular necrosis of the femoral head

Snapping hip
Trochanteric bursitis
Iliopsoas abscess
Iliofemoral venous thrombosis
Lumbar disk herniation
Obturator, femoral, or inguinal hernia
Osteomyelitis of the pubis
Compartment syndrome
Sexually transmitted disease
Muscle strain or contusion
Lateral cutaneous (femoral) nerve of the thigh entrapment

FIGURE 5-4 Potential causes of trochanteric, pubic, and thigh pain

constant pain with a specific motion or posture indicates an irritable structure.

- *Symptoms increased with minimal activity.* An irritable structure is one that requires very little to increase the symptoms.

- *Increased latent response of symptoms.* Symptoms that do not resolve within a few minutes following a movement or posture indicate an irritable structure.

If the behavior of the symptoms includes locking or giving way, the clinician must elicit further details about the causes of the hypomobility, hypermobility, or instability.

▶ *Frequency and duration.* The frequency and duration of the patient's symptoms can help the clinician to classify the injury according to its stage of healing: acute (inflammatory), subacute (migratory and proliferative), and chronic (remodeling).

- *Acute conditions:* present for 7 to 10 days

- *Subacute conditions:* present for 10 days to several weeks

- *Chronic conditions:* present for more than several weeks

In the case of a musculoskeletal injury that has been present without any formal intervention for a few months, there is a good possibility that adaptive shortening of the healing collagenous tissue has occurred, which may result in a failure to heal, and the persistence of symptoms.[95] The persistence of symptoms usually indicates a poorer prognosis, as it may indicate the presence of a chronic pain syndrome. Chronic pain syndromes have the potential to complicate the intervention process.[95]

If the frequency and duration of the patient's symptoms are reported to be increasing, it is likely the condition is worsening. Conversely, a decrease in the frequency and duration of the symptoms generally indicates that the condition is improving.

▶ *Aggravating and easing factors.* Of particular importance are the patient's chief complaint and the relationship of that complaint to specific aggravating activities or postures. Questions must be asked to determine whether the pain is sufficient to prevent sleep or to wake the patient at night and the effect that activities of daily living, work, sex, and so forth, have on the pain.

If no activities or postures are reported to aggravate the symptoms, the clinician needs to probe for more information. For example, if a patient complains of back pain, the clinician needs to determine the effect that walking, bending, sleeping position, prolonged standing, and sitting have on the symptoms. Nonmechanical events that provoke the symptoms could indicate a nonmusculoskeletal source for the pain[93]:

- *Eating.* Pain that increases with eating may suggest gastrointestinal involvement.

- *Stress.* An increase in overall muscle tension prevents muscles from resting.

- *Cyclical pain.* Cyclical pain can often be related to systemic events (e.g., menstrual pain).

If aggravating movements or positions have been reported, they should be tested at the end of the tests and measures portion of the examination to avoid any overflow of symptoms, which could confuse the clinician.

CLINICAL PEARL

Any relieving factors reported by the patient can often provide sufficient information to assist the clinician with the intervention plan.

▶ *Nature of the pain.* It is important to remember that pain perception is highly subjective and is determined by a number of factors. Certain characteristics of pain can give clues to its tissue of origin. For example, pain that arises from the somatic tissues such as the ligaments or joint capsule is often described as deep and aching, whereas pain from more superficial tissues may be described as

121

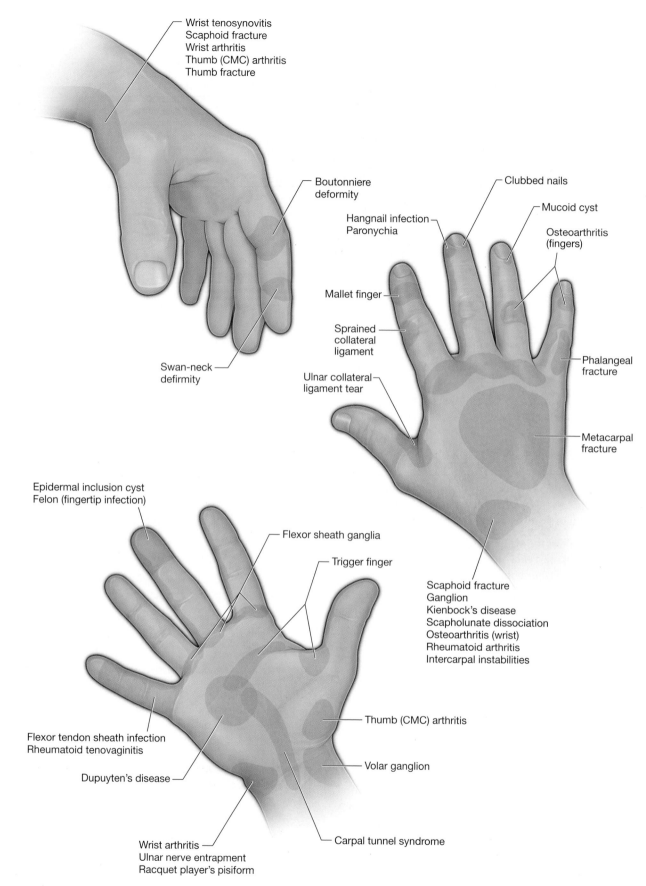

Wrist tenosynovitis
Scaphoid fracture
Wrist arthritis
Thumb (CMC) arthritis
Thumb fracture

Boutonniere
deformity

Clubbed nails

Mucoid cyst

Hangnail infection
Paronychia

Osteoarthritis
(fingers)

Mallet finger

Sprained
collateral
ligament

Ulnar collateral
ligament tear

Phalangeal
fracture

Swan-neck
deformity

Metacarpal
fracture

Epidermal inclusion cyst
Felon (fingertip infection)

Flexor sheath ganglia

Trigger finger

Scaphoid fracture
Ganglion
Kienbock's disease
Scapholunate dissociation
Osteoarthritis (wrist)
Rheumatoid arthritis
Intercarpal instabilities

Thumb (CMC) arthritis

Flexor tendon sheath infection
Rheumatoid tenovaginitis

Volar ganglion

Dupuyten's disease

Wrist arthritis
Ulnar nerve entrapment
Racquet player's pisiform

Carpal tunnel syndrome

FIGURE 5-5 Potential causes of wrist and hand pain

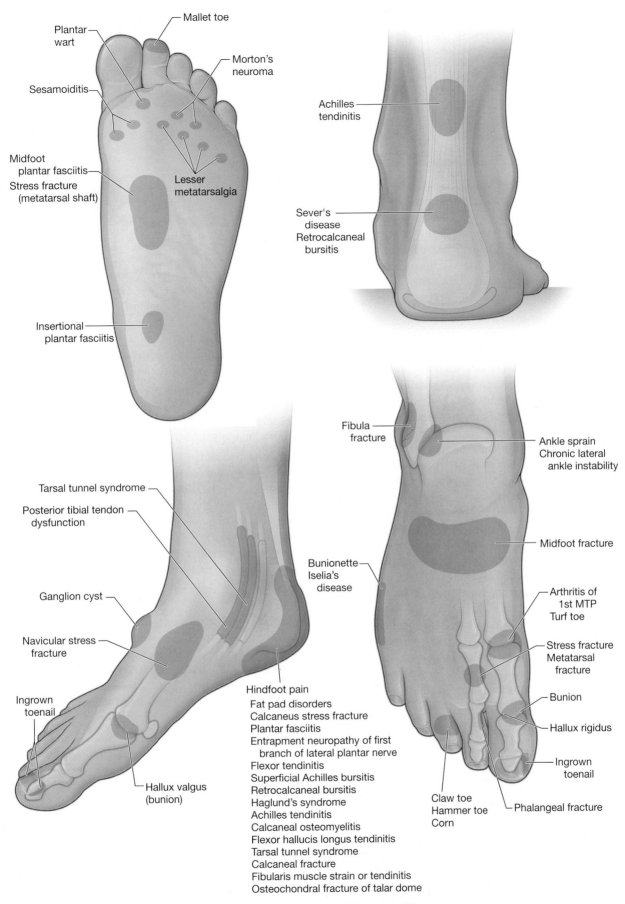

Plantar wart

Mallet toe

Morton's neuroma

Sesamoiditis

Midfoot plantar fasciitis

Stress fracture (metatarsal shaft)

Lesser metatarsalgia

Insertional plantar fasciitis

Achilles tendinitis

Sever's disease
Retrocalcaneal bursitis

Tarsal tunnel syndrome

Posterior tibial tendon dysfunction

Ganglion cyst

Navicular stress fracture

Ingrown toenail

Hallux valgus (bunion)

Fibula fracture

Ankle sprain
Chronic lateral ankle instability

Midfoot fracture

Bunionette
Iselia's disease

Arthritis of 1st MTP
Turf toe

Stress fracture
Metatarsal fracture

Bunion

Hallux rigidus

Ingrown toenail

Claw toe
Hammer toe
Corn

Phalangeal fracture

Hindfoot pain

Fat pad disorders
Calcaneus stress fracture
Plantar fasciitis
Entrapment neuropathy of first
  branch of lateral plantar nerve
Flexor tendinitis
Superficial Achilles bursitis
Retrocalcaneal bursitis
Haglund's syndrome
Achilles tendinitis
Calcaneal osteomyelitis
Flexor hallucis longus tendinitis
Tarsal tunnel syndrome
Calcaneal fracture
Fibularis muscle strain or tendinitis
Osteochondral fracture of talar dome

FIGURE 5-6 Potential causes of foot and ankle pain

sharp or electric. The nature of the pain depends on the type of receptor being stimulated:

- Stimulation of the cutaneous A-δ nociceptors leads to pricking pain.[96]
- Stimulation of the cutaneous C nociceptors results in burning or dull pain.[97]

▶ *Severity.* A description of pain is commonly sought from the patient. Because pain is variable in its intensity and quality, describing pain is often difficult for the patient. One of the simplest methods to quantify the intensity of pain is to use a 10-point visual analog scale (VAS). The VAS is a numerically continuous scale that requires the pain level be identified by making a mark on a 100-mm line, or by circling the appropriate number in a 1–10 series.[98] The patient is asked to rate his or her present pain compared with the worst pain ever experienced, with 0 representing no pain, 1 representing minimally perceived pain, and 10 representing pain that requires immediate attention.[99]

Interview. The interview is an important tool used to obtain information directly from the patient, family, caregiver, or other significant others. Ideally, the patient interview should be conducted in a quiet, well-lit room that offers a measure of privacy and safety. Cultural beliefs may necessitate that the patient be able to choose to work with a male or female clinician.

Listening with empathy involves understanding the ideas being communicated and the emotion behind the ideas. In essence, empathy is seeing another person's viewpoint, so that a deep and true understanding of what the person is experiencing can be obtained. The term *patient-centered* refers to an interviewing technique that provides a method to better understand the environment in which the patient resides, his or her worldview, and the unique conditions that affect his or her health. It is an approach that requires the clinician to become familiar with the personality beneath the presenting problem. Knowing the importance of each question is based on the didactic background of the clinician, as is the ability to convert the patient's responses into a working hypothesis. The interview style should be altered from patient to patient, as the level of understanding and answering ability varies between each individual. In general, the interview should flow as an active conversation, not as a question-and-answer session. The following points are recommended to make the interview process as effective as possible:

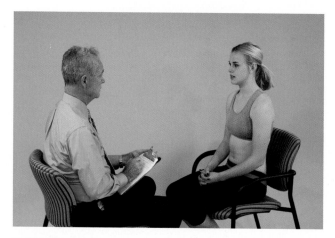

FIGURE 5-7 Correct clinician-patient positioning

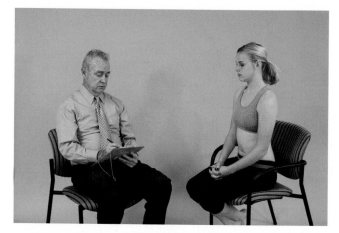

FIGURE 5-8 Incorrect clinician-patient positioning

▶ Eliminate physical barriers, such as desks and tables—the clinician and patient should be at a similar eye level, facing each other, with a comfortable space between them (approximately 3 feet) (Figure 5-7) so that the patient feels the clinician is interested and paying attention. Compare Figure 5-7 with Figure 5-8 and note the contrasting body language and degree of attention afforded to the patient.

▶ Explain the interviewing process to the patient. It is a good idea to obtain the patient's permission at the very beginning of the interview "to sometimes interrupt" and "ask a lot of questions."

▶ Make *content* and *process* observations. This skill involves being able to not focus solely on the words and questions (content) of what is being said—being able to read the nonverbal cues and gestures (process) made by the patient. For example, the patient may say "Everything is fine" (content) while fidgeting with his or her hands (process), to which the clinician might respond, "But you do seem a little nervous today." Thus, process observation is about "stating, not rating" behaviors, and using the observations as a springboard for inquiry and discussion.

▶ Use active and nonjudgmental listening. The clinician should ask questions that demonstrate that he or she has been listening to the patient by reflecting the patient's feelings. For example, stating "You seem worried or anxious about this" demonstrates to the patient that the clinician has some insight into the emotional overtones behind the words being spoken.

▶ Demonstrate a caring approach by conveying concern and support through both verbal responses and body language. Methods include maintaining eye contact, nodding at appropriate times, not moving around or being distracted, using encouraging verbalizations, mirroring body postures and language, and leaning forward.

A transfer of accurate information must occur between the patient and the clinician. A successful learning process requires the clinician to have patience, focus, and self-criticism.[92]

CLINICAL PEARL

Verbal communication skills can be enhanced by:

▶ Letting the patient do the talking.
▶ Keeping questions brief and simple.

TABLE 5-10 Contents of the History

History of Current Condition
Did the condition begin insidiously, or was trauma involved?
How long has the patient had the symptoms?
Where are the symptoms?
How does the patient describe the symptoms?
Reports about numbness and tingling suggest neurologic compromise. Reports of pain suggest a chemical or mechanical irritant. Pain needs to be carefully evaluated in terms of its site, distribution, quality, onset, frequency, nocturnal occurrence, aggravating factors, and relieving factors.

Past History of Current Condition
Has the patient had a similar injury in the past?
Was it treated, or did it resolve on its own? If it was treated, how was it treated, and did intervention help?
How long did the most recent episode last?

Past Medical/Surgical History
How is the patient's general health?
Does the patient have any allergies?

Medications Patient Is Presently Taking

Other Tests and Measures
Has the patient had any imaging tests such as x-ray, MRI, CT scan, bone scan?
Has the patient had an EMG test, or a nerve conduction velocity test, which would suggest compromise to muscle tissue and/or neurologic system?

Social Habits (Past and Present)
Does the patient smoke? If so, how many packs per day?
Does the patient drink alcohol? If so, how often and how much?
Is the patient active or sedentary?

Social History
Is the patient married, living with a partner, single, divorced, or widowed?
Is the patient a parent or single parent?

Family History
Is there a family history of the present condition?

Growth and Development
Is the patient right- or left-handed?
Were there any congenital problems?

Living Environment
What type of home does the patient live in with reference to accessibility?
Is there any support at home?
Does the patient use any extra pillows or special chairs to sleep?

Occupation/Employment/School
What does the patient do for work?
How long has he or she worked there?
What does the job entail in terms of physical requirements?
What level of education did the patient achieve?

Functional Status/Activity Level
How does the present condition affect the patient's ability to perform activities of daily living?
How does the present condition affect the patient at work?
How does the patient's condition affect sleep?
Is the patient able to drive? If so, for how long?

CT, computed tomography; EMG, electromyogram; MRI, magnetic resonance imaging.
Data from Clarnette RG, Miniaci A: Clinical exam of the shoulder. Med Sci Sports Exerc 30:1-6, 1998.

► Using language that is understandable to the patient— avoid acronyms and medical jargon if the patient is nonmedical.

► Giving the patient time to answer by asking one question at a time.

► Avoiding "how" or "why" questions, as they tend to be intimidating.

► Avoiding the use of clichés such as "Don't worry; it'll be all right."

► Avoiding interruptions to the patient's answers or thought processes.

Open-ended questions or statements, such as "Tell me why you are here," are used initially to encourage the patient to provide narrative information, to help determine the patient's chief complaint, and to decrease the opportunity for bias on the part of the clinician.[100] More specific questions, such as "How did this pain begin?" are asked as the examination proceeds (Table 5-10). The specific questions help to focus the examination and deter irrelevant information. The clinician should provide the patient with encouraging responses, such as a nod of the head, when the information is relevant and when needed to steer the patient into supplying necessary information. *Neutral* questions should be used whenever possible. These questions are structured in such a way so as to avoid leading the patient into giving a particular response. Leading questions, such as "Does it hurt more when you walk?" should be avoided. A more neutral question would be, "What activities make your symptoms worse?"

In addition to the foregoing, the clinician needs to determine the patient's age, gender, ethnicity, primary language, customs or religious beliefs that might affect care, cultural background, social/health habits, educational level, and family history. Formal questioning using a questionnaire helps to ensure that all of the important questions are asked. In the event that the patient is unable to provide the pertinent information, such information can also be obtained from the patient's family or caregiver.

Medical Record. The medical record provides detailed reports from other members of the healthcare team. Processing these reports requires an understanding of disease and injury, medical terminology and management, and the ability to interpret laboratory and other diagnostic tests. The types of data that may be generated from a patient history are outlined in Table 5-11.

TABLE 5-11	Data Generated from a Patient History
General demographics	Includes information about the patient's age, height, weight, and marital status and primary language spoken by the patient.[1]
Social history and social habits	Includes information about the patient's social history, including support systems, family and caregiver resources, and cultural beliefs and behaviors.[1] An individual's response to pain and dysfunction is, in large part, determined by his or her cultural background, social standing, educational and economical status, and anticipation of functional compromise.[2]
Occupation/employment	Includes information about the patient's occupation, employment, and work environment, including current and previous community and work activities.[1] The clinician must determine the patient's work demands, the activities involved, and the activities or postures that appear to be aggravating the condition or determine the functional demands of a specific vocational or avocational activity to which the patient is planning to return. Work-related low back injuries and repetitive motion disorders of the upper extremities are common in patients whose workplaces involve physical labor. Habitual postures may be the source of the problem in those with sedentary occupations. Patients who have sedentary occupations may also be at increased risk of overuse injuries when they are not at work, as a result of recreational pursuits (the *weekend warrior*).
Growth and development	Includes information about the patient's developmental background and hand or foot dominance. Developmental or congenital disorders that the clinician should note include such conditions as Legg–Calvé–Perthes disease, cerebral palsy, Down syndrome, spina bifida, scoliosis, and congenital hip dysplasia.
Living environment	The clinician should be aware of the living situation of the patient, including entrances and exits to the house, the number of stairs, and the location of bathrooms within the house.
Functional status and activity level	Includes information about the patient's current and prior level of function, with particular reference to the type of activities performed and the percentage of time spent performing those activities.
Past history of current condition	It is important for the clinician to determine whether the patient has had successive onsets of similar symptoms in the past, because recurrent injury tends to have a detrimental effect on the potential for recovery. If the patient's history indicates a recurrent injury, the clinician should note how often, and how easily, the injury has recurred and the success or failure of previous interventions.
Past medical/surgical history	Includes information with regard to allergies, childhood illnesses, and previous trauma. In addition, information on any health conditions, such as cardiac problems, high blood pressure, or diabetes, should be elicited, as these may affect exercise tolerance (cardiac problems and high blood pressure) and speed of healing (diabetes). If the surgical history is related to the current problem, the clinician should obtain as much detail about the surgery as possible from the surgical report, including any complications, precautions, or postsurgical protocols. Although this information is not always related to the presenting condition, it does afford the clinician some insight as to the potential impact or response the planned intervention may have on the patient.
Family history and general health status	Certain diseases, such as rheumatoid arthritis, diabetes, cardiovascular disease, and cancer, have familial tendencies. The general health status refers to a review of the patient's health perception and physical and psychological function, as well as any specific questions related to a particular body region or complaint.[1]

1. Guide to physical therapist practice. Phys Ther 81:S13-S95, 2001.

2. Judge RD, Zuidema GD, Fitzgerald FT: The medical history and physical, in Judge RD, Zuidema GD, Fitzgerald FT (eds): Clinical Diagnosis (ed 4). Boston, Little, Brown and Company, 1982, pp 9–19.

TABLE 5-12   Signs and Symptoms Requiring Immediate Medical Referral

Signs/Symptoms	Common Cause
Angina pain not relieved in 20 minutes	Myocardial infarction
Angina pain with nausea, sweating, and profuse sweating	Myocardial infarction
Bowel or bladder incontinence and/or saddle anesthesia	Cauda equina lesion
Anaphylactic shock	Immunological allergy or disorder
Signs/symptoms of inadequate ventilation	Cardiopulmonary failure
Patient with diabetes who is confused, is lethargic, or exhibits changes in mental function	Diabetic coma
Patient with positive McBurney's point or rebound tenderness	Appendicitis or peritonitis
Sudden worsening of intermittent claudication	Thromboembolism
Throbbing chest, back, or abdominal pain that increases with exertion accompanied by a sensation of a heartbeat when lying down and palpable pulsating abdominal mass	Aortic aneurysm or abdominal aortic aneurysm

Data from Goodman CC, Snyder TEK: Differential Diagnosis in Physical Therapy. Philadelphia: WB Saunders, 1990; Stowell T, Cioffredi W, Greiner A, et al: Abdominal differential diagnosis in a patient referred to a physical therapy clinic for low back pain. J Orthop Sports Phys Ther 35:755–764, 2005.

Systems Review

The information from the history and the systems review serves as a guide for the clinician in determining which structures and systems require further investigation. The systems review is the part of the examination that identifies possible health problems that require consultation with, or referral to, another healthcare provider (Table 5-12).[16] The systems review consists of a limited examination of the anatomic and physiologic status all systems (i.e., musculoskeletal, neurological, cardiovascular, pulmonary, integumentary, gastrointestinal [GI], urinary system [US], and genitoreproductive).[16] The systems review includes an assessment of the following components[16]:

► For the cardiovascular/pulmonary system, the assessment of heart rate, respiratory rate, blood pressure (see Chapter 9), and edema. Edema is an observable swelling from fluid accumulation in certain body tissues. Edema most commonly occurs in the feet and legs, where it is also referred to as peripheral edema. Swelling or edema may be localized at the site of the injury or diffused over a larger area. The more serious reasons for swelling include fracture, tumor, congestive heart failure, and deep vein thrombosis. However, in some cases, serious injuries produce very limited swelling.

► For the integumentary system, the assessment of skin integrity, skin color, and presence of scar formation. The integumentary system includes the skin, hair, and nails. Examination of the integumentary system may reveal manifestations of systemic disorders. The overall color of the skin should be noted. Cyanosis in the nails, hands, and feet may be a sign of a central (advanced lung disease, pulmonary edema, congenital heart disease, or low hemoglobin level) or peripheral (pulmonary edema, venous obstruction, or congestive heart failure) dysfunction.[101] Palpation of the skin, in general, should include assessment of temperature, texture, moistness, mobility, and turgor.[101] Skin temperature is best felt over

large areas using the back of the clinician's hand. An assessment should be made as to whether this is localized or generalized warmth[101]:

■ *Localized.* May be seen in areas of the underlying inflammation or infection.

■ *Generalized.* May indicate fever or hyperthyroidism.

Skin texture is described as smooth or rough (coarse). Skin mobility may be decreased in areas of edema or in scleroderma.

► For the musculoskeletal system, the assessment of gross symmetry, gross range of motion, gross strength, weight, and height.

► For the neuromuscular system, a general assessment of gross coordinated movement (e.g., balance, locomotion, transfers, and transitions). In addition, the clinician observes for peripheral and cranial nerve integrity and notes any indication of neurological compromise such as tremors or facial tics.

► For communication ability, affect, cognition, language, and learning style, the clinician notes whether the patient's communication level is age appropriate; whether the patient is oriented to person, place, and time; and whether the emotional and behavioral responses appear to be appropriate to his or her circumstances. It is important to verify that the patient can communicate his or her needs. The clinician should determine whether the patient has a good understanding of his or her condition, the planned intervention, and the prognosis. The clinician should also determine the learning style that best suits the patient.

Tests and Measures

The tests and measures component of the examination, which serves as an adjunct to the history and the systems review, involves the physical examination of the patient. Components of the tests and measures include the items listed in Table 5-13,

TABLE 5-13	Categories for Tests and Measures

Aerobic capacity and endurance
Anthropometric characteristics
Arousal, attention, and cognition
Assistive and adaptive devices
Circulation (arterial, venous, and lymphatic)
Cranial and peripheral nerve integrity
Environmental, home, and work (job, school, and play) barriers
Ergonomics and body mechanics
Gait, locomotion, and balance
Integumentary integrity
Joint integrity and mobility
Motor function (motor control and learning)
Muscle length
Muscle power and endurance
Neuromotor development and sensory integration
Orthotic, protective, and supportive devices
Pain
Prosthetic requirements
Reflex integrity
Self-care and home management (ADLs and IADLs)
Sensory integrity (including proprioception and kinesthesia)
Ventilation and respiration and gas exchange
Work, community, and leisure integration or reintegration

ADLs, activities of daily living; IADLs, instrumental activities of daily living.
Data from American Physical Therapy Association: Guide to Physical Therapist Practice. Phys Ther 81:S13-S95, 2001.

in addition to an assessment of posture, palpation, an assessment of a patient's range of motion using goniometry (see Chapter 11), an assessment of the patient's strength using manual muscle testing (see Chapter 12), and various tests designed to accurately determine the degree of specific function and dysfunction of the patient.

Posture. Postural development begins at a very early age. As the infant starts to activate the postural system, skeletal muscles develop according to their predetermined specific uses in various recurrent functions and movement strategies.[102] Jull and Janda[103,104] developed a system that characterized muscles based on common patterns of kinetic chain dysfunction, into two functional divisions (see Table 4-7 in Chapter 4):

▶ *Postural muscles.* These relatively strong muscles are designed to counter gravitational forces and provide a stable base for other muscles to work from, although they are likely to be poorly recruited, lax in appearance, and show an inability to perform inner range contractions over time.

▶ *Phasic muscles.* These muscles tend to function in a dynamically antagonistic manner to the postural muscles. Phasic muscles tend to become relatively weak compared to the postural muscles, are more prone to atrophy and adaptive shortening, and show preferential recruitment in synergistic activities. In addition, these muscles will tend to dominate movements and may alter posture by restricting movement.

On casual observation, the human body appears symmetrical, such that both sides of the body look the same. However, on closer examination, there is often a lack of symmetry. This

asymmetry may be the result of a limb length discrepancy, a right side versus left side dominance, a muscle imbalance between synergists and their respective antagonists, or a postural dysfunction, to name a few examples. Any lack of symmetry should prompt further examination to determine the cause and potential management strategies. It is important to remember that asymmetry does not necessarily equate with dysfunction. Indeed, it is only those inequalities or imbalances that produce pain and/or dysfunction that should concern the clinician. Confounding the issue is the fact that the body is capable of compensating for many imbalances. Although this may appear to be a satisfactory solution, these compensations can lead to further misalignment and eventual pathologic conditions. For example, a muscle maintained in a shortened or lengthened position will eventually adapt to its new position. Although this muscle initially is incapable of producing a maximal contraction in the newly acquired position,[105] changes at the sarcomere level eventually allow the muscle to produce maximal tension at the new length.[106] However, the changes in length produce changes in tension development, as well as changes in the angle of pull.[107] It is theorized that, if a muscle lengthens by way of compensation, it results in an alteration in the normal force–couple and arthrokinematic relationship of the area, thereby affecting the efficient and ideal operation of the movement system.[106,108–111] A common example occurs if the Achilles tendon is adaptively shortened to the point where it prevents any dorsiflexion. When this occurs, the tibia cannot advance forward over the fixed foot during gait, and the body's center of mass (COM) (see Chapter 14) is placed further behind the ankle, creating a greater torque and greater workload. To avoid this inefficiency, the body compensates by hyperextending the knee, which permits the body's COM to be closer to the fulcrum. Other compensations include a shortening of the hip flexors to tilt the pelvis anteriorly and incline the body forward, which in turn produces the compensations of increased lumbar lordosis, thoracic kyphosis, and cervical lordosis.

During the initial assessment of musculoskeletal imbalances, the clinician initially observes for any obvious asymmetries and determines whether they are structural or functional:

▶ *Structural:* An asymmetry that is present at rest. For example, torticollis and kyphosis can be structural deformities.

▶ *Functional:* An asymmetry that is the result of an assumed posture and which disappears when the posture is changed. For example, a functional scoliosis due to a leg length discrepancy should disappear when the patient bends forward.

Once an evaluation of the obvious asymmetries has been made, the focus of the examination switches to the more subtle asymmetries. This part of the examination requires an understanding of the etiology of imbalances and the resulting compensatory changes. Symmetrical alignment may be defined as "the optimal alignment of the patient's body that allows the neuromuscular system to perform actions requiring the least amount of energy to achieve the desired effect."[112] Postural alignment has important consequences, as each joint has a direct effect both on its neighboring joint and on the joints further away. A syndrome is a characteristic pattern of symptoms or dysfunctions. Abnormal, or *nonneutral*, alignment is defined as "positioning that deviates from the midrange position of function."[113] To be classified as abnormal or dysfunctional, the alignment must produce physical functional limitations. These functional limitations can occur anywhere along the kinetic chain, at adjacent or distal joints through compensatory motions or postures. The postural control system is the mechanism by which the body maintains balance and equilibrium and consists of several subsystems, namely, the vestibular, visual, and somatosensory subsystems.[114,115] In a multisegmented organism such as the human body, many postures are adopted throughout the course of a day. Nonneutral alignment, whether maintained statically or performed repetitively, appears to be a key precipitating factor in soft tissue and neurologic pain.[116] This may be the result of an alteration in joint load distribution or in the force transmission of the muscles. This alteration can result in a musculoskeletal imbalance.

The work of Jull and Janda[103] introduced the concept of postural patterns and described a lower quadrant syndrome called the *pelvic crossed syndrome*. In this syndrome, the erector spinae and iliopsoas are adaptively shortened (tight), and the abdominals and gluteus maximus are weak. This syndrome promotes an anterior pelvic tilt, an increased lumbar lordosis, and a slight flexion of the hip. The hamstrings frequently are adaptively shortened in this syndrome, and this may be a compensatory strategy to lessen the anterior tilt of the pelvis,[110] or because the glutei are weak. In addition to increasing the lumbar lordosis, an increased thoracic kyphosis and a compensatory increase in cervical lordosis to keep the head and eyes level occurs. Janda also described an upper quadrant syndrome called the *upper crossed syndrome*.[104] This syndrome involves adaptive shortening of the levator scapulae, upper trapezius, pectoralis major and minor, and sternocleidomastoid, and weakness of the deep neck flexors and lower scapular stabilizers. The syndrome produces elevation and protraction of the shoulder and rotation and abduction of the scapula, together with scapular winging. It also theoretically produces a forward head and hypermobility of the C4–5 and T4 segments.

More recently, Sahrmann[106] has stressed the importance of the relationship of neighboring joints along both directions of the kinetic chain to determine the mechanical cause of the symptoms.

Palpation. Palpation is a fundamental skill used in a number of the tests and measures. Both Gerwin and colleagues[117] and Njoo and Van der Does[118] found that training and experience are essential in performing reliable palpation tests. Palpation, which can play a central role in the performance of several manual therapy techniques,[119] is performed to[120,121]

▶ Check for any vasomotor changes such as an increase in skin temperature that might suggest an inflammatory process.

▶ Localize specific sites of swelling.

▶ Determine the presence of muscle tremors and/or fasciculations.

▶ Identify specific anatomic structures and their relationship to one another.

▶ Identify sites of point tenderness. Hyperalgic skin zones can be detected using skin drag, which consists of moving the pads of the fingertips over the surface of the skin and attempting to sense resistance or drag.

▶ Identify soft-tissue texture changes or myofascial restriction. Normal tissue is soft and mobile and moves equally in all directions. Abnormal tissue may feel hard, sensitive, or somewhat crunchy or stringy.[122]

▶ Locate changes in muscle tone resulting from trigger points, muscle spasm, hypertonicity, or hypotonicity. However, a study by Hsieh and colleagues[123] found that among nonexpert physicians, physiatrists, or chiropractors, trigger point palpation is not reliable for detecting taut band and local twitch response, and only marginally reliable for referred pain after training. The most useful diagnostic test to detect these changes is to create a fold in the tissue and to stretch it.[124] The tissue should be soft and supple, and there should be no resistance to the stretch.

▶ Determine circulatory status by checking distal pulses.

▶ Detect changes in the moisture of the skin.

The physical examination must be supported by as much science as possible, so that the decision about which test(s) to use during the examination should be based on their appropriateness relative to the patient's unique problems and the best available research evidence (see Chapter 3). Before proceeding with the tests and measures, the clinician must obtain a valid consent, and a full explanation must be provided to the patient as to what procedures are to be performed and the reasons for these. The tests used by the clinician must be based on the patient's history or presentation. At times, a complete examination cannot be performed. For example, if an area to be examined is too acutely inflamed, the clinician may defer some of the examinations to the subsequent visit. If problems arise that are not initially identified in the history or systems review, or if the data obtained are inconsistent, additional tests or measures may be indicated.[125]

EVALUATION

In contrast to the examination, an *evaluation* is the level of judgment necessary to make sense of the findings in order to identify a relationship between the symptoms reported and the signs of disturbed function.[126]

The evaluation is used to determine the diagnosis, prognosis, and plan of care, whereas the diagnosis guides the intervention. Before performing the examination, the clinician has some idea of the likelihood that the patient has the condition of interest, based on the history.[127] Once the examination is complete, the clinician should be able to add and subtract the various findings and determine the accuracy of the working hypothesis. During a patient examination, it is difficult to establish a relationship between impairment and functional limitations and determine which of those impairments are critical to the loss of function.[128] One way to circumnavigate such a problem is to focus on enablement perspectives using algorithms. An algorithm is a systematic process involving a finite number of steps that produces the solution to a problem. Algorithms used in healthcare allow for clinical decisions and adjustments to be made during the clinical reasoning and decision-making process because they are not prescriptive or protocol driven.[129] The most commonly used algorithm in physical therapy is the *hypothesis-oriented algorithm for clinicians* (HOAC) designed by Rothstein and Echternach.[130] The HOAC is designed to guide the clinician from evaluation to intervention planning with a logical sequence of activities. It requires the clinician to generate working hypotheses early in the examination process, a strategy often used by expert clinicians. The initial step in the HOAC process is to attempt to clarify the cause of functional movement problems, which requires the clinician to generate several alternative hypotheses about the potential causes. The next step is for the clinician to determine the crucial test(s) and their expected outcomes that would rule out one or more of the hypotheses. As these tests are carried out, the clinician continues the process of generating and testing hypotheses, which refines the clinician's understanding of the cause(s) of the problem. The keys to success of the HOAC process are determined by the generation of the correct hypothesis and the correct choice of the crucial test.

DIAGNOSIS

An accurate diagnosis depends on a properly constructed and tested classification scheme, based on evidence-informed practice, which can aid the clinician to select the best techniques and correctly identify, quantify, and classify the patient's condition.

Preferred Practice Patterns

The Guide[16] uses preferred practice patterns to group clusters of musculoskeletal impairments that occur together:

► Pattern 4B refers to conditions resulting from impaired posture.

► Pattern 4C refers to conditions resulting from impaired muscle performance.

► Pattern 4D refers to conditions resulting from impaired joint mobility, motor function, muscle performance, and range of motion associated with connective tissue dysfunction.

► Pattern 4E refers to conditions resulting from impaired joint mobility, motor function, muscle performance, and range of motion associated with localized inflammation.

► Pattern 4F refers to conditions resulting from impaired joint mobility, motor function, muscle performance, range of motion, and reflex integrity associated with spinal disorders.

► Pattern 4G refers to conditions resulting from impaired joint mobility, motor function, muscle performance, and range of motion associated with fracture.

► Pattern 4H refers to conditions resulting from impaired joint mobility, motor function, muscle performance, and range of motion associated with joint arthroplasty.

► Pattern 4I refers to conditions resulting from impaired joint mobility, motor function, muscle performance, and range of motion associated with bony or soft tissue surgery.

► Pattern 4J refers to conditions resulting from impaired motor function, muscle performance, range of motion, gait, locomotion, balance, and motor function associated with amputation.

► Pattern 5F refers to conditions resulting from impaired peripheral nerve integrity and muscle performance associated with peripheral nerve injury.

Each of these patterns represents a diagnostic or impairment classification. Impairments resulting primarily from pain are integrated in all of the preferred practice patterns. Pain can greatly influence an individual's ability to function, depending on its location and severity.

Differential Diagnosis

An important component of the Vision 2020 statement set forth by the American Physical Therapy Association (APTA)[1] is achieving direct access through independent, self-determined, professional judgment and action.[131] With the majority of states now permitting direct access to physical therapists, many physical therapists now have the primary responsibility for being the gatekeepers of healthcare and for making medical referrals. In light of the APTA's movement toward realizing "Vision 2020," an operational definition of *autonomous practice* and the related term *autonomous physical therapist practitioner* is given by the APTA's Board as follows:

► Autonomous physical therapist practice is practice characterized by independent, self-determined professional judgment and action.

► An autonomous physical therapist practitioner within the scope of practice defined by the *Guide to Physical Therapist Practice* provides physical therapy services to patients who have direct and unrestricted access to their services, and may refer as appropriate to other healthcare providers and other professionals and for diagnostic tests.[2]

Through history and physical examination, physical therapists diagnose and classify different types of information for use in their clinical reasoning and intervention.[132] For example, one of the most common types of information used is the location of the pain. Figures 5-3 through 5-6 provide the reader with some of the potential causes of pain with respect to different body areas.

The Guide clearly articulates the physical therapist's responsibility to recognize when a consultation with, or referral to, another healthcare provider is necessary.[16] This responsibility requires that the clinician have a high level of knowledge, including an understanding of the concepts of medical screening and differential diagnosis. The results of a number of studies have demonstrated that physical therapists can provide safe and effective care for patients with musculoskeletal conditions in a direct access setting.[133–135] Indeed, in a study by Childs and colleagues,[136] physical therapists demonstrated higher levels of knowledge in managing musculoskeletal conditions than medical students, physician interns and residents, and most physician specialists except for orthopaedists. In addition, physical therapist students enrolled in educational programs conferring the doctoral degree achieved higher scores than their peers enrolled in programs conferring the master's degree.[136] Furthermore, licensed physical therapists who were board certified achieved higher scores and passing rates than their colleagues who were not board certified.[136]

In an effort to aid in the differential diagnosis of musculoskeletal conditions commonly encountered by physical therapists, screening tools have been designed to help recognize and potential serious disorders (red or yellow flags).[137]

▶ Red Flag findings are symptoms or conditions that may require immediate attention and supersede physical therapy being the primary provider of service (see Table 5-12), as they are typically indicative of nonmechanical (nonneuromusculoskeletal) conditions or pathologies of visceral origin.

▶ Yellow flag findings are potential confounding variables that may be cautionary warnings regarding the patient's condition and that require further investigation. Examples include dizziness, abnormal sensation patterns, fainting, progressive weakness, and circulatory or skin changes.

Stith and colleagues[138] describe the red-flag findings found within a patient's history that indicate a need for referral to a physician. The presence of any of the following findings during the patient history, systems review, and/or scanning examination may indicate serious pathology requiring a medical referral:

▶ *Fevers, chills, or night sweats.* These signs and symptoms are almost always associated with a systemic disorder such as an infection.[139]

▶ *Recent unexplained weight changes.* An unexplained weight gain could be caused by congestive heart failure, hypothyroidism, or cancer.[93] An unexplained weight loss could be the result of a gastrointestinal disorder, hyperthyroidism, cancer, or diabetes.[93]

▶ *Malaise or fatigue.* These complaints, which can help to determine the general health of the patient, may be associated with a systemic disease.[139]

▶ *Unexplained nausea or vomiting.* This is never a good symptom or sign.[139]

▶ *Unilateral, bilateral, or quadrilateral paresthesias.* The distribution of neurologic symptoms can give the clinician clues as to the structures involved. Quadrilateral paresthesia always indicates the presence of central nervous system (CNS) involvement.

▶ *Shortness of breath.* Shortness of breath can indicate a myriad of conditions. These can range from anxiety and asthma to a serious cardiac or pulmonary dysfunction.[139]

▶ *Dizziness.* The differential diagnosis of dizziness can be quite challenging. Patients often use the word *dizziness* to refer to feelings of lightheadedness, various sensations of body orientation, blurry vision, or weakness in the legs.

▶ *Nystagmus.* Nystagmus is characterized by a rhythmic movement of the eyes, with an abnormal shifting away from fixation and rapid return.[140] Failure of any one of the main control mechanisms for maintaining steady gaze fixation (the vestibulo-ocular reflex and a gaze-holding system) results in a disruption of steady fixation.

▶ *Bowel or bladder dysfunction.* Bowel and bladder dysfunction may indicate involvement of the cauda equina. *Cauda equina syndrome* is associated with compression of the spinal nerve roots that supply neurologic function to the bladder and bowel. A massive disk herniation may cause spinal cord or cauda equina compression. One of the early signs of cauda equina

compromise is the inability to urinate while sitting down, because of the increased levels of pressure. The most common sensory deficit occurs over the buttocks, posterior–superior thighs, and perianal regions (the so-called saddle anesthesia), with a sensitivity of approximately 0.75.[141] Anal sphincter tone is diminished in 60% to 80% of cases.[141,142] Rapid diagnosis and surgical decompression of this abnormality is essential to prevent permanent neurologic dysfunction.

▶ *Severe pain.* This includes the presence of an insidious onset of severe pain with no specific mechanism of injury.

- Pain at night that awakens the patient from a deep sleep, usually at the same time every night, and which is unrelated to a movement. This finding may indicate the presence of a tumor.

- *Painful weakness.* The presence of a painful weakness almost always indicates serious pathology, including but not limited to a complete rupture of contractile tissue, or nerve palsy.

- A gradual increase in the intensity of the pain. This symptom typically indicates that the condition is worsening, especially if it continues with rest.

▶ *Radiculopathy.* Neurologic symptoms associated with more than two lumbar levels, or more than one cervical level. With the exception of central protrusions or a disk lesion at L4 through L5, disk protrusions typically only affect one spinal nerve root. Multiple-level involvement could suggest the presence of a tumor or other growth, or it may indicate symptom magnification. The presence or absence of objective findings should help determine the cause.

Performing a medical screen is an inherent step in making a diagnosis for the purpose of deciding whether a patient referral is warranted, but the medical screen performed by the physical therapist is not synonymous with differential diagnosis. Differential diagnosis involves the ability to quickly differentiate problems of a serious nature from those that are not, using the history and physical examination. Problems of a serious nature include, but are not limited to, visceral diseases, cancer, infections, fractures, and vascular disorders. The purpose of the medical screen is to confirm (or rule out) the need for physical therapy intervention; the appropriateness of the referral; whether there are any red-flag findings, red-flag risk factors, or clusters of red-flag signs and/or symptoms; and whether the patient's condition falls into one of the categories of conditions outlined by the Guide.[143] Boissonnault and Bass[144] noted that screening for medical disease includes communicating with a physician regarding a list or pattern of signs and symptoms that have caused concern, but not to suggest the presence of a specific disease.[132]

In clinical practice, physical therapists commonly use a combination of the location and type of symptoms, red flag findings, the scanning examination, and the systems review to detect medical diseases. The combined results provide the physical therapist with a method to gather and evaluate examination data, pose and solve problems, infer, hypothesize, and make clinical judgments, such as the need for a patient/client referral.[143]

Systemic dysfunction or disease can present with seemingly bizarre symptoms. These symptoms can prove to be very confusing to the inexperienced clinician. Complicating the scenario is that certain patients who are pursuing litigation can also present with equally bizarre symptoms. These patients may be subdivided into two groups:

1. Those patients with a legitimate injury and cause for litigation who genuinely want to improve.

2. Those patients who are merely motivated by the lure of the litigation settlement and who have no intention of showing signs of improvement until their case is settled. Termed *malingerers,* these patients are a frustrating group for clinicians to deal with, because they display exaggerated complaints of pain, tenderness, and suffering.

Malingering is defined as the intentional production of false symptoms or the exaggeration of symptoms that truly exist.[145] These symptoms may be physical or psychological but have in common the intention of achieving a certain goal. Any individual involved in litigation, whether the result of a motor vehicle accident, work injury, or accident, has the potential for malingering.[146] Malingering can be thought of as synonymous with faking, lying, or fraud, and it represents a frequently unrecognized and mismanaged medical diagnosis.[145] Unfortunately, because of the similarity between malingerers and genuine patients with nonorganic symptoms, this deception often causes a significant, negative response from the clinician toward malingerers and nonorganic patients alike.

It is most important that the clinician address any suspected deception in a structured and unemotional manner and that interactions with the patient be performed in a problem-oriented, constructive, and helpful fashion.[145]

CLINICAL PEARL

The diagnosis of malingering should be made based on the production of actions in the attainment of a known goal, without elaboration of those actions based on the negative emotional response of the clinician.[145]

With very few exceptions, patients in significant pain look and feel miserable, move extremely slowly, and present with consistent findings during the examination. In contrast, malingerers present with severe symptoms and exaggerated responses during the examination but can often be observed to be in no apparent distress at other times. This is particularly true if the malingering patient is observed in an environment outside of the clinic.

However, it cannot be stressed enough that all patients should be given the benefit of the doubt until the clinician, with a high degree of confidence, can rule out an organic cause for the pain.

PROGNOSIS

The prognosis is the predicted level of function that the patient will attain within a certain time frame. The prognosis represents a synthesis, based on an understanding of the extent of pathology, premorbid conditions, the ability of surrounding tissue structures to compensate in the short or long term,

the healing processes of the various tissues, the patient's age, foundational knowledge, theory, evidence, experience, and examination findings, and takes into account the patient's social, emotional, and motivational status.[66,147] This prediction helps guide the intensity, duration, and frequency of the intervention and aids in justifying the intervention. Knowledge of the severity of an injury, the age and physical status of a patient, and the healing processes of the various tissues involved are among the factors used in determining the prognosis.

PLAN OF CARE

The plan of care is organized around the patient's goals. The physical therapist plan of care consists of a blend of consultation, education, and intervention.

Patient Participation in Planning. The patient's aspirations and patient-identified problems, together with those problems identified by the clinician, determine the focus of the goals.[147] The patient and clinician should come to an agreement regarding the most important problems, around which care should be focused, and together establish relevant goals.[147] Patient education and patient responsibility become extremely important in determining the prognosis.

Anticipated Goals and Expected Outcomes. This includes the predicted positive effects on the:

▶ Disorder or condition

▶ Dysfunction

▶ Functional limitations and disabilities

▶ Prevention of future occurrences

▶ Health, fitness and wellness of the patient

▶ Patient/client satisfaction

Perhaps one of the most difficult aspects of documentation for the inexperienced clinician is the setting of short-term (anticipated) goals and long-term (expected outcomes) goals. The patient's aspirations and patient-identified problems, together with those problems identified by the clinician, determine the focus of the goals.[147]

CLINICAL PEARL

The most successful intervention programs are those that are custom designed from a blend of clinical experience and scientific data, with the level of improvement achieved being related to goal setting and the attainment of those goals.

The intervention is typically guided by short- and long-term goals, which are dynamic in nature, being altered as the patient's condition changes, and strategies with which to achieve those goals based on the stages of healing. The following information must be included within the POC based on the anticipated goals.

▶ Frequency of treatments, including how often the patient will be seen per day or per week.

- What interventions the patient will receive, including the use of any modalities, therapeutic exercise, and any specialized equipment.

- Plans for discharge, including patient and family education, equipment needs, and referral to other services as appropriate.

When writing goals, the clinician should use the following guidelines:

- *Who.* This refers to the individual involved. Almost always this is the patient, but it can be a family member.

- *What.* This refers to what the individual will accomplish functionally, and to the level of ability. For example, the patient will demonstrate independence with ambulation using a cane for a distance of 100 feet.

- *When.* This refers to an estimate of the time needed to accomplish the goal, which is usually expressed in days or weeks depending on the patient's diagnosis and general condition. This is a difficult task for inexperienced clinicians because it is difficult to predict how quickly a patient will respond or progress without experience. The time frame may be a function of the clinical setting. For example, in an acute care setting, where the patient may be seen for only 3 to 5 days, the focus will be on short-term goals. In contrast, in a long-term care setting, where the patient may be seen for months, more focus is placed on the long-term goals.

- *How.* This refers to the circumstances under which the functional task will be completed, or the circumstances necessary for the functional task to be completed. This includes the amount of assistance a patient requires to perform a task, or any assistive devices that are necessary.

The documented goals should be listed in order of priority with the most important or more vital functional activities listed first.

Short-term (Anticipated) Goals. Short-term goals are the interim steps along the way to achieving the long-term goals. The purposes of the short-term goals include:

- To set the priorities of an intervention.

- To direct the intervention based on the specific needs and problems of the patient.

- To provide a mechanism to measure the effectiveness of the intervention.

- To communicate with other healthcare professionals.

- To provide an explanation of the rationale behind the goal to third-party payers.

The time frame for short-term goals can be based on the next time the patient will be seen.

CLINICAL PEARL

Examples of short-term goals based on the facility (with and without using abbreviations):

- *Acute-care:* Indep. walker amb. on level surfaces 50% PWB on R LE for 50 ft w/i 3 d. Patient will ambulate independently with a walker for 50 feet with 50% partial weight bearing of the right lower extremity within three days.

- *Outpatient orthopedic clinic:* Pt. will ↑ R knee √ AROM to 0–90° within 2 d. to assist with amb. The patient will increase right knee flexion AROM to 0–90 degrees within two days to assist with ambulation.

Long-term (Expected Outcomes) Goals. Long-term goals are the final product of a therapeutic intervention. The purposes of long-term goals are the same as those for short-term goals. Long-term goals typically use functional terms rather than such items as degrees of range of motion, or grades of muscle strength. Examples of typical long-term goals would include:

- Patient will be independent with transfers on/off toilet, supine-sit, and sit-stand and with ambulation for 100 feet using an assistive device at time of discharge.

- Patient will be independent with ambulation on level and uneven surfaces and stair negotiation without assistive device at time of discharge.

Interventions

According to The Guide,[16] an intervention is "the purposeful and skilled interaction of the physical therapist and the patient/client and, when appropriate, with other individuals involved in the patient/client care, using various physical therapy procedures and techniques to produce changes in the condition consistent with the diagnosis and prognosis."

Components of the physical therapy interventions include:

- Coordination, communication, and documentation

- Patient/client-related instruction

- Procedural interventions

Coordination and Communication

Coordination and communication across all settings are critical responsibilities of a physical therapist and ensure that patient/client receives safe, appropriate, comprehensive, efficient, and effective care from initial evaluation through discharge.

These collaborative processes may include addressing advance directives, individualized educational programs (IEPs), or individualized family service plans (IFSPs); informed consent; mandatory communication and reporting; admission and discharge planning; case management; collaboration and coordination with agencies; communication across settings; cost-effective resource utilization; data collection, analysis, and reporting; documentation across settings; interdisciplinary teamwork; and referrals to other professionals or resources.[148]

Patient/Client Related Instruction

Patient/family/client-related instruction forms the cornerstone of every intervention and so the ability of the clinician to communicate with patients, family members, other practitioners, and coworkers is extremely important. During the physical therapy visits, the clinician and the patient work to alter the patient's perception of his or her functional capabilities. Together, the patient and clinician discuss the parts of the patient's life that he or she can and cannot control and then consider how to improve those parts that can be changed. It is imperative that the clinician spend time educating the patient about his or her condition, so that the patient can fully understand the importance of his or her role in the rehabilitation process and become an educated consumer. Educating the patient about strategies to adopt in order to prevent recurrences and to self-manage his or her condition is also very important. Discussions about intervention goals must continue throughout the rehabilitative process and must be mutually acceptable (see Patient Adherence and Compliance).

Often, the physician relies on the physical therapist to give a broader explanation about the condition and to answer questions and concerns related to the rehabilitative process. The aim of patient education is to create independence, not dependence, and to foster an atmosphere of learning in the clinic. A detailed explanation should be given to the patient in a language that he or she can understand. This explanation should include:

▶ The name of the structure(s) involved, the cause of the problem, and the effect of the biomechanics on the area. Whenever possible, an illustration of the offending structure should be shown to the patient. Anatomic models can be used to explain biomechanical principles in layperson's terms.

▶ Information about tests, diagnosis, and interventions that are planned.

▶ The prognosis of the problem and a discussion about the patient's functional goals. An estimation of healing time is useful for the patient, so that he or she does not become frustrated at a perceived lack of progress.

▶ What patients can do to help themselves. This includes the allowed use of the joint or area, a brief description about the relevant stage of healing, and the vulnerability of the various structures during the pertinent healing phase. This information makes the patient aware and more cautious when performing ADLs, recreational activities, and the home exercise program. Emphasis should be placed on dispelling the myth of "no pain, no gain," and patients should be encouraged to respect pain. Patients often have misconceptions about when to use heat and ice, and it is the role of the clinician to clarify such issues.

▶ Home exercise program. Before prescribing a home exercise program, the clinician should take into consideration the time that will be needed to perform the program. In addition, the level of tolerance and motivation for exercise varies among individuals and is based on their diagnosis and stage of healing. A short series of exercises, performed more frequently during the day, should be prescribed for patients with poor endurance or when the emphasis is on functional reeducation. Longer programs, performed less frequently, are aimed at building strength or endurance. Each home exercise program needs to be individualized to meet the patient's specific needs. Although two patients may have the same diagnosis, the examination may reveal different

positive findings and stages of healing, both of which may alter the intervention.

There are probably as many ways to teach as there are to learn. The clinician needs to be aware that people may have very different preferences for how, when, where, and how often to learn (see Chapter 7).

Procedural Interventions

Procedural interventions can be broadly classified into three main groups[125]:

▶ *Restorative interventions.* These are directed toward remediating or improving the patient's status in terms of impairments, functional limitations, and recovery of function. For example, a patient who has recently undergone a total knee arthroplasty can be assisted with locomotor training using a body-weight support mechanism.

▶ *Compensatory interventions.* These are directed toward promoting optimal function using residual abilities. For example, a patient with a right hemiplegia is taught how to dress using the left upper extremity.

▶ *Preventative interventions.* These are directed toward minimizing potential impairments, functional limitations, and disabilities. For example, the potential of developing pneumonia or a deep venous thrombosis can be minimized by using early resumption of upright activity following surgery.

The choice of interventions involves a series of decisions that will benefit the patient without doing any harm. Fortunately, most of the treatment options available to the physical therapist are not high risk. Indeed, the vast majority of physical therapy interventions involve a gradual progression of strengthening and flexibility exercises, while avoiding further damage to an already compromised structure.[149]

The most successful intervention programs are those that are custom designed from a blend of clinical experience and scientific data, with the level of improvement achieved being related to goal setting and the attainment of those goals (Table 5-14). The necessary knowledge to perform an intervention includes[66]:

▶ The temporal phases of tissue healing, common impairments in each phase, and stresses that tissues can safely tolerate during each phase

▶ Movement characteristics, including amount of range, control, and capacity required for various functional activities

▶ The range of available intervention strategies and procedures to promote these movement characteristics, and corresponding outcomes in varied patient populations

▶ Sequencing of various interventions to challenge appropriately involved tissues and the whole patient—for example, being able to recognize the underlying tissue healing and balance disorders in a patient status post hip fracture with diabetes mellitus, the need for aerobic conditioning in assessing patients with low back

TABLE 5-14	Key Questions for Intervention Planning

What is the stage of healing: acute, subacute, or chronic?

How long do you have to treat the patient?

What does the patient do for activities?

How compliant is the patient?

How much *skilled* physical therapy is needed?

What needs to be taught to prevent recurrence?

Are any referrals needed?

What has worked for other patients with similar problems?

Are there any precautions?

What is your skill level?

Data from Guide to physical therapist practice: Phys Ther 81:S13-S95, 2001.

dysfunction, and the importance of body mechanics education in prenatal and postnatal exercise classes

▶ Intervention strategies to promote health and prevent secondary dysfunction

CLINICAL PEARL

The goal of the intervention process is to achieve desired functional outcomes by reduction of existing impairments, prevention of secondary impairments, enhancement of functional ability, promotion of optimal health, and reduction of environmental challenges.[66,150]

Documentation

Documentation in healthcare includes any entry into the patient/client record. As the record of client care, documentation provides useful information for the clinician, other members of the healthcare team, and third-party payers. This documentation, considered a legal document, becomes a part of the patient's medical record. The process of clinical decision making includes examining the patient, evaluating the data from the examination, formulating a diagnosis and prognosis, and determining the plan of care.

▶ An initial note is written after the first patient visit and documents the results from the examination, the subsequent evaluation, diagnosis, prognosis, and plan of care.

▶ A progress note is written after each subsequent visit and documents the results of any reexamination and reevaluation and any change in the prognosis and plan of care as appropriate.

▶ A discharge note is written at the time that therapy is discontinued and occurs after the final examination and evaluation are performed.

Note Formats

Three types of format of commonly used for writing notes:

▶ POMR (problem-oriented medical record): a traditional form of documentation developed in the 1960s by

Dr. Lawrence Weed. The POMR has four phases: formation of a database which includes current and past information about the patient; development of a specific, current problem list which includes problems to be treated by various practitioners; identification of a specific treatment plan developed by each practitioner; and assessment of the effectiveness of the treatment plans.

▶ SOAP (subjective, objective, assessment, plan): a progression of the POMR note format used by each clinician involved in the patient's care to address each of the patient's problems. A number of variations of the SOAP format have been developed over the years.

▶ Patient/client management based on *The Guide to Physical Therapist Practice*, initially published in 1997, with the second edition publishing a Documentation Template for use in both inpatient and outpatient settings.

Purposes of Documentation

The purposes of documentation are as follows[151]:

▶ To document what the clinician is doing to manage the individual patient's case.

▶ To record examination findings, patient status, intervention provided, and the patient's response to treatment.

▶ To communicate with all other members of the healthcare team—this helps provide consistency among the services provided. This includes communication between the physical therapist (PT) and the physical therapist assistant (PTA).

▶ To provide information to third-party payers, such as Medicare and other insurance companies, who make decisions about reimbursement based on the quality and completeness of the physical therapy received and the documentation that verifies the intervention.

▶ To help the physical therapist organize his/her thought processes involved in patient care.

▶ To document the functional outcome or outcomes attained by the patient through the use of objective and measurable terms, language, or data. Strength and range-of-motion data should be linked to the person's ability to perform functional tasks such as dressing, lifting, reaching, eating, and personal hygiene.

▶ To be used for quality assurance and improvement purposes and for issues such as discharge planning.

▶ To serve as a source of data for quality assurance, peer and utilization review, and research.

SOAP Format

▶ *Subjective:* information about the condition from patient or family member

▶ *Objective:* measurement a clinician obtains during the physical examination

▶ *Assessment:* analysis of problem including the long and short-term goals

135

► *Plan:* a specific intervention plan for the identified problem

Patient/Client Management Format

► *Examination:* the information gathered during the examination is organized according to the nature of the data into History, Systems Review, and Tests and Measures.

► *Evaluation:* this information is divided into two sections: the Diagnosis and the Prognosis.

  ■ The diagnosis attempts to include a Preferred Practice Pattern from *The Guide to Physical Therapist Practice* and relates the patient's functional deficits to the patient's impairment.

  ■ The prognosis section includes an assessment of the predicted level of improvement (rehabilitation potential) that the patient will be able to achieve and the amount of time that it will take to achieve that level of improvement.

► *Plan of Care:* this section includes the Anticipated Goals (short-term goals), Expected Outcomes (long-term goals), any Interventions to be used to achieve these goals, an Education Plan, and a Discharge Plan.

CLINICAL PEARL

A clinician should never enter an endnote or sign an entry for someone else and should not ask someone else to perform such acts. Documentation is a mark of a clinician's credibility, honesty, and intent, and any breaches of documentation rules can lead to charges of incompetence, negligent behavior, or poor judgment.

Guidelines for Writing in a Medical Record

The emphasis in medical record entries is on brevity, clarity, and accuracy.

► *Brevity:* the clinician must learn to use concise sentences while adhering to the style of the clinical facility. Facility recognized abbreviations can be used to aid in brevity (see Medical Abbreviations and Terminology).

► *Clarity:* the clinician must learn to write legibly and in a style that makes the meaning of the documentation immediately clear. Facility-recognized abbreviations can be used to aid in clarity.

► *Accuracy:* the medical record is a permanent, legal document, and so the information contained within it must be accurate and factual. There should be no blank or empty lines between one entry and another. If an error is made, a felt marker, correction fluid, or tape should not be used. Instead, the clinician should put a line through the error (making certain that the deleted material remains legible), write the date, and place his or her initials above the error. In addition, in the margin, the clinician should state why the correction is necessary. Black ink should be used for all corrections and entries. Currently, there

are many software programs available for electronic documentation specific to rehabilitation that indicate when an entry has been altered and identify the person responsible for the entry.

CLINICAL PEARL

The use of punctuation within a clinical facility varies, and the following are just guidelines:

► Hyphens (-) should be used with care because of their confusion with the minus sign.

► The colon (:) can often be used instead of "is." For example, shoulder abduction: 0–110°

► The semicolon (;) can often be used to connect two related statements. For example, able to sleep on stomach; pain not felt during the night.

On occasion, a physician may give a verbal order to the treating therapist. In such instances, the therapist documents the date and time of the order as well as the details of the order—the abbreviation *v.o.* is typically used followed by the physician's name and the therapist's signature.

Every entry into the medical record must be signed using a legal signature followed by the initials that indicate the status of the clinician as a physical therapist (PT) or physical therapist assistant (PTA). The professional designator to be used after the therapist's signature is currently under debate. In the 1970s and 1980s, RPT (Registered Physical Therapist) or LPT (Licensed Physical Therapist) were used. It was then decided in the 1980s and early 1990s to just simply use PT—a physical therapist could not practice without being licensed or registered, making use of "R" or "L" redundant. Currently, there is debate as to whether to change the designator to DPT, although the same redundancy argument could be used for the letter "D."

Medical Abbreviations and Terminology

To be able to read and understand a medical record, the clinician must be familiar with the abbreviations and medical terminology commonly used. Many of the terms are derived from Greek or Latin words. A medical term is a word or phrase made up of elements to express a specific idea:

► *Root element:* the main subject or topic of a medical term, which is commonly a body part. For example, *osteo-* (bone).

► *Prefix element:* used at the beginning of a medical term to change the meaning of the medical term or make it more specific. For example, *hemi-* (half).

► *Suffix element:* used at the end of a medical term to describe a condition of a body part or an action to a body part. For example, *porosis* (a porous condition), as of the bones—osteoporosis.

Examples of these elements of medical terminology are provided in Table 5-15.

TABLE 5-15	Commonly Used Abbreviations			
A:	Assessment		CGA	Contact guard assist
AAA	Abdominal aortic aneurysm		c/o	Complains of
AAROM	Active assisted range of motion		CNS	Central nervous system
abd	Abduction		CO	Cardiac output
ABG	Arterial blood gases		COPD	Chronic obstructive pulmonary disease
AE	Above elbow		CP	Cerebral palsy
ACL	Anterior cruciate ligament		CPM	Continuous passive motion
add	Adduction		CR	Contract-relax
ADL	Activities of daily living		CRF	Chronic renal failure
Ad lib	At discretion		CTLSO	Cervical-thoracic-lumbar-sacral orthosis
afib	Atrial fibrillation		CTR	Carpal tunnel release
AFO	Ankle foot orthosis		CXR	Chest x-ray
AIDS	Acquired immunodeficiency syndrome		d/c (D/C)	Discontinued or discharged
AIIS	Anterior inferior iliac spine		DDD	Degenerative disk disease
AK	Above knee		DF	Dorsiflexion
ALS	Amyotrophic lateral sclerosis		DIP	Distal interphalangeal
amb	Ambulation		DJD	Degenerative joint disease
AMA	Against medical advice		DOB	Date of birth
ANS	Autonomic nervous system		DTR	Deep tendon reflex
A-P (AP)	Anterior-posterior		DVT	Deep venous thrombosis
ARF	Acute renal failure		Dx	Diagnosis
AROM	Active range of motion		EENT	Ear, eyes, nose, throat
ASAP	As soon as possible		EMG	Electromyogram
A-V	Arteriovenous		ER	External rotation or emergency room
AVM	Arteriovenous malformation		E-stim	Electrical stimulation
Bid (BID)	Twice a day		ex	Exercise
BK	Below knee		ext	Extension
BOS	Base of support		FES	Functional electrical stimulation
BP	Blood pressure		Flex	Flexion
bpm	Beats per minute		FUO	Fever, unknown origin
BR	Bed rest		FWB	Full weight-bearing
CA	Cancer		Fx	Fracture
CABG	Coronary artery bypass graft		GB	Gallbladder
CAD	Coronary artery disease		GI	Gastrointestinal
CC	Chief complaint		GSW	Gunshot wound
CF	Cystic fibrosis		HEP	Home exercise program
CHF	Congestive heart failure		HNP	Herniated nucleus pulposus

(continued)

TABLE 5-15   **Commonly Used Abbreviations (continued)**

HOB	Head of bed	PF	Plantarflexion
HP	Hot pack	PIP	Proximal interphalangeal
HR	Heart rate or hold-relax	PMH	Past medical history
HTN	Hypertension	PNF	Proprioceptive neuromuscular facilitation
Hx	History	Post op	Postoperative
IADL	Instrumental activities of daily living	PRE	Progressive resistive exercises
IDDM	Insulin-dependent diabetes mellitus	Prn	As needed
Ind	Independent	PROM	Passive range of motion
ICU	Intensive care unit	PWB	Partial weight-bearing
IR	Internal rotation	q	Every
IV	Intravenous	qd	Every day
JRA	Juvenile rheumatoid arthritis	qh	Every hour
Jt	Joint	qid	Four times a day
KAFO	Knee-ankle-foot orthosis	qn	Every night
LBP	Low back pain	RA	Rheumatoid arthritis
LCL	Lateral collateral ligament	reps	Repetitions
LE	Lower extremity	r/o	Rule out
LMN	Lower motor neuron	ROM	Range of motion
LOB	Loss of balance	RTC	Rotator cuff
LOC	Loss of consciousness	Rx	Treatment, prescription
LOS	Length of stay	SCI	Spinal cord injury
LTG	Long-term goal	SLR	Straight leg raise
MCL	Medial collateral ligament	SOB	Shortness of breath
MCP	Metacarpophalangeal	STG	Short-term goal
MI	Myocardial infarction	TB	Tuberculosis
MMT	Manual muscle test	TBI	Traumatic brain injury
MVA	Motor vehicle accident	TDWB	Touchdown weight-bearing
N/A	Not applicable	TENS	Transcutaneous electrical nerve stimulation
NIDDM	Non–insulin-dependent diabetes mellitus	THA	Total hip arthroplasty
NWB	Non–weight-bearing	Tid	Three times a day
OA	Osteoarthritis	TKA	Total knee arthroplasty
OOB	Out of bed	TKE	Terminal knee extension
OP	Outpatient	TMJ	Temporomandibular joint
OR	Operating room	TPR	Temperature, pulse, and respiration
ORIF	Open reduction and internal fixation	TTWB	Toe-touch weight-bearing
OT (OTR)	Occupational therapy	Tx	Traction
PCL	Posterior cruciate ligament	UE	Upper extremity

TABLE 5-15	Commonly Used Abbreviations (continued)			
US	Ultrasound	WBAT	Weight-bearing as tolerated
UTI	Urinary tract infection	WFL	Within functional limits
VC	Vital capacity	WNL	Within normal limits
v.o. (VO)	Verbal order	y/o	Year(s) old
WB	Weight-bearing		

Patient Adherence and Compliance

The clinician needs to be aware that people may have very different preferences for how, when, where, and how often to learn (see Chapter 7). Patient adherence and compliance are vitally important in the healing process. Whereas *compliance* can be defined as engaging in behavior as instructed or prescribed,[152] *adherence* can be defined as choosing to engage in behaviors. The latter term has gained more accep-tance because it indicates a more proactive approach from the patient. Both compliance and adherence are related to motivation. Motivation, a psychological feature that drives an organism toward a desired goal, is considered vital to maintaining behavior. Motivation has been classified as either intrinsic (internal) or extrinsic (external). A number of motivational theories have been proposed (Table 5-16).

Anecdotally, unmotivated patients may progress more slowly. Much literature has conceptualized or reported poor

TABLE 5-16	Motivational Theories	
Theory	**Proponents**	**Description**
Social cognitive	Bandura[1]	Individuals act as contributors to their own motivation, behavior, and development. Behavior and characteristics are modified by environment. Primary mediators include self-efficacy and the ability to self-regulate. Mastery is the best way to create a strong sense of efficacy.
Self-determination (SDT)	Lepper, Greene, and Nisbett[2]	Choices made are based on experiences, thoughts, contemplations, and interactions with others. Essential psychological needs include competence, relatedness, and autonomy. Composed of five mini-theories[3]: ▶ Cognitive Evaluation Theory (CET): intrinsic motivation is a lifelong creative wellspring. CET highlights the critical roles played by competence and autonomy in fostering intrinsic motivation. ▶ Organismic Integration Theory (OIT): extrinsic motivation is behavior that aims toward outcomes extrinsic to the behavior itself. Highlights supports for autonomy and relatedness as critical to internalization. ▶ Causality Orientations Theory (COT): describes individual differences in people's tendencies to orient toward environments and regulate behavior in various ways based on rewards, gains, and approval. ▶ Basic Psychological Needs Theory (BPNT): psychological well-being and optimal functioning are predicated on meeting the needs of autonomy, competence, and relatedness. ▶ Goal Contents Theory (GCT): Goals are seen as differentially affording basic need satisfactions and are thus differentially associated with well-being.
Health belief model	Ajzen[4] and Fishbein[5]	An individual's attitude, social norms, and perceived control are accurate predictors of behavioral intentions. Involves the theory of reasoned action (TRA) and the theory of planned behavior (TPB): ▶ TRA is most successful when applied to behavior under an individual's voluntary control. ▶ TPB theorizes that if an individual's perceived control, self-efficacy, or self-esteem are low, the perception and belief that he or she can influence behavior in a positive manner is undermined.
Humanistic	Maslow[6]	Based on the concept that there is a hierarchy of biogenic and psychogenic needs that humans must progress through. Hypothesizes that the higher needs in this hierarchy only come into focus once all the needs that are lower down are mainly or entirely satisfied.

(continued)

TABLE 5-16	Motivational Theories (continued)	
Theory	**Proponents**	**Description**
Trans-theoretical model (TTM)	Prochaska and DiClemente[7]	Describes five stages of change: ▶ Precontemplation: defined by a lack of intention to take action ▶ Contemplation: defined by the individual thinking about engaging in a behavior or activity in the near future ▶ Preparation: defined by the individual intending to take action in the immediate future ▶ Action: defined by the individual actively engaging in the behavior or change ▶ Maintenance: defined by an individual who has engaged in a behavior or change for longer than six months

1. Bandura A: Social foundations of thought and action: a social-cognitive theory. Upper Saddle River, NJ, Prentice Hall, 1986.

2. Lepper MK, Greene D, Nisbett R: Undermining children's intrinsic interest with extrinsic reward: A test of the "overjustification" hypothesis. J Personality Soc Psychol 28:129-137, 1973.

3. University of Rochester: Self determination theory: approach to human motivation and personality. Available at http://www.psych.rochester.edu/SDT/theory.php.

4. Ajzen I: From intentions to actions: a theory of planned behavior in Kuhl J, Beckmann J (eds): Action-Control: From Cognition to Behavior. Heidelberg, Springer, 1985, pp 11-39.

5. Ajzen I, Fishbein M: Understanding Attitudes and Predicting Social Behavior. Englewood Cliffs, NJ, Prentice Hall, 1980.

6. Maslow A: The Farther Reaches of Human Nature. New York, Viking Press, 1971.

7. Prochaska JO, DiClemente CC: Stages and processes of self-change of smoking: toward an integrative model of change. J Consult Clin Psychol 51:390-395, 1983.

motivation in rehabilitation as secondary to patient-related factors, including depression, apathy, cognitive impairment, low self-efficacy (e.g., low confidence in one's ability to successfully rehabilitate), fatigue, and personality factors.[153] Various studies have found that average compliance with medication regimens only occurs in 50% to 60% of patients, and compliance with physical therapy programs is approximately 40%.[154] Other reports have found that compliance was decreased if the physical therapist did not provide patients with positive feedback.[155]

Several factors can impact the level of compliance:

▶ The patient's age—older individuals tend to adhere to exercise programs more than younger individuals[156]

▶ The patient's marital status—singles tend to have lower rates of adherence to physical activity/exercise than married couples.[157]

▶ The patient's education—individuals with high levels of education show more compliance to exercise programs than those who are uneducated.[157]

▶ The patient's gender—males report greater levels of total and vigorous activity than females.[157]

▶ The patient's biomedical status—poorer health tends to lead to decreased adherence.[158]

▶ The patient's socioeconomic status—an individual's income bracket tends to influence the ability to access medical care, as well as exercise equipment and venues.[159–161]

▶ The patient's ethnicity—Caucasians appear to participate in more physical activities than other racial or ethnic groups, regardless of age.[157]

Finally, a number of factors have been outlined to improve compliance[162–164]:

▶ Involving the patient in the intervention planning and goal setting

▶ Realistic goal setting for both short- and long-term goals

▶ Promoting high expectations regarding final outcome

▶ Promoting perceived benefits

▶ Projecting a positive attitude

▶ Providing clear instructions and demonstrations with appropriate feedback

▶ Keeping the exercises pain free or with a low level of pain

▶ Encouraging patient problem solving

OUTCOMES

The purpose of the physical therapy intervention is to safely return a patient to their preinjury state, with as little risk of reinjury as possible and with the minimum amount of patient inconvenience. Throughout an episode of care and at the time of discharge, the physical therapist measures the impact of the physical therapy interventions to determine whether the patient has attained the desired level of function based on the initial stated goals and the intervention plan through the use of evidenced-based measurement tools. The most commonly used outcomes tools have been tested for reliability and validity and help provide an accurate assessment of the effectiveness of the physical therapy interventions.[148]

HEALTH PROMOTION, WELLNESS, AND PHYSICAL FITNESS

In 1996, the Surgeon General's report on physical activity and health highlighted the importance of engaging in an active lifestyle to prevent the insidious onset of chronic disease and illness.[165] Healthy People 2010 established goals for promoting a healthy lifestyle for individuals in the United States.[166]

The World Health Organization (WHO) has defined *health promotion* as "the process of enabling people to increase control over their health and its determinants, and thereby improve their health."*

The National Wellness Institute has delineated six components of wellness†:

▶ *Social*. This includes contributing to one's environment and community, and emphasizing the interdependence between others and nature.

▶ *Occupational*. This includes satisfaction and enriching life through work.

▶ *Spiritual*. This includes appreciation of the depth and expanse of life, and having meaning in one's life.

▶ *Physical*. This includes awareness of the need for regular physical activity, good diet and nutrition, and avoiding habits that are harmful to wellness.

▶ *Intellectual*. This includes being able to problem solve, expand knowledge and skills, and be open to new ideas.

▶ *Emotional*. This includes awareness and acceptance of one's feelings, and thinking of oneself positively.

Physical therapists serve as major providers of health promotion, wellness, and fitness by making patients and clients more aware of lifestyle changes, particularly in the areas of physical activity, lifelong health promotion, and creating an environment that supports health practices leading to a healthy lifestyle.[167] Evidence exists that when healthcare professionals counsel patients about risk reduction, those patients are more likely to change poor health habits, thus enhancing a healthier lifestyle.‡

The effects of physical activity and exercise on various physiologic and psychological parameters across the life span through the use of exercise prescriptions support their role in preventing disease and improving function and health. This is particularly relevant in promoting mobility and independence of the elderly, the older old, and the frail elderly.[167]

REFERENCES

1. National Council of State Boards of Nursing: Changes in Healthcare Professions' Scope of Practice: Legislative Considerations. Chicago, IL, National Council of State Boards of Nursing, 2009.
2. Guide to Physical Therapist Practice. Second Edition. American Physical Therapy Association. Phys Ther 81:9-746, 2001.
3. Verbrugge LM, Jette AM: The disablement process. Soc Sci Med 38:1-14, 1994.
4. Jette AM: Physical disablement concepts for physical therapy research and practice. Phys Ther 74:375-382, 1994.
5. Lawrence R, Jette A: Disentangling the disablement process. J Gerontol B Psychol Sci Soc Sci 51B:S173-S182, 1996.
6. Nagi S: Disability concepts revisited: implications for prevention, in Pope A, Tartov A (eds): Disability in America: Toward a National Agenda for Prevention. Washington, DC, National Academy Press, 1991, pp 309-327.
7. Pope A, Tartov A: Disability in America: Toward a National Agenda for Prevention. Washington DC, National Academy Press, 1991.
8. Salen BO, Spangfort EV, Nygren AL, et al: The disability rating index: an instrument for the assessment of disability in clinical settings. J Clin Epidemiol 47:1423-1434, 1994.
9. Simeonsson RJ, Leskinen M: Disability, secondary conditions and quality of life: conceptual issues, in Simeonsson RJ, McDevitt LN (eds): Issues in Disability and Health: The Role of Secondary Conditions and Quality of Life. Chapel Hill, University of North Carolina Press, 1999, pp 51-72.
10. Guide to physical therapist practice: revisions. American Physical Therapy Association. Phys Ther 79, 2001.
11. Brandt EN Jr, Pope AM: Enabling America: Assessing the role of rehabilitation science and engineering. Washington, DC: Institute of Medicine, National Academies Press, 1997.
12. Palisano RJ, Campbell SK, Harris SR: Evidence-based decision-making in pediatric physical therapy, in Campbell SK, Vander Linden DW, Palisano RJ (eds): Physical Therapy for Children. St Louis, Saunders, 2006, pp 3-32.
13. Nagi S: Some conceptual issues in disability and rehabilitation, in Sussman M (ed): Sociology and Rehabilitation. Washington DC, American Sociological Association, 1965, pp 100-113.
14. Guide to Physical Therapist Practice. Second Edition. American Physical Therapy Association. Phys Ther 81:1-746, 2001.
15. Goodman CC, Boissonnault WG: Pathology: Implications for the physical therapist. Philadelphia, WB Saunders, 1998.
16. Guide to physical therapist practice: Phys Ther 81:S13-S95, 2001.
17. American Medical Association: Guides to the Evaluation of Permanent Impairment (ed 5). Chicago, American Medical Association, 2001.
18. Randall KE, McEwen IR: Writing patient-centered goals. Phys Ther 80:1197-1203, 2000.
19. O'Neill DL, Harris SR: Developing goals and objectives for handicapped children. Phys Ther 62:295-298, 1982.
20. Badley EM, Wagstaff S, Wood PHN: Measures of functional ability (disability) in arthritis in relation to impairment of range of joint movement. Ann Rheum Dis 43:563-569, 1984.
21. Dijkers MPJM, Whiteneck G, El-Jaroudi R: Measures of social outcomes in disability. Arch Phys Med Rehabil 81(suppl 2):S63-S80, 2000.
22. McFarlane AC, Brooks PM: The assessment of disability and handicap in musculoskeletal disease. J Rheumatol 24:985-989, 1997.
23. Verbrugge LM: Disability. Rheum Dis Clin North Am 16:741-761, 1990.
24. Americans with Disabilities Act of 1989: 104 Stat 327.101-336, 42 USC 12101 s2 (a) (8), 1989.
25. Waddell G, Waddell H: A review of social influences on neck and back pain disability, in Nachemson AL, Jonsson E (eds): Neck and Back Pain: The Scientific Evidence of Causes, Diagnosis, and Treatment. Philadelphia, Lippincott Williams & Wilkins, 2000, pp 13-55.
26. Olkin R: Could you hold the door for me? Including disability in diversity. Cultur Divers Ethnic Minor Psychol 8:130-137, 2002.
27. Helmrich SP, Ragland DR, Leung RW, et al: Physical activity and reduced occurrence of non-insulin-dependent diabetes mellitus. N Engl J Med 325:147-152, 1991.
28. Manson JE, Rimm EB, Stampfer MJ, et al: Physical activity and incidence of non-insulin-dependent diabetes mellitus in women. Lancet 338:774-778, 1991.
29. Yassin AS, Beckles GL, Messonnier ML: Disability and its economic impact among adults with diabetes. J Occupat Environ Med 44:136-142, 2002.
30. Pinsky JL, Branch LG, Jette AM, et al: Framingham Disability Study: Relationship of disability to cardiovascular risk factors among persons free of diagnosed cardiovascular disease. Am J Epidemiol 122:644-656, 1985.
31. Ettinger WH Jr, Fried LP, Harris T, et al: Self-reported causes of physical disability in older people: The cardiovascular health study. J Am Geriatr Soc 42:1035-1044, 1994.
32. Lund JP, Donga R, Widmer CG, et al: The pain-adaptation model: A discussion of the relationship between chronic musculoskeletal pain and motor activity. Can J Physiol Pharmacol 69:683-694, 1991.
33. Raine S, Twomey LT: Attributes and qualities of human posture and their relationship to dysfunction or musculoskeletal pain. Crit Rev Phys Rehabil Med 6:409-437, 1994.
34. West CG, Gildengorin G, Haegerstrom-Portnoy G, et al: Is vision function related to physical functional ability in older adults? J Am Geriatr Soc 50:136-145, 2002.

---

*Available at http://w3.whosea.org/EN/Section1174/Section1458/Section2057 .htm, accessed September 2005.

†Available at www.nationalwellness.org/index.php?id=166&id_tier=81, accessed September 2005.

‡Available at www.healthwellness.org/archive/research/study5.htm, accessed November 2004.

35. Voight ML, Cook G: Impaired neuromuscular control: reactive neuromuscular training, in Prentice WE, Voight ML (eds): Techniques in Musculoskeletal Rehabilitation. New York, McGraw-Hill, 2001, pp 93-124.

36. Escalante A, del Rincon I: How much disability in rheumatoid arthritis is explained by rheumatoid arthritis? Arthritis Rheum 42:1712-1721, 1999.

37. Krause JS, Bell RB: Measuring quality of life and secondary conditions: Experiences with spinal cord injury, in Simeonsson RJ, McDevitt LN (eds): Issues in Disability and Health: The Role of Secondary Conditions and Quality of Life. Chapel Hill, University of North Carolina Press, 1999, pp 129-143.

38. Buchner DM, Beresford SAA, Larson E, et al: Effects of physical activity on health status in older adults. II: Intervention studies. Annu Rev Public Health 13:469-488, 1992.

39. Caspersen CJ, Powell KE, Christenson GM: Physical activity, exercise and physical fitness. Public Health Rep 100:125-131, 1985.

40. Gregg EW, Pereira MA, Caspersen CJ: Physical activity, falls, and fractures among older adults: a review of the epidemiologic evidence. J Am Geriatr Soc 48:883-893, 2000.

41. Lee I, Paffenbarger RS, Hsieh C: Physical activity and risk of developing colorectal cancer among college alumni. J Natl Cancer Inst 83:1324-1329, 1991.

42. Leon AS, Connett J, Jacobs DR Jr, et al: Leisure-time physical activity levels and risk of coronary heart disease and death: the Multiple Risk Factor Intervention trial. JAMA 258:2388-2395, 1987.

43. Paffenbarger RS, Wing AL, Hyde RT, et al: Physical activity and incidence of hypertension in college alumni. Am J Epidemiol 117:245-257, 1983.

44. Paffenbarger RS, Hyde RT, Wing AL, et al: Physical activity, all-cause mortality, and longevity of college alumni. N Engl J Med 314:605-613, 1986.

45. Powell KE, Thompson PD, Caspersen CJ, et al: Physical activity and the incidence of coronary heart disease. Annu Rev Public Health 8:253-287, 1987.

46. Fried LP, Guralnik JM: Disability in older adults: Evidence regarding significance, etiology, and risk. J Am Geriatr Soc 45:92-100, 1997.

47. Steultjens MP, Dekker J, Bijlsma JW: Avoidance of activity and disability in patients with osteoarthritis of the knee: the mediating role of muscle strength. Arthritis Rheum 46:1784-1788, 2002.

48. Elton D, Stanley G: Cultural expectations and psychological factors in prolonged disability. Adv Behav Med 2:33-42, 1982.

49. Zborowski M: Cultural components in responses to pain. J Soc Issues 8:16-30, 1952.

50. Nordin M, Hiebert R, Pietrek M, et al: Association of comorbidity and outcome in episodes of nonspecific low back pain in occupational populations. J Occupat Environ Med 44:677-684, 2002.

51. Callahan LF, Pincus T: Formal education level as a significant marker of clinical status in rheumatoid arthritis. Arthritis Rheum 31:1346-1357, 1988.

52. Nordin M: Education and return to work, in Gunzburg R, Szpalski M (eds): Whiplash Injuries: Current Concepts in Prevention, Diagnosis and Treatment of the Cervical Whiplash Syndrome. Philadelphia, Lippincott-Raven, 1998, pp 199-210.

53. Cavalieri F, Salaffi F, Ferraccioli GF: Relationship between physical impairment, psychological variables and pain in rheumatoid disability: an analysis of their relative impact. Clin Exp Rheumatol 9:47-50, 1991.

54. Encandela J: Social science and the study of pain since Zborowski: a need for a new agenda. Soc Sci Med 36:783-791, 1993.

55. Edwards RR, Doleys DM, Fillingim RB, et al: Ethnic differences in pain tolerance: clinical implications in a chronic pain population. Psychosomatic Medicine 63:316-323, 2001.

56. Lautenbacher S, Rollman GB: Sex differences in responsiveness to painful and non-painful stimuli are dependent upon the stimulation method. Pain 53:255-264, 1993.

57. Walker JS, Carmody JJ: Experimental pain in healthy human subjects: gender differences in nociception and in response to ibuprofen. Anesth Analg 86:1257-1262, 1998.

58. Ellermeier W, Westphal W: Gender differences in pain ratings and pupil reactions to painful pressure stimuli. Pain 61:435-439, 1995.

59. Aro S, Leino P: Overweight and musculoskeletal morbidity: A ten-year follow-up. Int J Obesity 9:267-275, 1985.

60. Deyo RA, Bass JE: Lifestyle and low-back pain. The influence of smoking and obesity. Spine 14:501-506, 1989.

61. Lilienfeld DE, Vlahov D, Tenney JH, et al: Obesity and diabetes as risk factors for postoperative wound infections after cardiac surgery. Am J Infect Control 16:3-6, 1988.

62. National Center for Health Statistics: Prevalence of overweight and obesity among adults: United States. Hyattsville, Md, 2000.

63. Groves JE: Taking care of the hateful patient. N Engl J Med 298:883-887, 1978.

64. Judge RD, Zuidema GD, Fitzgerald FT: Introduction, in Judge RD, Zuidema GD, Fitzgerald FT (eds): Clinical Diagnosis (ed 4). Boston, Little, Brown and Company, 1982, pp 3-8.

65. Cipriani DJ, Noftz II JB: The utility of orthopedic clinical tests for diagnosis, in Magee D, Zachazewski JE, Quillen WS (eds): Scientific Foundations and Principles of Practice in Musculoskeletal Rehabilitation. St Louis, Mo, WB Saunders, 2007, pp 557-567.

66. Sullivan PE, Puniello MS, Pardasaney PK: Rehabilitation program development: clinical decision-making, prioritization, and program integration, in Magee D, Zachazewski JE, Quillen WS (eds): Scientific Foundations and Principles of Practice in Musculoskeletal Rehabilitation. St Louis, Mo, WB Saunders, 2007, pp 314-327.

67. Tait RC, Chibnall JT, Krause S: The Pain Disability Index: psychometric properties. Pain 40:171-182, 1990.

68. Tait RC, Pollard CA, Margolis RB, et al: The Pain Disability Index: psychometric and validity data. Arch Phys Med Rehab 68:438-441, 1987.

69. Pollard CA: Preliminary validity study of Pain Disability Index. Percep Motor Skills 59:974, 1984.

70. Burkhardt CS: The use of the McGill Pain Questionnaire in assessing arthritis pain. Pain 19:305, 1984.

71. Melzack R: The McGill Pain Questionnaire: Major properties and scoring methods. Pain 1:277, 1975.

72. Pearce J, Morley S: An experimental investigation of the construct validity of the McGill Pain Questionnaire. Pain 115:115, 1989.

73. Fisher C, Dvorak M: Orthopaedic research: What an orthopaedic surgeon needs to know, Orthopaedic Knowledge Update: Home Study Syllabus. Rosemont, Ill, American Academy of Orthopaedic Surgeons, 2005, pp 3-13.

74. Delitto A: Subjective measures and clinical decision making. Phys Ther 69:580, 1989.

75. Denegar CR, Donley PB: Impairment due to pain: Managing pain during the rehabilitation process, in Voight ML, Hoogenboom BJ, Prentice WE (eds): Musculoskeletal Interventions: Techniques for Therapeutic Exercise. New York, McGraw-Hill, 2007, pp 99-110.

76. Dray A: Inflammatory mediators of pain. Br J Anaesth 75:125-31, 1995.

77. Wiener SL: Differential Diagnosis of Acute Pain by Body Region. New York, McGraw-Hill, 1993, pp 1-4.

78. Adams RD, Victor M: Principles of Neurology (ed 5). New York, McGraw-Hill, Health Professions Division, 1993.

79. Chusid JG: Correlative Neuroanatomy & Functional Neurology (ed 19). Norwalk, Conn, Appleton-Century-Crofts, 1985, pp 144-148.

80. Judge RD, Zuidema GD, Fitzgerald FT: Musculoskeletal system, in Judge RD, Zuidema GD, Fitzgerald FT (eds): Clinical Diagnosis (ed 4). Boston, Little, Brown and Company, 1982, pp 365-403.

81. Bonica JJ: Neurophysiological and pathological aspects of acute and chronic pain. Arch Surg 112:750-761, 1977.

82. Chaturvedi SK: Prevalence of chronic pain in psychiatric patients. Pain 29:231-237, 1987.

83. Dunn D: Chronic regional pain syndrome, Type 1: Part I. AORN J 72:421-424, 426, 428-432, 435, 437-442, 444-449, 452-458, 2000.

84. Bogduk N: The anatomy and physiology of nociception, in Crosbie J, McConnell J (eds): Key Issues in Physiotherapy. Oxford, Butterworth-Heinemann, 1993, pp 48-87.

85. Wright A, Zusman M: Neurophysiology of pain and pain modulation, in Boyling JD, Jull GA (eds): Grieve's Modern Manual Therapy: The Vertebral Column. Philadelphia, Churchill Livingstone, 2004, pp 155-171.

86. Sterling M, Jull G, Wright A: The effect of musculoskeletal pain on motor activity and control. J Pain 2:135-145, 2001.

87. Hides JA, Richardson CA, Jull GA: Multifidus muscle recovery is not automatic after resolution of acute, first-episode low back pain. Spine 21:2763-2769, 1996.

88. Hodges P, Richardson C: Inefficient muscular stabilisation of the lumbar spine associated with low back pain: A motor control evaluation of transversus abdominis. Spine 21:2540-2650, 1996.

89. Voight M, Weider D: Comparative reflex response times of the vastus medialis and the vastus lateralis in normal subjects and subjects with extensor mechanism dysfunction. Am J Sports Med 10:131-137, 1991.

INTRODUCTION TO PHYSICAL THERAPY AND PATIENT SKILLS

90. Dubner R, Ren K: Endogenous mechanisms of sensory modulation. Pain Suppl 6:S45-S53, 1999.

91. Grieve GP: The masqueraders, in Boyling JD, Palastanga N (eds): Grieve's Modern Manual Therapy (ed 2). Edinburgh, Churchill Livingstone, 1994, pp 841-856.

92. Maitland G: Vertebral Manipulation. Sydney, Butterworth, 1986.

93. Goodman CC, Snyder TEK: Differential Diagnosis in Physical Therapy. Philadelphia, WB Saunders, 1990.

94. Maitland G: Peripheral Manipulation (ed 3). London, Butterworth, 1991.

95. McKenzie R, May S: History, in McKenzie R, May S (eds): The Human Extremities: Mechanical Diagnosis and Therapy. Waikanae, New Zealand, Spinal Publications New Zealand Ltd, 2000, pp 89-103.

96. Konietzny F, Perl ER, Trevino D, et al: Sensory experiences in man evoked by intraneural electrical stimulation of intact cutaneous afferent fibers. Exp Brain Res 42:219-222, 1981.

97. Ochoa J, Torebjörk E: Sensations evoked by intraneural microstimulation of C nociceptor fibres in human skin nerves. J Physiol 415:583-599, 1989.

98. Huskisson EC: Measurement of pain. Lancet 2:127, 1974.

99. Halle JS: Neuromusculoskeletal scan examination with selected related topics, in Flynn TW (ed): The Thoracic Spine and Rib Cage: Musculoskeletal Evaluation and Treatment. Boston, Butterworth-Heinemann, 1996, pp 121-146.

100. Goodman CC, Snyder TK: Introduction to the interviewing process, in Goodman CC, Snyder TK (eds): Differential Diagnosis in Physical Therapy. Philadelphia, Saunders, 1990, pp 7-42.

101. Bailey MK: Physical examination procedures to screen for serious disorders of the low back and lower quarter, in Wilmarth MA (ed): Medical Screening for the Physical Therapist. Orthopaedic Section Independent Study Course 14.1.1 La Crosse, Wisc, Orthopaedic Section, APTA, Inc, 2003, pp 1-35.

102. Morris C, Chaitow L, Janda V: Functional examination for low back syndromes, in Morris C (ed): Low back syndromes: Integrated clinical management. New York, McGraw-Hill, 2006, pp 333-416.

103. Jull GA, Janda V: Muscle and motor control in low back pain, in Twomey LT, Taylor JR (eds): Physical Therapy of the Low Back: Clinics in Physical Therapy. New York, Churchill Livingstone, 1987, pp 258-278.

104. Janda V: Muscles and motor control in cervicogenic disorders: assessment and management, in Grant R (ed): Physical Therapy of the Cervical and Thoracic Spine. New York, Churchill Livingstone, 1994, pp 195-216.

105. Tardieu C, Tabary JC, Tardieu G, et al: Adaptation of sarcomere numbers to the length imposed on muscle, in Guba F, Marechal G, Takacs O (eds): Mechanism of Muscle Adaptation to Functional Requirements. Elmsford, NY, Pergamon Press, 1981, pp 99-114.

106. Sahrmann SA: Diagnosis and Treatment of Movement Impairment Syndromes. St Louis, Mo, Mosby, 2001.

107. Seidel-Cobb D, Cantu R: Myofascial Treatment, in Donatelli RA (ed): Physical Therapy of the Shoulder (ed 3). New York, Churchill Livingstone, 1997, pp 383-401.

108. Janda V: Muscle strength in relation to muscle length, pain and muscle imbalance, in Harms-Ringdahl K (ed): Muscle Strength. New York, Churchill Livingstone, 1993, pp 83-91.

109. Janda V: Muscle Function Testing. London, Butterworths, 1983.

110. Lewit K: Manipulative Therapy in Rehabilitation of the Motor System (ed 3). London, Butterworths, 1999.

111. Lewit K, Simons DG: Myofascial pain: relief by post-isometric relaxation. Arch Phys Med Rehabil 65:452-456, 1984.

112. Ayub E: Posture and the Upper Quarter, in Donatelli RA (ed): Physical Therapy of the Shoulder (ed 2). New York, Churchill Livingstone, 1991, pp 81-90.

113. Putz-Anderson V: Cumulative Trauma Disorders: A Manual for Musculoskeletal Diseases of the Upper Limbs. Bristol, PA, Taylor & Francis, 1988.

114. Johansson R, Magnusson M: Human postural dynamics. Crit Rev Biomed Eng 18:413-437, 1991.

115. Johansson R, Magnusson M: Determination of characteristic parameters of human postural dynamics. Acta Otolaryngol Suppl 468: 221-225, 1989.

116. Keller K, Corbett J, Nichols D: Repetitive strain injury in computer keyboard users: pathomechanics and treatment principles in individual and group intervention. J Hand Ther 11:9-26, 1998.

117. Gerwin RD, Shannon S, Hong C, et al: Interrater reliability in myofascial trigger point examination. Pain 17:591-595, 1997.

118. Njoo KH, Van der Does E: The occurrence and inter-rater reliability of myofascial trigger points in the quadratus lumborum and gluteus medius: A prospective study in non-specific low back patients and controls in general practice. Pain 58:317-321, 1994.

119. Farrell JP: Cervical passive mobilization techniques: The Australian approach. Phys Med Rehabil 4:309-334, 1990.

120. Dyson M, Pond JB, Joseph J, et al: The stimulation of tissue regeneration by means of ultrasound. Clin Sci 35:273-285, 1968.

121. Dyson M, Suckling J: Stimulation of tissue repair by ultrasound: a survey of the mechanisms involved. Physiotherapy 64:105-108, 1978.

122. Ramsey SM: Holistic manual therapy techniques. Prim Care 24:759-785, 1997.

123. Hsieh CY, Hong CZ, Adams AH, et al: Interexaminer reliability of the palpation of trigger points in the trunk and lower limb muscles. Arch Phys Med Rehabil 81:258-264, 2000.

124. Dvorak J, Dvorak V: General Principles of Palpation, in Gilliar WG, Greenman PE (eds): Manual Medicine: Diagnostics (ed 2). New York, Thieme Medical, 1990, pp 71-75.

125. O'Sullivan SB: Clinical decision-making, in O'Sullivan SB, Schmitz TJ (eds): Physical Rehabilitation (ed 5). Philadelphia, FA Davis, 2007, pp 3-24.

126. Grieve GP: Common Vertebral Joint Problems. New York, Churchill Livingstone, 1981.

127. Fritz JM, Wainner RS: Examining diagnostic tests: an evidence-based perspective. Phys Ther 81:1546-1564, 2001.

128. Shumway-Cook A, Woollacott MH: A conceptual framework for clinical practice, in Shumway-Cook A, Woollacott MH (eds): Motor Control—Translating Research into Clinical Practice. Philadelphia, Lippincott Williams & Wilkins, 2007, pp 137-153.

129. Hoogenboom BJ, Voight ML: Clinical reasoning: An algorithm-based approach to musculoskeletal rehabilitation, in Voight ML, Hoogenboom BJ, Prentice WE (eds): Musculoskeletal Interventions: Techniques for Therapeutic Exercise. New York, McGraw-Hill, 2007, pp 81-95.

130. Rothstein JM, Echternach JL: Hypothesis-oriented algorithm for clinicians. A method for evaluation and treatment planning. Phys Ther 66:1388-1394, 1986.

131. American Physical Therapy Association House of Delegates: Vision 2020, HOD 06-00-24-35. Alexandria, VA, American Physical Therapy Association, 2000.

132. DuVall RE, Godges J: Introduction to physical therapy differential diagnosis: The clinical utility of subjective examination, in Wilmarth MA (ed): Medical Screening for the Physical Therapist. Orthopaedic Section Independent Study Course 14.1.1 La Crosse, Wisc, Orthopaedic Section, APTA, Inc, 2003, pp 1-44.

133. Overman SS, Larson JW, Dickstein DA, et al: Physical therapy care for low back pain. Monitored program of first-contact nonphysician care. Phys Ther 68:199-207, 1988.

134. Weale AE, Bannister GC: Who should see orthopaedic outpatients—physiotherapists or surgeons? Ann R Coll Surg Engl 77:71-73, 1995.

135. Mitchell JM, de Lissovoy G: A comparison of resource use and cost in direct access versus physician referral episodes of physical therapy. Phys Ther 77:10-18, 1997.

136. Childs JD, Whitman JM, Sizer PS, et al: A description of physical therapists' knowledge in managing musculoskeletal conditions. BMC Musculoskelet Disord 6:32, 2005.

137. Fritz J, Flynn TW: Autonomy in physical therapy: less is more. J Orthop Sports Phys Ther 35:696-698, 2005.

138. Stith JS, Sahrmann SA, Dixon KK, et al: Curriculum to prepare diagnosticians in physical therapy. J Phys Ther Educ 9:50, 1995.

139. Stetts DM: Patient Examination, in Wadsworth C (ed): Current Concepts of Orthopaedic Physical Therapy—Home Study Course 11.2.2. La Crosse, Wisc, Orthopaedic Section, APTA, 2001.

140. Magee DJ: Head and Face, in Magee DJ (ed): Orthopedic Physical Assessment (ed 4). Philadelphia, WB Saunders, 2002, pp 67-120.

141. Kostuik JP, Harrington I, Alexander D, et al: Cauda equina syndrome and lumbar disc herniation. J Bone Joint Surg 68A:386-391, 1986.

142. O'Laoire SA, Crockard HA, Thomas DG: Prognosis for sphincter recovery after operation for cauda equina compression owing to lumbar disc prolapse. BMJ 282:1852-1854, 1981.

143. Boissonnault W, Goodman C: Physical therapists as diagnosticians: Drawing the line on diagnosing pathology. J Orthop Sports Phys Ther 36:351-353, 2006.

144. Boissonnault WG, Bass C: Medical screening examination: not optional for physical therapists. J Orthop Sports Phys Ther 14:241-242, 1991.

145. LoPiccolo CJ, Goodkin K, Baldewicz TT: Current issues in the diagnosis and management of malingering. Ann Med 31:166-174, 1999.

146. American Psychiatric Association: Diagnostic and Statistical Manual of Mental Disorders (ed 4). Washington, DC, American Psychiatric Association, 1994.

147. Schenkman M, Deutsch JE, Gill-Body KM: An integrated framework for decision making in neurologic physical therapist practice. Phys Ther 86:1681-1702, 2006.

148. American Physical Therapy Association: Today's Physical Therapist: A Comprehensive Review of a 21st-Century Health Care Profession. Alexandria, Va, American Physical Therapy Association, 2011.

149. Hungerford DS, Lennox DW: Rehabilitation of the knee in disorders of the patellofemoral joint: Relevant biomechanics. Orthop Clin North Am 14:397-444, 1983.

150. Jette DU, Grover L, Keck CP: A qualitative study of clinical decision making in recommending discharge placement from the acute care setting. Phys Ther 83:224-236, 2003.

151. Kettenbach G: Background Information, in Kettenbach G (ed): Writing SOAP Notes with Patient/Client Management Formats (ed 3). Philadelphia, FA Davis, 2004, pp 1-5.

152. Brawley LR, Culos-Reed SN: Studying adherence to therapeutic regimens: overview, theories, recommendations. Control Clin Trials 21:156S-163S, 2000.

153. Lenze EJ, Munin MC, Quear T, et al: The Pittsburgh Rehabilitation Participation Scale: reliability and validity of a clinician-rated measure of participation in acute rehabilitation. Arch Phys Med Rehabil 85:380-384, 2004.

154. Deyo RA: Compliance with therapeutic regimens in arthritis: Issues, current status, and a future agenda. Semin Arthritis Rheum 12:233-244, 1982.

155. Sluijs EM, Kok GJ, van der Zee J: Correlates of exercise compliance in physical therapy. Phys Ther 73:771-782; discussion 783-786, 1993.

156. Lee JY, Jensen BE, Oberman A, et al: Adherence in the training levels comparison trial. Med Sci Sports Exerc 28:47-52, 1996.

157. Keele-Smith R, Leon T: Evaluation of individually tailored interventions on exercise adherence. Western J Nurs Res 25:623-640; discussion 641-651, 2003.

158. Boyette LW, Lloyd A, Boyette JE, et al: Personal characteristics that influence exercise behavior of older adults. J Rehab Res Dev 39:95-103, 2002.

159. Cohen B, Vittinghoff E, Whooley M: Association of socioeconomic status and exercise capacity in adults with coronary heart disease (from the Heart and Soul Study). Am J Cardiol 101:462-466, 2008.

160. Wister AV: The effects of socioeconomic status on exercise and smoking: age-related differences. J Aging Health 8:467-488, 1996.

161. Clark DO: Age, socioeconomic status, and exercise self-efficacy. Gerontologist 36:157-164, 1996.

162. Blanpied P: Why won't patients do their home exercise programs? J Orthop Sports Phys Ther 25:101-102, 1997.

163. Chen CY, Neufeld PS, Feely CA, et al: Factors influencing compliance with home exercise programs among patients with upper extremity impairment. Am J Occup Ther 53:171-180, 1999.

164. Friedrich M, Cermak T, Madebacher P: The effect of brochure use versus therapist teaching on patients performing therapeutic exercise and on changes in impairment status. Phys Ther 76:1082-1088, 1996.

165. U.S. Department of Health and Human Services: Physical Activity and Health: A Report of the Surgeon General. Atlanta, National Center for Chronic Disease Prevention and Health Promotion, 1996.

166. U.S. Department of Health and Human Services: Office of Disease Prevention and Health Promotion—Healthy People 2010. NASNewsletter 15:3, 2000.

167. Moffat M: Clinicians' roles in health promotion, wellness, and physical fitness, in Magee D, Zachazewski JE, Quillen WS (eds): Scientific Foundations and Principles of Practice in Musculoskeletal Rehabilitation. St Louis, Mo, WB Saunders, 2007, pp 328-356.

CHAPTER 6

Movement Dysfunction

CHAPTER OBJECTIVES

At the completion of this chapter,
the reader will be able to:

1. List some of the various causes of movement dysfunction that have been considered over the years

2. Describe some of the musculoskeletal causes of movement dysfunction

3. Describe some of the neurologic causes of movement dysfunction

4. Describe some of the cardiovascular causes of movement dysfunction

5. Describe some of the respiratory causes of movement dysfunction

6. Describe some of the integumentary causes of movement dysfunction

7. Describe the systematic changes that occur with a pregnancy

OVERVIEW

The content of this chapter will likely seem overwhelming, but it's intent is to demonstrate how comprehensive the knowledge base needs to be for a practicing clinician. A qualified physical therapist is an expert in recognizing movement dysfunction, which makes an early introduction to the causes of movement dysfunction essential even at an early level of understanding.

Over the past hundred years, various causes of movement dysfunction have been considered[1]:

▶ *Peripheral neuromuscular dysfunction.* This early approach resulted from findings following war injuries and poliomyelitis (see Chapter 1). The physical therapy diagnosis was based on the results from manual muscle testing (MMT), and the focus of the treatment was to maintain range of motion through the use of stretching exercises and braces followed by exercises based on the results from the MMT, designed to strengthen the recovering and uninvolved muscles.

▶ *Central nervous system (CNS) dysfunction.* This approach was based on patients with stroke, brain or spinal cord injury, and cerebral palsy. As the previous focus on using MMT to determine the diagnosis was no longer effective, a number of new theories evolved to address the diagnosis and management of the patient with CNS dysfunction.

▶ *Joint dysfunction.* This approach incorporated the testing of accessory joint motions based on the belief that soft tissue or joint restrictions were the cause of dysfunction.

However, as outlined in Chapter 4, purposeful and skilled movement is a factor of the integration of many systems, many of which are vulnerable to compromise. Of particular importance are the musculoskeletal, neurologic, cardiovascular, respiratory, integumentary, and metabolic systems. Compromise to any one of these systems can result in movement dysfunction, either directly or indirectly. Thus, any approach that examines and treats each of these systems in isolation is clearly inadequate. Instead, the examination and treatment must incorporate all of these systems as appropriate, how they relate to one another, and how the clinical findings relate to the subjective complaints and any alteration in function.

Much of the detail provided in this chapter will be covered in depth layer in the curriculum, so this chapter can be revisited as each of these specialties are introduced. It is important that the reader become aware that the vast majority of conditions seen by physical therapists do not occur in isolation and that many are manifested by both direct and indirect (secondary) impairments. Although this is more obvious in the serious conditions such as a spinal cord injury, cerebrovascular accident, and traumatic brain injury, many so-called benign conditions can also have associated complications. For this reason, pregnancy is included at the end of the chapter. It serves as a good illustration of how a physical therapist must combine all of the findings from the examination in order to determine the best plan of care and not to treat each impairment as an individual entity.

MUSCULOSKELETAL CAUSES

Many studies have evaluated the effect of injury to the musculoskeletal system.[2–8] The musculoskeletal system undergoes continuous development as various parts of the body grow at different rates. This results in a change of bodily proportions over time. For example, a neonate's head is 70% of its adult size at birth, and then increases in size from birth to maturity, whereas the trunk grows the fastest during the first year of life, contributing about 60% of the increase in body length.

Two types of mechanical forces act on the musculoskeletal system and continually affect the development of movement (see Chapter 4):

► *Internal.* Internal forces include the center of mass (COM), the line of gravity, and the base of support (BOS).

► *External.* External forces include gravity, ground reaction, and inertia of the body segment.

The development of strength and endurance typically follows the development of movement as maintaining posture against gravity begins to play a greater role in function. As individuals age, repeated motions together with sustained postures begin to have an impact on function.

Structural Misalignment

Changes in the contours or orientation of the body shape can be so subtle that it often is impossible to isolate the structure involved, the movements affected, and the related joint dysfunction from observation alone.[9] For example, a change in a soft tissue contour as compared to the other side could indicate muscle atrophy or muscle hypertrophy.

CLINICAL PEARL

Postural deviations negatively affecting the location of the COM in relation to the BOS may result in patients complaining of pain and/or dysfunction when in sustained positions.

The ability to maintain correct musculoskeletal alignment appears to be related to a number of factors[10,11]:

► *Energy cost.*[11] The increase in metabolic rate over the basal rate when standing is so insignificant as to be negligible, compared with a metabolic cost of moving and exercising. This posture is one in which the knees are hyperextended, the hips are pushed forward to the limit of extension, the thoracic curve is increased, the head is projected forward, and the upper trunk is inclined backward in a posterior lean. In contrast, other postures, such as leaning the trunk forward, require greater energy expenditure.

► *Strength and flexibility.* Pathologic changes to the musculoskeletal system (e.g., excessive wearing of the articular surfaces of joints, the development of osteophytes and traction spurs, and maladaptive changes in the length-tension development and angle of pull of muscles and tendons) may be the result of the cumulative effect of repeated small stresses (microtrauma) over a long phase of time or of constant abnormal stresses (macrotrauma) over a short phase of time. Strong, flexible muscles are able to resist the detrimental effects of faulty

postures for longer periods and are able to unload the structures through a change of position. However, these changes in position are not possible if the joints are stiff (hypomobile) or too mobile (hypermobile), or if the muscles are weak, shortened, or lengthened.

► *Age.* As the human body develops from infancy to old age, several physical and neurologic factors may affect posture. At birth, a series of primary curves cause the entire vertebral column to be concave forward, or flexed, giving a kyphotic posture to the whole spine, although the overall contour in the coronal plane is straight. In contrast, the contour of the sagittal plane changes with growth. With development of the erect posture, secondary curves appear in the cervical and lumbar spines, producing a lordosis in these regions. The curves in the spinal column provide it with increased flexibility and shock-absorbing capabilities.[2] At the other end of the life span, the aging adult tends to alter posture in several ways. A common function of aging, at least in women, is the development of a stooped posture associated with osteoporosis with a resultant kyphosis of the thoracic spine. In addition degeneration of the lumbar spine tends to flatten the lumbar lordosis.

► *Psychological aspects.*[11] Not all posture problems can be explained in terms of physical causes. Atypical postures may be symptoms of personality problems or emotional disturbances.

► *Evolutionary and heredity influences.*[11] The transformation of the human race from arboreal quadrupeds to upright bipeds is likely related to the need of the male hominid to have the upper extremities available for carrying a wider variety of foods from fairly long distances.[12] This transformation from quadruped to biped was responsible not only for the changes in the weight-bearing parts of the musculoskeletal structures but also for adaptations in the upper extremities, which were now free for the development of a greater variety of manipulative skills.

CLINICAL PEARL

When attempting to correct an individual's posture, one must be realistic and accept the limits imposed by possible hereditary factors.

► *Structural deformities.* The normal coronal and sagittal alignment of the spine can be altered by many conditions, including leg-length inequality, congenital anomalies, developmental problems, or trauma.[13–15] For example, scoliosis represents a progressive disturbance of the intercalated series of spinal segments that produces a three-dimensional deformity (lateral curvature and vertebral rotation) of the spine. Scoliosis can be idiopathic, a result of congenital deformity, pain, or degeneration, or it can be associated with numerous neuromuscular conditions.

► *Disease.* The normal coronal alignment of the spine can be altered by many disease conditions, including joint pathology such as ankylosing spondylitis. Sagittal plane alignment can also be altered by disease and injury. Kyphosis, which is a condition of overcurvature of the thoracic vertebrae, can be the result of degenerative diseases (e.g., arthritis), developmental problems (e.g., Scheuermann's disease), osteoporosis with associated compression fractures of the vertebrae, or trauma. Respiratory conditions (e.g., emphysema), general weakness, excess weight, loss of proprioception, or muscle spasm (as seen in cerebral palsy or with trauma) may also lead to adaptive changes to posture.[16]

▶ *Habit.* The most common postural problem is poor postural habit and its associated adaptive changes. In particular, poor sitting posture is considered to be a major contributing factor in the development and perpetuation of shoulder, neck, and back pain.

It is difficult to determine why a particular posture becomes dysfunctional in one individual, yet not in another. Differing adaptive potentials of the tissues between individuals may be among the causes in addition to neurologic, neurodevelopmental, and neurophysiologic factors.

CLINICAL PEARL

The pain from any sustained position is thought to result from ischemia of the isometrically contracting muscles, localized fatigue, or an excessive mechanical strain on the structures. Intramuscular pressure can compress the blood vessels and prevent the removal of metabolites and the supply of oxygen, either of which can cause temporary pain.[17,18]

CLINICAL PEARL

Musculoskeletal imbalances involve the entire body, as should any corrections. It is important to remember that an appropriate examination must take place before any intervention.

Edema

Edema is an observable swelling resulting from the accumulation of fluid in certain body tissues. Edema occurs as a result of changes in the local circulation and an inability of the lymphatic system to maintain equilibrium, usually as a result of one or more of four basic physiologic events:

1. An increase in capillary pressure
2. A decrease in osmotic pressure
3. An increase in capillary permeability
4. An obstruction in the lymphatic system

Most of the body's fluids that are found outside of the cells are normally stored in two spaces: the blood vessels (referred to as blood volume) and the interstitial spaces (referred to as interstitial fluid). When functioning correctly, fluid leaks out of the arterial end of the capillaries and is reabsorbed at the venous end. However, because this exchange is not perfectly balanced, a small but significant net filtration of fluid into the interstitial spaces occurs. The drainage of this excess fluid occurs through the lymphatic system.

CLINICAL PEARL

In certain cases where muscle is tightly contained by bony or fascial surroundings, the accumulation of fluid, combined with compromise to the lymphatic drainage channels involved with venous return, results in a pressure increase—a compartment syndrome. Unless this pressure can be reduced quickly, severe muscle destruction can occur.

Two types of edema are recognized: local and general.

▶ Local edema is often associated with trauma to the musculoskeletal system. At the time of the injury, fluid leaks into intercellular spaces because of disrupted tissue and torn vessels, and then further edema occurs through the action of various chemicals released in the inflammatory process of healing, which act on the permeability of the capillary membranes. In general, the amount of swelling is related to the severity of the injury. However, in some cases, serious injuries produce very limited swelling. Similarly, minor injuries can cause significant swelling. A report of rapid joint swelling (within 2 to 4 hours) following a traumatic event may indicate bleeding into the joint. Swelling of a joint that is more gradual, occurring 8 to 24 hours after the trauma, is likely caused by an inflammatory process or synovial swelling.

▶ *General.* Generalized edema typically results from surgical, pharmaceutical, or pathologic causes. This type of edema most commonly occurs in the feet and legs, where it is also referred to as peripheral edema. In various diseases, such as peripheral vascular disease, excess fluid can accumulate in either one or both of the interstitial spaces or blood vessels. An edematous limb indicates poor venous return. Pitting edema is characterized by an indentation of the skin after the pressure has been removed.

CLINICAL PEARL

The more serious reasons for swelling include fracture, tumor, congestive heart failure, and deep vein thrombosis (DVT).

Impaired Muscle Performance

Clinical findings of weakness can have many causes. A distinction must be made among weakness that occurs throughout the range of motion (pathologic weakness), weakness that only occurs in certain positions (positional weakness), and weakness that only occurs in specific muscles or muscle groups (neurologic weakness). A finding of muscle weakness must also be differentiated from weakness due to fatigue. Muscle fatigue is a complex mix of objective and subjective sensations. The simplest definition of fatigue is the feeling of tiredness or exhaustion. Fatigue can also refer to the gradual or sudden inability of a tissue to perform the purpose for which it is designed.

As outlined in Chapter 4, all tissues demonstrate an upper limit of tolerance to loading, after which signs of fatigue or failure may occur. Whereas most connective tissues (bone, cartilage, ligament, and tendon) react to excessive loading by breaking down, muscle reacts by ceasing to function.

According to Cyriax,[19,20] strength testing can provide the clinician with the following findings:

▶ A weak and painless contraction may indicate palsy or a complete rupture of the muscle–tendon unit. The motor disorder of peripheral neuropathy is first manifested by weakness and diminished or absent tendon reflex[21]

▶ A strong and painless contraction indicates a normal finding.

▶ A weak and painful contraction. A study by Franklin[22] indicated that the conditions related to this finding need to be expanded to include not only serious pathology, such as a significant muscle tear or tumor, but relatively minor muscle damage and inflammation such as that induced by eccentric isokinetic exercise.[23]

▶ A strong and painful contraction indicates a grade I contractile lesion.

Pain that does not occur during the test, but occurs on the release of the contraction, is thought to have an articular source, produced by the joint glide that occurs following the release of tension.

Range of Motion and Flexibility

In order for a joint to function normally, both the osteokinematic and arthrokinematic motions have to occur fully (see Chapter 4). It, therefore, follows that if a joint is not functioning completely, either the physiologic range of motion is limited compared with the expected norm or there is no passive range of motion (ROM) available between the physiologic barrier and the anatomic barrier. In general, the physiologic motion is controlled by the contractile tissues, whereas the accessory motion is controlled by the integrity of the joint surfaces and the noncontractile (inert) tissues. This guideline may change in the case of a joint that has undergone degenerative changes, which can result in a decrease in the physiologic motions (capsular pattern of restriction).

A decrease in ROM and/or in the flexibility of one joint can affect the entire kinetic chain (see Chapter 4). For example, a decrease in ROM or flexibility at the shoulder can affect the function of the entire upper extremity. To provide a treatment for a loss of motion, the clinician must make the determination as to the specific cause—that is, a loss of ROM or a decrease in flexibility. For example, a determination must be made as to whether the specific cause is due to joint effusion, adaptive shortening of the connective tissue structures, a change in bony architecture, or an alteration in the alignment of the articular surfaces.

Normal flexibility and ROM are necessary for efficient movement. Joint movement may be viewed as a combination of the amount of joint ROM and the arthrokinematic glide that occurs at the joint surfaces (referred to as *joint play*), whereas flexibility is a factor of the degree of extensibility of the periarticular and connective tissues that cross the joint. A number of anatomic factors can limit the ability of a joint to move through a full, unrestricted range of motion. These include:

▶ Muscles and their tendons
▶ Connective tissue
▶ Bone
▶ Adipose tissue
▶ Skin
▶ Neural tissue

Central Control Dysfunction

A loss of active control of muscle function can result in a loss of force output, which in turn can produce aberrant movement patterns, ineffective force production, or a change in the timing of the onset of muscle activity in one of the partners or synergists of the movement. Thus, if muscle control is poor, joint strain and pain may result.[25,26]

Trauma to tissues that contain mechanoreceptors may result in involvement of the nervous system, which can include partial deafferentation, proprioceptive deficits, and altered joint function.[27,28] For example, in addition to the mechanical restraint provided by ligaments, it has been observed that ligaments provide neurologic feedback that directly mediates reflex muscle contractions about a joint.[27,29]

A normal muscle at rest has some resistance to passive lengthening, whereas a muscle affected by neurologic injury demonstrates an alteration to this characteristic resistance in one of two ways:

▶ Increased resistance to passive lengthening and poor active muscle control combine to hold joints rigidly immobile in positions that favor contracture formation.

▶ Decreased resistance to passive lengthening results in flaccidity that, accompanied by a lack of active muscle control, can result in a general vascular and fluid status in the involved area that predisposes the segment to edema formation and eventual contracture development.

Aging

The musculoskeletal changes associated with aging affect all of the soft tissues, including skeletal muscle, articular cartilage, and intervertebral disks. Many of these changes are associated with a decrease in physical activity and the subsequent loss of strength due to disuse. In addition, many diseases can cause degeneration of the connective tissues, including myopathies, neuropathies, neoplasms, and a host of rheumatic diseases. Aging is the accumulation of diverse adverse changes that increase the risk of death.[30] The rate of aging, that is, the rate at which aging changes occur, normally varies from individual to individual, resulting in differences in the age of death, the onset of various diseases, and the impact of aging on function.[30] Changes as the result of aging can be attributed to a combination of development, genetic defects, the environment, disease, and the aging process. A number of sequential alterations that accompany advancing age increase the probability of experiencing a chronic debilitating disease.[30] This increase in the incidence of chronic conditions with advancing age occurs largely because aging is often accompanied by several comorbidities, such as cardiovascular disorders, osteoporosis, arthritis, and diabetes, which increase the vulnerability of the geriatric patient.

Musculoskeletal impairments are among the most prevalent and symptomatic health problems of middle and old age.[31] The gradual loss of strength and motion, and increasing pain, that accompany the aging process prevent elderly individuals from making full use of their abilities and from participating in the regular physical activity necessary to maintain optimum mobility, general health, and, in some cases, independence.[32]

CLINICAL PEARL

The history and physical examination of the geriatric patient must differentiate between the effects of aging, inactivity, and disease on the underlying impairments and functional limitations that result in movement dysfunction.[33] For example, mild impairments in range of motion may be due to the increased stiffness associated with aging that occurs in the tendinous or ligamentous structures around a joint, or it could be due to acute immobilization, or chronic inactivity and reduced demands on a particular joint for full range of motion.[34]

Muscle size can decrease an average of 30% to 40% over one's lifetime and affects the lower extremities more than the upper extremities.[35] Fiber loss appears to be more accelerated in type II muscle fibers, which decrease from an average of 60% of total muscle fiber type in sedentary young men to below 30% after the age of 80.[36] Type II fibers are used primarily in activities requiring more power, such as sprinting or strength training, and are not stimulated by normal activities of daily living.[32] In addition, a loss of range in the lower extremities can have a negative impact on functional activities such as gait (see Chapter 14).

CLINICAL PEARL

Three musculoskeletal conditions that can severely affect function in the geriatric population are osteoporosis, osteoarthritis, and hip fractures.

Studies have noted that individuals over 65 tend to walk with a slower self-selected gait speed, a shorter stride width, an increase in double support time, and with increased gait variability. Some of these changes are the inevitable effects of aging, whereas others are due to pathology or disuse. For example, elderly individuals tend to go through a decreased range of dorsiflexion during midstance.[37,38] However, significant changes in gait are not noted unless multiple joints are involved or there are impairments in other systems such as loss of strength or motor control.

CLINICAL PEARL

Bloem and colleagues,[39] in a study of individuals aged over 88, noted that 20% of the subjects exhibited unimpaired gait. Another study demonstrated that those who exhibit senile gait disorders are more likely to go on to develop dementia and die earlier than age-matched individuals who walk normally.[40] This raises the enticing possibility that gait changes associated with aging may actually be an early manifestation of pathologies such as subtle white matter changes, vestibular dysfunction, musculoskeletal disorders, or visual changes.[40] What is known is that sensory system impairments have a tremendous impact on gait and that training to improve proprioception can improve gait parameters and safety.[41]

Fractures commonly occur among seniors and can have a significant impact on the morbidity, mortality, and functional dependence of this population.

CLINICAL PEARL

Fracture of the hip can have devastating consequences in the elderly—the mortality rate is 20%.[42-44] About 50% of patients will not resume their premorbid level of function after a hip fracture.[45,46]

Most commonly, such fractures include pathologic fractures, proximal femur fractures, stress fractures, distal radius fractures, proximal humerus fractures, and compression fractures of the spine.

It is estimated that up to 5% of all stress fractures involve the femoral neck, with another 5% involving the femoral head.[47]

Fractures in the elderly have their own set of problems:

- The fractures heal more slowly.
- Older adults are prone to secondary complications, including:
  - Pneumonia if the fracture causes a period of immobility or bed rest
  - Changes in mental status due to adverse reaction to anesthesia
  - Pressure ulcers
  - Comorbidities
  - Falls due to decreased vision and poor balance

It is important to remember that frailty is not a natural consequence of aging and that the performance of physical activity throughout the aging years can produce a number of physiologic benefits:

- Substantial improvements can be made in almost all aspects of cardiovascular functioning.
- Individuals of all ages can benefit from muscle-strengthening exercises. In particular, resistance training can have a significant impact on the maintenance of independence in old age.
- Regular activity helps prevent and/or postpone the age-associated declines in flexibility, balance, and coordination.

Conversely, disuse exacerbates the aging process and negatively affects the physiologic reserve in the face of disease and injury.

NEUROLOGIC CAUSES

With the exception of pain (see Chapter 5), the vast majority of the neurologic causes of movement dysfunction are the result of trauma, a congenital or developmental disorder of the nervous system, or disease involving compromise to either the central nervous system (CNS) or the peripheral nervous system (PNS).

Motor Neuron Dysfunction

This group of conditions involves compromise to the anterior horn cells, which contain the motor neurons that control the axial muscles (the muscles of the head of the trunk). Compromise to these cells can result from trauma or mechanical disruption (avulsion of the anterior root from the cord), inflammation (poliomyelitis), degeneration (amyotrophic lateral sclerosis), genetic defect (spinal muscular atrophy), infections, and chemical imbalances. As these conditions progress, speaking, breathing, and swallowing become negatively affected, producing progressive disability and death.

Axonal Dysfunction

These dysfunctions primarily fall into two categories:

- *Segmental demyelination.* Segmental demyelination involves a destructive loss of myelin (see Chapter 4) at the segments of the axons they cover. This loss of myelin removes the ability of the nerve to communicate using salutatory conduction (see Chapter 4), thereby slowing the velocity. Examples of demyelination diseases of the PNS include Guillain-Barré syndrome and Charcot-Marie-Tooth disease. Examples of demyelination diseases of the central nervous system include multiple sclerosis and tabes dorsalis.
- *Involvement of both the axon and the myelin.* This type, which is often caused by trauma, involves Wallerian degeneration. Wallerian degeneration, which occurs after axonal injury in both the PNS and CNS, involves degeneration of the entire axon and the myelin sheath distal to the site of lesion. This results in the loss of both sensory and motor functions. Regeneration in the PNS is rapid, occurring at rates of up to 1 millimeter a day of regrowth. Regeneration in the CNS is not as rapid. An example of axonal dysfunction of the PNS includes a traumatic transection of the radial nerve resulting in paralysis of the wrist extensors and loss of sensation of the thumb in the posterior-lateral surface of the hand.

Neuromuscular Junction Diseases

The function of the neuromuscular junction (NMJ) is described in Chapter 4. Dysfunction of the NMJ is usually the result of a chemical imbalance that results either in a decreased amount of released neurotransmitter, or in various substances competing with the neurotransmitter for the membrane receptor site. An example of an NMJ disease is myasthenia gravis, which is manifested by fluctuating muscle weakness and fatigability.

Motor Neuron Lesions

Motor neuron lesions are generally of two types:

- *Upper motor neuron (UMN).* Upper motor neurons are located in the white columns of the spinal cord and the cerebral hemispheres. A UMN lesion, also known as a central palsy, is a lesion of the neural pathway above the anterior horn cell or motor nuclei of the cranial nerves. These lesions are characterized by spastic paralysis or paresis, little or no muscle atrophy, hyper-reflexive muscle stretch (deep tendon) reflexes in a nonsegmental distribution, and the presence of pathologic signs (e.g., spasticity) and pathologic reflexes (e.g., Babinski).
- *Lower motor neuron (LMN).* The lower motor neuron begins at the α motor neuron and includes the posterior (dorsal) and anterior (ventral) roots, spinal nerve, peripheral nerve, neuromuscular junction, and muscle–fiber complex.[48] The LMN consists of a cell body located in the anterior gray column and its axon, which travels to a muscle by way of the cranial or peripheral nerve. Lesions to the LMN can occur in the cell body or anywhere along the axon.

An LMN lesion is also known as a peripheral palsy. These lesions can be the result of direct trauma, toxins, infections, ischemia, or compression. The characteristics of an LMN lesion include muscle atrophy and hypotonus, diminished or absent muscle stretch (deep tendon) reflex of the areas served by a spinal nerve root or a peripheral nerve, and absence of pathologic signs or reflexes.

Vascular Diseases

Cerebrovascular Accident

A cerebrovascular accident (CVA) or stroke syndrome encompasses a heterogeneous group of pathophysiologic causes, including thrombosis, embolism, and hemorrhage, that result in a sudden loss of circulation to an area of the brain, resulting in a corresponding loss of neurologic function.

CLINICAL PEARL

Any process that disrupts blood flow to a portion of the brain unleashes an ischemic cascade, leading to the death of neurons and cerebral infarction.

Strokes currently are classified as either hemorrhagic or ischemic, although the two can coexist.

- *Hemorrhagic:* account for only 10% to 15% of all strokes but are associated with higher mortality rates than the ischemic variety.[49] This type results from abnormal bleeding into the extravascular areas of the brain. Causes include, but are not limited to, intracranial aneurysm, hypertension, arteriovenous malformation (AVM), and anticoagulant therapy.
- *Ischemic*[50–54]: the most common type, affecting about 80% of individuals with stroke. This type results when a clot blocks or impairs blood flow. Risk factors for ischemic stroke include advanced age (the risk doubles every decade), hypertension, smoking, heart disease (coronary artery disease, left ventricular hypertrophy, chronic atrial fibrillation), and hypercholesterolemia. Ischemic strokes most often are caused by extracranial embolism or intracranial thrombosis.
  - Emboli may arise from the heart, the extracranial arteries, or rarely, the right-sided circulation (paradoxical emboli). The sources of cardiogenic emboli include valvular thrombi (e.g., in mitral stenosis, endocarditis, prosthetic valves); mural thrombi (e.g., in myocardial infarction [MI], atrial fibrillation, dilated cardiomyopathy); and atrial myxomas.
  - Lacunar infarcts, which are cystic cavities that form after an infarct, commonly occur in patients with small-vessel disease such as diabetes and hypertension.
  - *Thrombosis:* the most common sites of thrombotic occlusion are cerebral artery branch points, especially in the distribution of the internal carotid artery. Arterial stenosis, atherosclerosis, and platelet adherence cause the formation of blood clots that either embolize or occlude the artery. Less common causes of thrombosis include polycythemia and sickle-cell anemia.

CLINICAL PEARL

Any process that causes dissection of the cerebral arteries also can cause thrombotic stroke (e.g., trauma, thoracic aortic dissection, arteritis).

Common symptoms of a stroke include an abrupt onset of hemiparesis, monoparesis, or quadriparesis; monocular or binocular visual loss; visual field deficits; diplopia; dysarthria; ataxia; vertigo; aphasia; or sudden decrease in the level of consciousness.

CLINICAL PEARL

A stroke should be considered in any patient presenting with an acute neurologic deficit (focal or global) or altered level of consciousness.

A stroke is largely preventable. Potentially modifiable risk factors include smoking, obesity, physical inactivity, diet, and excess alcohol consumption. The major neuroanatomic stroke syndromes are caused by disruption of their respective cerebrovascular distributions.

Trauma

Traumatic Brain Injury

Traumatic brain injury (TBI) is a nondegenerative, noncongenital insult to the brain caused by an external mechanical force, which can lead to permanent or temporary impairments of cognitive, physical, and psychosocial functions with an associated diminished or altered state of consciousness.[55–67] TBI is the major cause of death related to injury among Americans. The risk of TBI is highest for individuals aged 15 to 24 years.

CLINICAL PEARL

- In individuals aged 75 years and older, falls are the most common cause of TBI.
- Motor vehicle accidents (MVAs) are the leading cause of TBI in the general population.

TBI can manifest clinically from concussion to coma and death. Injuries are divided into a number of categories:

- *Focal injuries:* tend to be caused by contact forces.
- *Hypoxic-ischemic injury:* results from a lack of oxygenated blood flow to the brain tissue.
- *Increased intracranial pressure (ICP):* can lead to cerebral hypoxia, cerebral ischemia, cerebral edema, hydrocephalus, and brain herniation.
- *Diffuse injuries:* likely to be caused by noncontact, acceleration-deceleration, or rotational forces. A diffuse

axonal injury (DAI), caused by forces associated with acceleration-deceleration and rotational injuries, such as high-impact collisions of MVAs, contact sports, and shaken-baby syndrome. Impact loading (i.e., collision of the head with a solid object at a tangible speed) causes brain injury through a combination of contact forces and inertial forces:

- Inertial force ensues when the head is set in motion with or without any contact force, leading to acceleration of the head.

- Coup contusions occur at the area of direct impact to the skull and occur because of the creation of negative pressure when the skull, distorted at the site of impact, returns to its normal shape.

- Contrecoup contusions are similar to coup contusions but are located opposite the site of direct impact. Cavitation in the brain, from negative pressure due to translational acceleration impacts from inertial loading, may cause contrecoup contusions as the skull and dura matter start to accelerate before the brain on initial impact. The three basic types of tissue deformation include the following:

  - Compressive—tissue compression
  - Tensile—tissue stretching
  - Shear—tissue distortion produced when tissue slides over other tissue.

- Impulsive loading (i.e., sudden motion without significant physical contact)

Complications associated with TBI include:

▶ *Epidural hematoma:* occurs from impact loading to the skull with associated laceration of the dural arteries or veins with subsequent neurologic deterioration. More often, a tear in the middle meningeal artery causes this type of hematoma.

▶ *Subdural hematoma:* tends to occur in patients with injuries to the cortical veins or pial artery in severe TBI.

▶ *Intracerebral hemorrhage:* occurs within the cerebral parenchyma secondary to lacerations or contusion of the brain with injury to larger deeper cerebral vessels with extensive cortical contusion.

▶ *Subarachnoid hemorrhage:* may occur in cases of TBI in a manner other than secondary to ruptured aneurysms caused by lacerations of the superficial microvessels in the subarachnoid space.

▶ *Increased intracranial pressure (ICP):*

  - *Cerebral edema:* Edema may be caused by effects of neurochemical transmitters and by increased ICP.

  - *Hydrocephalus:* The communicating type of hydrocephalus is more common in TBI than the noncommunicating type.

  - *Brain herniation:* Supratentorial herniation is attributable to direct mechanical compression by an accumulating mass or to increased intracranial pressure.

Direct impairments associated with TBI include:

▶ Cognitive impairments (Table 6-1)
▶ Behavioral impairments
▶ Communication impairments
▶ Visual-perceptual impairments
▶ Swallowing impairments

Secondary impairments include soft tissue contractures, skin breakdown, deep vein thrombosis, heterotropic ossification, decreased bone density, muscle atrophy, decreased endurance, infection, and pneumonia.

A number of clinical rating scales exist that can be used to evaluate change in the patient over time. Two of the more commonly used scales are the Glasgow Coma Scale (GCS), which defines severity of TBI within 48 hours of injury (Table 6-2), and the Ranchos Los Amigos Cognitive Functioning Scale (Table 6-3), which can be used to determine the severity of deficit in cognitive functioning.

TABLE 6-1	Levels of Consciousness—a Continuum of Physiologic Readiness for Activity
Term	**Description**
Alert	A quality of mind characterized by attentiveness to normal levels of stimulation, self-awareness, subjectivity, sapience, and sentience.
Lethargic	The patient appears drowsy and may fall asleep if not stimulated in some way. Patient has difficulty in focusing or maintaining attention on the question or task.
Obtunded	A state of consciousness characterized by a state of sleep, reduced alertness to arousal, and delayed responses to stimuli.
Stupor (semicoma)	The patient responds only to strong, generally noxious stimuli and returns to the unconscious state when stimulation is stopped. When aroused, the patient is unable to interact with the clinician.
Vegetative state (unresponsive vigilance)	Absence of the capacity for self-aware mental activity due to overwhelming damage or dysfunction of the cerebral hemispheres with sufficient sparing of the diencephalon and brain stem to preserve autonomic and motor reflexes as well as normal sleep/wake cycles. Characterized by a lack of cognitive responsiveness but with the return of sleep/wake cycles, and normalization of vegetative functions (respiration, heart rate, blood pressure, digestion).
Coma	The patient is unarousable and unresponsive, and any response to repeated stimuli is only primitive avoidance reflexes; in profound coma, all brainstem and myotatic reflexes may be absent.

TABLE 6-2	Glasgow Coma Scale (GCS)			
	Test	**Patient Response**	**Score**
Eye-opening	Spontaneous	Opens eyes	4
	To speech	Opens eyes	3
	To pain	Opens eyes	2
	To pain	Doesn't open	1
Best verbal response	Speech	Conversation carried out correctly	5
		Confused, disoriented	4
		Inappropriate words	3
		Unintelligible sounds only	2
		Mute	1
Best motor response	Commands	Follows simple commands	6
	To pain	Pulls examiner's hand away	5
	To pain	Pulls part of body away	4
	To pain	Flexes body to pain	3
	To pain	Decerebrates	2
	To pain	No motor response	1

Spinal Cord Injury

Patients with spinal cord injury (SCI) usually have permanent and often devastating neurologic deficits and disability. The extent and seriousness of the consequences depends on the location and severity of the lesion.

CLINICAL PEARL

Injuries below L1 are not considered SCIs because they involve the segmental spinal nerves and/or cauda equina. Spinal injuries proximal to L1, above the termination of the spinal cord, often involve a combination of spinal cord lesions and segmental root or spinal nerve injuries.

▶ Injury to the corticospinal tract or posterior columns, respectively, results in ipsilateral paralysis or loss of sensation of light touch, proprioception, and vibration.

▶ Injury to the lateral spinothalamic tract causes contralateral loss of pain and temperature sensation.

▶ Because the anterior spinothalamic tract also transmits light touch information, injury to the posterior columns may result in complete loss of vibration sensation and proprioception, but only partial loss of light touch sensation.

Spinal cord injuries can be categorized as complete or incomplete. A complete cord syndrome is characterized clinically as complete loss of motor and sensory function below the level of the traumatic lesion.

CLINICAL PEARL

▶ *Tetraplegia* refers to complete paralysis of all four extremities and trunk, including the respiratory muscles, and results from lesions of the cervical cord.

▶ *Paraplegia* refers to complete paralysis of all or part of the trunk and both lower extremities resulting from lesions of the thoracic or lumbar spinal cord or cauda equina.

Incomplete cord syndromes have variable neurologic findings with partial loss of sensory and/or motor function below the level of injury.

CLINICAL PEARL

The term *sacral sparing* refers to an incomplete lesion of the spinal cord where some of the innermost (long) tracts with the sacral fibers remain intact and innervated. Signs and symptoms of sacral sparing include sensation of the saddle area, movement of the toe flexors, and rectal sphincter contraction.

A spinal cord concussion is characterized by a transient neurologic deficit localized to the spinal cord that fully recovers without any apparent structural damage.

CLINICAL PEARL

The neurologic level is defined as the most caudal level of the spinal cord with normal motor and sensory function on both the left and right sides of the body.

▶ *Motor level:* the most caudal segment of the spinal cord with normal motor function bilaterally.

▶ *Sensory level:* the most caudal segment of the spinal cord with normal sensory function bilaterally.

For example, a patient with C5 quadriplegia has, by definition, abnormal motor and sensory function from C6 down.

Complications associated with a SCI include:

▶ *Autonomic dysreflexia (AD).* AD is a syndrome of massive imbalanced reflex sympathetic discharge occurring in patients with SCI above the T5-T6 level.[68-74] Progressively higher spinal cord lesions or injuries cause increasing

TABLE 6-3	Modified Rancho Los Amigos Cognitive Functioning Scale	
Level I	No Response: Total Assistance	Complete absence of observable change in behavior when presented visual, auditory, tactile, proprioceptive, vestibular, or painful stimuli.
Level II	Generalized Response: Total Assistance	Demonstrates generalized reflex response to painful stimuli. Responds to repeated auditory stimuli with increased or decreased activity. Responds to external stimuli with physiological changes and/or generalized gross body movement but not purposeful vocalization. Responses noted above may be same regardless of type and location of stimulation. Responses may be significantly delayed.
Level III	Localized Response: Total Assistance	Demonstrates withdrawal or vocalization to painful stimuli. Turns toward or away from auditory stimuli. Blinks when strong light crosses visual field. Follows moving object passed within visual field. Responds to discomfort by pulling tubes or restraints. Responds inconsistently to simple commands. Responses directly related to type of stimulus. May respond to some persons (especially family and friends) but not to others.
Level IV	Confused/Agitated: Maximal Assistance	Alert and in heightened state of activity. Purposeful attempts to remove restraints or tubes or crawl out of bed. May perform motor activities such as sitting, reaching and walking but without any apparent purpose or upon another's request. Very brief and usually non-purposeful moments of sustained alternatives and divided attention. Absent short-term memory. May cry out or scream out of proportion to stimulus even after its removal. May exhibit aggressive or flight behavior. Mood may swing from euphoric to hostile with no apparent relationship to environmental events. Unable to cooperate with treatment efforts. Verbalizations are frequently incoherent and/or inappropriate to activity or environment.
Level V	Confused, Inappropriate Non-Agitated: Maximal Assistance	Alert, not agitated but may wander randomly or with a vague intention of going home. May become agitated in response to external stimulation, and/or lack of environmental structure. Not oriented to person, place or time. Frequent brief periods, non-purposeful sustained attention. Severely impaired recent memory, with confusion of past and present in reaction to ongoing activity. Absent goal directed, problem solving, self-monitoring behavior. Often demonstrates inappropriate use of objects without external direction. May be able to perform previously learned tasks when structured and cues provided. Unable to learn new information. Able to respond appropriately to simple commands fairly consistently with external structures and cues. Responses to simple commands without external structure are random and non-purposeful in relation to command. Able to converse on a social, automatic level for brief periods of time when provided external structure and cues. Verbalizations about present events become inappropriate and confabulatory when external structure and cues are not provided.
Level VI	Confused, Appropriate: Moderate Assistance	Inconsistently oriented to person, time and place. Able to attend to highly familiar tasks in non-distracting environment for 30 minutes with moderate redirection. Remote memory has more depth and detail than recent memory. Vague recognition of some staff. Able to use assistive memory aide with maximum assistance. Emerging awareness of appropriate response to self, family and basic needs. Moderate assist to problem solve barriers to task completion. Supervised for old learning (e.g., self-care). Shows carryover for relearned familiar tasks (e.g., self-care). Maximum assistance for new learning with little or no carryover. Unaware of impairments, disabilities and safety risks. Consistently follows simple directions. Verbal expressions are appropriate in highly familiar and structured situations.

TABLE 6-3	Modified Rancho Los Amigos Cognitive Functioning Scale (continued)	
Level VII	**Automatic, Appropriate: Minimal Assistance for Daily Living Skills**	Consistently oriented to person and place, within highly familiar environments. Moderate assistance for orientation to time. Able to attend to highly familiar tasks in a non-distraction environment for at least 30 minutes with minimal assist to complete tasks. Minimal supervision for new learning. Demonstrates carryover of new learning. Initiates and carries out steps to complete familiar personal and household routine but has shallow recall of what he/she has been doing. Able to monitor accuracy and completeness of each step in routine personal and household ADLs and modify plan with minimal assistance. Superficial awareness of his/her condition but unaware of specific impairments and disabilities and the limits they place on his/her ability to safely, accurately and completely carry out his/her household, community, work and leisure ADLs. Minimal supervision for safety in routine home and community activities. Unrealistic planning for the future. Unable to think about consequences of a decision or action. Overestimates abilities. Unaware of others' needs and feelings. Oppositional/uncooperative. Unable to recognize inappropriate social interaction behavior.
Level VIII	**Purposeful, Appropriate: Stand-By Assistance**	Consistently oriented to person, place, and time. Independently attends to and completes familiar tasks for 1 hour in distracting environments. Able to recall and integrate past and recent events. Uses assistive memory devices to recall daily schedule, "to do" lists and record critical information for later use with stand-by assistance. Initiates and carries out steps to complete familiar personal, household, community, work and leisure routines with stand-by assistance and can modify the plan when needed with minimal assistance. Requires no assistance once new tasks/activities are learned. Aware of and acknowledges impairments and disabilities when they interfere with task completion but requires stand-by assistance to take appropriate corrective action. Thinks about consequences of a decision or action with minimal assistance. Overestimates or underestimates abilities. Acknowledges others' needs and feelings and responds appropriately with minimal assistance. Depressed. Irritable. Low frustration tolerance/easily angered. Argumentative. Self-centered. Uncharacteristically dependent/independent. Able to recognize and acknowledge inappropriate social interaction behavior while it is occurring and takes corrective action with minimal assistance.
Level IX	**Purposeful, Appropriate: Stand-By Assistance on Request**	Independently shifts back and forth between tasks and completes them accurately for at least two consecutive hours. Uses assistive memory devices to recall daily schedule, "to do" lists and record critical information for later use with assistance when requested. Initiates and carries out steps to complete familiar personal, household, work, and leisure tasks independently and unfamiliar personal, household, work, and leisure tasks with assistance when requested. Aware of and acknowledges impairments and disabilities when they interfere with task completion and takes appropriate corrective action but requires stand-by assist to anticipate a problem before it occurs and takes action to avoid it. Able to think about consequences of decisions or actions with assistance when requested. Accurately estimates abilities but requires stand-by assistance to adjust to task demands. Acknowledges others' needs and feelings and responds appropriately with stand-by assistance. Depression may continue. May be easily irritable. May have low frustration tolerance. Able to self-monitor appropriateness of social interaction with stand-by assistance.

(continued)

TABLE 6-3	Modified Rancho Los Amigos Cognitive Functioning Scale (continued)
Level X — Purposeful, Appropriate: Modified Independent	Able to handle multiple tasks simultaneously in all environments but may require periodic breaks.
	Able to independently procure, create and maintain own assistive memory devices.
	Independently initiates and carries out steps to complete familiar and unfamiliar personal, household, community, work and leisure tasks but may require more than usual amount of time and/or compensatory strategies to complete them.
	Anticipates impact of impairments and disabilities on ability to complete daily living tasks and takes action to avoid problems before they occur but may require more than usual amount of time and/or compensatory strategies.
	Able to independently think about consequences of decisions or actions but may require more than usual amount of time and/or compensatory strategies to select the appropriate decision or action.
	Accurately estimates abilities and independently adjusts to task demands.
	Able to recognize the needs and feelings of others and automatically respond in appropriate manner.
	Periodic periods of depression may occur.
	Irritability and low frustration tolerance when sick, fatigued and/or under emotional stress.
	Social interaction behavior is consistently appropriate.

Data from Malkmus D, Stenderup K: Rancho Los Amigos Cognitive Scale Revised, Rancho Los Amigos Hospital, 1972.

degrees of autonomic dysfunction. Typical clinical manifestations include

- A sudden significant rise in both systolic and diastolic blood pressures, usually associated with bradycardia
- Profuse sweating above the level of lesion, especially in the face, neck, and shoulders
- Complaints of a headache (caused by vasodilation of pain sensitive intracranial vessels)
- Piloerection (goose bumps) above, or possibly below, the level of the lesion
- Flushing of the skin above the level of the lesion, especially in the face, neck, and shoulders
- Visual disturbances

The potential triggers for AD are numerous and include:

- Bladder distention/urinary catheter blockage from twisting
- Urinary tract infection
- Bowel distention or impaction
- Hemorrhoids
- Deep vein thrombosis
- Pulmonary emboli
- Pressure ulcers
- Ingrown toenail

CLINICAL PEARL

Physical therapists who treat SCI patients need to have a good understanding of AD and be familiar with the signs and symptoms of this potentially life-threatening condition, and be familiar with established protocols for medical management within his/her particular setting. If the patient becomes hypertensive during therapy, he/she should be placed in an upright position immediately, rather than remain in a supine or reclining position, before completing a careful inspection to identify the source of painful stimuli (e.g., catheter, restrictive clothing, leg bag straps, abdominal supports, orthoses).

- *Spinal/neurogenic shock.* Spinal shock is associated with autonomic dysfunction and is characterized by hypotension, relative bradycardia, peripheral vasodilation, and hypothermia.
- *Spasticity.* Spasticity, which occurs when there is damage to the spinal cord or CNS, involves altered skeletal muscle performance in muscle tone resulting in hypertonia. Supraspinal and interneuronal mechanisms appear to be responsible for spasticity. In general, spasticity develops because of an imbalance between the excitatory and inhibitory input to α motor neurons such that the reflex arc to the muscle remains anatomically intact despite the loss of cerebral innervation and control via the long tracts. Spasticity is manifested by a quite forceful, increased resistance to passive motion when an involved muscle is moved with speed and/or is stretched.

CLINICAL PEARL

It must be remembered that not all spasticity is problematic—it can be harnessed for transfers, ambulation, prevention of osteopenia, and improvement of bowel and bladder continence.

- *Heterotopic ossification (HO).* HO is a process by which bone tissue forms outside of the skeleton. Heterotopic ossification often begins as a painful palpable mass that gradually becomes nontender and smaller but firmer to palpation.
- *Orthostatic hypotension.* Orthostatic hypotension results from an inability to control all or most of the sympathetic nervous system (SNS) function. It is common following an upper thoracic or cervical SCI, especially with complete injuries. Orthostatic hypertension is manifested by a rapid increase in blood pressure, cutaneous vasodilatation, lack of sympathetic vasoconstrictor activity, and absent sympathetic input to the heart.

- Pressure ulcers (see Integumentary Causes).[76–88]
- *Deep vein thrombosis (DVT).* Factors predisposing individuals with acute SCI to DVT (see Cardiovascular Causes) include venous stasis secondary to muscle paralysis.[89–92]
- *Impaired temperature control.* After damage to the spinal cord, the hypothalamus can no longer control the cutaneous blood flow or the level of sweating.[93] This lack of sweating is often associated with excessive compensatory diaphoresis above the level of the lesion.[93]
- *Respiratory impairment.* Respiratory function varies considerably, depending on the level of the lesion. Between C1 and C3, phrenic nerve innervation and spontaneous respiration are significantly impaired or lost.[93]
- *Bladder/bowel and sexual dysfunction.* Urinary tract infections are among the most frequent medical complications during the initial medical-rehabilitation period.[93]

One of two types of bladder conditions can develop, depending on location of the lesion:

- *Spastic or reflex (automatic) bladder:* lesions that occur within the spinal cord above the conus medullaris.
- *Flaccid or nonreflex (autonomous) bladder:* a lesion of the conus medullaris or cauda equina.

As with the bladder, the neurogenic bowel condition that develops can be of two types:

- *Spastic or reflex (automatic) bowel:* lesion that occurs within the spinal cord above the conus medullaris.
- *Flaccid or nonreflex (autonomous) bowel:* a lesion of the conus medullaris or cauda equina.

As with bowel and bladder function, sexual capabilities are broadly divided between UMN and LMN lesions.

Congenital and Developmental Disorders

Cerebral Palsy

Cerebral palsy (CP), which is the neurologic condition most frequently encountered by pediatric physical therapists, is generally considered to be a nonprogressive defect or lesion in single or multiple locations in the immature brain.[94–140] CP is diagnosed when a child does not reach motor milestones and exhibits abnormal muscle tone or qualitative differences in movement patterns such as asymmetry. Despite advances in neonatal care, CP remains a significant clinical problem. In most cases of CP the exact cause is unknown but is most likely multifactorial (intracranial hemorrhage, intrauterine infection, birth asphyxia, multiple births, early prenatal, perinatal, or postnatal injury due to vascular insufficiency, or CNS malformation).

CP has been classified in a number of ways. A classification based on the area of the body exhibiting motor impairment yield the designations of monoplegia (one limb), diplegia (lower limbs), hemiplegia (upper and lower limbs on one side of the body), and quadriplegia (all limbs). Another classification is based on the most obvious movement abnormality resulting from common brain lesions: spastic, athetoid, ataxic, low tone, or a combination (Tables 6-4 and 6-5). Impairments in CP are problems of the neuromuscular and skeletal systems that are either an immediate result of the existing pathophysiologic process or an indirect consequence that has developed over time:

- *Primary impairments of the muscular system:* insufficient force generation, spasticity, abnormal extensibility, and exaggerated or hyperactive reflexes.
- *Primary impairments of the neuromuscular system:* Poor selected control of muscle activity, poor regulation of activity in muscle groups in anticipation of postural changes and body movement (anticipatory regulation), and decreased ability to learn unique movements.
- *Secondary impairments of the skeletal system:* misalignment such as torsion or hip deformities.

Syringomyelia

Syringomyelia is the development of a fluid-filled cavity or syrinx within the spinal cord (hydromyelia is a dilatation of the central canal by cerebrospinal fluid [CSF] and may be included within the definition of syringomyelia).[141-145] Although many mechanisms for syrinx formation have been postulated, the exact pathogenesis is still unknown. Syringomyelia usually progresses slowly; the course may extend over many years. The condition may have a more acute course, especially when the brainstem is affected (i.e., syringobulbia). Syringomyelia usually involves the cervical area. Clinical manifestations include the following:

- *Dissociated sensory loss:* a loss of pain and temperature sensibility, while light touch, vibration, and position senses are preserved.
- *Motor changes:* diffuse muscle atrophy that begins in the hands and progresses proximally to include the forearms and shoulder girdles.
- Upper extremity muscles stretch (deep tendon) reflexes are diminished early in the clinical course.
- Lower extremity spasticity, which may be asymmetrical, appears with paraparesis, hyperreflexia, and extensor plantar responses.
- Respiratory insufficiency, which usually is related to changes in position, may occur.

TABLE 6-4	**Cerebral Palsy Classifications and Manifestations**			
	Spastic	**Athetoid**	**Ataxic**	**Hypotonic**
Muscle stiffness	Excessively stiff and taut, especially during attempted movement	Low		Diminished resting muscle tone and decreased ability to generate voluntary muscle force
Posture	Abnormal postures and movements with mass patterns of flexion/extension	Poor functional stability especially in proximal joint	Low postural tone with poor balance	
Visual tracking	Some deficits	Poor visual tracking	Poor visual tracking, nystagmus	
Muscle tone	Increased in antigravity muscles. Imbalance of tone across joints that can cause contractures and deformities	Fluctuates, but generally decreased—floppy baby syndrome	Slightly decreased	Minimal to none
Initiating movement	Difficult	No problems	No problems	Difficult
Sustaining movement	Able to in some	Unable	No problems	Unable
Terminating movement	Unable		No problems	Uncontrolled
Muscle coactivation	Abnormal	Poorly timed	No problems	None
ROM limitations	Passive ROM, overall decreased	Hypermobile	In spine	Hypermobile

Spina Bifida

Spina bifida includes a continuum of congenital anomalies of the spine due to insufficient closure of the neural tube and failure of the vertebral arches to fuse.[146–152] Spina bifida is classified into aperta (visible or open) and occulta (not visible or hidden). The three main types of spina bifida are listed in Table 6-6. Spina bifida aperta is often used interchangeably with myelomeningocele, which is an open spinal cord defect that usually protrudes dorsally. The neurologic complications associated with spina bifida are outlined in Table 6-7.

TABLE 6-5	**Physical Attributes of Different Types of Cerebral Palsy**
Type	**Attributes**
Spastic (i.e., pyramidal)	Constitutes 75% of patients with cerebral palsy. Patients have signs of upper motor neuron involvement, including hyperreflexia, clonus, extensor Babinski response, persistent primitive reflexes, and overflow reflexes (i.e., crossed adductor). Cognitive impairment is present in approximately 30% of spastic diplegic patients, but most patients with spastic quadriplegia have some cognitive impairment.
Dyskinesia (i.e., extrapyramidal)	Characterized by extrapyramidal movement patterns, abnormal regulation of tone, abnormal postural control, and coordination deficits. Athetosis, chorea, and choreoathetoid or dystonic movements can be seen. Patients often have pseudobulbar involvement with dysarthria, swallowing difficulties, drooling, oromotor difficulties, and abnormal speech patterns. Generally, the child is hypotonic at birth with abnormal movement patterns emerging at 1 to 3 years. The arms are usually more involved than the legs. Abnormal movement patterns may increase with stress or purposeful activity. Muscle tone is normal during sleep. Intelligence is normal in 78% of patients with athetoid cerebral palsy. A high incidence of sensorineural hearing loss is reported.
Spastic diplegia	Patients with often have a period of hypotonia followed by extensor spasticity in the lower extremities with little or no functional limitation of the upper extremities. Patients have a delay in developing gross motor skills. Spastic muscle imbalance often causes persistence of infantile coxa valga and femoral anteversion. Scissoring gait (i.e., hips flexed and adducted, knees flexed with valgus stress, equinus ankles) is observed.
Hemiplegia	Characterized by weak hip flexion and ankle dorsiflexion, overactive posterior tibialis, hip hiking/circumduction, supinated foot in stance, upper extremity posturing (e.g., often held with shoulder adducted, elbow flexed, forearm pronated, wrist flexed, hand clenched in a fist with the thumb in the palm), impaired sensation, impaired 2-point discrimination, and/or impaired position sense. Some cognitive impairment is found in about 28% of these patients.

TABLE 6-6	Types of Spina Bifida
Type	**Description**
Spina bifida occulta	*Occulta* means "hidden," and the defect is not visible. Rarely linked with complications or symptoms. Usually discovered accidentally during an x-ray or MRI for some other reason.
Meningocele (spina bifida aperta)	The membrane that surrounds the spinal cord may enlarge, creating a lump or "cyst." This is often invisible through the skin and causes no problems. If the spinal canal is cleft, or "bifid," the cyst may expand and come to the surface. In such cases, because the cyst does not enclose the spinal cord, the cord is not exposed. The cyst varies in size, but it can almost always be removed surgically if necessary, leaving no permanent disability.
Myelomeningocele (spina bifida cystica)	The most complex and severe form of spina bifida. Usually involves neurologic problems that can be very serious or even fatal. A section of the spinal cord and the nerves that stem from the cord are exposed and visible on the outside of the body; or, if there is a cyst, it encloses part of the cord and the nerves. This condition accounts for 94% of cases of true spina bifida. The most severe form of spina bifida cystica is myelocele, or myeloschisis, in which the open neural plate is covered secondarily by epithelium and the neural plate has spread out onto the surface.

TABLE 6-7	The Neurologic Complications Associated with Spina Bifida
Complication	**Description**
Syringomeningocele	The Greek word *syrinx*, meaning tube or plate, is combined with *meninx* (membrane) and *kele* (tumor); the term thus describes a hollow center with the spinal fluid connecting with the central canal of the cord enclosed by a membrane with very little cord substance.
Syringomyelocele	Protrusion of the membranes and spinal cord lead to increased fluid in the central canal, attenuating the cord tissue against a thin-walled sac.
Diastematomyelia	From the Greek root *diastema* (interval) and *myelon* (marrow); is accompanied by a bony septum in some cases.
Myelodysplasia	From the Greek term *myelos*, meaning spinal cord, with *dys* for difficult and *plasi* for molding. This is a defective development of any part of the cord.
Arnold-Chiari deformity	Malformation of the cerebellum, with elongation of the cerebellar tonsils. The cerebellum is drawn into the fourth ventricle. The condition also is characterized by smallness of the medulla and pons and internal hydrocephalus. In fact, all patients with spina bifida cystica (failure to close caudally) have some form of Arnold-Chiari malformation (failure to close cranially). The Chiari II malformation is a complex congenital malformation of the brain, nearly always associated with myelomeningocele. This condition includes downward displacement of the medulla, fourth ventricle, and cerebellum into the cervical spinal canal, as well as elongation of the pons and fourth ventricle, probably due to a relatively small posterior fossa. Signs and symptoms include stridor, apnea, irritability, cerebellar ataxia, and hypertonia.
Craniorachischisis (total dysraphism)	A condition in which the brain and spinal cord are exposed. This often results in early spontaneous abortion, often associated with malformations of other organ systems.
Tethered cord	A longitudinal stretch of the spinal cord that occurs with growth resulting in progressive loss of sensory and motor function, long tract signs, and changes in posture and gait. Presence may be signaled by foot deformities previously braced easily, new onset of hip dislocation, or worsening of a spinal deformity, particularly scoliosis. Progressive neurologic defects in growing children may suggest a lack of extensibility of the spine, or that it is tethered and low-lying in the lumbar canal, with the potential for progressive irreversible neurologic damage and requiring surgical release.
Hydrocephalus	Characterized by a tense, bulging fontanel and increased occipital frontal circumference. Signs and symptoms include decreased upper extremity coordination, disturbed balance, strabismus, and ocular problems. Medical intervention involves placement of a shunt between ventricle and heart/abdomen.
Neurogenic bowel and bladder	Incontinence.

Data from Shaer CM, Chescheir N, Erickson K, et al: Obstetrician-gynecologists' practice and knowledge regarding spina bifida. Am J Perinatol 23:355-362, 2006; Woodhouse CR: Progress in the management of children born with spina bifida. Eur Urol 49:777-778, 2006; Verhoef M, Barf HA, Post MW, et al: Functional independence among young adults with spina bifida, in relation to hydrocephalus and level of lesion. Dev Med Child Neurol 48:114-119, 2006; Ali L, Stocks GM: Spina bifida, tethered cord and regional anaesthesia. Anaesthesia 60:1149-1150, 2005; Spina bifida. Nurs Times 101:31, 2005; Mitchell LE, Adzick NS, Melchionne J, et al: Spina bifida. Lancet 364:1885-1895, 2004; Dias L: Orthopaedic care in spina bifida: past, present, and future. Dev Med Child Neurol 46:579, 2004.

Aging

A wide variety of neurologic disorders and diseases can affect the aging population, including cerebrovascular accident; Parkinson's disease; cerebellar dysfunction; neuropathies; cognitive, psychological, and sensory problems (depression, fear, and anxiety); pain; and impaired vision. Age-related changes in the brain start at around age 60. Normal, nonprogressive, and negligible declines among the aged do not dramatically affect daily functioning (until the early 1980s), but the more serious disorders/diseases can significantly affect cognitive function in old age. Not all cognitive disorders are irreversible, but many require timely identification and intercession to offset permanent dysfunction.

▶ *Dementia.* Primarily a disease of the elderly, dementia is a generic term most often applied to geropsychological problems applying broadly to a progressive, persistent loss of cognitive and intellectual functions. Dementia presents with a history of chronic, steady decline in short- and long-term memory and is associated with difficulties in social relationships, work, and activities of daily life. In contrast to delirium, the patient's perception is clear. However, delirium can be superimposed on an underlying dementing process. Earlier stages of dementia may present subtly, and patients may minimize or attempt to hide their impairments. Patients at this stage often have associated depression. The typical end result of dementia is impairment of cognition that affects some or all of the following: alertness, orientation, emotion, behavior, memory, perception, language, praxis (applying knowledge), problem solving, judgment, and psychomotor activity.

▶ *Balance dysfunction.* Age-related balance dysfunctions can occur through a loss of sensory elements such as degenerative changes in the vestibular apparatus of the inner ear, an inability to integrate sensory information, and muscle weakness. Diseases common in aging populations lead to further deterioration in balance function in some patients (Ménière's disease, benign paroxysmal positional vertigo [BPPV], cerebrovascular disease, vertebrobasilar artery insufficiency, cerebellar dysfunction, and cardiac disease). Balance disorders can be associated with a number of other causes, including:

- Cardiac abnormalities
- Medications
- Postural hypotension
- Sensory loss
- Visual/auditory deficits

CARDIOVASCULAR CAUSES

The cardiovascular system (see Chapter 4) plays an important role in allowing muscle activity to continue over a sustained period by providing vascular support to the working muscles. The maximum work capacity of the cardiorespiratory system is a factor of the maximal amount of oxygen that can be taken in and used by the body, or VO$_2$ max, whereas the capacity of the neuromuscular system is a factor of the maximum tension that can be developed by the working muscle, or muscles—the maximal voluntary contraction. Assessment of the cardiovascular system provides the clinician with the justification for monitoring or not monitoring activities during a patient's rehabilitation or providing modifications in the exercise prescription.[153]

Physical therapists often examine and treat patients with one or more chronic medical conditions that are the inherent cause of dependence, dysfunction, and disability and/or increase the risk of other pathologic conditions.

▶ Comorbidity[154,155]

- *Atherosclerosis:* a major contributing factor to coronary heart disease, including angina pectoris and myocardial infarction.[156]
- *Hypertension:* causes mechanical damage to vascular endothelium resulting in areas that are stripped of normal endothelial cells. Associated with increased thrombus and plaque formation, intracerebral aneurysms and hemorrhage, and left ventricular hypertrophy.[157,158]
- *Hyperlipidemia* (high blood cholesterol).[159]
- *Diabetes:* a complex mix of physiologic abnormalities that accelerates the development of atherosclerosis and leads to many cardiovascular complications.[160–162]
- *Osteoporosis:* can be associated with classic spinal deformities including increased kyphosis with loss of height, thoracic vertebral body fractures, back pain, and decreased vital capacity.
- *Ankylosing spondylitis:* pulmonary involvement including nonspecific fibrosis, dilated bronchi, stiffening, and straightening of the spine, and decreased intestinal compliance, the last of which increases the potential for pneumothorax, atelectasis, and aspiration.
- *Idiopathic scoliosis:* the lateral curve plus the rotation of the involved thoracic vertebrae around a vertical axis causes a decrease in lung function.
- *Pectus deformities:* includes pectus excavatum (funnel chest) and pectus carinatum (pigeon breast).
- *Sarcoidosis:* a systemic disease that primarily affects the lungs and the lymphatic system.
- *Systemic lupus erythematosus (SLE):* affects the pulmonary system more frequently than any other collagen vascular disease. SLE can be associated with pleuritis, pneumonitis, pulmonary interstitial fibrosis, and pulmonary hypertension.

▶ Neurologic disease

- *Cerebrovascular accident:* cardiovascular disease is the most common cause of death in long-term survivors of stroke.[163–166]
- *Spinal cord injury:* stimulation of the cardiopulmonary system is impaired due to lack of innervation to the autonomic nervous system, thereby reducing the ability to support higher rates of aerobic metabolism.[167,168]

- *Multiple sclerosis:* the loss of myelin reduces the speed of nerve conduction, thus interfering with smooth, rapid, and coordinated movement.[169]
- *Parkinson's disease:* associated with bradykinesia, slow and shuffling gait, freezing, kyphotic posture, and overall flexed posture.[170]

▶ *Medications.* Aspirin resistance may increase the risk of major adverse cardiac events (MACE) more than threefold in patients with stable coronary artery disease (CAD).[171]

▶ *Lifestyle:* cigarette smoking substantially increases the risk for cardiovascular disease in addition to other diseases, notably chronic obstructive pulmonary disease and lung cancer.[172]

▶ *Obesity:* many of the effects of obesity appear to be mediated through other risk factors including diabetes and hypertension.[173]

▶ *Physical inactivity:* physical inactivity may exert much of its influence through other risk factors.[174] However, numerous public health and medical associations have identified physical inactivity as a significant risk factor for cardiovascular and other diseases.[175]

▶ *Race.* African American women have the highest risk of death from heart disease; Native Americans, particularly those living in North Dakota and South Dakota, also have a higher risk.[176]

▶ *Gender:* CAD is the number one killer of women, surpassing all forms of cancer, including breast cancer, combined.[177] At the onset of menopause, women's CAD risk begins to approach that of men.[177,178]

▶ *Family history:* family history is considered positive if myocardial infarction or sudden cardiac death occurred in a primary male relative, age 55 or less, or in a primary female relative, age 65 or less.[179]

▶ *Psychosocial factors:* an individual's response to stress can be a determinant factor in the development of CAD. Depression, social isolation, and chronic stress have all been shown to be associated with CAD.[180]

Poor Cardiac Function

Heart failure is the pathophysiologic state in which the heart fails to pump blood at a rate commensurate with the requirements of the metabolizing tissues.[181]

Congestive Heart Failure

CHF can be categorized as forward or backward ventricular failure:

▶ Forward ventricular failure is secondary to reduced forward flow into the aorta and systemic circulation.

▶ Backward failure is secondary to elevated systemic venous pressure.

Heart failure can also be subdivided into systolic and diastolic dysfunction.

▶ *Systolic (left heart) failure:* decrease in stroke volume, which leads to activation of peripheral and central baroreflexes and chemoreflexes that are capable of eliciting marked increases in sympathetic nerve activity. This in turn produces a temporary improvement in systolic blood pressure and

tissue perfusion. Signs and symptoms of left-sided heart failure include progressive severity of (1) exertional dyspnea, (2) orthopnea, (3) paroxysmal nocturnal dyspnea, (4) dyspnea at rest, and (5) acute pulmonary edema (termed congestive heart failure). Systolic failure can be further categorized as ischemic or nonischemic heart failure:

- *Ischemic:* the breakdown of the heart muscle because of lack of blood flow to the coronary vessels that may occur with or without myocardial infarction.
- *Nonischemic:* results from any process other than coronary artery disease (CAD).

▶ *Diastolic (right heart) failure:* a decrease in stroke volume with the same outcome as with systolic failure but through different mechanisms. The altered relaxation of the ventricle (due to a delay in calcium uptake and a delay in calcium efflux) occurs in response to an increase in ventricular afterload (pressure overload). This impaired relaxation of the ventricle leads to impaired diastolic filling of the left ventricle. Signs and symptoms of left-sided heart failure include ascites, congestive hepatomegaly, and anasarca (generalized edema).

Regardless of the etiology of classification, heart failure is characterized by the inability of the heart to meet the demands of the body—the finite adaptive mechanisms that may be adequate to maintain the overall contractile performance of the heart at relatively normal levels become maladaptive when trying to sustain adequate cardiac performance at higher levels. This results in the hallmark symptom of heart failure: exercise intolerance. The New York Heart Association uses the following functional classification:

▶ Class I describes a patient who is not limited with normal physical activity by symptoms.

▶ Class II occurs when ordinary physical activity results in fatigue, dyspnea, or other symptoms.

▶ Class III is characterized by a marked limitation in normal physical activity.

▶ Class IV is defined by symptoms at rest or with any physical activity.

A normal exercise response requires the coordination of multiple systems, including the cardiac, pulmonary, vascular, and musculoskeletal. During exercise, cardiac output should be able to increase to four to six times its resting level. Patients with heart failure can often only achieve half this normal increase in cardiac output during exercise.[182–184]

CLINICAL PEARL

The central hemodynamic characteristics of heart failure that contribute to exercise intolerance include:

▶ Abnormal pressures within the heart

▶ Reduced left ventricular ejection fraction

▶ Reduced cardiac output

▶ Increased pulmonary capillary wedge pressure

▶ Increased production of angiotensin II, which increases heart rate, impairs cardiac filling, and increases coronary vasoconstriction and peripheral vascular resistance

The medical intervention for heart failure focuses on improving central hemodynamics through three main goals: (1) preload reduction, (2) reduction of systemic vascular resistance (afterload reduction) through administration of vasodilators, and (3) inhibition of both the renin-angiotensin-aldosterone systems and the vasoconstrictor neurohumoral factors (inotropic support) produced by the sympathetic nervous system in patients with heart failure.

Cor Pulmonale

Cor pulmonale is defined as an alteration in the structure and function of the right ventricle caused by a disorder of the respiratory system, including pulmonary hypertension or a wide variety of cardiopulmonary disease processes.[185-189] Although cor pulmonale commonly has a chronic and slowly progressive course, acute onset or worsening cor pulmonale with life-threatening complications can occur. Clinical manifestations of cor pulmonale include complaints of fatigue, exertional dyspnea/chest pain, syncope with exertion, and hemoptysis.

Cardiac Impulse Abnormalities

A rhythm is either regular or irregular. Arrhythmias are a group of conditions that affect the cardiac nervous system. Arrhythmias (dysrhythmias) are usually classified according to their origin (ventricular, or supraventricular [atrial]), pattern (fibrillation or flutter), or the speed or rate at which they occur (tachycardia or bradycardia). Causes include congenital defects, hypertrophy of the heart muscle fibers, valvular heart disease, degeneration of conductive tissue, ischemic conditions of the myocardium, electrolyte imbalance, chemical imbalances, hypoxemia, hypertension, emotional stress, drugs, alcohol, and caffeine.[190]

Cardiomyopathies

Cardiomyopathy is part of a group of conditions affecting the heart muscle itself so that the fibers involved with contraction and relaxation of the myocardial muscle are impaired. Causes include CAD (see later), valvular disorders, hypertension, congenital defects, and pulmonary vascular disorders. Heart problems that occur secondary to impairment of the valves may be caused by infection such as endocarditis, congenital deformity, or disease.

CLINICAL PEARL

It is the closing of the valves that produces the familiar beating sounds of the heart, commonly referred to as the "lub-dub" sound—due to the closing of the semilunar and atrioventricular valves.

Coronary Artery Disease

Coronary artery disease (CAD) is a complex disease involving a narrowing of the lumen of one or more of the arteries that encircle and supply the heart, resulting in ischemia to the myocardium. Injury to the endothelial lining of arteries, an inflammatory reaction, thrombosis, calcification, and hemorrhage all contribute to arteriosclerosis or scarring of an artery wall.

Atherosclerosis

Atherosclerosis, the most common form of arteriosclerosis, is a chronic thickening of the arterial wall of medium and large sized vessels, through the accumulation of lipids, macrophages, T-lymphocytes, smooth muscle cells, extracellular matrix, calcium, and necrotic debris. Atherosclerosis primarily affects the lower extremities. When the arteries of the heart are affected it is referred to as coronary artery disease (CAD) or coronary heart disease (CHD); when the arteries to the brain are affected, cerebrovascular disease (CVD) develops.[191] Common symptoms of atherosclerosis include:

▶ Decreased or absent peripheral pulses.

▶ Skin color: pale on elevation, dusky red on dependency.

▶ Intermittent claudication (early stages): pain is described as burning, searing, aching, tightness, or cramping.

▶ In the later stages, patients exhibit ischemia and rest pain; ulcerations and gangrene, trophic changes.

Risk factors for CAD are classified as modifiable or unmodifiable.

▶ Modifiable risk factors include smoking, exposure to second-hand smoke, hypertension, hyperlipidemia, high cholesterol (total or LDL-C) levels, low HDL-C levels, high triglyceride levels, diabetes, abdominal obesity, and a sedentary lifestyle.

▶ Unmodifiable risk factors include age, male sex, race, and family history.

The clinical symptoms of CAD include any symptoms that may represent cardiac ischemia, such as an ache, pressure, pain, other discomfort, or possibly just decreased activity tolerance due to fatigue, shortness of breath, or palpitations.

Angina Pectoris

Angina pectoris is the result of myocardial ischemia caused by an imbalance between myocardial blood supply and oxygen demand, which causes myocardial cells to switch from aerobic to anaerobic metabolism, with a progressive impairment of metabolic, mechanical, and electrical functions.[192]

Most patients with angina pectoris complain of retrosternal chest discomfort rather than frank pain. The former is usually described as a pressure, heaviness, squeezing, burning, or choking sensation in the epigastrium, back, neck, or jaw. Typical locations for radiation of pain are the arms, shoulders, and neck (C8-T4 dermatomes). Typically, exertion, eating, exposure to cold, or emotional stress precipitate angina. Episodes typically last for approximately 1 to 5 minutes and are relieved by rest or by taking nitroglycerin.

The New York Heart Association classification (see Congestive Heart Failure) may be used to quantify the functional limitation imposed by patients' symptoms.

Myocardial Infarction

Myocardial infarction (MI) is the rapid development of myocardial necrosis caused by a critical imbalance between the oxygen supply and demand of the myocardium.[193] This usually results from plaque rupture with thrombus formation in a coronary vessel, resulting in an acute reduction of blood supply to a portion of the myocardium.

▶ Atherosclerotic causes of MI are the most common cause and result from a plaque rupture with subsequent exposure of the basement membrane that results in platelet aggregation, thrombus formation, fibrin accumulation, hemorrhage into the plaque, and varying degrees of vasospasm. MI occurs most frequently in persons older than 45 years.

▶ Nonatherosclerotic causes of MI include coronary vasospasm, coronary emboli from sources such as an infected heart valve, occlusion of the coronaries due to vasculitis, or other causes leading to mismatch of oxygen supply and demand, such as acute anemia from GI bleeding.

Signs and symptoms of MI include:

▶ Chest pain, typically described as tightness, pressure, or squeezing, located across the anterior precordium. Pain may radiate to the jaw, neck, arms, back, and epigastrium. The left arm is affected more frequently; however, pain may be felt in both arms.

▶ Dyspnea, which may accompany chest pain or occur as an isolated complaint (especially in an elderly person or the diabetic patient).

▶ Nausea and/or abdominal pain often are present in infarcts involving the inferior or posterior wall.

▶ Anxiety.

▶ Lightheadedness with or without syncope.

▶ Cough.

▶ Nausea with or without vomiting.

▶ Diaphoresis.

▶ Wheezing.

CLINICAL PEARL

As many as half of MIs are clinically silent in that they do not cause the classic symptoms. This is particularly true with elderly patients and those with diabetes who may have particularly subtle presentations—complaints of fatigue, syncope, or weakness. The elderly may also present with only altered mental status.

Vascular System Abnormalities

Arterial Disease

Arterial diseases can include the following:

▶ *Arteriosclerosis.* Arteriosclerosis is a group of diseases characterized by thickening and loss of elasticity of the arterial wall, often referred to as hardening of the arteries.

▶ *Arteriovenous malformation (AVM).* AVMs are congenital vascular malformations of the cerebral vasculature—the result of localized poor development of the primitive

vascular plexus of the heart. AVMs vary in size and location and therefore in clinical presentation. Early diagnosis can reduce the chance of hemorrhage.

▶ *Aneurysm.* An aneurysm is an abnormal stretching in the wall of an artery, a vein, or the heart with a diameter that is at least 50% greater than normal.[194] Aneurysms are named according to the specific site of formation. Aortic aneurysms can form a thoracic aneurysm (involving the ascending, transverse, or first half of the descending portion of the aorta) or an abdominal aneurysm (involving the aorta between the renal arteries and iliac branches). The underlying causes of aortic aneurysms are associated with many factors, including atherosclerosis, hypertension, medial degeneration of an arterial wall and aging, aortitis, congenital abnormalities, trauma, smoking, cellular enzyme dysfunction, and hyperlipidemia.[195]

CLINICAL PEARL

Acute aortic dissection, which is characterized by the onset of intense pain in the chest, back, and abdomen and decreased or absent distal pulses, is a potentially life-threatening condition requiring immediate transport of the patient to an emergency department.[195]

▶ *Arteritis.* Arteritis (giant cell arteritis, cranial or temporal arteritis) is a vasculitis primarily involving multiple sites of temporal and cranial arteries. Early diagnosis is important to prevent blindness.

▶ *Thromboangiitis obliterans.* Thromboangiitis obliterans (Buerger's disease) is a chronic, inflammatory vasculitis affecting the peripheral blood vessels (small arteries and veins), which occurs commonly in young adults, largely male, who smoke heavily. Risk of ulceration, gangrene, and amputation if left untreated. The condition usually progresses proximally in both upper and lower extremities, accompanied by a thrombus formation and vasospasm. Patients exhibit paresthesias or pain, cyanotic cold extremity, diminished temperature sensation, or fatigue (intermittent claudication) due to occlusion of the arteries.

CLINICAL PEARL

The differential diagnosis of paresthesias and peripheral neuropathy is difficult. Peripheral neuropathies can be caused by entrapment syndromes, trauma, diabetes, hypothyroidism, vitamin B_{12} deficiency, alcoholism, inflammatory conditions, connective tissue disorders, toxic injury, hereditary conditions, malignancy, infections, and miscellaneous causes.[196] Peripheral neuropathy can also be mimicked by myelopathy, syringomyelia, or dorsal column disorders, such as tabes dorsalis.[197] Hysterical symptoms can sometimes mimic a neuropathy. Many medications can cause a peripheral neuropathy.[197]

▶ *Raynaud's disease.* Raynaud's disease or phenomenon results in intermittent spasms of small arteries and arterioles, causing temporary pallor and cyanosis of the digits, usually exacerbated by exposure to cold or emotional stress.

- ■ Abnormal vasoconstrictor reflex results in pallor, cyanosis, numbness and tingling of digits (fingertips more often than toes).
- ■ Affects largely females.
- ■ Occlusive disease is not usually a factor.

▶ *Hypertension.* Hypertension (hypertensive vascular disease) includes hypertensive heart disease, pulmonary hypertension, and pulmonary heart disease.

▶ *Hypotension.* Blood pressure that is too low is known as hypotension. Low blood pressure may be a sign of severe disease and requires more urgent medical attention. When blood pressure and blood flow are very low, the perfusion of the brain may be critically decreased (i.e., the blood supply is not sufficient), causing lightheadedness, dizziness, weakness, and fainting. Sometimes the blood pressure drops significantly when a patient stands up from sitting—orthostatic hypotension (see next). Other causes of low blood pressure include:

- ■ Sepsis.
- ■ Hemorrhage.
- ■ Toxins including toxic doses of blood pressure medicine.
- ■ Hormonal abnormalities, such as Addison's disease.
- ■ *Shock.* Shock is a complex condition that leads to critically decreased blood perfusion. The usual mechanisms are loss of blood volume, pooling of blood within the veins reducing adequate return to the heart, and/or low effective heart pumping. Low blood pressure, especially low pulse pressure, is a sign of shock and contributes to/reflects decreased perfusion.

▶ *Orthostatic hypotension.* Orthostatic hypotension, in addition to being a complication of a spinal cord injury (see Neurologic Causes) can occur in all age groups and populations, but is more common in the elderly, especially in persons who are sick and frail. In cases of suspected orthostatic hypotension, the clinician should position the patient in the supine position, take a blood pressure measurement, and then repeat the blood pressure measurement at 1 and 3 minutes after the patient assumes a standing or sitting position.

CLINICAL PEARL

Instances of orthostatic hypotension should be reported to the patient's physician because of its association with several diagnoses and conditions, including an increased rate of falls, and a history of myocardial infarction or transient ischemic attack; it also may be predictive of ischemic stroke.[198]

Venous Insufficiency

In venous insufficiency states, venous blood escapes from its normal antegrade path of flow and refluxes backward down the veins into an already congested leg. Venous insufficiency

syndromes are caused by valvular incompetence in the high-pressure deep venous system, low-pressure superficial venous system, or both. Physical examination alone is not a reliable means of assessing the venous system—diagnostic testing nearly always is necessary to rule out deep venous obstruction, to assess the paths of reflux, and to guide treatment planning.

Deep Venous Insufficiency

Deep venous insufficiency occurs when the valves of the deep veins are damaged as a result of deep venous thrombosis (DVT)—see Deep Vein Thrombophlebitis. With no valves to prevent deep system reflux, the hydrostatic venous pressure in the lower extremity increases dramatically. This condition is often referred to as a postphlebitic syndrome.

Superficial Venous Insufficiency

Superficial venous incompetence is the most common form of venous disease. In superficial venous insufficiency, the deep veins are normal, but venous blood escapes from a normal deep system and flows backwards through dilated superficial veins in which the valves have failed. Most cases of superficial vein valve failure occur after a single point of high-pressure leakage develops between the deep system and the superficial system. High pressure causes secondary valve failure when otherwise normal superficial veins become so widely dilated that the thin flaps of the venous valves can no longer make contact in the lumen of the vessel. Over time, these incompetent superficial veins become visibly dilated and tortuous, at which point they are recognized as varicose veins.

Patients with venous insufficiency often report subjective symptoms that are typically bothersome early in the disease, become less severe in the middle phases, and then worsen again with advancing age. Common symptoms include the following:

- ▶ Burning
- ▶ Swelling
- ▶ Throbbing
- ▶ Cramping
- ▶ Aching
- ▶ Heaviness
- ▶ Restless legs
- ▶ Leg fatigue

Pain caused by venous insufficiency often is improved by walking or by elevating the legs.

Thrombophlebitis

Microscopic thrombosis is a normal part of the dynamic balance of hemostasis. There are two types of venous thrombosis: superficial vein thrombophlebitis and deep vein thrombophlebitis. Both types share the same pathophysiology, pathogenesis, and risk factors.

Superficial Vein Thrombophlebitis

Superficial vein thrombophlebitis may occur spontaneously or as a complication of medical or surgical interventions. Patients with superficial thrombophlebitis often give a history of a gradual onset of localized tenderness, followed by the appearance of an area of erythema along the path of a superficial vein. There may be a history of local trauma, prior similar episodes, varicose veins, prolonged travel, or enforced stasis. Swelling may result from acute venous obstruction (as in deep vein thrombosis) or from deep or superficial venous reflux, or it may be caused by an unrelated disease condition such as hepatic insufficiency, renal failure, cardiac decompensation, infection, trauma, or environmental effects. Palpation of a painful or tender area may reveal a firm, thickened, thrombosed vein.

Deep Vein Thrombophlebitis

Deep venous thrombosis (DVT) and its sequela, pulmonary embolism, are the leading causes of preventable in-hospital mortality in the United States.[199] The Virchow triad, as first formulated (i.e., venous stasis, vessel wall injury, hypercoagulable state), is still the primary mechanism for the development of venous thrombosis.[199] Hypercoagulable states include:

▶ *Genetic:* includes antithrombin C deficiency, protein C deficiency, and protein S efficiency

▶ *Acquired:* includes postoperative, postpartum, prolonged bed rest or immobilization, severe trauma, cancer, congestive heart failure, obesity, and prior thromboembolism

CLINICAL PEARL

Patients who undergo total hip arthroplasty or total knee arthroplasty are at high risk for DVT. If no prophylaxis is used, DVT occurs in 40% to 80% of these patients, and the proximal DVT occurs in 15% to 50%.[200]

The signs and symptoms of DVT are related to the degree of obstruction to venous outflow and inflammation of the vessel wall. No single physical finding or combination of symptoms and signs is sufficiently accurate to establish the diagnosis of DVT.[199] The following is a list outlining the most sensitive and specific physical findings in DVT[199,201–203]:

▶ Edema, principally unilateral.

▶ Tenderness, if present, is usually confined to the calf muscles or over the course of the deep veins in the thigh.

▶ Pain and/or tenderness away from these areas is not consistent with venous thrombosis and usually indicates another diagnosis.

▶ Fever: Patients may have a fever, usually low grade. High fever is usually indicative of an infectious process such as cellulitis or lymphangitis.

CLINICAL PEARL

In the event of a suspected DVT, the clinician should hold the therapeutic interventions and inform the physician. The patient should be positioned in non–weight-bearing on the affected lower extremity.

Aging

The patient admitted to a rehabilitation program may not have been physically active for some time, and the level of fitness may have declined considerably. Age-related anatomic and physiologic changes of the heart and blood vessels, which can either be mitigated or exacerbated with activity level, typically result in reduced capacity for oxygen transport at rest and in response to situations imposing an increase in metabolic demand for oxygen.[32] In addition, maximal oxygen consumption (PO_2 max), an index of maximal cardiovascular function, decreases 5% to 15% per decade after the age of 25 years.[204] As a result, at submaximal exercise, heart rate responses such as cardiac output and stroke volume are lower in older adults at the same absolute work rates, whereas blood pressures tends to be higher.[204] It is very important that elderly patients have a physician's evaluation of their cardiovascular status before engaging in a rehabilitation program. In addition, the patient should be carefully monitored for cardiovascular response and tolerance to exercise during rehabilitation sessions. HR, BP, and RPE (rate of perceived exertion) should be assessed before, during, and after exercise, and the physician should be notified of any abnormal or unusual findings. In addition to the normal aging changes, a number of complications can occur in the elderly, acute inactivity, such as that which occurs with hospitalization, can significantly reduce VO_2 max and increase blood viscosity and venous status, which increases the risk of thromboembolic disease.[34] Immobility is a common pathway by which a host of diseases and problems in the elderly produce further disability. Persons who are chronically ill, aged, or disabled are particularly susceptible to the adverse effects of prolonged bed rest, immobilization, and inactivity. Common causes for immobility in the elderly include arthritis, osteoporosis, fractures (especially hip and femur), podiatric problems, and neurologic disorders and diseases.

RESPIRATORY CAUSES

An individual's ability to move is based on the capacity of the pulmonary and vascular systems (Table 6-8) to deliver oxygen and nutrients to the exercising muscles (Table 6-9). Patients with heart or lung disease or dysfunction are unable to supply or transport nutrients or eliminate waste products and can therefore suffer from generalized fatigue during motor activities.

Inflammation of Respiratory Structures

Cystic Fibrosis

Cystic fibrosis (CF) is an autosomal recessive disorder of exocrine gland function, involving multiple organ systems (lungs, liver, intestine, pancreas) and chiefly resulting in chronic respiratory infections, pancreatic enzyme insufficiency, and associated complications in young patients. The failure of epithelial cells to conduct chloride and the associated water transport abnormalities result in viscous secretions in the respiratory tract, pancreas, gastrointestinal tract, sweat glands, and other exocrine tissues. The increased viscosity of these secretions makes them difficult to clear.

The clinical characteristics of CF are listed in Table 6-10. Sweat chloride analysis is critical to distinguish CF from other causes of severe pulmonary and pancreatic insufficiencies and to define patients who require further analysis.[205]

TABLE 6-8	Segments and Branches of the Aorta	
Segment of Aorta	**Arterial Branch**	**General Region or Organ Served**
Ascending portion of aorta	Right and left coronary aa.	Heart
Aortic arch	Brachiocephalic trunk	
	▶ Right common carotid a.	Right side of head and neck
	▶ Right subclavian a.	Right shoulder and right upper extremity.
	Left common carotid a.	Left side of head and neck
	Left subclavian a.	Left shoulder and left upper extremity
Thoracic portion of aorta	Pericardial aa.	Pericardium of heart
	Posterior intercostal aa.	Intercostal and thoracic muscles and pleurae
	Bronchial aa.	Bronchi of lungs
	Superior phrenic aa.	Superior surface of diaphragm
	Esophageal aa.	Esophagus
Abdominal portion of aorta	Inferior phrenic aa.	Inferior surface of diaphragm
	Celiac trunk	
	▶ Common hepatic a.	Liver, upper pancreas, and duodenum
	▶ Left gastric a.	Stomach and esophagus
	▶ Splenic a.	Spleen, pancreas, and stomach
	Superior mesenteric a.	Small intestine, pancreas, cecum, appendix, ascending colon, and transverse colon
	Suprarenal aa.	Adrenal (suprarenal) glands
	Lumbar aa.	Muscles and spinal cord of lumbar region
	Renal aa.	Kidneys
	Gonadal aa.	
	▶ Testicular aa.	Testes
	▶ Ovarian aa.	Ovaries
	Inferior mesenteric a.	Transverse colon, descending colon, sigmoid colon, and rectum
	Common iliac aa.	
	▶ External iliac aa.	Lower extremities
	▶ Internal iliac aa.	Genital organs and gluteal muscles

aa. = arteries; a. = artery

Data from Van de Graaff KM, Fox SI: Circulatory system, in Van de Graaff KM, Fox SI (eds): Concepts of Human Anatomy and Physiology. New York, WCB/McGraw-Hill, 1999, pp 610-691.

CLINICAL PEARL

▶ The quantitative pilocarpine iontophoresis test (QPIT) collects sweat and performs a chemical analysis of its chloride content.

▶ The sweat chloride reference value is less than 40 mEq/L, and a value of more than 60 mEq/L of chloride in the sweat is consistent with a diagnosis of CF (40–60 mEq/L are considered borderline).[205]

Asthma (Hyperreactive Airway Disease)

Asthma is a chronic inflammatory disorder of the airways. In susceptible individuals, the inflammation (acute, subacute, or chronic) causes an airway inflammation, intermittent airflow obstruction, and an associated increase in the existing bronchial responsiveness to a variety of stimuli.

Asthma is characterized by (particularly at night, or in the early morning) recurrent episodes of wheezing, breathless-ness, chest tightness, and coughing. The medical intervention for asthma may include pharmacologic therapy.

CLINICAL PEARL

Exercise-induced asthma (EIA), or exercise-induced bronchospasm, is an asthma variant defined as a condition in which exercise or vigorous physical activity triggers acute bronchospasm in persons with heightened airway reactivity to numerous exogenous and endogenous stimuli.

Chronic Bronchitis

Chronic bronchitis is a clinical diagnosis—a persistent productive cough that produces sputum for more than three months per year for at least two consecutive years in the absence of another definable medical cause.[206] Chronic bronchitis produces inflammation and eventual scarring of the

TABLE 6-9	Ventilation Terminology
Term	**Definition**
Air spaces	Alveolar ducts, alveolar sacs, and alveoli.
Airways	Structures that conduct air from the mouth and nose to the respiratory bronchioles.
Alveolar ventilation	Removal and replacement of gas in pulmonary alveoli; equal to the tidal volume minus the volume of dead space times the ventilation rate.
Anatomical dead space	Volume of the conducting airways to the zone where gas exchange occurs.
Apnea	Cessation of breathing.
Dyspnea	Unpleasant subjective feeling of difficult or labored breathing.
Eupnea	Normal, comfortable breathing at rest.
Hyperventilation	Alveolar ventilation that is excessive in relation to metabolic rate; results in abnormally low alveolar CO_2.
Hypoventilation	An alveolar ventilation that is low in relation to metabolic rate; results in abnormally high alveolar CO_2.
Physiological dead space	Combination of anatomical dead space and underventilated or underperfused alveoli that do not contribute normally to blood-gas exchange.
Pneumothorax	Presence of gas in the intrapleural space (the space between the visceral and parietal pleurae), causing lung collapse.
Torr	Unit of pressure very nearly equal to the millimeter of mercury (760 mm Hg = 760 torr).

Data from Van de Graaff KM, Fox SI: Respiratory system, in Van de Graaff KM, Fox SI (eds): Concepts of Human Anatomy and Physiology. New York, WCB/McGraw-Hill, 1999, pp 728-777.

TABLE 6-10	Clinical Manifestations of Cystic Fibrosis
System	**Signs and Symptoms**
Gastrointestinal tract	Intestinal, pancreatic, and hepatobiliary. Meconium ileus. Recurrent abdominal pain and constipation. Diabetes. Patients may present with a history of jaundice or gastrointestinal tract bleeding. Minimal weight gain—failure to thrive (FTT).
Integumentary	Salty perspiration ("Kiss your Baby week" for early detection). Clubbing of nail beds. Central and peripheral cyanosis.
Respiratory tract	Wheezing, rales, or rhonchi. Chronic or recurrent cough, which can be dry and hacking at the beginning and can produce mucoid (early) and purulent (later) sputum. Recurrent pneumonia, atypical asthma, pneumothorax, hemoptysis are all complications and may be the initial manifestation. Dyspnea on exertion, history of chest pain, recurrent sinusitis, nasal polyps, and hemoptysis may occur. Pulmonary artery hypertension. Cor pulmonale. Bronchospasm.
Urogenital tract	Males are frequently sterile because of the absence of the vas deferens. Undescended testicles or hydrocele may exist.

Data from: Lucas SR, Platts-Mills TA: Physical activity and exercise in asthma: relevance to etiology and treatment. J Allergy Clin Immunol 115:928-934, 2005; Mintz M: Asthma update: part I. Diagnosis, monitoring, and prevention of disease progression. Am Fam Physician 70:893-898, 2004; Ram FS, Robinson SM, Black PN, et al: Physical training for asthma. Cochrane Database Syst Rev:CD001116, 2005; Welsh L, Kemp JG, Roberts RG: Effects of physical conditioning on children and adolescents with asthma. Sports Med 35:127-141, 2005.

lining of the bronchial tubes. Presenting symptoms (patients are sometimes referred to as *blue bloaters*) include[207,208]:

▶ Patient may be obese.

▶ Chronic cough with frequent clearing of the throat.

▶ Low-grade fever.

▶ Increased mucus.

▶ Dyspnea on exertion.

▶ Use of accessory muscles for breathing.

▶ Coarse rhonchi and wheezing may be heard on auscultation.

▶ May have signs of right heart failure (i.e., cor pulmonale), such as edema and cyanosis.

Pneumonia

Pneumonia is an inoculation of the respiratory tract by infectious organisms that leads to an acute inflammatory response of the alveoli and terminal airspaces in response to invasion by an infectious agent that is introduced into the lungs through hematogenous spread or inhalation.[209–218] The inflammatory response differs according to the type of

infectious agent present. A large variety of organisms cause pneumonia. Bacterial, viral, mycoplasmal, chlamydial, fungal, and mycobacterial infections are relatively common. The infectious agents have predilections for certain age groups (Table 6-11).

CLINICAL PEARL

Aspiration has been clearly identified as a common contributing factor to the development of pneumonia.[206] Aspiration is associated with malnutrition, tube feeding, contracture of cervical extensors, and use of depressant medications.[219]

The typical clinical presentation for pneumonia includes fever and a productive cough with sputum production that is usually yellowish-green or rust-colored.[206] Fatigue, weight loss, dyspnea, and tachycardia may also be present, depending on the extent of the disease.[206] Identifying the infectious agent is the most valuable piece of information in managing

TABLE 6-11	Predilections of Pneumonia in Certain Age Groups
Age Group	**Type of Pneumonia**
Newborns (aged 0–30 days)	Bacterial pneumonia with group B *Streptococcus, Listeria monocytogenes*, or gram-negative rods (e.g., *Escherichia coli, Klebsiella pneumoniae*) are a common cause.
	Pneumocystis jirovecii pneumonia (PCP): an opportunistic infection that occurs in immunosuppressed populations, primarily patients with advanced human immunodeficiency virus infection. The classic presentation of nonproductive cough, shortness of breath, and fever.
	Community-acquired viral infections: The most commonly isolated virus is respiratory syncytial virus (RSV).
Infants and toddlers	Viruses are the most common cause of pneumonia. RSV is the most common viral pathogen, followed by parainfluenza types 1, 2, 3, and influenza A or B.
	Bacterial infections in this age group are uncommon and attributable to *Streptococcus pneumoniae, Haemophilus influenzae* type B, or *Staphylococcus aureus*.
Children younger than 5 years	Children enrolled in day care or those with frequent ear infections are at increased risk for invasive pneumococcal disease and infection with resistant pneumococcal strains.
Children aged 5 years, ready to start school	*Mycoplasma pneumoniae* is the most common cause of community-acquired pneumonia. *Chlamydia pneumoniae* is also fairly common in this age group and presents similarly.
School-aged children and adolescents	Bacterial pneumonia (10%) is common, and these children are often febrile and look ill. Tuberculosis (TB) pneumonia in children warrants special mention. These children may present with fever, night sweats, chills, cough, and weight loss. If TB is not treated in the early stages of infection, approximately 25% of children younger than 15 years develop extrapulmonary disease.
	Viral pneumonias are still common in this age group and are usually mild and self-limited, although they are occasionally severe and can rapidly progress to respiratory failure.

Data from: Coughlin AM: Combating community-acquired pneumonia. Nursing 37:61-63, 2007; Clark JE, Donna H, Spencer D, et al: Children with pneumonia—how do they present and how are they managed? Arch Dis Child 29:29, 2007; Parienti JJ, Carrat F: Viral pneumonia and respiratory sepsis: association, causation, or it depends? Crit Care Med 35:639-640, 2007; Hospital-acquired pneumonia. J Hosp Med 1:26-27, 2006; Community-acquired pneumonia. J Hosp Med 1:16-17, 2006; Flaherty KR, Martinez FJ: Nonspecific interstitial pneumonia. Semin Respir Crit Care Med. 27:652-658, 2006; Lynch JP 3rd, Saggar R, Weigt SS, et al: Usual interstitial pneumonia. Semin Respir Crit Care Med 27:634-651, 2006; Leong JR, Huang DT: Ventilator-associated pneumonia. Surg Clin North Am 86:1409-1429, 2006; Agusti C, Rano A, Aldabo I, et al: Fungal pneumonia, chronic respiratory diseases and glucocorticoids. Med Mycol 44 Suppl:207-211, 2006; Scannapieco FA: Pneumonia in nonambulatory patients: The role of oral bacteria and oral hygiene. J Am Dent Assoc 137 Suppl:21S-25S, 2006.

a complicated pneumonia. Several diagnostic studies are available:

- Sputum culture.
- *Bronchoscopy:* most useful in immunocompromised patients or patients who are severely ill.
- *Blood culture:* rarely positive in the presence of pneumonia.
- Lung aspirate.
- *Thoracentesis:* performed for diagnostic and therapeutic purposes in children with pleural effusions.
- Serology.
- *Radiography:* This is the primary imaging study used to confirm the diagnosis of pneumonia.

Once the diagnosis of pneumonia is made, antibiotic decisions are made based on the likely organism, bearing in mind the age of the patient, the history of exposure, the possibility of resistance, and other pertinent history.

Pneumoconiosis

Coal worker's pneumoconiosis (CWP) can be defined as the accumulation of coal dust in the lungs and the tissue's reaction to its presence.[220] Inhaled coal dust enters the terminal bronchioles, and the carbon pigment is engulfed by alveolar and interstitial macrophages.[221] Phagocytosed coal particles are transported by macrophages up the mucociliary elevator and are expelled in the mucus or through the lymphatic system.[222] When this system becomes overwhelmed, the dust-laden macrophages accumulate in the alveoli and may trigger an immune response.[221,222]

Certain jobs within coal mining require more exposure to respirable dust. For example, most dust is found at the coal-face where the cutting machine operator works.

Interstitial Lung Disease/Pulmonary Fibrosis

Interstitial lung disease (ILD), also referred to as idiopathic pulmonary fibrosis and interstitial pulmonary fibrosis, is a general term that includes a variety of chronic lung disorders.

The initial injury appears to damage the alveolar and epithelial cells. The damage causes inflammatory cells to release cytokines, tumor necrosis factor, and platelet-derived growth factor.

CLINICAL PEARL

- When inflammation involves the bronchioles, it is called bronchiolitis.
- When inflammation involves the alveoli, it is called alveolitis.
- When inflammation involves the small blood vessels, it is called vasculitis.
- When scarring of the lung tissue takes place, the condition is called pulmonary fibrosis.

The inflammatory chemicals result smooth muscle proliferation, degradation of the alveoli, and the proliferation of fibroblasts and collagen deposition.[223] Fibrosis, or scarring of the lung tissue, results in permanent loss of that tissue's ability to transport oxygen.

The insidious onset of breathlessness and a nonproductive cough can be the first symptoms of these diseases. The patient may also complain of systemic symptoms of low-grade fever, malaise, arthralgias, weight loss, and clubbing of the fingers and toenails.[223]

The patient history should investigate environmental and occupational factors, hobbies, legal and illegal drug use, arthritis, and risk factors for diseases that affect the immune system. Specific tests include bronchoalveolar lavage (BAL), a test, performed during bronchoscopy, which permits removal and examination of cells from the lower respiratory tract and open lung biopsy.

CLINICAL PEARL

Collagen vascular diseases that demonstrate features of interstitial lung disease include systemic lupus erythematosus, rheumatoid arthritis, progressive systemic sclerosis (see later), dermatomyositis and polymyositis, ankylosing spondylitis, Sjögren syndrome, and mixed connective tissue disease. Interstitial lung diseases associated with collagen vascular diseases are diverse and include nonspecific interstitial pneumonia, usual interstitial pneumonia, bronchiolitis obliterans organizing pneumonia, apical fibrosis, diffuse alveolar damage, and lymphocytic interstitial pneumonia.

Structural Abnormalities

Emphysema

Emphysema begins insidiously with the destruction of alveoli in the lungs, the walls of which become thin and fragile. Damage is irreversible and results in permanent destruction of the acini.* As the acini are destroyed, the lungs are able to transfer less and less oxygen to the bloodstream, causing shortness of breath/hyperinflation, and compensatory changes of the chest wall. Hyperinflation causes shortening of the inspiratory muscles and flattening of the diaphragm with loss of sarcomeres.[206] The end result is a loss of diaphragmatic excursion, a decline in the mechanical effectiveness of the diaphragm, and other respiratory muscles to support the increased demand of ventilation.[224] Signs and symptoms of emphysema (patients are sometimes referred to as *pink puffers*) include:

- In later stages of the disease, the patient becomes emaciated and may adopt the tripod sitting position.
- Barrel chest (enlarged anterior-posterior dimension), with an increased rib angle.
- The presence of a chronic cough and sputum production will vary and depend on the infectious history of the patient.
- Diminished breath sounds and wheezing.
- Shortness of breath, especially with exertion (dyspnea on exertion) assisted by pursed lips and use of accessory respiratory muscles, the latter of which may be hypertrophied through overuse.
- Heart sounds appear very distant.

---

*Each acinus, the functional unit of the lung for gas exchange, is composed of one of three respiratory bronchioles and the alveolar ducts and sacs.

Diagnosis is made by pulmonary function tests, chest x-ray (reveals hyperinflation with flattened diaphragm, decreased vascular markings, and possibly enlargement of the right side of the heart), along with the patient's history and physical examination.

There are a number of treatment options for the care of patients with emphysema:

- Smoking cessation is instrumental.
- Pharmacology (bronchodilators, anticholinergic drugs, corticosteroids).
- Long-term oxygen therapy, including the use of BiPap ventilation.
- *Bullectomy:* a bulla is a large airspace that is the result of destruction of the parenchyma, and which no longer participates in gas exchange or diffusion.
- Lung volume reduction surgery.
- *Lung transplantation (single or double):* for those patients with end-stage disease who have maximized medical intervention.

Idiopathic Scoliosis

Scoliosis represents a disturbance of the intercalated series of spinal segments that produces a three-dimensional deformity (lateral curvature and vertebral rotation) of the spine.[225–238] Despite an extensive amount of research devoted to discovering the cause of idiopathic scoliosis, the mechanics and specific etiology are not clearly understood. It is known, however, that there is a familial prevalence of idiopathic scoliosis.

Using the James classification system, scoliosis has three age distinctions. These distinctions, though seemingly arbitrary, have prognostic significance.

- *Infantile idiopathic:* children diagnosed when they are younger than 3 years, usually manifesting shortly after birth. This type accounts for less than 1% of all cases. In the most common curve pattern (right thoracic), the right shoulder is consistently rotated forward and the medial border of the right scapula protrudes posteriorly.
- *Juvenile idiopathic:* children diagnosed when they are aged 3–9 years.
- *Adolescent idiopathic:* manifesting at or around the onset of puberty and accounting for approximately 80% of all cases of idiopathic scoliosis.

The following are the main factors that influence the probability of progression in the skeleton of the immature patient:

1. The younger the patient at diagnosis, the greater the risk of progression.
2. Double-curve patterns have a greater risk for progression than single-curve patterns.
3. Curves with greater magnitude are at a greater risk to progress.
4. Risk of progression in females is approximately 10 times that of males with curves of comparable magnitude.
5. Greater risk of progression is present when curves develop before menarche.

TABLE 6-12	Risser Grades
Grade	Interpretation
0	Absence of ossification
1	25% ossification of the iliac apophysis
2	50% ossification of the iliac apophysis
3	75% ossification of the iliac apophysis
4	100% ossification of the iliac apophysis
5	The iliac apophysis has fused to the iliac crest after 100% ossification

Data from: Biondi J, Weiner DS, Bethem D, et al: Correlation of Risser sign and bone age determination in adolescent idiopathic scoliosis. J Pediatr Orthop 5:697-701, 1985; Little DG, Sussman MD: The Risser sign: a critical analysis. J Pediatr Orthop 14:569-575, 1994.

Scoliosis is generally described by the location of the curve or curves. One should also describe whether the convexity of the curve points to the right or left. If there is a double curve, each curve must be described and measured. The magnitude of a rib hump is quantified using a scoliometer (an inclinometer) with the forward bending test. Radiographs, which are usually only considered when a patient has a curve that might require treatment or could progress to a stage requiring treatment (usually 40° to 100°), can be used to determine location, type, and magnitude of the curve (using the Cobb method), as well as skeletal age. Skeletal maturity is determined using the Risser sign, which is defined by the amount of calcification present in the iliac apophysis, measuring the progressive ossification from anterolaterally to posteromedially (Table 6-12). Children can progress from a Risser grade 1 to a grade 5 over a two-year period.

CLINICAL PEARL

If scoliosis is neglected, the curves may progress dramatically, creating significant physical deformity and even cardiopulmonary problems with especially severe curves.

Most curves can be treated nonoperatively through observation with appropriate intermittent radiographs to check for the presence or absence of curve progression. However, 60% of curvatures in rapidly growing prepubertal children will progress and may require bracing (Boston, or custom thoracolumbosacral [TLSO]) or surgery. The primary goal of scoliosis surgery is to achieve a solid bony fusion. Even in the setting of adequate correction and solid fusion, up to 38% of patients still have occasional back pain.

CLINICAL PEARL

Scoliosis screening is done in schools across the United States. Generally, curvatures less than 30° will not progress after the child is skeletally mature.

Ankylosing Spondylitis

Ankylosing spondylitis (AS, also known as Bekhterev's or Marie–Strümpell disease) is a chronic rheumatoid disorder. Thoracic involvement in AS occurs almost universally. The patient is usually between 15 and 40 years of age.[239] Although males are affected more frequently than females, mild courses of AS are more common in the latter.[240]

The disease includes involvement of the anterior longitudinal ligament and ossification of the vertebral disk, thoracic zygapophyseal joints, costovertebral joints, and manubriosternal joint. In time, AS progresses to involve the whole spine and results in spinal deformities, including flattening of the lumbar lordosis, kyphosis of the thoracic spine, and hyperextension of the cervical spine. As the disease progresses, the pain and stiffness can spread up the entire spine, pulling it into forward flexion, so that the patient adopts the typical stooped-over position. The patient gazes downward, the entire back is rounded, the hips and knees are semiflexed, and the arms cannot be raised beyond a limited amount at the shoulders.[241]

The most characteristic feature of the back pain associated with AS is pain at night.[242] Patients often awaken in the early morning (between 2 and 5 AM) with back pain and stiffness, and usually either take a shower or exercise before returning to sleep.[240] Backache during the day is typically intermittent irrespective of exertion or rest.[240]

Calin and colleagues[243] describe five screening questions for AS:

1. Is there morning stiffness?
2. Is there improvement in discomfort with exercise?
3. Was the onset of back pain before age 40 years?
4. Did the problem begin slowly?
5. Has the pain persisted for at least 3 months?

Using at least four positive answers to define a "positive" result, the sensitivity of these questions was 0.95 and specificity, 0.85.[243] A human leukocyte antigen (HLA) haplotype association (HLA-B27) has been found with ankylosing spondylitis and remains one of the strongest known associations of disease with HLA-B27, but other diseases are also associated with the antigen.[240]

Peripheral arthritis is uncommon in AS, but when it occurs, it is usually late in the course of the arthritis.[244] The arthritis usually occurs in the lower extremities in an asymmetric distribution, with involvement of the "axial" joints, including shoulders and hips, more common than involvement of more distal joints.[240,245]

Chronic Obstructive Pulmonary Disease

Chronic obstructive pulmonary disease (COPD) is a generic term that refers to lung diseases that result in air trapping in the lungs (Table 6-13), causing hyperinflation of the lungs and a barrel chest deformity.[206] COPD is characterized by airway narrowing, parenchymal destruction, and pulmonary vascular thickening. COPD can be subdivided into:

► Nonseptic obstructive pulmonary diseases, including such diseases as asthma, chronic bronchitis, emphysema, and α_1 antitrypsin (α_1 ATD) deficiency.

TABLE 6-13	Diseases or Conditions That May Be Associated with Obstruction to Airflow
Lower airway obstruction:	Asthma Chronic bronchitis Emphysema Cystic fibrosis Sarcoidosis
Upper airway obstruction:	Croup Laryngotracheobronchitis Epiglottitis Various tumors and foreign bodies that may involve the upper airway

► Septic obstructive pulmonary diseases, including cystic fibrosis and bronchiectasis.

Risk factors for the development of COPD include both host factors and environmental factors:

► *Host factors:* hyperreactivity of the airways, overall lung growth, and genetics.

► *Environmental factors:* Smoking is the primary risk factor for COPD, with approximately 80% to 90% of COPD deaths caused by smoking.[246] Other risk factors of COPD include air pollution, second-hand smoke, history of childhood respiratory infections, and heredity.[247–249] Occupational exposure to certain industrial pollutants also increases the odds for COPD.[250] The quality of life for a person suffering from COPD diminishes as the disease progresses. At the onset, there is minimal shortness of breath, but as the disease progresses, these people may eventually require supplemental oxygen and may have to rely on mechanical respiratory assistance.[251]

Neurologic Compromise

Paralysis of the diaphragm can result from a number of conditions that compromise the phrenic nerve. Phrenic nerve involvement has been described in several neuropathies, including critical illness, polyneuropathy, Guillain-Barré syndrome, brachial neuritis, and hereditary motor and sensory neuropathy type 1.[252,253] The symptoms depend largely on the degree of involvement and whether one or both of the nerves are involved.[254]

► Unilateral paralysis of the diaphragm causes few or no symptoms except with heavy exertion.

► Bilateral paralysis of the diaphragm may be well tolerated if the person is in the upright position and is not engaged in heavy exercise, and if the other respiratory muscles are intact. However, because the vital capacity has been decreased by 25% to 50%, these patients become severely short of breath if lying supine for even 15 to 20 seconds.

In quadriplegia, the muscles of respiration may be weakened or paralyzed. Fortunately, the phrenic nerve exits the spinal cord at a high level (C3-C5) so can be spared, but the intercostal abdominal muscles are often paralyzed, requiring the use of abdominal binders to ensure proper diaphragmatic positioning in the upright posture.

Burns

An individual who has been burned in a closed space is likely to have an inhalation injury. Signs of an inhalation injury include facial burns, singed nasal hairs, harsh cough, hoarseness, abnormal breath sounds, respiratory distress, and carbonaceous sputum and/or hypoxemia.[255,256] The primary complications associated with this injury are carbon monoxide poisoning, tracheal damage, upper airway obstruction, pulmonary edema, and pneumonia.[255] Thermal damage to the lower respiratory tract can be caused by steam inhalation or by inhalation of hot gases, which produces immediate upper airway obstruction. Burns can affect the respiratory system in one of two ways:

1. *An inhalation injury.* Thermal damage to the respiratory tract can result from:

   ▶ Inhalation of hot gases/steam, which produces immediate upper airway obstruction.

   ▶ Inhaling toxic products (e.g., cyanide, carbon monoxide) generated by burning material (e.g., wood, plastics) may result in thermal injuries to the pharynx and upper airway as well as in ventilation injuries. Chemical injury to small airway alveolar capillaries can cause delayed progressive respiratory failure.

   ▶ Inhalation of carbon monoxide, which binds to hemoglobin, greatly reducing O_2 transport.

2. An increased demand in metabolic rate and energy metabolism. Because thermal injury results in more loss of body mass than any other disease, continued demands are placed on the metabolic system for the significant healing process. Metabolic acidosis may result from poor tissue perfusion due to hypovolemia (monitored through urine output) or to heart failure.

INTEGUMENTARY CAUSES

The integumentary system consists of the dermal and epidermal layers of the skin, hair follicles, nails, sebaceous glands, and sweat glands. The integument or skin is the largest organ system of the body and constitutes 15% to 20% of the body weight.[255]

Anatomically, the skin consists of two distinct layers of tissue: the epidermis and the dermis. A third layer involved in the anatomic consideration of the skin is the subcutaneous fat cell layer directly under the dermis and above muscle fascial layers.[255] The epidermis serves as the superficial, protective layer. All but the deepest layers of the epidermis are composed of dead cells, which contain no blood vessels. The dermis, considered the "true" skin because it contains blood vessels, lymphatics, nerves, collagen, and elastic fibers, is deeper and thicker than the epidermis.[255] This inner layer of the dermis is composed primarily of collagen and elastin fibrous connective tissue. The amount of elastin decreases with age. The dermis also contains sebaceous and sweat glands.

The extent to which the integumentary system can cause movement dysfunction is based on the size or amount of body surface area that is involved, and the extent or depth of injury. A significant injury to the integumentary system causes pain, edema, and tissue destruction.

▶ *Pain.* Superficial skin damage generally results in more pain than deeper injuries because the free endings are not destroyed in the former. However, as the nerve endings regenerate following damage to the deeper layers, intense pain may result. Pain is the major deterrent in preventing burn patients from participating in exercises and positioning following a burn injury, which in turn can cause contractures and joint dysfunction.

▶ *Edema.* The buildup of edema occurs as joints try to accommodate to a position that allows maximum space for fluid accumulation and distributes the fluid pressure. This position, which is often the so-called open position of the joint, is the position of maximal comfort but is also a position that encourages contractures if maintained for a prolonged period.

▶ *Tissue destruction.* Damage to the integumentary system can occur in many ways, including causative agents (e.g., electricity, chemicals, and heat), continued pressure to the skin resulting in ischemia, or excessive scar formation (eschar). Eschars can form in an organized manner termed *normotrophic* scarring, or in a disorganized manner such as that seen with hypertrophic or keloid scars.

▶ *Infection.* An infection, which can occur when the skin's bacterial barrier is compromised by an organism, is a major source of mortality and the most significant cause of loss of function and cosmetic appearance. A number of factors play a role in the development of an infection:

  ■ Vasoconstriction leading to peripheral hypoperfusion, particularly in the burned areas, creates a major defect in local host defense, enhancing bacterial invasion.

  ■ Dead tissue, warmth, peripheral hypoperfusion, and moisture are ideal for bacterial growth.

  ■ Streptococci and staphylococci usually predominate shortly after a burn, and gram-negative bacteria after 5 to 7 days; mixed flora is always present.

▶ *Critical:* 10% of body with third-degree burns and 30% or more with second-degree; complications such as respiratory involvement, smoke inhalation.

▶ *Moderate:* less than 10% with third-degree burns and 15% to 30% with second-degree.

▶ *Minor:* less than 2% with third-degree burns and 15% with second-degree burns.

▶ *Breakdown due to pressure.* The terms *pressure ulcer* and *decubitus ulcer* often are used interchangeably. Because the common denominator of all such ulcerations is pressure, pressure ulcer is the better term to describe this condition. Pressure ulcers result from sustained or prolonged pressure at levels greater than the level of the capillary filling pressure on the tissue (approximately 32 mm Hg) resulting in localized ischemia and/or tissue necrosis.[76-88] Most pressure ulcers can be avoided by anticipating and avoiding conditions that promote them. Prevention of pressure ulcers involves multiple members of the healthcare team (Table 6-14). The groups of patients most susceptible include elderly individuals, those who are neurologically impaired, and those who are acutely hospitalized (Table 6-15). Pressure against the skin over a bony prominence increases the risk for the development of necrosis and ulceration (Table 6-16). Bacterial contamination from improper skin care or urinary or fecal incontinence, although not truly an etiologic factor, is an important factor to consider in the treatment of pressure sores and can delay wound healing. Other contributing factors to pressure ulcers include shear, friction, heat, maceration (softening associated with excessive moisture), medication, malnutrition, and muscle atrophy (Table 6-17). Pressure ulcers can be graded using a staging system (Table 6-18). The clinician must

TABLE 6-14	Pressure Ulcer Prevention
Prevention Technique	**Suggested Strategies**
Proper positioning in bed and in wheelchair	Bony prominences protected and pressure distributed equally over large surface areas. Use of pressure distribution equipment such as wheelchair cushions, custom mattresses, and alternating pressure mattress pads.
Frequent changes in position	Every two hours when in bed. Every 15 to 20 minutes when seated.
Keep skin clean and dry	Good bowel and bladder care with immediate cleansing after episode of incontinence. Current cleansing and drying of skin at least once daily. Inspect skin for areas of redness in AM and PM.
Nutrition	Diet with adequate calories, protein, vitamins, and minerals. Sufficient water intake.
Clothing	Avoid clothes that are either too tight or too loose fitting. Avoid clothes with thick seams, buttons, or zippers in areas of pressure.
Activity	Regular cardiovascular exercise. Gradual buildup of skin tolerance for new activities, equipment, and positions. Avoid movements that rub, drag, or scratch the skin.

Data from Spangler LL: Nonprogressive spinal cord disorders, in Cameron MH, Monroe LG (eds): Physical Rehabilitation: Evidence-Based Examination, Evaluation, and Intervention. St Louis, MO, Saunders/Elsevier, 2007, pp 538-579.

TABLE 6-15	The Norton Score for Anticipating Pressure Ulcers	
General physical condition	1. Poor 2. Fair 3. Good 4. Excellent	Score:_____
Mobility	1. Immobilized 2. Tubes and restraints 3. Tubes or restraints 4. No impairment	Score:_____
Activity	1. Bedridden 2. Bed to chair 3. Walk with assist 4. Up at liberty	Score:_____
Mental status	1. Stuporous 2. Withdrawn 3. Confused 4. Alert and oriented	Score:_____
Continence	1. Doubly incontinent 2. Frequently incontinent of urine 3. Occasionally incontinent 4. Fully continent	Score:_____
Grading	Add the scores for all five categories. If cumulative score is greater than 15, there is little risk for pressure sore development; if cumulative score is less than 15, then there is a significant risk for pressure sore development.	

Data from: 1. Sever R, Gold A, Segal O, et al: Admission Norton scale scores (ANSS) are associated with post-operative complications following spine fracture surgery in the elderly. Arch Gerontol Geriatr 55:177-180, 2012; Gold A, Sever R, Lerman Y, et al: Admission Norton scale scores (ANSS) and postoperative complications following hip fracture surgery in the elderly. Arch Gerontol Geriatr 55:173-176, 2012; Guy N, Lerman Y, Justo D: Admission Norton scale scores (ANSS) correlate with rehabilitation outcome and length in elderly patients with deconditioning. Arch Gerontol Geriatr 54:381-384, 2012; Lewko J, Demianiuk M, Krot E, et al: Assessment of risk for pressure ulcers using the Norton scale in nursing practice. Rocz Akad Med Bialymst 50 Suppl 1:148-151, 2005; Norton D: Calculating the risk: reflections on the Norton Scale. 1989. Adv Wound Care 9:38-43, 1996.

remember when staging a healing ulcer that the staging system is not reversible. For example, a healing stage III ulcer cannot be documented as a stage II ulcer, because the healing involves the laying down of granulation tissue rather than replacement of the lost muscle, fat, and dermal tissues. Instead, pressure ulcer healing is documented in terms of improvement in the various characteristics of the wound, including size, depth, and tissue type.

Because the integumentary system is closely related to the cardiovascular, renal, pulmonary, metabolic, musculoskeletal, and nervous systems, damage to the integumentary system often results in involvement of one or more of these systems.

▶ *Cardiovascular and renal systems.* In cases of severe damage to the integumentary system, leaking of the intravascular substances results in depletion of the circulating cardiovascular volume, which can ultimately compromise cardiac output and kidney function.

▶ *Pulmonary system* (see Respiratory Causes).

▶ *Metabolic system.* A significant thermal injury can result in a substantial increase in metabolic activity as a result of a loss of the skin's ability to regulate body temperature and control evaporation, and because of the enormous healing process that is necessary. How an individual responds to the increased energy demands often dictates recovery.

TABLE 6-16	Bony Prominences Associated with Pressure Ulcers		
Supine	**Prone**	**Sidelying**	**Seated**
Occiput	Forehead	Ears	Spine of scapula
Spine of scapula	Anterior portion of the acromion process	Lateral portion of acromion process	Vertebral spinous processes
Inferior angle of scapula	Anterior head of humerus	Lateral head of humerus	Ischial tuberosities
Vertebral spinous processes	Sternum	Lateral epicondyle of humerus	
Medial epicondyle of humerus	Anterior superior iliac spine	Greater trochanter	
Posterior iliac crest	Patella	Head of fibula	
Sacrum	Dorsum of foot	Lateral malleolus	
Coccyx		Medial malleolus	

TABLE 6-17	Risk Factors Associated with Pressure Ulcers

Emaciation
Obesity
Elderly patient
Immobilization
Decrease in activity level
Diabetes
Circulatory disorders
Incontinence
Decreased mental status

▶ *Musculoskeletal system.* An integumentary system compromise that is significant enough to prevent movement for a prolonged period may result in muscle atrophy, contracture formation, and compensations by other parts of the body. If the level of destruction is high, amputation of the affected areas may be necessary.

CLINICAL PEARL

Contractures are especially likely to develop if wounds are not closed promptly. If a body part is left immobile for a protracted period of time, capsular contraction and shortening of tendon and muscle groups (which cross the joints) occur. This rapid process can be prevented by a program of passive ROM, antideformity positioning, and splinting. The general rule for splinting is to position the affected joint in the opposite direction from which it will contract.

▶ *Nervous system.* Any imbalance in tissue perfusion can result in dysfunction of the central nervous system. Early signs and symptoms that the clinician should be aware of include lethargy, disorientation, and episodes of confusion. Direct trauma to the integumentary system can result in damage to the peripheral motor and sensory nerves.

SYSTEMIC CAUSES

There are many conditions that affect many systems. Pregnancy, which spans approximately 40 weeks from conception to delivery, is a state of wellness despite the number of physiologic changes that occur during pregnancy and the postpartum period within the various body systems. These changes can occur within the endocrine, musculoskeletal, neurologic, gastrointestinal, respiratory, cardiovascular, metabolic, renal, and urologic systems.

Endocrine System

Changes that occur in the endocrine system include, but are not limited to, the following:

▶ The adrenal, thyroid, parathyroid, and pituitary glands enlarge.

▶ Hormone levels increase to support the pregnancy and the placenta, and to prepare the mother's body for labor.

Musculoskeletal System

The recommended weight gain during pregnancy is 25 to 27 pounds.[257] Pregnancy can produce a number of changes within the musculoskeletal system, including:

▶ The abdominal muscles are stretched and weakened as pregnancy develops.

▶ The development of relative ligamentous laxity, both capsular and extracapsular. During pregnancy, a female hormone (relaxin) is released that assists in the softening of the pubic symphysis so that during delivery, the female pelvis can expand sufficiently to allow birth. However, these hormonal changes are also thought to induce a greater laxity in all joints.[258,259] This can result in increased susceptibility to musculoskeletal injury.

▶ The rib cage circumference increases, increasing the subcostal angle and the transverse diameter. This results in an increase in tidal volume and minute ventilation—a

TABLE 6-18	National Pressure Ulcer Advisory Panel (NPUAP) Pressure Ulcers Stages
Stage	**Characteristics**
Stage I	An observable pressure related alteration of intact skin whose indicators as compared to an adjacent or opposite area of the body may include changes in skin color, skin temperature (warm or cool), tissue consistency (firm or boggy) and/or sensation (pain, itching).
Stage II	A partial thickness tissue loss that involves the epidermis and/or dermis. The ulcer is superficial and presents clinically as an abrasion, a blister, or shallow crater.
Stage III	A full thickness tissue loss that involves damage or necrosis of subcutaneous tissue that may extend down to, but not through, underlying fascia. The ulcer presents clinically as a deep crater with or without undermining adjacent tissue.
Stage IV	A full thickness tissue loss with extensive destruction, tissue necrosis or damage to muscle, bone or supporting structures (e.g., tendon, joint capsule). Undermining or sinus tracts may be present.
Unstageable	A full thickness tissue loss where the base of the ulcer is covered by slough and/or eschar so that its depth cannot be determined.

Data from Pressure ulcer prevention and treatment following spinal cord injury: a clinical practice guideline for health-care professionals. J Spinal Cord Med 24 Suppl 1:S40-S101, 2001.

natural state of hyperventilation to meet the oxygen demands.

▸ *Pelvic floor weakness.* The term *pelvic floor muscles* primarily refers to the levator ani, a muscle group composed of the pubococcygeus, puborectalis, and iliococcygeus. The levator ani muscles join the coccygeus muscles to complete the pelvic floor. Pelvic floor weakness can develop with advanced pregnancy and childbirth because of the increased weight and pressure directly over these muscles they must sustain—the pelvic floor drops as much as 2.5 cm (1 inch) as a result of pregnancy.[260] This can result in a condition called stress incontinence. The pelvic floor muscles can also become stretched or torn during childbirth, producing an even greater risk of urinary incontinence.

▸ Postural changes related to the weight of growing breasts, and the uterus and fetus, result in a shift in the woman's center of gravity in an anterior and superior direction, resulting in the need for postural compensations to maintain stability and balance. Although never substantiated, postural changes have often been implicated as a major cause of back pain in pregnant women.[261,262] The relationship between posture and the back pain experienced during pregnancy is unclear. This may be because significant skeletal alignment changes that are related to back pain are occurring at the pelvis during pregnancy but may not be directly measured by postural assessments, such as lumbar lordosis, sacral base angle, and pelvic tilt. Moore et al[263] found a significant relationship ($r = 0.49$) between change in lordosis during 16–24 and 34–42 weeks of pregnancy and an increase in low back pain. Ostgaard et al[264] found that abdominal sagittal diameter ($r = 0.15$), transverse diameter ($r = 0.13$), and depth of lordosis ($r = 0.11$) were related to the development of back pain during pregnancy. Bullock et al,[262] in the only study that used a validated and reliable posture assessment instrument, found no relationship between spinal posture (thoracic kyphosis, lumbar lordosis, and pelvic tilt) magnitude or changes during pregnancy and back pain. The results from a study by Franklin and Conner-Kerr[265] suggest that from the first to the third trimester of pregnancy, lumbar lordosis, posterior head position, lumbar angle, and pelvic tilt increase; however, the magnitudes and the changes of these posture variables are not related to back pain.

In advanced pregnancy, the patient develops a wider base of support and increased external rotation at the hips and has increased difficulty with walking, stair climbing, and rapid changes in position. Specific postural changes include[263]:

■ Increased thoracic kyphosis with scapular retraction

■ Increased cervical lordosis and forward head

■ Increased lumbar lordosis

These changes in posture do not automatically correct postpartum and can become habitual.

CLINICAL PEARL

Pregnant women should be taught correct body mechanics and postural exercises to stretch, strengthen, and train postural muscles.

▸ *Symphysis pubis dysfunction (SPD).*[266–269] SPD can occur during pregnancy or, more commonly, as a result of trauma during vaginal delivery. On examination, the patient typically demonstrates an antalgic, waddling gait. Subjectively, the patient reports pain with any activity that involves lifting one leg at a time or parting the legs. Lifting the leg to put on clothes, getting out of a car, bending over, turning over in bed, sitting down or getting up, walking up stairs, standing on one leg, lifting heavy objects, and walking in general are all painful. Palpation reveals anterior pubic symphyseal tenderness. Occasional clicking can be felt or heard. The amount of symphyseal separation does not always correlate with severity of symptoms or the degree of disability. Therefore, the intervention is based on the severity of symptoms rather than the degree of separation as measured by imaging studies.[270]

CLINICAL PEARL

Symphysis pubis dysfunction (SPD) should always be considered when treating patients in the postpartum period who are experiencing suprapubic, sacroiliac, or thigh pain.

▸ *Low back pain.*[261–264,271–275] Low back pain (LBP) is said to occur in 50% to 70% of pregnant women.[276] However, it is not clear whether the LBP is the result of the shift in the center of gravity and concomitant postural changes in the spinal curvature. Because the annulus is a ligamentous structure, and therefore softens with the release of relaxin, it could be postulated that the LBP may be related to structural changes in the intervertebral disk. However, frank disk herniations are no more common during pregnancy than at other times. Thus, the pain is likely mechanical in nature.

CLINICAL PEARL

It is worth remembering that complaints of low back pain in this population may be because of a kidney or urinary tract infection.

▸ *Peripartum posterior pelvic pain.* More than 50% of women experience peripartum posterior pelvic pain (PPPP) during pregnancy, with one third of these women experiencing severe pain.[275,277,278] The etiology of PPPP has been linked to the physiologic adaptation of the pelvis in preparation for childbirth, which is accomplished through softening of connective tissue structures around the pelvis, pubic symphysis, and sacroiliac joint.[279] Patients with PPPP typically complain of weight-bearing LBP with symptoms referred below the level of the buttocks (with no findings suggesting nerve root involvement) and with the first episode of pain occurring during pregnancy.

▸ *Coccydynia.*[280–284] Coccygeal pain, pain in and around the region of the coccyx, is relatively common postpartum. Symptoms include pain with sitting. The patient should be provided with seating adaptation (donut cushion) to lessen the weight on the coccyx and to support the lumbar lordosis.

- *Diastasis recti abdominis (DRA).* A DRA, which is common in the pre- and postpartum phases, refers to a split between the two rectus abdominis muscles to the extent that the linea alba may split under strain. Predisposing factors for a DRA in women include obesity, a narrow pelvis, multiparity, multiple births, excess uterine fluid, large babies, and weak abdominals before pregnancy. It is believed that a DRA may hinder the abdominal wall function related to posture, trunk stability and strength, respiration, visceral support, diminished pelvic floor facilitation, and delivery of the fetus. An umbilical hernia may result as well. A DRA is also believed to contribute to chronic pelvic pain and LBP. According to Noble,[285] exercises for the abdominals to prevent, decrease, and/or eliminate a DRA should be prescribed. Proper exercise intensity is essential, and intervention should occur as soon as possible.

Neurologic

Swelling and increased fluid volume can cause symptoms of thoracic outlet syndrome due to compression of the brachial plexus, carpal tunnel syndrome due to median nerve compression, or meralgia paresthetica, which is compression of the lateral femoral cutaneous nerve of the thigh.[286-288]

Pregnancy-related depression and postpartum depression may occur. Postnatal depression has been documented to occur in 5% to 20% of all postpartum mothers,[289-291] but can also occur in fathers.[292] Depressive postpartum disorders range from "postpartum blues," which occurs from one to five days after birth and lasts for only a few days, to postpartum depression and postpartum psychosis. The latter two are more serious conditions and require medical or social intervention to avoid serious ramifications for the family unit.[293-295]

Gastrointestinal

Nausea and vomiting may occur in early pregnancy. They are generally confined to the first 16 weeks but occasionally remain throughout the entire pregnancy (hyperemesis gravidarum).[293,296-299] The causes of hyperemesis gravidarum are largely unknown. Indications that the patient may have this condition include persistent and excessive nausea and vomiting throughout the day and an inability to keep down any solids or liquids. If the condition is prolonged, the patient may also report[296,299]:

- Fatigue, lethargy
- Headache
- Faintness

Various degrees of dehydration may be present: skin may be pale, there may be dark circles under eyes, eyes may appear sunken, mucous membranes may be dry, and skin flexibility may be poor.[296,299]

Other changes related to the gastrointestinal system include[296-299]:

- A slowing of intestinal motility.
- The development of constipation, abdominal bloating, and hemorrhoids.
- Esophageal reflux.

- Heartburn (pyrosis)—50% to 80% of women report heartburn during pregnancy, with its incidence peaking in the third trimester.[293]
- An increase in the incident and symptoms of gallbladder disease.

Respiratory System

Adaptive changes that occur in the pulmonary system during pregnancy include:

- The diaphragm elevates with a widening of the thoracic cage. This results in a predominance of costal versus abdominal breathing.
- Mild increases in oxygen consumption, which is caused by increased respiratory center sensitivity and drive due to the increased oxygen requirement of the fetus.[300] With mild exercise, pregnant women have a greater increase in respiratory frequency and oxygen consumption to meet their greater oxygen demand.[300] As exercise increases to moderate and maximal levels, however, pregnant women demonstrate decreased respiratory frequency and maximal oxygen consumption.[300]

Cardiovascular System

The pregnancy-induced changes in the cardiovascular system develop primarily to meet the increased metabolic demands of the mother and fetus. These include:

- Increased blood volume: increases progressively beginning at 6 to 8 weeks' gestation (pregnancy) and reaches a maximum at approximately 32 to 34 weeks, with little change thereafter.[301] The increased blood volume serves two purposes[302,303]:
  - It facilitates maternal and fetal exchanges of respiratory gases, nutrients, and metabolites.
  - It reduces the impact of maternal blood loss at delivery. Typical losses of 300–500 ml for vaginal births and 750–1000 ml for cesarean sections are thus compensated by the so-called autotransfusion of blood from the contracting uterus.
- Increased plasma volume (40% to 50%) is relatively greater than that of red cell mass (20%-30%) resulting in hemodilution and a decrease in hemoglobin concentration (intake of supplemental iron and folic acid is necessary to restore hemoglobin levels to normal [12 g/dl]).[302,304,305]
- Increased cardiac output: increases to a similar degree as the blood volume.[302,303] During the first trimester cardiac, output is 30% to 40% higher than in the nonpregnant state.[304] During labor, further increases are seen. The heart is enlarged by both chamber dilation and hypertrophy.

CLINICAL PEARL

Hypertensive disorders complicating pregnancy are the most common medical risk factor responsible for maternal morbidity and death related to pregnancy.[293]

Changes in blood pressure during pregnancy include:

▶ Systemic arterial pressure should not increase during normal gestation.

▶ Pulmonary arterial pressure also maintains a constant level.

▶ Vascular tone is more dependent on sympathetic control than in the nonpregnant state, so that hypotension develops more readily and more markedly.

▶ Central venous and brachial venous pressures remain unchanged during pregnancy, but femoral venous pressure is progressively increased because of mechanical factors.

During pregnancy, a condition called supine hypotension (also known as inferior vena cava syndrome) may develop in the supine position, especially after the first trimester. The decrease in blood pressure is thought to be caused by the occlusion of the aorta and inferior vena cava by the increased weight and size of the uterus. Spontaneous recovery usually occurs on change of maternal position. However, patients should not be allowed to stand up quickly to decrease the potential for orthostatic hypotension. Signs and symptoms of this condition include:

▶ Bradycardia

▶ Shortness of breath

▶ Syncope (fainting)

▶ Dizziness

▶ Nausea and vomiting

▶ Sweating or cold, clammy skin

▶ Headache

▶ Numbness in extremities

▶ Weakness

▶ Restlessness

In general, limiting the time the patient spends in supine to approximately 5 minutes helps to minimize the effects of this problem. Alternative positions include left sidelying (best position for minimizing compression), right sidelying, supine reclined, or supine with a small wedge under the right hip.

Metabolic System

Because of the increased demand for tissue growth, insulin is elevated from plasma expansion, and blood glucose is reduced for a given insulin load. Fats and minerals are stored for maternal use. The metabolic rate increases during both exercise and pregnancy, resulting in greater heat production. Fetoplacental metabolism generates additional heat, which maintains fetal temperature at 0.5 to 1.0°C (0.9 to 1.8°F) above maternal levels.[306-308]

Gestational diabetes is defined as carbohydrate intolerance of variable severity, with onset or first recognition during pregnancy. After the birth, blood sugars usually return to normal levels; however, frank diabetes often develops later in life. Typical causes include:

▶ Genetic predisposition.

▶ High-risk populations include people of Aboriginal, Hispanic, Asian or African descent.

▶ Family history of diabetes, gestational diabetes, or glucose intolerance.

▶ Increased tissue resistance to insulin during pregnancy, due to increased levels of estrogen and progesterone.

Current risk factors include:

▶ Maternal obesity (>20% above ideal weight).

▶ Excessive weight gain during pregnancy.

▶ Low level of high-density-lipoprotein (HDL) cholesterol (<0.9 mmol/L) or elevated fasting level of triglycerides (>2.8 mmol/L).

▶ Hypertension or preeclampsia (risk for gestational diabetes is increased to 10% to 15% when hypertension is diagnosed).

▶ Maternal age >25 years.

Most individuals with gestational diabetes are asymptomatic. However, subjectively the patient may complain of:

▶ Polydipsia

▶ Polyuria

▶ Polyphagia

▶ Weight loss

Renal and Urologic Systems

During pregnancy, the renal threshold for glucose drops because of an increase in the glomerular filtration rate, and there is an increase in sodium and water retention.[293] Anatomic and hormonal changes during pregnancy place the pregnant woman at risk for both lower and upper urinary tract infections and for urinary incontinence.[293] As the fetus grows, stress on the mother's bladder can occur. This can result in urinary incontinence.

REFERENCES

1. Sahrmann SA: Introduction, in Sahrmann SA (ed): Movement Impairment Syndromes. St Louis, Mosby, 2001, pp 1-8.
2. Barrack RL, Skinner HB, Cook SD, et al: Effect of articular disease and total knee arthroplasty on knee joint position sense. J Neurophysiol 50:684-687, 1983.
3. Barrack RL, Skinner HB, Buckley SL: Proprioception in the anterior cruciate deficient knee. Am J Sports Med 17:1-6, 1989.
4. Corrigan JP, Cashman WF, Brady MP: Proprioception in the cruciate deficient knee. J Bone Joint Surg 74-B:247-250, 1992.
5. Fremerey RW, Lobenhoffer P, Zeichen J, et al: Proprioception after rehabilitation and reconstruction in knees with deficiency of the anterior cruciate ligament: a prospective, longitudinal study. J Bone Joint Surg [Br] 82:801-806, 2000.
6. Payne KA, Berg K, Latin RW: Ankle injuries and ankle strength, flexibility and proprioception in college basketball players. J Athl Training 32:221-225, 1997.
7. Sell S, Zacher J, Lack S: Disorders of proprioception of arthrotic knee joint. Z Rheumatol 52:150-155, 1993.
8. Voight M, Blackburn T: Proprioception and balance training and testing following injury, in Ellenbecker TS (ed): Knee Ligament Rehabilitation. Philadelphia, Churchill Livingstone, 2000, pp 361-385.
9. Vasilyeva LF, Lewit K: Diagnosis of muscular dysfunction by inspection, in Liebenson C (ed): Rehabilitation of the Spine: A Practitioner's Manual. Baltimore, Lippincott Williams & Wilkins, 1996, pp 113-142.

10. Darnell MW: A proposed chronology of events for forward head posture. J Craniomandib Prac 1:49-54, 1983.

11. Hamilton N, Luttgens K: The Standing Posture, in Hamilton N, Luttgens K (eds): Kinesiology: Scientific Basis of Human Motion (ed 10). New York, McGraw-Hill, 2002, pp 399-411.

12. Lovejoy CO: Evolution of human walking. Sci Am 259:118-125, 1988.

13. Korr IM, Wright HM, Thomas PE: Effects of experimental myofascial insults on cutaneous patterns of sympathetic activity in man. J Neural Transm 23:330-355, 1962.

14. Travell JG, Simons DG: Myofascial Pain and Dysfunction—The Trigger Point Manual. Baltimore, Williams & Wilkins, 1983.

15. Beal MC: The short leg problem. JAOA 76:745-751, 1977.

16. Magee DJ: Assessment of posture, in Magee DJ (ed): Orthopedic Physical Assessment. Philadelphia, WB Saunders, 2002, pp 873-903.

17. Smith A: Upper limb disorders—Time to relax? Physiotherapy 82:31-38, 1996.

18. Wilder DG, Pope MH, Frymoyer JW: The biomechanics of lumbar disc herniation and the effect of overload and instability. J Spinal Disord 1:16, 1988.

19. Cyriax J: Textbook of Orthopaedic Medicine, Diagnosis of Soft Tissue Lesions (ed 8). London, Bailliere Tindall, 1982.

20. Cyriax JH, Cyriax PJ: Illustrated Manual of Orthopaedic Medicine. London, Butterworth, 1983.

21. Rowland LP: Diseases of the motor unit, in Kandel ER, Schwartz JH, Jessell TM (eds): Principles of Neural Science (ed 4). New York, McGraw-Hill, 2000, pp 695-712.

22. Franklin ME: Assessment of exercise induced minor lesions: The accuracy of Cyriax's diagnosis by selective tissue tension paradigm. J Orthop Sports Phys Ther 24:122, 1996.

23. White DJ: Musculoskeletal examination, in O'Sullivan SB, Schmitz TJ (eds): Physical Rehabilitation (ed 5). Philadelphia, FA Davis, 2007, pp 159-192.

24. Williams PL, Warwick R, Dyson M, et al: Gray's Anatomy (ed 37). London, Churchill Livingstone, 1989.

25. Panjabi MM: The stabilizing system of the spine. Part 1. Function, dysfunction adaption and enhancement. J Spinal Disord 5:383-389, 1992.

26. Panjabi M, Hult EJ, Crisco J, III, et al: Biomechanical studies in cadaveric spines, in Jayson MIV (ed): The Lumbar Spine and Back Pain. New York, Churchill Livingstone, 1992, pp 133-135.

27. Lephart SM, Pincivero DM, Giraldo JL, et al: The role of proprioception in the management and rehabilitation of athletic injuries. Am J Sports Med 25:130-137, 1997.

28. Schutte MJ, Happel RT: Joint innervation in joint injury. Clin Sports Med 9:511-517, 1990.

29. Kennedy JC, Alexander IJ, Hayes KC: Nerve supply of the human knee and its functional importance. Am J Sports Med 10:329-335, 1982.

30. Harman D: Aging: Phenomena and theories. Ann N Y Acad Sci 854:1-7, 1998.

31. Jette AM, Branch LG, Berlin J: Musculoskeletal impairments and physical disablement among the aged. J Gerontol 45:M203-M208, 1990.

32. Voight C: Rehabilitation considerations with the geriatric patient, in Prentice WE Jr, Voight ML (eds): Techniques in Musculoskeletal Rehabilitation. New York, McGraw-Hill, 2001, pp 679-696.

33. Lewis CB, Bottomley JM: Geriatric Physical Therapy: A Clinical Approach. Norwalk, Conn, Appleton & Lange, 1994.

34. Bennett JL, Shoemaker MJ: Rehabilitation considerations for the geriatric patient, in Voight ML, Hoogenboom BJ, Prentice WE (eds): Musculoskeletal Interventions: Techniques for Therapeutic Exercise. New York, McGraw-Hill, 2007, pp 783-802.

35. Gallagher D, Visser M, De Meersman RE, et al: Appendicular skeletal muscle mass: effects of age, gender, and ethnicity. J Appl Physiol 83:229-239, 1997.

36. Larsson L, Sjodin B, Karlsson J: Histochemical and biochemical changes in human skeletal muscle with age in sedentary males, age 22-65 years. Acta Physiol Scand 103:31-39, 1978.

37. Nigg BM, Fisher V, Allinger TL, et al: Range of motion of the foot as a function of age. Foot Ankle 13:336-343, 1992.

38. Kegelmeyer D: Stability of gait and fall prevention, in Hughes C (ed): Movement Disorders and Neuromuscular Interventions for the Trunk and Extremities—Independent Study Course 18.2.6. La Crosse, Wisc, Orthopaedic Section, APTA, Inc, 2008, pp 1-20.

39. Bloem BR, Haan J, Lagaay AM, et al: Investigation of gait in elderly subjects over 88 years of age. J Geriatr Psychiatr Neurol 5:78-84, 1992.

40. Snijders AH, van de Warrenburg BP, Giladi N, et al: Neurological gait disorders in elderly people: Clinical approach and classification. Lancet Neurol 6:63-74, 2007.

41. van Hedel HJ, Dietz V: The influence of age on learning a locomotor task. Clin Neurophysiol 115:2134-2143, 2004.

42. Howard L, Kirkwood G, Leese M: Risk of hip fracture in patients with a history of schizophrenia. Br J Psychiatry 190:129-134, 2007.

43. Liporace FA, Egol KA, Tejwani N, et al: What's new in hip fractures? Current concepts. Am J Orthop 34:66-74, 2005.

44. Woolf AD, Pfleger B: Burden of major musculoskeletal conditions. Bull World Health Organ 81:646-56, 2003.

45. Van Balen R, Essink-Bot ML, Steyerberg E, et al: Quality of life after hip fracture: a comparison of four health status measures in 208 patients. Disabil Rehabil 25:507-519, 2003.

46. Braithwaite RS, Col NF, Wong JB: Estimating hip fracture morbidity, mortality and costs. J Am Geriatr Soc 51:364-370, 2003.

47. Clough TM: Femoral neck stress fracture: the importance of clinical suspicion and early review. Br J Sports Med 36:308-309, 2002.

48. Jermyn RT: A nonsurgical approach to low back pain. JAOA 101 (suppl 2):S6–S11, 2001.

49. Locksley HB: Hemorrhagic strokes. Principal causes, natural history, and treatment. Med Clin North Am 52:1193-1212, 1968.

50. Khealani BA, Syed NA, Maken S, et al: Predictors of ischemic versus hemorrhagic strokes in hypertensive patients. J Coll Physicians Surg Pak 15:22-25, 2005.

51. Leys D, Lamy C, Lucas C, et al: Arterial ischemic strokes associated with pregnancy and puerperium. Acta Neurol Belg 97:5-16, 1997.

52. Ryglewicz D, Hier DB, Wiszniewska M, et al: Ischemic strokes are more severe in Poland than in the United States. Neurology 54:513-515, 2000.

53. Sagui E, M'Baye PS, Dubecq C, et al: Ischemic and hemorrhagic strokes in Dakar, Senegal: a hospital-based study. Stroke 36:1844-1847, 2005.

54. Yahia AM, Kirmani JF, Xavier AR, et al: Characteristics and predictors of aortic plaques in patients with transient ischemic attacks and strokes. J Neuroimaging 14:16-22, 2004.

55. Agha A, Phillips J, Thompson CJ: Hypopituitarism following traumatic brain injury (TBI). Br J Neurosurg 21:210-216, 2007.

56. Kokiko ON, Hamm RJ: A review of pharmacological treatments used in experimental models of traumatic brain injury. Brain Inj 21:259-274, 2007.

57. Zehtabchi S, Sinert R, Soghoian S, et al: Identifying traumatic brain injury in patients with isolated head trauma: are arterial lactate and base deficit as helpful as in polytrauma? Emerg Med J 24:333-335, 2007.

58. Hartl R: Back to basics, or the evolution of traumatic brain injury management since Scipione Riva-Rocci. Crit Care Med 35:1196-1197, 2007.

59. Irdesel J, Aydiner SB, Akgoz S: Rehabilitation outcome after traumatic brain injury. Neurocirugia (Astur) 18:5-15, 2007.

60. Teasell R, Bayona N, Lippert C, et al: Post-traumatic seizure disorder following acquired brain injury. Brain Inj 21:201-214, 2007.

61. Scherer M: Gait rehabilitation with body weight-supported treadmill training for a blast injury survivor with traumatic brain injury. Brain Inj 21:93-100, 2007.

62. Pressman HT: Traumatic brain injury rehabilitation: Case management and insurance-related issues. Phys Med Rehabil Clin North Am 18:165-174, viii, 2007.

63. Young JA: Pain and traumatic brain injury. Phys Med Rehabil Clin North Am 18:145-63, vii-viii, 2007.

64. Yen HL, Wong JT: Rehabilitation for traumatic brain injury in children and adolescents. Ann Acad Med Singapore 36:62-66, 2007.

65. Chua KS, Ng YS, Yap SG, et al: A brief review of traumatic brain injury rehabilitation. Ann Acad Med Singapore 36:31-42, 2007.

66. Ducrocq SC, Meyer PG, Orliaguet GA, et al: Epidemiology and early predictive factors of mortality and outcome in children with traumatic severe brain injury: Experience of a French pediatric trauma center. Pediatr Crit Care Med 7:461-467, 2006.

67. Chesnut RM: The evolving management of traumatic brain injury: Don't shoot the messenger. Crit Care Med 34:2262; author reply 2262-2263, 2006.

68. Osgood SL, Kuczkowski KM: Autonomic dysreflexia in a parturient with spinal cord injury. Acta Anaesthesiol Belg 57:161-162, 2006.

69. Wu KP, Lai PL, Lee LF, et al: Autonomic dysreflexia triggered by an unstable lumbar spine in a quadriplegic patient. Chang Gung Med J. 28:508-511, 2005.

70. Adiga S: Further lessons in autonomic dysreflexia. Arch Phys Med Rehabil 86:1891; author reply 1891, 2005.

71. Sullivan-Tevault M: Autonomic dysreflexia in spinal cord injury. Emerg Med Serv 34:79-80, 85, 2005.
72. Jacob C, Thwaini A, Rao A, et al: Autonomic dysreflexia: the forgotten medical emergency. Hosp Med 66:294-296, 2005.
73. Bycroft J, Shergill IS, Chung EA, et al: Autonomic dysreflexia: a medical emergency. Postgrad Med J 81:232-235, 2005.
74. Taylor AG: Autonomic dysreflexia in spinal cord injury. Nurs Clin North Am 9:717-25, 1974.
75. Bailey MK: Physical examination procedures to screen for serious disorders of the low back and lower quarter, in Wilmarth MA (ed): Medical Screening for the Physical Therapist. Orthopaedic Section Independent Study Course 14.1.1 La Crosse, Wisc, Orthopaedic Section, APTA, Inc, 2003, pp 1-35.
76. Thomas DR: Prevention and management of pressure ulcers. Mo Med 104:52-57, 2007.
77. Evans J, Stephen-Haynes J: Identification of superficial pressure ulcers. J Wound Care 16:54-56, 2007.
78. McNees P, Meneses KD: Pressure ulcers and other chronic wounds in patients with and patients without cancer: a retrospective, comparative analysis of healing patterns. Ostomy Wound Manage 53:70-78, 2007.
79. Stewart TP, Magnano SJ: Burns or pressure ulcers in the surgical patient? Adv Skin Wound Care 20:74, 77-78, 80 passim, 2007.
80. Spilsbury K, Nelson A, Cullum N, et al: Pressure ulcers and their treatment and effects on quality of life: hospital inpatient perspectives. J Adv Nurs 57:494-504, 2007.
81. Whitney J, Phillips L, Aslam R, et al: Guidelines for the treatment of pressure ulcers. Wound Repair Regen 14:663-679, 2006.
82. Dini V, Bertone M, Romanelli M: Prevention and management of pressure ulcers. Dermatol Ther 19:356-364, 2006.
83. Rycroft-Malone J, McInnes L: The prevention of pressure ulcers. Worldviews Evid Based Nurs 1:14614-9, 2004.
84. Effective methods for preventing pressure ulcers. J Fam Pract 55:942, 2006.
85. Benbow M: Guidelines for the prevention and treatment of pressure ulcers. Nurs Stand 20:42-4, 2006.
86. Cullum N, Nelson EA, Nixon J: Pressure ulcers. Clin Evid 15:2592-2606, 2006.
87. Reddy M, Gill SS, Rochon PA: Preventing pressure ulcers: a systematic review. JAMA 296:974-984, 2006.
88. Baranoski S: Pressure ulcers: a renewed awareness. Nursing 36:36-41; quiz 42, 2006.
89. Czell D, Schreier R, Rupp R, et al: Influence of passive leg movements on blood circulation on the tilt table in healthy adults. J Neuroengineering Rehabil 1:4, 2004.
90. Jacobs PL, Mahoney ET, Robbins A, et al: Hypokinetic circulation in persons with paraplegia. Med Sci Sports Exerc 34:1401-1407, 2002.
91. Houtman S, Colier WN, Oeseburg B, et al: Systemic circulation and cerebral oxygenation during head-up tilt in spinal cord injured individuals. Spinal Cord 38:158-163, 2000.
92. Johnson RH, Spaulding JM: Disorders of the autonomic nervous system. Chapter 7. Some disorders of regional circulation. Contemp Neurol Ser:114-128, 1974.
93. Fulk GD, Schmitz TJ, Behrman AL: Traumatic spinal cord injury, in O'Sullivan SB, Schmitz TJ (eds): Physical Rehabilitation (ed 5). Philadelphia, FA Davis, 2007, pp 937-996.
94. Witt P, Parr C: Effectiveness of Trager psychophysical integration in promoting trunk mobility in a child with cerebral palsy, a case report. Phys Occup Ther Pediatr 8:75-94, 1988.
95. Gage JR, Deluca PA, Renshaw TS: Gait analysis: Principles and applications with emphasis on its use with cerebral palsy. Inst Course Lect 45:491-507, 1996.
96. Abel MH, Damiano DL, Pannunzio M, et al: Muscle-tendon surgery in diplegic cerebral palsy: functional and mechanical changes. J Pediatr Orthop 19:366-375, 1999.
97. Blair E, Stanley F: Issues in the classification and epidemiology of cerebral palsy. Mental Retard Devel Disab Res Rev 3:184-193, 1997.
98. Davids JR, Foti T, Dabelstein J, et al: Voluntary (normal) versus obligatory (cerebral palsy) toe-walking in children: a kinematic, kinetic, and electromyographic analysis. J Pediatr Orthop 19:461-469, 1999.
99. Gage JR: Gait Analysis in Cerebral Palsy. London, MacKeith Press, 1991.
100. Mayston M: Evidence-based physical therapy for the management of children with cerebral palsy. Dev Med Child Neurol 47:795, 2005.
101. Harris SR, Roxborough L: Efficacy and effectiveness of physical therapy in enhancing postural control in children with cerebral palsy. Neural Plast 12:229-243, 2005.
102. Palisano RJ, Snider LM, Orlin MN: Recent advances in physical and occupational therapy for children with cerebral palsy. Semin Pediatr Neurol 11:66-77, 2004.
103. Wilton J: Casting, splinting, and physical and occupational therapy of hand deformity and dysfunction in cerebral palsy. Hand 5Clin 19:573-84, 2003.
104. Engsberg JR, Ross SA, Wagner JM, et al: Changes in hip spasticity and strength following selective dorsal rhizotomy and physical therapy for spastic cerebral palsy. Dev Med Child Neurol 44:220-226, 2002.
105. Engsberg JR, Ross SA, Park TS: Changes in ankle spasticity and strength following selective dorsal rhizotomy and physical therapy for spastic cerebral palsy. J Neurosurg 91:727-732, 1999.
106. Barry MJ: Physical therapy interventions for patients with movement disorders due to cerebral palsy. J Child Neurol 11 (Suppl 1):S51–S60, 1996.
107. Campbell SK, Gardner HG, Ramakrishnan V: Correlates of physicians' decisions to refer children with cerebral palsy for physical therapy. Dev Med Child Neurol 37:1062-1074, 1995.
108. Harryman SE: Lower-extremity surgery for children with cerebral palsy: physical therapy management. Phys Ther 72:16-24, 1992.
109. Mayo NE: The effect of physical therapy for children with motor delay and cerebral palsy. A randomized clinical trial. Am J Phys Med Rehabil 70:258-267, 1991.
110. Stine SB: Therapy—physical or otherwise—in cerebral palsy. Am J Dis Child 144:519-520, 1990.
111. Campbell SK, Anderson JC, Gardner HG: Use of survey research methods to study clinical decision making: referral to physical therapy of children with cerebral palsy. Phys Ther 69:610-615, 1989.
112. Bower E: The effects of physical therapy on cerebral palsy. Dev Med Child Neurol 31:266, 1989.
113. Harris SR: Commentary on "The effects of physical therapy on cerebral palsy: a controlled trial in infants with spastic diplegia." Phys Occup Ther Pediatr 9:1-4, 1989.
114. Horton SV, Taylor DC: The use of behavior therapy and physical therapy to promote independent ambulation in a preschooler with mental retardation and cerebral palsy. Res Dev Disabil 10:363-375, 1989.
115. Physical therapy for cerebral palsy. N Engl J Med 319:796-797, 1988.
116. Palmer FB, Shapiro BK, Wachtel RC, et al: The effects of physical therapy on cerebral palsy. A controlled trial in infants with spastic diplegia. N Engl J Med 318:803-808, 1988.
117. Sommerfeld D, Fraser BA, Hensinger RN, et al: Evaluation of physical therapy service for severely mentally impaired students with cerebral palsy. Phys Ther 61:338-344, 1981.
118. Sussman MD, Cusick B: Preliminary report: the role of short-leg, tone-reducing casts as an adjunct to physical therapy of patients with cerebral palsy. Johns Hopkins Med J 145:112-114, 1979.
119. Abdel-Salam E, Maraghi S, Tawfik M: Evaluation of physical therapy techniques in the management of cerebral palsy. J Egypt Med Assoc 61:531-541, 1978.
120. Marx M: Integrating physical therapy into a cerebral palsy early education program. Phys Ther 53:512-514, 1973.
121. Mathias A: Management of cerebral palsy. Physical therapy in relation to orthopedic surgery. Phys Ther 47:473-482, 1967.
122. Stroumbou-Alamani S: Current concepts in the medical treatment of cerebral palsy. Physical therapy. Arch Ital Pediatr Pueric 25:113-120, 1967.
123. D'Wolf N, Donnelly E: Physical therapy and cerebral palsy. Clin Pediatr (Phila) 5:351-355, 1966.
124. Footh WK, Kogan KL: Measuring the Effectiveness of Physical Therapy in the Treatment of Cerebral Palsy. J Appl Toxicol 43:867-873, 1963.
125. Paine RS: Physical therapy in the management of cerebral palsy. Dev Med Child Neurol 5:193, 1963.
126. Gelperin A, Payton O: Evaluation of equanil as adjunct to physical therapy for children with severe cerebral palsy. Phys Ther Rev 39:383-388, 1959.
127. Schwartz FF: Physical therapy for children with cerebral palsy. J Int Coll Surg 21:84-87, 1954.
128. Brooks W, Callahan M, Schleich-Korn J: Physical therapy and the adult with cerebral palsy; report of a conference on vocational guidance. Phys Ther Rev 33:426-428, 1953.
129. Bailey LA: Physical therapy in the treatment of cerebral palsy. Phys Ther Rev 30:230-231, 1950.
130. Grogan DP, Lundy MS, Ogden JA: A method for early postoperative mobilization of the cerebral palsy patient using a removable abduction bar. J Pediatr Orthop 7:338-340, 1987.

131. Katz K, Arbel N, Apter N, et al: Early mobilization after sliding Achilles tendon lengthening in children with spastic cerebral palsy. Foot Ankle Int 21:1011-1014, 2000.

132. Palisano R, Rosenbaum P, Walter S, et al: Development and reliability of a system to classify gross motor function in children with cerebral palsy. Dev Med Child Neurol 39:214-223, 1997.

133. Prechtl HF: State of the art of a new functional assessment of the young nervous system. An early predictor of cerebral palsy. Early Hum Dev 50:1-11, 1997.

134. Olney SJ, Wright MJ: Cerebral Palsy, in Campbell SK, Vander Linden DW, Palisano RJ (eds): Physical Therapy for Children. St Louis, Saunders, 2006, pp 625-664.

135. Rosenbaum P: Cerebral palsy: what parents and doctors want to know. BMJ 326:970-974, 2003.

136. Lepage C, Noreau L, Bernard PM: Association between characteristics of locomotion and accomplishment of life habits in children with cerebral palsy. Phys Ther 78:458-469, 1998.

137. Sterba JA: Does horseback riding therapy or therapist-directed hippotherapy rehabilitate children with cerebral palsy? Dev Med Child Neurol 49:68-73, 2007.

138. Westberry DE, Davids JR, Jacobs JM, et al: Effectiveness of serial stretch casting for resistant or recurrent knee flexion contractures following hamstring lengthening in children with cerebral palsy. J Pediatr Orthop 26:109-114, 2006.

139. Hoare B, Wasiak J, Imms C, et al: Constraint-induced movement therapy in the treatment of the upper limb in children with hemiplegic cerebral palsy. Cochrane Database Syst Rev 2:CD004149, 2007.

140. Casady RL, Nichols-Larsen DS: The effect of hippotherapy on ten children with cerebral palsy. Pediatr Phys Ther 16:165-172, 2004.

141. Greitz D: Unraveling the riddle of syringomyelia. Neurosurg Rev 29:2512-63; discussion 264, 2006.

142. Milhorat TH: Classification of syringomyelia. Neurosurg Focus 8:E1, 2000.

143. Pearce JM: Syringes and syringomyelia. Eur Neurol 54:243, 2005.

144. Todor DR, Mu HT, Milhorat TH: Pain and syringomyelia: a review. Neurosurg Focus 8:E11, 2000.

145. Wollman DE: Syringomyelia: an uncommon cause of myelopathy in the geriatric population. J Am Geriatr Soc 52:1033-1034, 2004.

146. Shaer CM, Chescheir N, Erickson K, et al: Obstetrician-gynecologists' practice and knowledge regarding spina bifida. Am J Perinatol 23:355-362, 2006.

147. Woodhouse CR: Progress in the management of children born with spina bifida. Eur Urol 49:777-778, 2006.

148. Verhoef M, Barf HA, Post MW, et al: Functional independence among young adults with spina bifida, in relation to hydrocephalus and level of lesion. Dev Med Child Neurol 48:114-119, 2006.

149. Ali L, Stocks GM: Spina bifida, tethered cord and regional anaesthesia. Anaesthesia 60:1149-1150, 2005.

150. Spina bifida. Nurs Times 101:31, 2005.

151. Mitchell LE, Adzick NS, Melchionne J, et al: Spina bifida. Lancet 364:1885-1895, 2004.

152. Dias L: Orthopaedic care in spina bifida: past, present, and future. Dev Med Child Neurol 46:579, 2004.

153. Haykowsky MJ, Hillegass EA: Integration of the cardiovascular system in assessment and interventions in musculoskeletal rehabilitation, in Magee D, Zachazewski JE, Quillen WS (eds): Scientific Foundations and Principles of Practice in Musculoskeletal Rehabilitation. St Louis, MI, WB Saunders, 2007, pp 414-431.

154. Cay S, Metin F, Korkmaz S: Association of renal functional impairment and the severity of coronary artery disease. Anadolu Kardiyol Derg 7:44-48, 2007.

155. Junnila JL, Runkle GP: Coronary artery disease screening, treatment, and follow-up. Prim Care 33:863-885, vi, 2006.

156. Sbarsi I, Falcone C, Boiocchi C, et al: Inflammation and atherosclerosis: the role of TNF and TNF receptors polymorphisms in coronary artery disease. Int J Immunopathol Pharmacol 20:145-154, 2007.

157. Ask the doctors. I recently read that patients with coronary artery disease ought to have their blood pressure reduced to less than 120/80. I thought 120/80 was normal blood pressure, so why would you want blood pressure to be lower than normal? Heart Advis 10:8, 2007.

158. Dzielinska Z, Januszewicz A, Demkow M, et al: Cardiovascular risk factors in hypertensive patients with coronary artery disease and coexisting renal artery stenosis. J Hypertens 25:663-670, 2007.

159. DeFaria Yeh D, Freeman MW, Meigs JB, et al: Risk factors for coronary artery disease in patients with elevated high-density lipoprotein cholesterol. Am J Cardiol 99:1-4, 2007.

160. Carneiro AV: Coronary heart disease in diabetes mellitus: risk factors and epidemiology. Rev Port Cardiol 23:1359-1366, 2004.

161. Graner M, Syvanne M, Kahri J, et al: Insulin resistance as predictor of the angiographic severity and extent of coronary artery disease. Ann Med 39:137-144, 2007.

162. Orchard TJ, Costacou T, Kretowski A, et al: Type 1 diabetes and coronary artery disease. Diabetes Care 29:2528-2538, 2006.

163. Pepine CJ, Kowey PR, Kupfer S, et al: Predictors of adverse outcome among patients with hypertension and coronary artery disease. J Am Coll Cardiol 47:547-551, 2006.

164. Hennessey JV, Westrick E: Coronary artery disease and cerebrovascular disease prevention in diabetes mellitus: early identification and aggressive modification of risk factors. Med Health R I 81:350-352, 1998.

165. Sukhija R, Aronow WS, Yalamanchili K, et al: Prevalence of coronary artery disease, lower extremity peripheral arterial disease, and cerebrovascular disease in 110 men with an abdominal aortic aneurysm. Am J Cardiol 94:1358-1359, 2004.

166. Ness J, Aronow WS: Prevalence of coronary artery disease, ischemic stroke, peripheral arterial disease, and coronary revascularization in older African-Americans, Asians, Hispanics, whites, men, and women. Am J Cardiol 84:932-933, A7, 1999.

167. Lee CS, Lu YH, Lee ST, et al: Evaluating the prevalence of silent coronary artery disease in asymptomatic patients with spinal cord injury. Int Heart J 47:325-330, 2006.

168. Bauman WA, Spungen AM, Raza M, et al: Coronary artery disease: metabolic risk factors and latent disease in individuals with paraplegia. Mt Sinai J Med 59:163-168, 1992.

169. White LJ, McCoy SC, Castellano V, et al: Effect of resistance training on risk of coronary artery disease in women with multiple sclerosis. Scand J Clin Lab Invest 66:351-355, 2006.

170. Steffens DC, O'Connor CM, Jiang WJ, et al: The effect of major depression on functional status in patients with coronary artery disease. J Am Geriatr Soc 47:319-322, 1999.

171. Pamukcu B, Oflaz H, Onur I, et al: Clinical relevance of aspirin resistance in patients with stable coronary artery disease: a prospective follow-up study (PROSPECTAR). Blood Coagul Fibrinolysis 18:187-192, 2007.

172. Ludvig J, Miner B, Eisenberg MJ: Smoking cessation in patients with coronary artery disease. Am Heart J 149:565-572, 2005.

173. Schooling CM, Lam TH, Leung GM: Effect of obesity in patients with coronary artery disease. Lancet 368:1645; author reply 1645-1646, 2006.

174. Lundberg GD: A new aggressive approach to screening and early intervention to prevent death from coronary artery disease. MedGenMed 8:22, 2006.

175. Boekholdt SM, Sandhu MS, Day NE, et al: Physical activity, C-reactive protein levels and the risk of future coronary artery disease in apparently healthy men and women: the EPIC-Norfolk prospective population study. Eur J Cardiovasc Prev Rehabil 13:970-976, 2006.

176. Prayaga S: Asian Indians and coronary artery disease risk. Am J Med 120:e15; author reply e19, 2007.

177. Chambers TA, Bagai A, Ivascu N: Current trends in coronary artery disease in women. Curr Opin Anaesthesiol 20:75-82, 2007.

178. Turhan S, Tulunay C, Gulec S, et al: The association between androgen levels and premature coronary artery disease in men. Coron Artery Dis 18:159-162, 2007.

179. Saghafi H, Mahmoodi MJ, Fakhrzadeh H, et al: Cardiovascular risk factors in first-degree relatives of patients with premature coronary artery disease. Acta Cardiol 61:607-613, 2006.

180. Ahmed A, Lefante CM, Alam N: Depression and nursing home admission among hospitalized older adults with coronary artery disease: a propensity score analysis. Am J Geriatr Cardiol 16:76-83, 2007.

181. Zevitz ME: Heart failure. Available at: http://www.emedicine.com/med/topic3552.htm, 2005.

182. Rees K, Taylor RS, Singh S, et al: Exercise based rehabilitation for heart failure. Cochrane Database Syst Rev 3:CD003331, 2004.

183. Pina IL, Daoud S: Exercise and heart failure. Minerva Cardioangiol 52:537-546, 2004.

184. Pina IL, Apstein CS, Balady GJ, et al: Exercise and heart failure: A statement from the American Heart Association Committee on exercise, rehabilitation, and prevention. Circulation 107:1210-1225, 2003.

185. Budev MM, Arroliga AC, Wiedemann HP, et al: Cor pulmonale: an overview. Semin Respir Crit Care Med 24:233-244, 2003.

186. Weitzenblum E: Chronic cor pulmonale. Heart 89:225-230, 2003.

187. Lehrman S, Romano P, Frishman W, et al: Primary pulmonary hypertension and cor pulmonale. Cardiol Rev 10:265-278, 2002.

188. Romano PM, Peterson S: The management of cor pulmonale. Heart Dis 2:431-437, 2000.

189. Missov ED, De Marco T: Cor Pulmonale. Curr Treat Options Cardiovasc Med 2:149-158, 2000.

190. DeTurk WE, Cahalin LP: Electrocardiography, in DeTurk WE, Cahalin LP (eds): Cardiovascular and pulmonary physical therapy: an evidence-based approach. New York, McGraw-Hill, 2004, pp 325-359.

191. Roffe C: Aging of the heart. Br J Biomed Sci 55:136-148, 1998.

192. Alaeddini J, Alimohammadi B: Angina pectoris. Available at: http://www.emedicine.com/med/topic133.htm, 2006.

193. Fenton DE, Stahmer S: Myocardial infarction. Available at: http://www.emedicine.com/EMERG/topic327.htm, 2006.

194. Goodman CC: The cardiovascular system, in Goodman CC, Boissonnault WG, Fuller KS (eds): Pathology: Implications for the Physical Therapist (ed 2). Philadelphia, Saunders, 2003, pp 367-476.

195. Nauer K, A.: Acute dissection of the aorta: a review for nurses. Crit Care Nurs Q 23:20-27, 2000.

196. McKnight JT, Adcock BB: Paresthesias: a practical diagnostic approach. Am Fam Physician 56:2253-2260, 1997.

197. Poncelet AN: An algorithm for the evaluation of peripheral neuropathy. Am Fam Physician 57:755-764, 1998.

198. Gillette PD: Exercise in aging and disease, in Placzek JD, Boyce DA (eds): Orthopaedic Physical Therapy Secrets. Philadelphia, Hanley & Belfus, 2001, pp 235-242.

199. Motsch J, Walther A, Bock M, et al: Update in the prevention and treatment of deep vein thrombosis and pulmonary embolism. Curr Opin Anaesthesiol 19:52-58, 2006.

200. Garmon RG: Pulmonary embolism: incidence, diagnosis, prevention, and treatment. J Am Osteopath Assoc 85:176-185, 1985.

201. Bounameaux H, Reber-Wasem MA: Superficial thrombophlebitis and deep vein thrombosis: a controversial association. Arch Intern Med 157:1822-1824, 1997.

202. Gorman WP, Davis KR, Donnelly R: ABC of arterial and venous disease. Swollen lower limb—1: general assessment and deep vein thrombosis. BMJ 320:1453-1456, 2000.

203. Aschwanden M, Labs KH, Engel H, et al: Acute deep vein thrombosis: early mobilization does not increase the frequency of pulmonary embolism. Thromb Haemost 85:42-46, 2001.

204. Heath GW, Hagberg JM, Ehsani AA, et al: A physiological comparison of young and older endurance athletes. J Appl Physiol 51:634-640, 1981.

205. Shah U, Moatter T: Screening for cystic fibrosis: the importance of using the correct tools. J Ayub Med Coll Abbottabad 18:7-10, 2006.

206. Wells C: Pulmonary pathology, in DeTurk WE, Cahalin LP (eds): Cardiovascular and Pulmonary Physical Therapy: an Evidence-Based Approach. New York, McGraw-Hill, 2004, pp 151-188.

207. Chang AB, Masters IB, Everard ML: Re: membranous obliterative bronchitis: a proposed unifying model. Pediatr Pulmonol 41:904; author reply 905-906, 2006.

208. Wang JS, Tseng HH, Lai RS, et al: Sauropus androgynus–constrictive obliterative bronchitis/bronchiolitis—histopathological study of pneumonectomy and biopsy specimens with emphasis on the inflammatory process and disease progression. Histopathology 37:402-410, 2000.

209. Coughlin AM: Combating community-acquired pneumonia. Nursing 37:64hn1-3, 2007.

210. Clark JE, Donna H, Spencer D, et al: Children with pneumonia—how do they present and how are they managed? Arch Dis Child 29:29, 2007.

211. Parienti JJ, Carrat F: Viral pneumonia and respiratory sepsis: association, causation, or it depends? Crit Care Med 35:639-640, 2007.

212. Hospital-acquired pneumonia. J Hosp Med 1:26-27, 2006.

213. Community-acquired pneumonia. J Hosp Med 1:16-17, 2006.

214. Flaherty KR, Martinez FJ: Nonspecific interstitial pneumonia. Semin Respir Crit Care Med 27:652-658, 2006.

215. Lynch JP, 3rd, Saggar R, Weigt SS, et al: Usual interstitial pneumonia. Semin Respir Crit Care Med 27:634-651, 2006.

216. Leong JR, Huang DT: Ventilator-associated pneumonia. Surg Clin North Am 86:1409-1429, 2006.

217. Agusti C, Rano A, Aldabo I, et al: Fungal pneumonia, chronic respiratory diseases and glucocorticoids. Med Mycol 44 Suppl:207-11, 2006.

218. Scannapieco FA: Pneumonia in nonambulatory patients: The role of oral bacteria and oral hygiene. J Am Dent Assoc 137 Suppl:21S–25S, 2006.

219. Medina-Walpole AM, Katz PR: Nursing home-acquired pneumonia. J Am Geriatr Soc 47:1005-1015, 1999.

220. Tang WK, Lum CM, Ungvari GS, et al: Health-related quality of life in community-dwelling men with pneumoconiosis. Respiration 73:203-208, 2006.

221. Chong S, Lee KS, Chung MJ, et al: Pneumoconiosis: comparison of imaging and pathologic findings. Radiographics 26:59-77, 2006.

222. Attfield MD, Kuempel ED: Pneumoconiosis, coalmine dust and the PFR. Ann Occup Hyg 47:525-529, 2003.

223. Nicod LP: Recognition and treatment of idiopathic pulmonary fibrosis. Drugs 55:555-562, 1998.

224. Poole DC, Sexton WL, Farkas GA, et al: Diaphragm structure and function in health and disease. Med Sci Sports Exer. 29:738-54, 1997.

225. Patrick C: Spinal conditions, in Campbell SK, Vander Linden DW, Palisano RJ (eds): Physical Therapy for Children. St Louis, Saunders, 2006, pp 337-358.

226. McKenzie RA: Manual correction of sciatic scoliosis. N Z Med J 76:194-199, 1972.

227. Blum CL: Chiropractic and Pilates therapy for the treatment of adult scoliosis. J Manipulative Physiol Ther 25:E3, 2002.

228. Miller NH: Genetics of familial idiopathic scoliosis. Clin Orthop Rel Res 401:60-64, 2002.

229. Kane WJ: Scoliosis prevalence: A call for a statement of terms. Clin Orthop 126:43-46, 1977.

230. Miller NH: Cause and natural history of adolescent idiopathic scoliosis. Orthop Clin North Am 30:343-352, vii, 1999.

231. Dobbs MB, Weinstein SL: Infantile and juvenile scoliosis. Orthop Clin North Am 30:331-41, vii, 1999.

232. Greiner KA: Adolescent idiopathic scoliosis: radiologic decision-making. Am Fam Physician 65:1817-1822, 2002.

233. Lonstein JE, Winter RB: Adolescent idiopathic scoliosis. Nonoperative treatment. Orthop Clin North Am 19:239-246, 1988.

234. Lenke LG: Lenke classification system of adolescent idiopathic scoliosis: treatment recommendations. Instr Course Lect 54:537-542, 2005.

235. Lenke LG, Edwards CC, 2nd, Bridwell KH: The Lenke classification of adolescent idiopathic scoliosis: how it organizes curve patterns as a template to perform selective fusions of the spine. Spine 28:S199-S207, 2003.

236. Weinstein SL, Ponseti IV: Curve progression in idiopathic scoliosis. J Bone Joint Surg Am 65:447-455, 1983.

237. Ponseti IV, Pedrini V, Wynne-Davies R, et al: Pathogenesis of scoliosis. Clin Orthop Relat Res (120):268-280, 1976.

238. Ponseti IV, Friedman B: Prognosis in idiopathic scoliosis. J Bone Joint Surg Am 32A:381-395, 1950.

239. Gladman DD, Brubacher B, Buskila D, et al: Differences in the expression of spondyloarthropathy: a comparison between ankylosing spondylitis and psoriatic arthritis: genetic and gender effects. Clin Invest Med 16:1-7, 1993.

240. Haslock I: Ankylosing spondylitis. Baillieres Clin Rheumatol 7:99, 1993.

241. Turek SL: Orthopaedics—Principles and Their Application (ed 4). Philadelphia, JB Lippincott, 1984.

242. Gran JT: An epidemiologic survey of the signs and symptoms of ankylosing spondylitis. Clin Rheumatol 4:161-169, 1985.

243. Calin A, Porta J, Fries JF, et al: Clinical history as a screening test for ankylosing spondylitis. JAMA 237:2613-2614, 1977.

244. Cohen MD, Ginsurg WW: Late onset peripheral joint disease in ankylosing spondylitis. Arthritis Rheum 26:186-90, 1983.

245. Gladman DD: Clinical aspects of the spondyloarthropathies. Am J Med Sci 316:234-238, 1998.

246. Solak ZA, Goksel T, Telli CG, et al. "Success of a smoking cessation program among smoking relatives of patients with serious smoking-related pulmonary disorders." European addiction research 11(2): 57-61, 2005.

247. Mahler DA, Barlow PB, Matthay RA: Chronic obstructive pulmonary disease. Clin Geriatr Med 2:285-312, 1986.

248. Mulroy J: Chronic obstructive pulmonary disease in women. Dimens Crit Care Nurs 24:1-18; quiz 19-20, 2005.

249. Ong KC, Ong YY: Cardiopulmonary exercise testing in patients with chronic obstructive pulmonary disease. Ann Acad Med Singapore 29:648-652, 2000.

250. Balmes JR: Occupational contribution to the burden of chronic obstructive pulmonary disease. J Occup Environ Med 47:154-60, 2005.

251. Man SF, McAlister FA, Anthonisen NR, et al: Contemporary management of chronic obstructive pulmonary disease: clinical applications. JAMA. 290:2313-6, 2003.

252. Carter GT, Kilmer DD, Bonekat HW, et al: Evaluation of phrenic nerve and pulmonary function in hereditary motor and sensory neuropathy type 1. Muscle Nerve 15:459-456, 1992.

253. Bolton CF: Clinical neurophysiology of the respiratory system. Muscle Nerve 16:809-818, 1993.

254. Chusid JG: Correlative Neuroanatomy & Functional Neurology (ed 19). Norwalk, Conn, Appleton-Century-Crofts, 1985, pp 144-148.

255. Richard RL, Ward RS: Burns, in O'Sullivan SB, Schmitz TJ (eds): Physical Rehabilitation (ed 5). Philadelphia, FA Davis, 2007, pp 1091-1115.

256. Cioffi WG: Inhalation injury, in Carrougher GJ (ed): Burn care and therapy. St Louis, CV Mosby, 1998, p 35.

257. Wiles R: The views of women of above average weight about appropriate weight gain in pregnancy. Midwifery 14:254-260, 1998.

258. Lee HY, Zhao S, Fields PA, et al: Clinical use of relaxin to facilitate birth: reasons for investigating the premise. Ann N Y Acad Sci 1041:351-366, 2005.

259. Lubahn J, Ivance D, Konieczko E, et al: Immunohistochemical detection of relaxin binding to the volar oblique ligament. J Hand Surg [Am] 31:80-84, 2006.

260. Stephenson R, O'Connor L: Obstetric and Gynecologic Care in Physical Therapy (ed 2). Thorofare, NJ, Charles B Slack, 2000.

261. Berg G, Hammar M, Moller-Nielsen J, et al: Low back pain during pregnancy. Obstet Gynecol 71:71-75, 1988.

262. Bullock JE, Jull GA, Bullock MI: The relationship of low back pain to postural changes during pregnancy. Aust J Physiother 33:10-17, 1987.

263. Moore K, Dumas GA, Reid JG: Postural changes associated with pregnancy and their relationship with low back pain. Clin Biomech (Bristol, Avon) 5:169-174, 1990.

264. Ostgaard HC, Andersson GBJ, Schultz AB, et al: Influence of some biomechanical factors on low back pain in pregnancy. Spine 18:61-65, 1993.

265. Franklin ME, Conner-Kerr T: An analysis of posture and back pain in the first and third trimesters of pregnancy. J Orthop Sports Phys Ther 28:133-138, 1998.

266. Depledge J, McNair PJ, Keal-Smith C, et al: Management of symphysis pubis dysfunction during pregnancy using exercise and pelvic support belts. Phys Ther 85:1290-1300, 2005.

267. Leadbetter RE, Mawer D, Lindow SW: Symphysis pubis dysfunction: a review of the literature. J Matern Fetal Neonatal Med 16:349-354, 2004.

268. Owens K, Pearson A, Mason G: Symphysis pubis dysfunction—a cause of significant obstetric morbidity. Eur J Obstet Gynecol Reprod Biol 105:143-146, 2002.

269. Allsop JR: Symphysis pubis dysfunction. Br J Gen Pract 47:256, 1997.

270. Snow RE, Neubert AG: Peripartum pubic symphysis separation: a case series and review of the literature. Obstet Gynecol Surv 52:438-443, 1997.

271. Whitman JM: Pregnancy, low back pain, and manual physical therapy interventions. J Orthop Sports Phys Ther 32:314-317, 2002.

272. Mogren IM, Pohjanen AI: Low back pain and pelvic pain during pregnancy: prevalence and risk factors. Spine 30:983-991, 2005.

273. Pool-Goudzwaard AL, Slieker ten Hove MC, Vierhout ME, et al: Relations between pregnancy-related low back pain, pelvic floor activity and pelvic floor dysfunction. Int Urogynecol J Pelvic Floor Dysfunct 16:468-474, 2005.

274. Wang SM, Dezinno P, Maranets I, et al: Low back pain during pregnancy: prevalence, risk factors, and outcomes. Obstet Gynecol 104:65-70, 2004.

275. Fast A, Weiss L, Ducommun EJ, et al: Low back pain in pregnancy. Abdominal muscles, sit-up performance and back pain. Spine 15:28-30, 1990.

276. Nilsson-Wikmar L, Holm K, Oijerstedt R, et al: Effect of three different physical therapy treatments on pain and activity in pregnant women with pelvic girdle pain: a randomized clinical trial with 3, 6, and 12 months follow-up postpartum. Spine 30:850-856, 2005.

277. Hall J, Cleland JA, Palmer JA: The effects of manual physical therapy and therapeutic exercise on peripartum posterior pelvic pain: Two case reports. J Man Manipulative Ther 13:94-102, 2005.

278. Fast A, Shapiro D, Ducommun EJ, et al: Low-back pain in pregnancy. Spine 12:368-371, 1987.

279. Hainline B: Low-back pain in pregnancy. Adv Neurol 64:65-76, 1994.

280. Hodges SD, Eck JC, Humphreys SC: A treatment and outcomes analysis of patients with coccydynia. Spine J 4:138-140, 2004.

281. Ryder I, Alexander J: Coccydynia: a woman's tail. Midwifery 16:155-160, 2000.

282. Maigne JY, Lagauche D, Doursounian L: Instability of the coccyx in coccydynia. J Bone Joint Surg Br 82:1038-1041, 2000.

283. Boeglin ER, Jr.: Coccydynia. J Bone Joint Surg Br 73:1009, 1991.

284. Wray CC, Easom S, Hoskinson J: Coccydynia. Aetiology and treatment. J Bone Joint Surg Br 73:335-338, 1991.

285. Noble E: Essential Exercises for the Childbearing Year (ed 4). Harwich, Mass, New Life Images, 1995.

286. Noronha A: Neurologic disorders during pregnancy and the puerperium. Clin Perinatol 12:695-713, 1985.

287. Godfrey CM: Carpal tunnel syndrome in pregnancy. Can Med Assoc J 129:928, 1983.

288. Graham JG: Neurological complications of pregnancy and anaesthesia. Clin Obstet Gynaecol 9:333-350, 1982.

289. Lee DT, Chung TK: Postnatal depression: an update. Best Pract Res Clin Obstet Gynaecol 21: 183-191, 2006 .

290. Howard L: Postnatal depression. Clin Evid:1919-1931, 2006.

291. Howard L: Postnatal depression. Clin Evid:1764-1775, 2005.

292. Cox J: Postnatal depression in fathers. Lancet 366:982, 2005.

293. Boissonnault JS, Stephenson R: The obstetric patient, in Boissonnault WG (ed): Primary Care for the Physical Therapist: Examination and Triage. St Louis, Elsevier Saunders, 2005, pp 239-270.

294. Hanley J: The assessment and treatment of postnatal depression. Nurs Times 102:24-26, 2006.

295. Mallikarjun PK, Oyebode F: Prevention of postnatal depression. J R Soc Health 125:221-226, 2005.

296. Lamondy AM: Managing hyperemesis gravidarum. Nursing 37:66-68, 2007.

297. Dodds L, Fell DB, Joseph KS, et al: Outcomes of pregnancies complicated by hyperemesis gravidarum. Obstet Gynecol 107:285-292, 2006.

298. Fell DB, Dodds L, Joseph KS, et al: Risk factors for hyperemesis gravidarum requiring hospital admission during pregnancy. Obstet Gynecol 107:277-284, 2006.

299. Loh KY, Sivalingam N: Understanding hyperemesis gravidarum. Med J Malaysia 60:394-399; quiz 400, 2005.

300. Wise RA, Polito AJ, Krishnan V: Respiratory physiologic changes in pregnancy. Immunol Allergy Clin North Am 26:1-12, 2006.

301. Sadaniantz A, Kocheril AG, Emaus SP, et al: Cardiovascular changes in pregnancy evaluated by two-dimensional and Doppler echocardiography. J Am Soc Echocardiogr 5:253-258, 1992.

302. Atkins AF, Watt JM, Milan P, et al: A longitudinal study of cardiovascular dynamic changes throughout pregnancy. Eur J Obstet Gynecol Reprod Biol 12:215-224, 1981.

303. Chesley LC: Cardiovascular changes in pregnancy. Obstet Gynecol Annu 4:71-97, 1975.

304. Capeless EL, Clapp JF: Cardiovascular changes in early phase of pregnancy. Am J Obstet Gynecol 161:1449-1453, 1989.

305. Walters WA, Lim YL: Changes in the maternal cardiovascular system during human pregnancy. Surg Gynecol Obstet 131:765-784, 1970.

306. Urman BC, McComb PF: A biphasic basal body temperature record during pregnancy. Acta Eur Fertil 20:371-372, 1989.

307. Grant A, Mc BW: The 100 day basal body temperature graph in early pregnancy. Med J Aust 46:458-460, 1959.

308. Siegler AM: Basal body temperature in pregnancy. Obstet Gynecol 5:830-832, 1955.

Correcting Movement Dysfunction

CHAPTER 7

CHAPTER OBJECTIVES

*At the completion of this chapter,
the reader will be able to:*

1. List the factors that, when dysfunctional, can have a negative impact on movement

2. Describe the various methods by which physical therapy can have a positive impact on movement dysfunction

3. List three stages of learning according to Fitts and Posner

4. Describe the differences between an open skill and a closed skill

5. Describe the differences among the various types of practices

6. Describe the types of feedback that can be provided by a patient and the advantages and disadvantages of each

7. Discuss the importance of measuring functional outcomes

8. Apply the various principles behind the provided patient example in a variety of situations

OVERVIEW

The correction of movement dysfunction requires a detailed analysis of the various components of movement. As described in Chapter 4, the production of movement is a complex process involving a number of interrelated systems and normal development of those systems. Each of these systems controls a number of critical components that work together to allow normal movement to occur. As described in Chapter 6, these critical components are subject to breakdown, resulting in movement dysfunction. These components include, but are not limited to:

▶ Strength

▶ Range of motion

▶ Flexibility

▶ Coordination

▶ Proprioception

▶ Pain

▶ Balance

▶ Cardiovascular endurance

All of the listed components can be viewed as separate entities, with each having the potential to have a negative impact on movement if dysfunctional. The focus of physical therapy is to view the body as a whole and to determine the sum effect of each component breakdown on an individual's function. Movement without purpose and control is both inefficient and ineffective. Skilled performance requires cooperation among strength, endurance, speed, and accuracy. In addition, skilled performance is dependent on practice or experience.

CLINICAL PEARL

A physical therapist can be viewed as an expert in both the detection and correction of abnormal movement.

A trained physical therapist can observe a patient and determine a working hypothesis for the reason behind every abnormal movement observed. Once the diagnosis is correct, the intervention consists of methods to rehabilitate and retrain the dysfunctional structures.

As the physical therapy student progresses through his or her studies, a wide array of tools and techniques will be learned that will enable the student to correctly diagnose a condition and then design an appropriate treatment plan. The goal of a therapeutic intervention is to maximize function and thereby minimize disability; however, accomplishing this goal requires an understanding of the path from disease to disability.[1] Planning for the intervention begins with role performance, considering the best combination of remediation, adaptation, and compensation in order to promote the patient/client-identified level of functioning to fulfill desired roles. Recovery of the patient/client can occur:

▶ Spontaneously, without the benefit of any intervention

▶ By force, where the functional gains occur through therapeutic intervention

▶ Through adaptation attained by altering the methods or contexts within which the patient/client accomplishes a task

The purpose of this chapter is to begin building a conceptual framework for a clinical approach to diagnosing and treating movement dysfunction.

PHYSICAL THERAPY IMPACT

The Guide has defined physical therapy as including *"restoration, maintenance, and promotion of optimal physical function, optimal fitness and wellness, and optimal quality of life as it relates to movement and health."* The purpose of the physical therapy intervention process is to achieve desired functional outcomes by reduction of existing impairments, prevention of secondary impairments, enhancement of functional ability, promotion of optimal health, and reduction of environmental challenges.[2,3] Normally, this is achieved with a gradual progression of functional training and exercises, while avoiding further damage to an already-compromised structure.[4] Decisions about the intervention to restore functional homeostasis are custom designed from a blend of clinical experience and scientific data, and the answers to a few key questions (Table 7-1).

Physical therapists have at their disposal a battery of physical agents, electrotherapeutic modalities, and techniques for use during the various stages of healing. The necessary knowledge to perform an intervention includes[3]:

▶ The temporal phases of tissue healing, common impairments in each phase, and stresses that tissues can safely tolerate during each phase

▶ Movement characteristics, including amount of range, control, and capacity required for various functional activities

▶ The range of available intervention strategies and procedures to promote these movement characteristics, and corresponding outcomes in varied patient populations

▶ Sequencing of various interventions to challenge appropriately involved tissues and the whole patient: for example, being able to recognize the underlying tissue healing and balance disorders in a patient with diabetes mellitus and a recent hip fracture; the need for aerobic conditioning in assessing patients with low back

TABLE 7-1	Key Questions for Intervention Planning
What is the stage of healing: acute, subacute, or chronic?	
How long do you have to treat the patient?	
What does the patient do for activities?	
How compliant is the patient?	
How much *skilled* physical therapy is needed?	
What needs to be taught to prevent recurrence?	
Are any referrals needed?	
What has worked for other patients with similar problems?	
Are there any precautions?	
What is your skill level?	

Data from Guide to physical therapist practice. Phys Ther 81:S13-S95, 2001.

dysfunction; and the importance of body mechanics education in prenatal and postnatal exercise classes

▶ Intervention strategies to promote health and prevent secondary dysfunction

The intervention is typically guided by short- and long-term goals (see Chapter 5), which are dynamic, being altered as the patient's condition changes, and strategies with which to achieve those goals based on the stages of healing. Intervention strategies can be subdivided into active (direct) or passive (indirect), with the goal being to make the intervention as active as possible at the earliest opportunity.

In general, the majority of goals for the patient fall into one of the following categories:

▶ Decrease pain

▶ Correct a structural imbalance

▶ Improve muscle performance

▶ Increase range of motion and flexibility

▶ Improve balance

▶ Minimize the effects of aging

Physical Therapy Impact—Pain

Physical therapists can use several therapeutic interventions to manage pain. These include:

▶ *Transcutaneous electrical nerve stimulation (TENS).* TENS has been used effectively for many years as a safe, noninvasive, drug-free method of treatment for various chronic and acute pain syndromes. It was first introduced in the early 1950s to determine the suitability of patients with pain as candidates for the implantation of posterior (dorsal) column electrodes. Depending on the parameters of electrical stimuli applied, there are several modes of therapy, resulting in different contributions of hyperemic, muscle-relaxing, and analgesic components of TENS. TENS has been shown to be effective in providing pain relief in the early stages of healing following surgery[5-10] and in the remodeling phase and is frequently used to treat a number of pain conditions, including back pain, osteoarthritis, and fibromyalgia.[11-14]

The percentage of patients who benefit from short-term TENS pain intervention has been reported to range from 50% to 80%, and good long-term results with TENS have been observed in 6% to 44% of patients.[11,13,15,16] However, most of the TENS studies rely solely on subjects' pain reports to establish efficacy and rarely on other outcome measures such as activity, socialization, or medication use.

TENS units typically deliver symmetric or balanced asymmetric biphasic waves of 100- to 500-millisecond pulse duration, with zero net current to minimize skin irritation,[17] and may be applied for extended periods.

Three modes of action are theorized for the efficacy of this modality:

1. *Gate control mechanism.* Spinal gating control through stimulation of the large, myelinated A-alpha fibers inhibits transmission of the smaller pain transmitting unmyelinated C fibers and myelinated A-delta fibers.[9,18]

2. *Endogenous opiate control.* When subjected to certain types of electrical stimulation of the sensory nerves, there may be a release of enkephalin from local sites within the central nervous system and the release of β-endorphin from the pituitary gland into the cerebrospinal fluid.[17,19,20] A successful application can produce an analgesic effect that lasts for several hours.

3. *Central biasing.* Intense electrical stimulation, approaching a noxious level, of the smaller C or pain fibers produces a stimulation of the descending neurons.

▶ *Interferential current.* Clinically, interferential current therapy is beneficial for treating painful conditions such as osteoarthritic pain. The potential mechanisms behind this pain control include an increase in blood flow, and the same mechanisms as TENS—segmental inhibition and activation of descending inhibitory pathways.

▶ *Thermal modalities.* These include moist heat packs, continuous ultrasound, and warm whirlpools. Thermal modalities generally involve the transfer of thermal energy. Five types of heat transfer exist:

1. *Convection* occurs when a liquid or gas moves past a body part. An example of this type of heat transfer is a therapeutic whirlpool.

2. *Evaporation* occurs when there is a change in state of a liquid to a gas and a resultant cooling takes place. An example of this type of heat transfer occurs during spray and stretch techniques.

3. *Conversion* occurs when one form of energy is converted into another form. Examples of this type of heat transfer include ultrasound, long and shortwave diathermy.

4. *Radiation* occurs when there is a transmission and absorption of electromagnetic waves. Examples include magnetic field therapy, microwave diathermy and infrared ray therapy.

5. *Conduction* occurs when heat is transferred between two objects that are in contact with each other. An example of this type of heat transfer occurs with hydrocollator heating packs.

Thermotherapy is used in the later stages of healing, because the deep heating of structures during the acute inflammatory stage may destroy collagen fibers and accelerate the inflammatory process.[21] However, in the later stages of healing, an increase in blood flow to the injured area is beneficial.

The physiologic effects of a local heat application include the following[22–26]:

■ *Dissipation of body heat.* This effect occurs through selective vasodilation and shunting of blood via reflexes in the microcirculation and regional blood flow.[27]

■ *Decreased muscle spasm.*[27–30] The muscle relaxation probably results from a decrease in neural excitability on the sensory nerves, and hence gamma input.

■ *Increased capillary permeability*, cell metabolism, and cellular activity, which have the potential to increase the delivery of oxygen and chemical nutrients to the area, while decreasing venous stagnation.[23,31]

■ Increased analgesia through hyperstimulation of the cutaneous nerve receptors.

■ *Increased tissue extensibility.*[27] This effect has obvious implications for the application of stretching techniques. The best results are obtained if heat is applied during the stretch and if the stretch is maintained until cooling occurs after the heat has been removed.

CLINICAL PEARL

For a heat application to have a therapeutic effect, the amount of thermal energy transferred to the tissue must be sufficient to stimulate normal function, without causing damage to the tissue.[32]

▶ *Cryotherapy.* These include cold packs and ice massage. The use of ice, or cryotherapy, by itself[33] or in conjunction with compression,[34–37] has been demonstrated to be effective in minimizing the amount of exudate. Cryotherapy, which removes heat from the body, thereby decreasing the temperature of the body tissues, is the most commonly used modality for the intervention of acute musculoskeletal injuries.[38–61] Hocutt and colleagues[34] demonstrated that cryotherapy started within 36 hours of injury was statistically better than heat for complete and rapid recovery. Patients using cryotherapy within 36 hours of injury reached full activity in an average of 13.2 days compared with an average 30.4 days for those initiating cryotherapy more than 36 hours after injury. Individuals who used heat required 33.3 days for return to full activity.[34]

The physiologic effects of a local cold application are principally the result of vasoconstriction, reduced metabolic function,[62] and reduced motor and sensory conduction velocities.[63,64] These effects include the following:

■ *A decrease in muscle and intra-articular temperature.* This decrease in muscle temperature[65] and intra-articular structures[66–68] occurs because of a decrease in local blood flow[57,59,61,69,70] and appears to be most marked between the temperatures of 40°C and 25°C.[71] Temperatures below 25°C, which typically occur after 30 minutes of cooling therapy, actually result in an increase in blood flow,[71] with a consequent detrimental increase in hemorrhage and an exaggerated acute inflammatory response.[64] The decrease in muscle and intra-articular temperature is maintained for several hours after removal of the cooling agent.[72] A prolonged application of cold, however, can result in a sympathetically mediated reflex vasodilation in an attempt to rewarm the area, which may actually worsen the swelling.[72,73]

■ *Local analgesia.*[30,33,38–42] The four stages of analgesia achieved by cryotherapy are, in order of appearance, cold sensation, burning or aching, local analgesia, and then deep tissue vasodilation.[34] It is worth remembering that the timing of the stages depends on the depth of penetration and varying thickness of adipose tissue.[43] The patient should be advised as to these various stages, especially in light of the fact that the burning or aching phase occurs before the therapeutic phases.

- *Decreased muscle spasm.*[36,38,44-46]
- *Decrease in swelling.*[38,47,48]
- *Decrease in nerve conduction velocity.*[49]

▸ *Manual therapy.* Manual therapy techniques can range from simple massage to specific joint mobilizations. MT techniques have traditionally been used to produce a number of therapeutic alterations in pain and soft-tissue extensibility through the application of specific external forces.[50-53] Although it is generally agreed that manual techniques are beneficial for specific impairments, such as a restricted joint glide and adaptively shortened connective tissue, there is less agreement on which technique is the most effective. The decision about which approach or technique to use has traditionally been based on the clinician's belief, level of expertise, and decision-making processes.

CLINICAL PEARL

There are numerous concerns with determining the validity of studies addressing the efficacy of manual techniques:

▸ The selection of a particular technique is typically made on an ad hoc basis.

▸ A strong placebo effect is associated with the laying on of hands.

▸ Many musculoskeletal conditions are self-limiting so that patients may improve with time regardless of the intervention.

▸ It is difficult to blind clinicians and subjects to the intervention the subjects are receiving.

▸ Clear-cut definitions as to when one technique is more efficacious than another are lacking.

▸ Overreliance on MT techniques to improve a patient's status is a passive approach in an era when patient independence is stressed.

▸ *Exercise.* The hierarchy of exercise includes passive range of motion (PROM), active assisted range of motion (AAROM), active range of motion (AROM), and resisted exercises. To help relieve pain, PROM and AAROM exercises are typically used.

▸ *Patient education.* Patients can be educated on pain management techniques (relaxation, cognitive behavioral approaches, and biofeedback), positions and activities to avoid, and positions and activities to adopt.

Physical Therapy Impact—Malalignment

The focus of a therapeutic intervention for posture and movement impairment syndromes is to alleviate symptoms and to play a significant role in educating the patient against habitual abuse. Interestingly, despite the widespread inclusion of postural correction in therapeutic interventions, there are limited experimental data to support its effectiveness. Therapeutic exercise programs for the correction of muscle imbalances traditionally focus on regaining the normal length of a muscle, so that good movement patterns can be achieved. The intervention of any muscle imbalance is divided into three stages:

1. *Restoration of normal length of the muscles.* If the muscle activity is inhibited, the muscle should be stretched in the inhibitory phase. If the muscle is hypertonic, muscle energy techniques may be used to produce minimal facilitation and a minimal stretch. With true adaptive shortening of the muscle, stronger resistance is used to activate the maximum number of motor units, followed by vigorous stretching of the muscle.

2. *Strengthening of the muscles that have become inhibited and weak.* Vigorous strengthening should be initially avoided to prevent substitutions and the reinforcement of poor patterns of movement.

3. *Establishing optimal motor patterns to secure the best possible protection to the joints and the surrounding soft tissues.*

In addition to using specific techniques to stretch and strengthen muscles, muscle energy, proprioceptive neuromuscular facilitation (PNF), and the incorporation of a more "wholistic" approach can often have a beneficial effect on postural dysfunction and movement impairment.

CLINICAL PEARL

Proprioceptive neuromuscular facilitation (PNF), a manual technique that promotes the response of the neuromuscular mechanism through stimulation of the proprioceptor, was developed at the Kabat Kaiser Institute by Herman Kabat and Margaret Knott during the late 1940s and early 1950s.[54] Initially, the approach was developed as a method of treatment for muscles that were neurologically weak because of anterior poliomyelitis. The techniques were later expanded for use in general muscle strengthening, joint mobilizations, and the stretching of adaptively shortened muscles.[55]

There is a growing interest in the field of integrative care—the blending of complementary or *wholistic* therapies with conventional medical practice. Wholistic approaches provide whole-person care—addressing people rather than diseases, caring rather than curing, using all possible therapeutic modalities rather than a limited few, and empowering patients wherever possible to use self-care approaches and to be active participants in decisions regarding their health.

Examples of these wholistic approaches, currently used in association with physical therapy, include the Alexander technique, Feldenkrais method, Trager psychophysical integration (TPI), Pilates, tai chi chuan (TCC), and yoga.

Physical Therapy Impact—Muscle Performance

Before initiating an exercise program, it is necessary to conduct a needs analysis to evaluate the physical requirements and physical attributes of the patient. Determining the selection of exercise is dependent on the goals and objectives and the needs analysis. As with prescriptions for medications, a successful exercise prescription requires the correct balance between the dose (exercise variables) and the response (specific health or fitness adaptations).[56] The *dosage* of an exercise refers to each particular patient's exercise capability and is determined by a number of variables (Table 7-2).[57] For these

TABLE 7-2	Resistive Exercise Variables
Resistance (load or weight)	
Duration	
Training frequency (weekly, daily)	
Point of application	
Bouts (timed sessions of exercise)	
Sets and repetitions	
Training volume	
Mode (type of contraction)	
Rests	

TABLE 7-3	Possible Benefits of a Warmup before Physical Activity
Increased blood flow to muscles	
Increased oxyhemoglobin breakdown, with increased oxygen delivery to muscles	
Increased circulation leading to decreased vascular resistance	
Increased release of oxygen from myoglobin	
Enhanced cellular metabolism	
Reduced muscle viscosity leading to smoother muscle contraction and increased mechanical efficiency	
Increased speed of nerve impulses	
Increased sensitivity of nerve receptors	
Decreased activity of alpha fibers and sensitivity of muscles to stretch	
Decreased number of injuries due to increased range of motion	
Decreased stiffness of connective tissue leading to decreased likelihood of tears	
Increased cardiovascular response to sudden strenuous exercise	
Increased relaxation and concentration	

Data from Bahr R: Principles of injury prevention. In: Brukner P, Khan K (eds): Clinical Sports Medicine (ed 3). Sydney, McGraw-Hill, 2007, pp 78-101; Stewart IB, Sleivert GG: The effect of warm-up intensity on range of motion and anaerobic performance. J Orthop Sports Phys Ther 27:154-161, 1998; Rosenbaum D, Hennig EM: The influence of stretching and warm-up exercises on Achilles tendon reflex activity. J Sports Sci 13:481-490, 1995; Green JP, Grenier SG, McGill SM: Low-back stiffness is altered with warm-up and bench rest: Implications for athletes. Med Sci Sports Exerc 34:1076-1081, 2002.

variables to be effective, the patient must be compliant and be able to train without exacerbating the condition.[58] Depending on the specific program design, resistance training is known to enhance muscular strength, power, or endurance and can provide a potent stimulus to the neuromuscular system. Other variables such as speed, balance, coordination, jumping ability, flexibility, and other measures of motor performance have also been positively enhanced by resistance training.[59] It is worth remembering that when the individual trains for two different types of adaptations (e.g., aerobic fitness and strength), the training stimuli can interfere with one another and result in less improvement in one or both of the effects. For example, when strength loads are combined with aerobic training, the aerobic adaptation is not detrimentally affected, but there is a negative impact on strength development.[60,61]

Each exercise session should include a 5- to 15-minute warmup and a 5- to 15-minute cooldown period.

▶ Warmup
  ▪ Includes low-intensity cardiorespiratory activities
  ▪ Prevents the heart and circulatory system from being suddenly overloaded and prepares the soft tissues and joints

▶ Cooldown
  ▪ Includes low-intensity cardiorespiratory activities and flexibility exercises
  ▪ Helps prevent abrupt physiologic alterations that can occur with sudden cessation of strenuous exercise

The type of exercise prescribed determines the type of warmup.[62] The possible benefits of a warmup before physical activity are listed in Table 7-3. The most effective warmup consists of both general (walking, biking, jogging, and gentle resistive exercises) and specific (movements that are appropriate for the particular activity to be undertaken) exercises.[62] The length of the warmup and cooldown sessions may need to be longer for deconditioned or older individuals.

Once the warmup is completed, it is recommended that a flexibility program be incorporated to increase joint movement and muscle extensibility.

The initial exercise is prescribed at a level that the patient can perform, before progressing in difficulty. The early goals of exercise are concerned with increasing circulation, preventing atrophy, increasing protein synthesis, and reducing the level of metabolites.[58]

The following factors should be considered with exercise prescriptions.

▶ *Frequency.* Training frequency refers to the number of times exercise sessions are completed in a given period (e.g., the number of workouts per week). Optimal training frequency depends on several factors such as experience, training volume and status, intensity (see later), exercise selection, level of conditioning, recovery ability, and the number of muscle groups trained per workout session.

▶ *Repetitions.* Initial selection of a starting resistance may require some trial and error to find the correct number of repetitions. For any given exercise, the amount of resistance selected should be sufficient to allow 3 to 9 repetitions per exercise for three sets with a recovery period between sets of 60 to 90 seconds. The American College of Sports Medicine recommends 8 to 12 repetitions per set to elicit improvements in muscular strength and endurance as well as muscle hypertrophy.[63]

▶ *Duration.* Duration refers to the length of the exercise session. Physical conditioning occurs over a period of 15 to 60 minutes depending on the level of intensity. Average conditioning time is 20 to 30 minutes for moderate-intensity exercise. However, individuals who are severely compromised are more likely to benefit from a series of short exercise sessions (3 to 10 minutes) spaced throughout the day.

▶ *Rest periods.* In most functional exercises, fatigue of the muscle being exercised is the goal. However, fatigue may also occur because of lack of coordination, insufficient balance, poor motivation, or the addition of compensatory movements. In addition, fatigue may also be associated with specific clinical diseases, such as multiple sclerosis, cardiac disease, peripheral vascular dysfunction, and pulmonary diseases. Because fatigue is detrimental to performance, rest is an important component of any exercise progression. The rest period must be sufficient to allow for muscular recuperation and development while alleviating the potential for overtraining.[64] In general, the heavier the loads lifted, the longer the rest period between sets. The rest period between sets can be determined by the time the breathing rate, or pulse, of the patient returns to the steady state.

CLINICAL PEARL

One of the biggest challenges for a physical therapist is to find a balance between achieving a maximum training effect and alleviating fatigue. Fortunately, fatigue has a much faster decay time in the training effect. Thus, to remove the fatigue, the volume of training should be reduced while maintaining the training effect by holding the intensity of the training load constant.[65]

▶ *Intensity.* Intensity refers to the power output (rate of performing work) or how much effort is required to perform the exercise. In clinical terms, intensity refers to the weight or resistance lifted by the patient. It is now recognized that an individual's perception of effort (relative perceived exertion or RPE) is closely related to the level of physiologic effort.[66,67] The Borg Scale is commonly used to help determine a patient's rate of perceived exertion (RPE), as an individual's perception of effort (relative perceived exertion) is closely related to the level of physiologic effort—a high correlation exists between a person's RPE multiplied by 10, and their actual heart rate.[66,67] For example, if a person's RPE is 15, then $15 \times 10 = 150$; so the heart rate should be approximately 150 beats per minute. A cardiorespiratory training effect can be achieved at a rating of "somewhat hard" or "hard" (13 to 16). Note that this calculation is only an approximation of heart rate, and the actual heart rate can vary quite a bit depending on age and physical condition. The original scale introduced by Borg[67] rated exertion on a scale of 6 to 20, but a more recent one designed by Borg included a category (C) ratio (R) scale, the Borg CR10 Scale (Table 7-4).

TABLE 7-4	Rating of Perceived Exertion	
Traditional Scale	Verbal Rating	Revised 10-Grade Scale
6	No exertion at all	0
7	Very, very light	0.5
8		
9	Very light	1.0
10		
11	Light	
12	Fairly light	2.0
13	Moderate	3.0
14	Somewhat hard	4.0
15	Hard (heavy)	5.0
16		6.0
17	Very hard	7.0
18		8.0
19	Very, very (extremely) hard	9.0
20	Maximal (exhaustion)	10.0

Data from Borg GAV: Psychophysical basis of perceived exertion. Med Sci Sports Exerc 14:377–381, 1992; Borg's Perceived Exertion and Pain Scales. Champaign, IL: Human Kinetics; 1998.

▶ *Speed of exercise.* The speed of the exercise should depend on the imposed demands of an individual. In some cases, increasing the speed of an exercise following the initial phase of learning a particular exercise and developing proficiency in the performance of the exercise is beneficial.[68] In addition, higher-velocity training appears to improve peak power measures.[59]

▶ *Variation.* Variation in training is a fundamental principle that supports the need for alterations in one or more program variables over time to allow for the training stimulus to remain optimal (Table 7-5).[59] The concept of variation has been rooted in program design universally for many years. The most commonly examined resistance training theory is periodization. Periodization is the systematic process of planned variations in a resistance-training program over a specified training cycle to prevent overtraining and to perform at peak or optimum levels at the right time.[69]

Physical Therapy Impact—ROM and Flexibility

A variety of stretching techniques can be used to increase the extensibility of the soft tissues.

TABLE 7-5	Types of Training That Incorporate Variation
Circuit training	Circuit training or cross-training incorporates a wide variety of modes of training and uses high repetitions and low weight to provide a more general conditioning program aimed at improving body composition, muscular strength, and cardiovascular fitness.
Interval training	Interval training includes an exercise period followed by a prescribed rest interval. It is perceived to be less demanding than continuous training and tends to improve strength and power more than endurance.
	With appropriate spacing of work and rest intervals, a significant amount of high-intensity work can be achieved and is greater than the amount of work accomplished with continuous training.
	The longer the work interval, the more the anaerobic system is stressed. The duration of the rest period is not important.
	In a short work interval, a work recovery ratio of 1:1 or 1:5 is appropriate to stress the aerobic system.

TABLE 7-6	Static Stretching Guidelines

Heat should be applied to increase intramuscular temperature prior to, and during, stretching. This heat can be achieved with either through low-intensity warm-up exercise, or through the use of thermal modalities. The application of a cold pack following the stretch is used to take advantage of the thermal characteristics of connective tissue, by lowering its temperature and thereby theoretically prolonging the length changes—the elasticity of a muscle diminishes with cooling.

Effective stretching, in the early phase, should be performed every hour, but with each session lasting only a few minutes.

With true muscle shortness, stronger resistance is used to activate the maximum number of motor units, followed by vigorous stretching of the muscle.

Stretching should be performed at least three times a week using:

- ▶ Low force, avoiding pain
- ▶ Prolonged duration
- ▶ Rapid cooling of the muscle while it is maintained in the stretched position

Data from Assmussen E, Bonde-Peterson F: Storage of elastic energy in skeletal muscle in man. Acta Physiol Scand 91:385-392, 1974; Bosco C, Komi PV: Potentiation of the mechanical behavior of the human skeletal muscle through prestretching. Acta Physiol Scand 106:467-472, 1979; Cavagna GA, Saibene FP, Margaria R: Effect of negative work on the amount of positive work performed by an isolated muscle. J Appl Physiol 20:157, 1965; Cavagna GA, Disman B, Margarai R: Positive work done by a previously stretched muscle. J Appl Physiol 24:21-32, 1968.

Static Stretching. Static stretching involves the application of a steady force for a sustained period (Table 7-6). The stretch should be performed at the point just shy of the pain, although some discomfort may be necessary to achieve results.[70] Small loads applied for long periods produce greater residual lengthening than heavy loads applied for short periods.[71] Weighted traction or pulley systems may be used for this type of stretching. It is important for the patient to realize that the initial session of stretching may increase symptoms.[72] However, this increase in symptoms should be temporary, lasting for a couple of hours at most.[73,74]

Dynamic Stretching. Dynamic stretching involves stretching using joint motions to increase or decrease the joint angle where the muscle crosses, thereby elongating the musculotendinous unit as the end ROM is obtained.[75] Dynamic stretching is a specific warmup using activity-specific movements to prepare the muscles by taking them through the movements used in a particular sport.[75] Dynamic stretching does not incorporate end-range ballistic movements but rather controlled movements through a normal range of motion.[75]

There is some debate as to whether the static or dynamic method is better to stretch a muscle. Static stretching is considered the gold standard in flexibility training.[76] However, recent studies have found that static stretching is not an effective way to reduce injury rates[77,78] and may actually inhibit athletic performance.[79] This is likely because the nature of static stretching is passive and does nothing to warm a muscle.[80] More dynamic methods of stretching involve either a contraction of the antagonist muscle group, thus allowing the agonist to elongate naturally in a relaxed state, or eccentrically training a muscle through a full range of motion.[76] The latter method would appear to address the problem that most injuries occur in the eccentric phase of activity.[77] A study by Nelson[76] that compared the immediate effect of static stretching, eccentric training, and no stretching/training on hamstring flexibility in high school and college athletes (75 subjects) found the flexibility gains in the eccentric training group to be significantly greater than in the static stretch group.

Proprioceptive Neuromuscular Facilitation. The PNF techniques of contract-relax (CR), an agonist contraction

(AC), or a contract-relax-agonist contraction sequence (CRAC) can be used to actively stretch soft tissues[81]:

- ▶ *Contract-relax.* CR stretching begins, as does static stretching, in that the clinician supports the patient and brings the limb to the end of range of motion until gentle stretching is felt. At that point, the clinician asks the patient to provide an isometric contraction of the muscle being stretched (the antagonist) for approximately 2 to 5 seconds, after which the patient is asked to relax the muscle. The clinician moves the limb passively into the new range until a limitation is again felt and repeats the procedure two to four times.

- ▶ *Agonist contraction.* AC stretching uses the principle of reciprocal inhibition. The clinician moves the limb to the position of gentle stretch and asks the patient for a contraction of the muscle opposite the muscle being stretched (the antagonist). For example, when stretching the hamstring muscles, a simultaneous contraction of the quadriceps muscles can facilitate the stretch of the hamstrings. The contraction is held for 2 to 5 seconds, and the technique is repeated two to four times.

- ▶ *Contract-relax-agonist contraction.* This technique combines the CR and AC stretches. The clinician takes the limb to the point of gentle stretch and performs a CR sequence (i.e., resistance applied against the muscle being stretched). After contracting the muscle being stretched, the patient is asked to relax this muscle while contracting the opposing muscle group (antagonist), thus facilitating the stretch. For example, when stretching the hamstring muscles, the hamstrings are brought to a position stretch, the hamstrings are contracted against resistance and then relaxed, and the quadriceps are contracted.

The majority of studies have shown the PNF techniques to be the most effective for increasing ROM through muscle lengthening when compared to the static or slow sustained and the ballistic or bounce techniques,[82–86] although one study found them to be not necessarily better.[87]

Other techniques that can assist in lengthening of contractile tissue through relaxation include the following:

- The application of heat, which increases the extensibility of the shortened tissues, will allow the muscles to relax and lengthen more easily, reducing the discomfort of stretching. Heat without stretching has little or no effect on long-term improvement in muscle flexibility, whereas the combination of heat and stretching produces greater long-term gains in tissue length than stretching alone.
- Massage, which increases local circulation to the muscle and reduces muscle spasm and stiffness.
- Biofeedback, which teaches the patient to reduce the amount of tension in a muscle.

Ballistic Stretching. This technique of stretching uses bouncing movements to stretch a particular muscle. The muscle is stretched by momentum created from the bouncing movement of the body supplying the tensile force used for the stretch.[75] The patient quickly relaxes the muscle when reaching the end of range of motion. This is performed in a cyclical bouncing motion and repeated several times, thus engaging the neurologic component called active resistance—the contraction of muscles that resist elongation in the form of muscle reflex activity.[75,88] In comparisons of the ballistic and static methods, two studies[89,90] have found that both produce similar improvements in flexibility. However, the ballistic method appears to cause more residual muscle soreness or muscle strain than do techniques that incorporate relaxation.[91–93]

Further research is needed to determine the appropriate type of stretching for long-lasting changes in flexibility. Researchers have reported that techniques using cyclic and sustained stretching for 15 minutes on five consecutive days increased hamstring muscle length, and that a significant percentage of the increased length was retained one week post-treatment.[94] Other researchers have reported that using four consecutive knee flexor static stretches of 30 seconds, the new knee ROM was maintained for three minutes but had returned to prestretch levels after six minutes.[95] A similar study using a sequence of five modified hold-relax stretches reported producing significantly increased hamstring flexibility that lasted six minutes after the stretching protocol ended.[96] The specific duration, frequency, and number of stretching repetitions vary in the literature. Evidence to date has shown that stretches are generally held anywhere from 10 to 60 seconds, with the research recommending that stretches be held between 15 and 30 seconds.[75,97,98] In contrast, little research has been conducted on the number of repetitions of a stretch in an exercise session, although it has been determined that 80% of the length changes occur in the first four stretches of 30 seconds each.[75,99] Current American College of Sports Medicine Guidelines recommend three to five repetitions for each stretching exercise.[100]

Physical Therapy Impact—Central Control

Central control (see Chapter 6) refers to the regulation of the neuromusculoskeletal system. Central control provides the ability to perform voluntary, purposeful, and skilled movements or functional activities. Without central control, an individual is vulnerable to a number of secondary complications. The goals of the physical therapy intervention for such an individual include[101]:

- *The prevention of secondary impairments:* proper positioning both in bed and in a chair/wheelchair is essential to prevent skin breakdown and contractures, improve pulmonary hygiene and circulation, and help modify muscle tone.[102,103] The patient should be turned every two hours when in bed.
- *Improving arousal through sensory stimulation:* multisensory stimulation involves the presentation of sensory stimulation in a highly structured and consistent manner.[101] The following sensory systems are systematically stimulated: auditory, olfactory, gustatory, visual, tactile, kinesthetic, and vestibular.[101]
- *Patient and family education:* to teach the family about the stages of recovery and what can be expected in the future.
- *Managing the effects of abnormal tone and spasticity:* a wide variety of methods are available to the therapist to treat the adverse effects of abnormal tone.
- *Early transition to sitting postures:* as soon as medically stable, the patient should be transferred to a sitting position and out of bed to wheelchair or chair. This transition may require the use of a tilt table.

Neuromuscular rehabilitation (NMR) is a method of training the enhancement of unconscious motor responses, by stimulating both the afferent signals and the central mechanisms responsible for dynamic joint control.[104] The aims of NMR are to improve the ability of the nervous system to generate a fast and optimal muscle-firing pattern, to increase joint stability, to decrease joint forces, and to relearn movement patterns and skills.[104] Before a neuromuscular training program is developed, the faulty movement pattern or absent motor skill must be identified.[105] In addition, before beginning a neuromuscular training program, individuals must have adequate muscle strength to perform training exercises correctly. If weaknesses are present, training activities must begin at a more baseline level that includes weight training, technique instruction, and performing single-plane versus multiplanar movements.[105]

Physical Therapy Impact—Aging

Although aging is inevitable, its consequences are not necessarily inevitable. Intervention strategies to prevent disability from immobility should include the following, while monitoring vital signs:

- Minimize duration of bed rest. Avoid strict bed rest unless absolutely necessary.
- Be aware of possible adverse effects of medications.
- Encourage the continuation of daily activities that the patient is able to perform as tolerated while avoiding overexertion.
  - Bathroom privileges or bedside commode
- Let patient stand 30 to 60 seconds during transfers (bed to chair).
- Encourage sitting up at a table for meals.
- Encourage getting dressed in street clothes each day.
- Encourage daily exercises as a basis of good care. Exercises should emphasize:
  - Balance and proprioception
  - Strength and endurance

- Coordination and equilibrium
- Aerobic capacity
- Posture

▶ Design possible ways to enhance mobility through the use of assistive devices (e.g., walking aids, wheelchairs) and making the home accessible.

▶ Ensure that a sufficient fluid intake is being maintained (1.5 to 2 liters fluid intake per day as possible), and adequate nutritional levels.

▶ Encourage socialization with family, friends, or caregivers.

▶ If the patient is bed-bound, maintain proper body alignment and change positions every few hours. Pressure padding and heel protectors may be used to provide comfort and prevent pressure sores. An assessment should be made of the following:

- Skin integrity
- Protective sensations
- Discriminatory sensations

PATIENT INVOLVEMENT

When designing a plan of care, it is important to consider the patient's stage of learning, the best approach in terms of the structure of the tasks, the type of practice to be used, and the type of feedback to be given.

CLINICAL PEARL

A patient cannot succeed in functional and recreational activities if his or her neuromuscular system is not prepared to meet the demands of the specific activities.[106]

Stages of Motor Learning

Fitts and Posner[107] described three stages of motor learning: cognitive, associative, and autonomous.

▶ *Cognitive:* this stage begins when the patient is first introduced to the motor task and is instructed on what to do. This stage requires great concentration, and performance is variable and filled with errors because the patient must determine the objective of the skill as well as the relational and environmental cues to control and regulate the movement. During this stage, the patient has a general idea of the movement required for the task but is not quite sure how to execute the task. In other words, the patient is concerned with what to do and how to do it. During this stage, the clinician should provide frequent and explicit positive feedback using a variety of forms of feedback (verbal, tactile, visual), and allow trial and error to occur within safe limits. During this stage, the patient often requires lots of assistance and may need to verbalize components of the task before performing it.

▶ *Associative:* during this stage, the patient is less concerned about every detail of the task but is more concerned on

how to do it. There is greater consistency with performance and fewer errors and conscious decisions about what to do become more automatic and less rushed. During this phase, the clinician should begin to increase the complexity of the task and should emphasize problem solving and learning from errors through internal feedback. Learning from errors is thought to promote generalization to similar motor tasks. In general the clinician gives less visual feedback and only moderate assistance.

▶ *Autonomous:* the focus of this stage is how to perform the task well and is thus characterized by an efficient and nearly automatic kind of performance. At this stage, the motor skill has been learned and little cognitive effort is required to execute it, such that a motor skill can be performed while engaging in another task. For example, a patient is able to walk and talk without conscious thought. During this phase, the clinician should set up a series of progressively more difficult activities the patient can do independently, such as increasing the speed, distance, and complexity of the task.

CLINICAL PEARL

Most patients in rehabilitation are often in the associative stage because they are familiar with the skills they need to perform. The movement for a particular skill may be altered and need to be learned because of neuromuscular dysfunction.[105]

Litzinger and Osif[108] organized individuals into four main types of learners, based on instructional strategies:

1. *Accommodators.* This type looks for the significance of the learning experience. These learners enjoy being active participants in their learning and will ask many questions, such as, "What if?" and "Why not?"

2. *Divergers.* This type is motivated to discover the relevancy of a given situation and prefers to have information presented in a detailed, systematic, and reasoned manner.

3. *Assimilators.* This type is motivated to answer the question, "What is there to know?" These learners like accurate, organized delivery of information, and they tend to respect the knowledge of the expert. They are perhaps less instructor intensive than some other types of learners and will carefully follow prescribed exercises, provided a resource person is clearly available and able to answer questions.

4. *Convergers.* This type is motivated to discover the relevancy, or "how," of a situation. The instructions given to this type of learner should be interactive, not passive.

Another way of classifying learners that is frequently used incorporates three common learning styles:

1. *Visual.* As the name suggests, the visual learner assimilates information by observation, using visual cues and information such as pictures, anatomic models, and physical demonstrations. Written materials can be used to provide detailed information but are made more user friendly with the inclusion of diagrams and illustrations.

2. *Auditory.* Auditory learners prefer to learn by having things explained to them verbally. When providing verbal instructions, it is important to choose the vocabulary that is appropriate for the patient. The use of layman's terms are often preferable to using medical vocabulary.

3. *Tactile.* Tactile learners, who learn through touch and interaction, are the most difficult of the three groups to teach. Close supervision is required with this group until they have demonstrated to the clinician that they can perform the exercises correctly and independently. PNF techniques, with their emphasis on physical and tactile cues, often work well with this group.

A patient's learning style can be identified by asking how he or she prefers to learn. For example, some patients will prefer a simple handout with pictures and instructions; others will prefer to see the exercises demonstrated and then be supervised while they perform the exercises. Some may want to know why they are doing the exercises, which muscles are involved, why they are doing three sets of a particular exercise, and so on. Others will require less explanation. Whatever method is preferred, it is important that the clinician provide the information at a pace that the patient can digest. The most critical information should be provided first.

If the clinician is unsure about the patient's learning style, it is recommended that each exercise first be demonstrated by the clinician, and then by the patient. The rationale and purpose behind each of the exercises must be given, as well as the frequency and intensity expected. Feedback is a critical component of learning (see Feedback), as is patient adherence to the program (see Chapter 5).

Task Structure

As outlined in Chapter 4, motor learning is contingent on the type of task to be learned and can be categorized as discrete, continuous, or serial[109,110]:

▶ *Discrete:* involves a task with a recognizable beginning and end—for example, throwing a ball, or opening a door.

▶ *Serial:* involves a series of discrete movements that are combined in a particular sequence—for example, getting dressed.

▶ *Continuous:* involves repetitive, uninterrupted movements that have no distinct beginning and ending. Examples include walking and cycling.

Tasks can also be classified as open versus closed. An open skill involves temporal and spatial factors in an unpredictable environment. A closed skill also involves spatial factors, but only in a predictable environment. Using sports as an example, a closed skill could include shooting a foul shot in basketball. An everyday example of a closed skill is drinking from a cup. An example of an open skill in everyday life would be stepping onto a moving walkway, whereas in sports an open skill would involve throwing a touchdown pass. Whereas closed skills allow an individual to evaluate the environment and perform the movement without much modification, open skills require more cognitive processing and decision making in choosing and adjusting the movement.[105] Open and closed skills can be viewed as a one-dimensional continuum,

where the perceptual and habitual nature of a task determines how closed or open a task is.

Gentile[111] expanded the popular one-dimensional classification system of open and closed skills to combine an environmental context with the function of the action[110,112]:

▶ The environmental (closed or open) context in which the task is performed. Regulatory conditions (other people, objects) in the environment may be either stationary (closed skills) or in motion (open skills).

▶ The intertrial variability (absent or present) of the environment that is imposed on the task. When the environment in which a task is set is unchanging from one performance of a task to the next, intertrial variability is absent—the environmental conditions are predictable. For example, walking on a flat surface involves predictable environmental conditions. Intertrial variability is present when the demands change from one attempt or repetition of the task to the next. For example, walking over varying terrain involves unpredictable environmental conditions.

▶ The need for a person's body to remain stationary (stable) or to move (transport) during the task. Skills that require body transport are more complex than skills that require no body transport, as there are more variables to consider. For example, a body transport task could include walking in a crowded shopping mall.

▶ The presence or absence of manipulation of objects during the task. When a person must manipulate an object, the skill increases in complexity because the person must do two things at once—manipulate the object correctly, and adjust the body posture to fit the efficient movement of the object.

Practice

Practice, repeatedly performing a movement or series of movements in a task, is probably the single most important variable in learning a motor skill.[110,112] The rate of improvement during any part of practice is linearly related on a logarithmic scale to the amount left to improve.[109] This means that in the early phases of practice of a new task, performance improves rapidly, whereas after much practice, it improves more slowly. The various types of practice conditions for motor learning are as follows[110]:

▶ Part versus whole practicing involves breaking a task down into interim steps before attempting the whole task.

■ *Part practice.* A task is broken down into separate components, and the individual components (usually the more difficult ones) are practiced. After mastery of the individual components, the components are combined in a sequence so that the whole task can be practiced. Although learning parts of a task may be helpful during early stages of learning, this approach does not facilitate learning the skill in the context in which it will be used.[113,114]

- *Whole practice.* The entire task is performed from beginning to end and is not practiced in separate components. Research has shown that part versus whole training results in different kinematic profiles, with better movement quality obtained in whole-task practice conditions.[115]

▶ Blocked versus random.

- *Blocked.* The same task, or series of tasks, is performed repeatedly under the same conditions and in a predictable order. For example, a patient could practice walking in a straight line along a flat surface.

- *Random.* Variations of the same task are performed in random order. For example, a patient could practice walking on a variety of walking surfaces and in different directions. Random practice offers greater retention and transfer of skills.

▶ Massed versus distributed.

- *Massed.* Involves participation in a long bout of practice, where substantially less time is spent in rest compared to time spent practicing during the practice period. The disadvantages of this type of practice are that there is more potential for fatigue and an increased likelihood of a slight detriment for learning.[109]

- *Distributed.* This type of practice, in which the amount of rest between trials is equal to or greater than the amount of time for a trial, involves participation in a series of practices throughout the day. The advantage of this type of practice is that the patient is able to reflect on his or her performance between practices. Distributed practice is considered superior to massed practice in contributing to motor learning.

Feedback

Second only to practice, feedback is considered the next most important variable that influences learning. The various types of feedback associated with motor learning are as follows[110]:

▶ Intrinsic versus extrinsic (augmented).

- *Intrinsic.* Intrinsic feedback is a natural part of a task.[109] It can take the form of a sensory cue (proprioceptive, kinesthetic, tactile, visual, or auditory), or set of cues, inherent in the execution of the motor task. The feedback arises from within the learner and is derived from performance of the task. This type of feedback may immediately follow completion of a task, or may occur even before the task has been completed. This type of feedback is not under conscious control, but the clinician can facilitate it by structuring the task and environment to support effective movement patterns.

- *Extrinsic.* Extrinsic feedback is supplemental feedback that is not normally an inherent part of the task. This

type of feedback can include sensory cues from an external source (verbal, visual, or auditory). Unlike intrinsic feedback, the clinician can control the type, timing, and frequency of extrinsic feedback.

Feedback about performance can be provided at a variety of times:

▶ Continuous versus intermittent.

- *Continuous:* is ongoing. This type of feedback improves skill acquisition more quickly during the initial stage of learning than intermittent feedback.

- *Intermittent:* occurs irregularly and randomly. Intermittent feedback has been shown to promote learning more effectively than continuous feedback.

▶ Immediate, delayed, and summary.

- *Immediate:* is given directly after a task is completed. This type of feedback is used most frequently during the cognitive (initial) stage of learning.

- *Delayed:* is given after an interval of time elapses, allowing the learner to reflect on how well or poorly a task was done. This type of feedback promotes retention and the generalization of the learned skills.

- *Summary:* is given about the average performance of several repetitions of the movement or task. This type of feedback is used most frequently during the associative stage of learning.

Two other points, related to feedback and motor learning, are knowledge of results (KR) and knowledge of performance (KP):

▶ *KR:* immediate, posttask, extrinsic feedback about the outcome of a motor task. This type of feedback is primarily reserved for instances when individuals are unable to generate this type of information for themselves, or when the information may serve as a motivational tool.[109]

▶ *KP:* feedback given about the nature or quality of the performance of the motor task. This type of feedback better facilitates motor skill learning than KR.

CLINICAL PEARL

Based on the motor control and learning principles outlined in Chapter 4, the chosen therapeutic activities should have the following characteristics:

▶ Variability, to enhance learning transferability.

▶ A schedule and structure of practice that enhances the patient's active participation while considering motor control and learning principles.

▶ An environmental setup that includes all of the factors that might regulate a specific task practice

▶ The availability of appropriate feedback (in terms of timing and amount) to enhance the motor learning or relearning processes.

The use of the above requires knowledge and skills of task analysis of the necessary targeted activities to be performed.[116]

MEASUREMENT OF FUNCTIONAL OUTCOMES

Outcomes measurement is a process that describes a systematic method to gauge the effectiveness and efficiency of an intervention in daily clinical practice.[117] Effectiveness in this context refers to the outcome of an intervention during the rigors of ordinary and customary care delivery.[117] The efficiency of an intervention is a factor of utilization (number of outpatient visits, length of inpatient stay) with the costs of care and outcome. The trend in using outcome measures in the decision-making process is consistent with evidence-informed practice and represents the final step in the evaluation of clinical performance.[118] The clinician should be able to evaluate and choose the appropriate outcome measure for a specific patient population, because the caliber of information that an outcome measurement provides is a function of the sophistication, predictability, and accuracy of the tools or instruments used.[119] Sensitivity and specificity are used to describe the accuracy of diagnostic tests (see Chapter 3). Sensitivity is the ability of the test to pick up what it is testing for, and specificity is the ability of the test to reject what it is not testing for.

CLINICAL PEARL

▶ Sensitivity represents the proportion of patients with a disorder who test positive. A test that can correctly identify every person who has the disorder has a sensitivity of 1.0. *SnNout* is an acronym for when *sensitivity* of a symptom or sign is high, a *negative* response rules *out* the target disorder. Thus, a so-called highly sensitive test helps rule out a disorder. The positive predictive value is the proportion of patients with positive test results who are correctly diagnosed.

▶ Specificity is the proportion of the study population without the disorder that test negative.[120] A test that can correctly identify every person who does not have the target disorder has a specificity of 1.0. *SpPin* is an acronym for when *specificity* is extremely high, a *positive* test result rules *in* the target disorder. Thus, a so-called highly specific test helps rule in a disorder or condition. The negative predictive value is the proportion of patients with negative test results who are correctly diagnosed.

Measurement instruments must be able to detect change when it has occurred and to remain stable when change has not occurred.[121] The more sophisticated, predictable, and accurate the measurement tool, the less chance there is for errors in measurement that make it difficult to ascertain whether true progress has occurred. In an effort to counteract the potential for these measurement errors, the term minimal detectable change has been introduced. Minimum detectable change (MDC) is defined as the minimum amount of change that exceeds measurement error.[121] The MDC is a statistical measure of meaningful change and is related to an instrument's reliability.[121] Although various methods for calculating the MDC have been proposed, consensus has yet to be reached as to what is the optimal method.[122] Unfortunately, statistically significant change using the MDC may

not indicate that the change is clinically relevant. The minimum clinically important difference (MCID) is a measure of clinical relevance and indicates the amount of change in scale points that must occur before the change may be considered meaningful.[123] The sensitivity of the MCID is represented by the number of patients the outcome measure correctly identifies as having changed an important amount divided by all of the patients who truly changed an important amount.[124] The specificity of the MCID is represented by the number of patients the outcome measure correctly identifies as not having changed an important amount divided by all of the patients who truly did not change an important amount.[124] Although it is tempting to make the assumption that the minimum level of statistical change (MDC) would be less than or equal to the MCID, the relationship between the MDC and the MCID scores has yet to be determined.[123]

In addition to these clinical and statistical measures, the success of an intervention is based on the perspective of the stakeholder.[121,125] For example, to the patient, success may be considered as the relief of symptoms. To the payers of healthcare, a successful outcome is likely viewed as one that involved cost-efficient patient management.[121] Physical therapists tend to define good outcomes as the learning of long-term management strategies, relief of symptoms, and improved function.[125]

Part of the problem in designing a functional measurement tool is that function is highly individual, with multiple levels of difficulty and a high degree of specificity. The traditional outcome measurements have been divided into those that assess upper extremity function, those that assess lower extremity function, and those that measure the performance of basic and instrumental activities of daily living (BADLs and IADLs). Functional measurement tools for the upper extremity have involved an assessment of coordination and dexterity measurements, whereas functional measurements for the lower extremity have included the ability of the patient to perform sit-to-stand transfers, standing balance, ambulation, and stair negotiation. Some of the measurement tools that have been devised to assess the performance of BADLs and IADLs include:

▶ *Physical Performance Test (PPT).*[126] The PPT is a performance-based measure of both BADLs and IADLs that has been used to describe and monitor physical performance. The PPT takes about 10 minutes to administer. Scoring is based on the time taken to complete a series of usual daily tasks, such as writing a sentence, simulated eating, donning and doffing a jacket, turning 360° when standing, lifting a book, picking up a penny from the floor, and walking 50 feet.

▶ *Functional Status Questionnaire (FSQ).*[127] The FSQ is a self-report measure of physical, psychologic, and social role functions in patients who are ambulatory. The test takes about 15 minutes and has been found to have both construct and convergent reliability.[127]

▶ *Sickness Impact Profile (SIP).*[128] The SIP is a widely used health status measure. It measures both physical and psychosocial outcomes from the patient's perspective. The SIP is composed of 136 items that address the following areas: ambulation, mobility, body care and movement, social interaction, communication, alertness, emotional behavior, sleep and rest, eating, work, home management, and recreation and pastime activities. The SIP questionnaire has been extensively and successfully tested for its internal consistency, external validity, responsiveness to changes over time, and test-retest reliability in a wide range of clinical situations.[129]

▶ *The FIM+FAM* (Table 7-7). The Functional Independence Measure (FIM) is an 18-item, seven level ordinal scale intended to be sensitive to change in an individual over the course of a comprehensive inpatient medical rehabilitation program. The 12 items of the Functional Assessment Measure (FAM), not be confused with the Functional Rating Index,[130] were developed as an adjunct to the FIM to specifically address the major functional areas that are relatively less emphasized in the FIM, including measures of cognition, such as community integration, emotional status, orientation, attention, reading and writing skills, and employability.

The FIM+FAM scale was originally intended for patients with brain injury, but is useful in all rehabilitation settings.

▶ *Patient-Specific Functional Scale (PSFS)*[131] (Table 7-8). The PSFS is a patient-specific outcome measure, which investigates functional status by asking the patient to nominate activities that are difficult to perform based on his or her condition and rate the level of limitation with each activity.[132] The PSFS has been shown to be valid and responsive to change for patients with various clinical conditions, including knee pain,[133] low back pain,[131] neck pain,[134] and cervical radiculopathy.[132]

▶ *Short Musculoskeletal Function Assessment (SMFA)*[135] (Table 7-9). The SMFA consists of a 46-item questionnaire (see Table 7-9). The first 34 items refer to activities of daily living. The patient ranks his or her perceived difficulty or problems with these tasks to provide a *dysfunction index*.

TABLE 7-7   The FIM+FAM

Self-care	Sphincters	Mobility
1. Eating	1. Bladder management	1. Transfers: bed/chair/wheelchair
2. Grooming	2. Bowel management	2. Transfers: toilet
3. Bathing/showering		3. Transfers: bathtub/shower
4. Dressing upper body		4. Transfers: car*
5. Dressing lower body		5. Locomotion: walking/wheelchair
6. Toileting		6. Locomotion: stairs
7. Swallowing*		7. Community mobility*

Communication	Psychosocial	Cognition
1. Expression	1. Social interaction	1. Problem solving
2. Comprehension	2. Emotional status*	2. Memory
3. Reading*	3. Adjustment to limitations*	3. Orientation*
4. Writing*	4. Employability*	4. Attention*
5. Speech intelligibility*		5. Safety judgment*

*FAM items.

Seven levels for each item

Level Description

7 Complete independence. Fully independent
6 Modified independence. Requiring the use of a device but no physical help
5 Supervision. Requiring only standby assistance or verbal prompting or help with set-up
4 Minimal assistance. Requiring incidental hands-on help only (subject performs > 75% of the task)
3 Moderate assistance. Subject still performs 50–75% of the task
2 Maximal assistance. Subject provides less than half of the effort (25–49%)
1 Total assistance. Subject contributes < 25% of the effort or is unable to do the task.

▶ Do not leave any score blank.
▶ Score 1 if the subject does not perform the activity at all, or if no information is available.
▶ If function is variable, use the lower score

Data from: Dickson, H. G. and F. Kohler (1999). "Functional independence measure (FIM)." Scand J Rehabil Med. 31(1): 63–64;

Hamilton BB, Granger CV, Sherwin FS, et al. A uniform national data system for medical rehabilitation. In: Fuhrer MJ, editor. Rehabilitation Outcomes: analysis and measurement. Baltimore, MD: Brookes; 1987. pp. 137–47.

Stineman MG, Jette A, Fiedler R, et al. Impairment-specific dimensions within the Functional Independence Measure. Arch Phys Med Rehabil. 1997;78: 636–43.

Hall KM, Mann N, High WM, et al. Functional measures after traumatic brain injury: ceiling effects of FIM, FIM+FAM, DRS and CIQ. J Head Trauma Rehabil. 1996; 11: 27–39.

Turner-Stokes L, Nyein K, Turner-Stokes T, et al. The UK FIM+FAM: development and evaluation. Clin Rehabil. 1999; 13: 277–87.

TABLE 7-8	The Patient-Specific Functional Scale. This Useful Questionnaire Can Be Used to Quantify Activity Limitation and Measure Functional Outcome for Patients with any Orthopedic Condition.

Clinician to read and fill in below: Complete at the end of the history and prior to physical examination.

Initial Assessment:
I am going to ask you to identify up to three important activities that you are unable to do or are having difficultly with as a result of your problem. Today, are there any activities that you are unable to do or having difficulty with because of your problem? (Clinician: show scale to patient and have the patient rate each activity).

Follow-up Assessments:
When I assessed you on (state previous assessment date), you told me that you had difficulty with (read all activities from list at a time). Today, do you still have difficulty with: (read and have patient score each item in the list)?

Patient-specific activity scoring scheme (Point to one number):

0   1   2   3   4   5   6   7   8   9   10

Unable to perform activity

Able to perform activity at the same level as before injury or problem

(Date and Score)

Activity	Initial						
1.							
2.							
3.							
4.							
5.							
Additional							
Additional							

The 12 remaining items are ranked according to how much they bother the patient and provide the clinician with a *bother index*.

Although these tests measure some of the components of function, they are not multidimensional. For example, they do not always address the patient's value system or the patient's overall physical performance in his or her own environment. It is very difficult to extrapolate examination results from the clinical outcomes of pain, strength, and range of motion to specific and meaningful changes in function and quality of life.

It is now commonly agreed that a satisfactory outcome measure should include both subjective and objective measures of quality-of-life issues. *Health-related quality of life* (HRQOL) represents the total effect of individual and environmental factors on an individual's function and health status, including physical, mental, pain, function, and satisfaction. The term *health-related quality of life* is often used interchangeably with the terms *functional status*, *health status*, and *health outcomes*. The definitions of these terms however, might range from negatively valued aspects of life, such as death, to more positively valued aspects, such as social functioning or happiness.[136–142]

Traditionally HRQOL outcomes have been regarded as soft measures, as they have been perceived as subjective and easily influenced by a patient who exaggerates symptoms or disability. These patient influences are not limited to questionnaires, because mood, motivation, and other psychosocial issues can prejudice physiologic measurements such as range of motion, strength, and the ability to perform functional tasks.[143] There are three general psychometric criteria that should be established in HRQOL measures before they are endorsed: reliability, validity, and responsiveness (the ability of the questionnaire to detect clinically relevant changes or differences, which varies depending on the type of question in the patient population being evaluated).

Generic instruments have been designed in an attempt to evaluate HRQOL. The major advantage of generic instruments is that they deal with a variety of areas in any population regardless of the underlying disease.[143] The SF-36 is perhaps the most well-known of these generic tools:

▶ *36-Item Short-Form Health Survey (SF-36)*.[144] The SF-36 is a general measure of health status, using a self-report with eight subscales of health. The acute version of the test takes about 7 to 10 minutes to complete, is moderately easy to score, and asks questions about physical, social, emotional role, and physical role function; mental health; energy; pain; and general health perception. Previous research has shown that, compared with other

TABLE 7-9   Short Musculoskeletal Function Assessment (SMFA)

INSTRUCTIONS

We are interested in finding out how you are managing with your injury or arthritis this week. We would like to know about any problems you may be having with your daily activities because of your injury or arthritis.

   Please answer each question by putting a check in the box corresponding to the choice that best describes you.

   These questions are about how much difficulty you may be having *this week* with your daily activities because of your injury or arthritis.

	Not at All Difficult	A Little Difficult	Moderately Difficult	Very Difficult	Unable to Do
1. How difficult is it for you to get in or out of a low chair?	☐	☐	☐	☐	☐
2. How difficult is it for you to open medicine bottles or jars?	☐	☐	☐	☐	☐
3. How difficult is it for you to shop for groceries or other things?	☐	☐	☐	☐	☐
4. How difficult is it for you to climb stairs?	☐	☐	☐	☐	☐
5. How difficult is it for you to make a tight fist?	☐	☐	☐	☐	☐
6. How difficult is it for you to get in or out of the bathtub or shower?	☐	☐	☐	☐	☐
7. How difficult is it for you to get comfortable sleep?	☐	☐	☐	☐	☐
8. How difficult is it for you to bend or kneel down?	☐	☐	☐	☐	☐
9. How difficult is it for you to use buttons, snaps, hooks, or zippers?	☐	☐	☐	☐	☐
10. How difficult is it for you to cut your own fingernails?	☐	☐	☐	☐	☐
11. How difficult is it for you to dress yourself?	☐	☐	☐	☐	☐
12. How difficult is it for you to walk?	☐	☐	☐	☐	☐
13. How difficult is it for you to get moving after you have been sitting or lying down?	☐	☐	☐	☐	☐
14. How difficult is it for you to go out by yourself?	☐	☐	☐	☐	☐
15. How difficult is it for you to drive?	☐	☐	☐	☐	☐
16. How difficult is it for you to clean yourself after going to the bathroom?	☐	☐	☐	☐	☐
17. How difficult is it for you to turn knobs or levers (for example, to open doors or to roll down car windows)?	☐	☐	☐	☐	☐
18. How difficult is it for you to write or type?	☐	☐	☐	☐	☐
19. How difficult is it for you to pivot?	☐	☐	☐	☐	☐
20. How difficult is it for you to do your usual physical recreational activities, such as bicycling, jogging, or walking?	☐	☐	☐	☐	☐
21. How difficult is it for you to do your usual leisure activities, such as hobbies, crafts, gardening, card-playing, or going out with friends?	☐	☐	☐	☐	☐
22. How much difficulty are you having with sexual activity?	☐	☐	☐	☐	☐
23. How difficult is it for you to do *light* housework *or* yard work, such as dusting, washing dishes, or watering plants?	☐	☐	☐	☐	☐
24. How difficult is it for you to do *heavy* housework *or* yard work; such as washing floors, vacuuming, or mowing lawns?	☐	☐	☐	☐	☐
25. How difficult is it for you to do your usual work, such as a paid job, housework, or volunteer activities?	☐	☐	☐	☐	☐

The following questions ask how often you are experiencing problems *this week* because of your injury or arthritis.

	Not at All	A Little of the Time	Some of the Time	Most of the Time	All of the Time
26. How often do you walk with a limp?	☐	☐	☐	☐	☐
27. How often do you avoid using your painful limb(s) or back?	☐	☐	☐	☐	☐
28. How often does your leg lock or give way?	☐	☐	☐	☐	☐
29. How often do you have problems with concentration?	☐	☐	☐	☐	☐
30. How often does doing too much in one day affect what you do the next day?	☐	☐	☐	☐	☐
31. How often do you act irritable toward those around you (for example, snap at people, give sharp answers, or criticize easily)?	☐	☐	☐	☐	☐
32. How often are you tired?	☐	☐	☐	☐	☐
33. How often do you feel disabled?	☐	☐	☐	☐	☐
34. How often do you feel angry or frustrated that you have this injury or arthritis?	☐	☐	☐	☐	☐

These questions are about how much you are bothered by problems you are having *this week* because of your injury or arthritis.

	Not at All Bothered	A Little Bothered	Moderately Bothered	Very Bothered	Extremely Bothered
35. How much are you bothered by problems using your hands, arms, or legs?	☐	☐	☐	☐	☐
36. How much are you bothered by problems using your back?	☐	☐	☐	☐	☐
37. How much are you bothered by problems doing work around your home?	☐	☐	☐	☐	☐
38. How much are you bothered by problems with bathing, dressing, toileting, or other personal care?	☐	☐	☐	☐	☐
39. How much are you bothered by problems with sleep and rest?	☐	☐	☐	☐	☐
40. How much are you bothered by problems with leisure or recreational activities?	☐	☐	☐	☐	☐
41. How much are you bothered by problems with your friends, family, or other important people in your life?	☐	☐	☐	☐	☐
42. How much are you bothered by problems with thinking, concentrating, or remembering?	☐	☐	☐	☐	☐
43. How much are you bothered by problems adjusting or coping with your injury or arthritis?	☐	☐	☐	☐	☐
44. How much are you bothered by problems doing your usual work?	☐	☐	☐	☐	☐
45. How much are you bothered by problems with feeling dependent on others?	☐	☐	☐	☐	☐
46. How much are you bothered by problems with stiffness and pain?	☐	☐	☐	☐	☐

Data from Swiontkowski MF, Engelberg R, Martin DP, et al: Short musculoskeletal function assessment questionnaire: validity, reliability, and responsiveness. J Bone Joint Surg 81A:1256-1258, 1999.

generic instruments, the SF-36 is a reliable and valid generic measure of the health of patients.[145] Although this test is a good tool for overall function, it is not specific to functional problems at specific joints, and it is recommended that it be used in conjunction with tests that are specific to the patient's dysfunctional joint.[145]

Disease-specific measures are questionnaires that concentrate on a region of primary interest that is generally relevant to the patient and clinician.[143] As a result of this focus on a regional disease state, the likelihood of increased responsiveness is higher. Some examples of the primary focus of these instruments include populations (rheumatoid arthritis), symptoms (back pain), and function (activities of daily living).[143] The disadvantage of a disease-specific outcome is that general information is lost, and therefore, it is generally recommended that when evaluating patient outcomes, both a disease-specific and generic outcome measure should be used.[143]

Felce and Perry[139] have proposed a model of HRQL that integrates subjective and objective indicators, reflecting a broad range of life domains, through an individual ranking of the relative importance of each domain (Figure 7-1). These domains are physical well-being, material well-being, social well-being, development and activity, and emotional well-being. The Felce and Perry model[139] is designed to address the concern that objective data should not be interpreted without reference to personal autonomy, preferences, and concerns. It is critical that the outcome measures chosen by the physical therapist evaluate functional improvement as perceived by the patient.

Another example of a HQROL is Patrick's model of health promotion for people with disabilities,[136] which depicts four broad planes of outcome: total environment, opportunity, disabling process, and quality of life (Figure 7-2).

▶ *Total environment.* This plane includes the individual's biologic and genetic makeup, demographic characteristics (race, gender, age), lifestyle behaviors (smoking, exercise, diet, risk-taking), health and social care systems, and physical and social characteristics of the environment.

▶ *Opportunity.* This plane represents outcomes related to independent living, economic self-sufficiency, equality of rights or status, and full participation in community life. Opportunity represents the interaction between the total environment of the individual at his or her particular stage of life course, and the disabling process.

▶ *Disabling process.* This plane represents the theoretical progression from disease or injury to the restriction of activities. The disablement outcomes represented in this plane include disease or injury, impairment, functional limitation, and activity restriction or disability.

▶ *Quality of life.* This plane represents a distinct outcome that includes people's perceptions of their position in life in the context of their particular culture and value system and in relation to their personal goals, expectations, standards, and concerns.

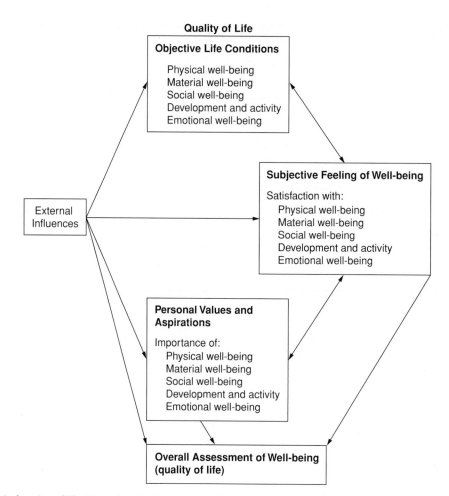

Quality of Life

Objective Life Conditions

Physical well-being
Material well-being
Social well-being
Development and activity
Emotional well-being

Subjective Feeling of Well-being

Satisfaction with:
Physical well-being
Material well-being
Social well-being
Development and activity
Emotional well-being

External Influences

Personal Values and Aspirations

Importance of:
Physical well-being
Material well-being
Social well-being
Development and activity
Emotional well-being

Overall Assessment of Well-being (quality of life)

FIGURE 7-1 A model of quality of life. (Reproduced with permission from Felce D, Perry J: Quality of life: Its definition and measurement. *Res Dev Disabil* 16:51-74, 1995.)

According to Patrick, the elements within these planes do not constitute a linear or temporal process, in that they do not occur in an entirely unilateral direction.[136] Patrick suggests that quality-of-life outcomes are influenced by the other three planes, and that the disabling process may be halted or reversed at any of the interaction points in the model. Under such a model, the intervention includes the restoration or maintenance of functional status, the promotion of opportunity, and alterations to the patient's environment and individual behavior.[136]

PATIENT EXAMPLE—PUTTING IT ALL TOGETHER

Essential to any patient progression is a correct diagnosis and evaluation. It is a common belief in physical therapy that arriving at a correct diagnosis is more complicated and complex than designing an intervention plan. That said, intervention planning is not always a simple process, as there are many factors to consider based on the principles of motor development and motor learning. For example, the following have to be considered:

▶ Practice schedule

▶ Amount of practice

▶ Type of task

▶ Stage of the learner

▶ Amount and type of feedback

▶ Environmental influences

This can be overwhelming for the novice physical therapist and can often deter the application of these theories into an intervention program. In addition, the conventional therapeutic objectives such as increasing flexibility and muscle strength and using appropriate postures are important, because contractures, weakness, and inadequate postural control all can be major obstacles to functional movement. However, rather than address these impairments as individual entities, they should be addressed according to how they affect participation in meaningful activities. For example, strengthening can be accomplished using one's body weight for resistance. Embedding repeated practice of standing up and sitting down into task-related activities (e.g., standing at the sink, applying makeup, attending a yoga class) leads to increased strength, skill, and decreased muscle stiffness.

The following framework for goal-directed training, based on the one designed by Mastos et al,[146] is recommended to give the novice some guidance:

▶ The first component of goal-directed training is the selection of a meaningful goal.

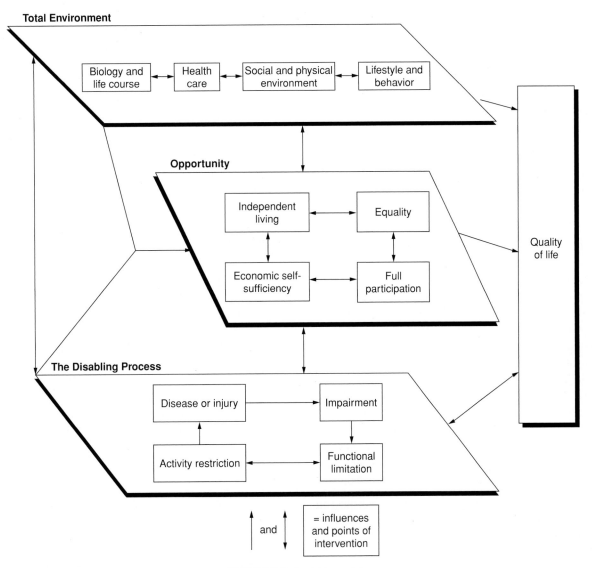

Total Environment

Biology and life course → Health care → Social and physical environment → Lifestyle and behavior

Opportunity

Independent living ↔ Equality

Economic self-sufficiency ↔ Full participation

Quality of life

The Disabling Process

Disease or injury → Impairment

Activity restriction → Functional limitation

↑ and ↕ = influences and points of intervention

FIGURE 7-2 Patrick's model.

► The second component of goal-directed training is to assess baseline performance.

► The third component of goal-directed training is to perform a task analysis.

► The fourth component of goal directed training is to design an intervention.

► The fifth component of goal-directed training is to evaluate the outcome of the therapy goal.

To best illustrate the application of these theories, the following patient example uses the preceding framework[113]:

A 14-year-old patient presents with a history of an acquired brain injury (ABI) from a motor vehicle accident (MVA) 4 years previously. The medical diagnosis on the prescription is given as "Moderate ABI."

The patient history reveals that the patient is living at home and is receiving school-based consultation from a physical therapist.

The examination reveals that the patient has left-sided spastic hemiplegia as a result of the ABI but is fortunately right-handed; he requires the use of a powered wheelchair for community-based activities.

The patient and his parents are concerned that he seldom plays with classmates or friends, in part because of his limited motor skills. Based on these concerns, the patient and his parents, together with the school physical therapist, identified the functional goal of increasing the patient's playtime with appropriate friends in his neighborhood (first component of goal-directed training). The patient's specific goal was to learn how to bowl so that he could go bowling with a group of neighborhood friends.

To assess baseline performance (second component of goal-directed training), the school physical therapist analyzed the patient's functional abilities with his right upper extremity (person), while sitting in his wheelchair in the bowling alley (environment), and performing the desired task (bowling). Because the patient had no difficulty grasping the bowling ball by inserting his fingers into the three holes but did have trouble releasing it, the therapist performed a task analysis of the motor skills required (third component of goal-directed training) to release the ball in order to propel it down the lane. As it was also determined that there were no specific environmental constraints caused by the patient's wheelchair or with accessibility to the bowling alleys and lanes, the physical therapist decided to develop a motor-learning-based intervention program to assist with developing the ability to release the bowling ball. To accomplish this, the physical therapist developed the following initial therapy objective: "While sitting in his wheelchair in a specified 'practice lane' at the local bowling alley, the patient will release the bowling ball onto the lane independently four out of five times within an eight-minute period with physical assistance and verbal cueing from his physical therapist."

The intervention (fourth component of goal-directed training) was based on Fitts and Posner's[107] three stages of motor learning:

- In the first or cognitive stage, the physical therapist asked the patient to try to problem solve, or think through the necessary skills required to release the bowling ball. The physical therapist then provided both physical cueing and verbal instructions to facilitate the release of the ball.

- In the second or associative stage, the physical therapist asked the patient to release the ball on the bowling alley without any added physical assistance from the physical therapist but with continued verbal cueing. The patient was allowed to make errors and to learn from those errors as he repeatedly attempted (practiced) releasing the ball onto the alley.

- During the third stage of learning, the autonomous stage, the patient was able to consistently release the ball onto the alley without the need for verbal cueing from the physical therapist.

The outcome of the initial specific therapy objective (fifth component of goal-directed training) was evaluated independently by the physical therapist.

THE FUTURE

In the current era of increasing accountability for healthcare services, the issues of quality and access to healthcare are of overriding importance. Improvements in accountability must clearly include indicators of efficiency.[143] The correct selection and application of standardized outcome measurement instruments is a fundamental component of the clinical decision-making process. and Dobrzykowski[121] recommend the following guidelines to assist the clinician in their selection:

1. Select an instrument with known reliability, validity, and demonstrated sensitivity to change.

2. Administer the instrument on intake, reassessment, and on discharge, and know the suggested time frame for repeat administration.

3. Be familiar with the scoring procedure for the chosen instrument.

4. Complete the scoring accurately.

5. Document the health-related quality of life (HRQOL) at intake, discharge, and when change in scores occur on the patient record.

6. Understand the clinical meaning of the range of scores.

7. Be familiar with the minimum detectable change (MDC) and the minimum clinically important difference (MCID) for the scale.

8. Establish a treatment goal for change of the HRQOL score that is greater than the MDC or MCID for the instrument, if these are known.

9. Assess changes in HRQOL scores and compare to the known MDC for the instrument to determine if true change has been made.

10. Analyze outcomes to evaluate treatment effectiveness and efficiency.

REFERENCES

1. Shumway-Cook A, Woollacott MH: A conceptual framework for clinical practice, in Shumway-Cook A, Woollacott MH (eds): Motor control—Translating research into clinical practice. Philadelphia, Lippincott Williams & Wilkins, 2007, pp 137-153.
2. Jette DU, Grover L, Keck CP: A qualitative study of clinical decision making in recommending discharge placement from the acute care setting. Phys Ther 83:224-236, 2003.
3. Sullivan PE, Puniello MS, Pardasaney PK: Rehabilitation program development: clinical decision-making, prioritization, and program integration, in Magee D, Zachazewski JE, Quillen WS (eds): Scientific foundations and principles of practice in musculoskeletal rehabilitation. St Louis, WB Saunders, 2007, pp 314-327.
4. Hungerford DS, Lennox DW: Rehabilitation of the knee in disorders of the patellofemoral joint: Relevant biomechanics. Orthop Clin North Am 14:397-444, 1983.
5. Smith MJ: Electrical stimulation for the relief of musculoskeletal pain. Phys Sports Med 11:47-55, 1983.
6. Goth RS, al. e: Electrical stimulation effect on extensor lag and length of hospital stay after total knee arthroplasty. Arch Phys Med Rehabil 75:957, 1994.
7. Magora F, Aladjemoff L, Tannenbaum J, et al: Treatment of pain by transcutaneous electrical stimulation. Acta Anaesthesiol Scand 22:589-592, 1978.
8. Mannheimer JS, Lampe GN: Clinical Transcutaneous Electrical Nerve Stimulation. Philadelphia, FA Davis, 1984, pp 440-445.
9. Woolf CF: Segmental afferent fiber-induced analgesia: transcutaneous electrical stimulation (TENS) and vibration, in Wall PD, Melzack R (eds): Textbook of Pain. New York, Churchill Livingstone, 1989, pp 884-896.
10. Smith MJ, Hutchins RC, Hehenberger D: Transcutaneous neural stimulation use in post-operative knee rehabilitation. Am J Sports Med 11:75-82, 1983.
11. Long DM: Fifteen years of transcutaneous electrical stimulation for pain control. Stereotact Funct Neurosurg 56:2-19, 1991.
12. Fried T, Johnson R, McCracken W: Transcutaneous electrical nerve stimulation: its role in the control of chronic pain. Arch Phys Med Rehabil 65:228-31, 1984.
13. Eriksson MBE, Sjölund BH, Nielzen S: Long-term results of peripheral conditioning stimulation as an analgesic measure in chronic pain. Pain 6:335-347, 1979.
14. Fishbain DA, Chabal C, Abbott A, et al: Transcutaneous electrical nerve stimulation (TENS) treatment outcome in long term users. Clin J Pain 12:201-214, 1996.
15. Ishimaru K, Kawakita K, Sakita M: Analgesic effects induced by TENS and electroacupuncture with different types of stimulating electrodes on deep tissues in human subjects. Pain 63:181-187, 1995.
16. Eriksson MBE, Sjölund BH, Sundbärg G: Pain relief from peripheral conditioning stimulation in patients with chronic facial pain. J Neurosurg 61:149-155, 1984.
17. Murphy GJ: Utilization of transcutaneous electrical nerve stimulation in managing craniofacial pain. Clin J Pain 6:64-69, 1990.
18. Melzack R: The gate theory revisited, in LeRoy PL (ed): Current Concepts in the Management of Chronic Pain. Miami, Symposia Specialists, 1977, pp 43-65.
19. Salar G: Effect of transcutaneous electrotherapy on CSF beta-endorphin content in patients without pain problems. Pain 10:169-172, 1981.

20. Clement-Jones V: Increased beta endorphin but not metenkephalin levels in human cerebrospinal fluid after acupuncture for recurrent pain. Lancet 8:946-948, 1980.
21. Feibel A, Fast A: Deep heating of joints: A reconsideration. Arch Phys Med Rehabil 57:513-514, 1976.
22. Clark D, Stelmach G: Muscle fatigue and recovery curve parameters at various temperatures. Res Q 37:468-479, 1966.
23. Baker R, Bell G: The effect of therapeutic modalities on blood flow in the human calf. J Orthop Sports Phys Ther 13:23, 1991.
24. Knight KL, Aquino J, Johannes SM, et al: A re-examination of Lewis' cold induced vasodilation in the finger and ankle. Athl Training 15:248-250, 1980.
25. Zankel H: Effect of physical agents on motor conduction velocity of the ulnar nerve. Arch Phys Med Rehabil 47:197-199, 1994.
26. Abramson DI, Bell B, Tuck S: Changes in blood flow, oxygen uptake and tissue temperatures produced by therapeutic physical agents: effect of indirect or reflex vasodilation. Am J Phys Med 40:5-13, 1961.
27. Frizzell LA, Dunn F: Biophysics of ultrasound, in Lehman JF (ed): Therapeutic Heat and Cold (ed 3). Baltimore, Williams & Wilkins, 1982, pp 353-385.
28. Lehman JF, Masock AJ, Warren CG, et al: Effect of therapeutic temperatures on tendon extensibility. Arch Phys Med Rehabil 51:481-487, 1970.
29. Kalenak A, Medlar CE, Fleagle SB, et al: Athletic injuries: heat vs cold. Am Fam Physician 12:131-34, 1975.
30. Michlovitz SL: The use of heat and cold in the management of rheumatic diseases, in Michlovitz SL (ed): Thermal Agents in Rehabilitation. Philadelphia, FA Davis, 1990, pp 158-174.
31. Barcroft H, Edholm OS: The effect of temperature on blood flow and deep temperature in the human forearm. J Physiol 102:5-20, 1943.
32. Griffin JG: Physiological effects of ultrasonic energy as it is used clinically. J Am Phys Ther Assoc 46:18, 1966.
33. Knight KL: Cryotherapy: Theory, Technique, and Physiology. Chattanooga, TN, Chattanooga Corp, 1985.
34. Hocutt JE, Jaffee R, Rylander R, et al: Cryotherapy in ankle sprains. Am J Sports Med 10:316-319, 1982.
35. Quillen WS, Rouillier LH: Initial management of acute ankle sprains with rapid pulsed pneumatic compression and cold. J Orthop Sports Phys Ther 4:39-43, 1981.
36. Starkey JA: Treatment of ankle sprains by simultaneous use of intermittent compression and ice packs. Am J Sports Med 4:142-143, 1976.
37. Wilkerson GB: Treatment of ankle sprains with external compression and early mobilization. Phys Sports Med 13:83-90, 1985.
38. McMaster WC, Liddle S, Waugh TR: Laboratory evaluation of various cold therapy modalities. Am J Sports Med 6:291-294, 1978.
39. Daniel DM, Stone ML, Arendt DL: The effect of cold therapy on pain, swelling, and range of motion after anterior cruciate ligament reconstructive surgery. Arthroscopy 10:530-533, 1994.
40. Konrath GA, Lock T, Goitz HT, et al: The use of cold therapy after anterior cruciate ligament reconstruction. A prospective randomized study and literature review. Am J Sports Med 24:629-633, 1996.
41. Speer KP, Warren RF, Horowitz L: The efficacy of cryotherapy in the postoperative shoulder. J Shoulder Elbow Surg 5:62-68, 1996.
42. Knight KL: Cryotherapy in Sports Injury Management. Champaign, Ill, Human Kinetics, 1995.
43. Kellett J: Acute soft tissue injuries: a review of the literature. Med Sci Sports Exerc 18:5, 1986.
44. McMaster WC: A literary review on ice therapy in injuries. Am J Sports Med 5:124-126, 1977.
45. Hartviksen K: Ice therapy in spasticity. Acta Neurol Scand 3(Suppl): 79-84, 1962.
46. Basset SW, Lake BM: Use of cold applications in the management of spasticity. Phys Ther Rev 38:333-334, 1958.
47. Lamboni P, Harris B: The use of ice, air splints, and high voltage galvanic stimulation in effusion reduction. Athl. Training 18:23-25, 1983.
48. McMaster WC: Cryotherapy. Phys Sports Med 10:112-119, 1982.
49. Waylonis GW: The physiological effects of ice massage. Arch Phys Med Rehabil 48:42-47, 1967.
50. Threlkeld AJ: The effects of manual therapy on connective tissue. Phys Ther 72:893-902, 1992.
51. Maitland G: Vertebral Manipulation. Sydney, Butterworth, 1986.
52. Kaltenborn FM: Manual Mobilization of the Extremity Joints: Basic Examination and Treatment Techniques (ed 4). Oslo, Olaf Norlis Bokhandel, Universitetsgaten, 1989.
53. Jull GA, Janda V: Muscle and motor control in low back pain, in Twomey LT, Taylor JR (eds): Physical Therapy of the Low Back: Clinics in Physical Therapy. New York, Churchill Livingstone, 1987, pp 258-278.
54. Voss DE, Ionta MK, Myers DJ: Proprioceptive Neuromuscular Facilitation: Patterns and Techniques (ed 3). Philadelphia, Harper & Row, 1985, pp 1-342.
55. Pollard H, Ward G: A study of two stretching techniques for improving hip flexion range of motion. J Man Physiol Ther 20:443-447, 1997.
56. Rhea MR, Alvar BA, Burkett LN, et al: A meta-analysis to determine the dose response for strength development. Med Sci Sports Exerc 35:456-64, 2003.
57. Albert M: Concepts of muscle training, in Wadsworth C (ed): Orthopaedic Physical Therapy: Topic—Strength and Conditioning Applications in Orthopaedics—Home Study Course 98A. La Crosse, Wisc, Orthopaedic Section, APTA, Inc, 1998.
58. Grimsby O, Power B: Manual therapy approach to knee ligament rehabilitation, in Ellenbecker TS (ed): Knee Ligament Rehabilitation. Philadelphia, Churchill Livingstone, 2000, pp 236-251.
59. Pollock ML, Gaesser GA, Butcher JD, et al: The recommended quantity and quality of exercise for developing and maintaining cardiorespiratory and muscular fitness, and flexibility in healthy adults: American College of Sports Medicine Position Stand. Med Sci Sports Exerc 30:975-991, 1998.
60. Sporer BC, Wenger HA: Effects of aerobic exercise on strength performance following various periods of recovery. J Strength Cond Res 17:638-644, 2003.
61. Wenger HA, McFadyen PF, Middleton L, et al: Physiological principles of conditioning for the injured and disabled, in Magee D, Zachazewski JE, Quillen WS (eds): Scientific Foundations and Principles of Practice in Musculoskeletal Rehabilitation. St Louis, WB Saunders, 2007, pp 357-374.
62. Bahr R: Principles of injury prevention, in Brukner P, Khan K (eds): Clinical Sports Medicine (ed 3). Sydney, McGraw-Hill, 2007, pp 78-101.
63. Fleck SJ, Kraemer WJ: Designing resistance training programs (ed 2). Champaign, Ill, Human Kinetics Books, 1997.
64. Simoneau GG, Bereda SM, Sobush DC, et al: Biomechanics of elastic resistance in therapeutic exercise programs. J Orthop Sports Phys Ther 31:16-24, 2001.
65. Shepley B, MacDougall JD, Cipriano N, et al: Physiological effects of tapering in highly trained athletes. J Appl Physiol 72:706-711, 1992.
66. Borg GAV: Psychophysical basis of perceived exertion. Med Sci Sports Exerc 14:377-381, 1992.
67. Borg GAV: Perceived exertion as an indicator of somatic stress. Scand J Rehabil Med 2:92-98, 1970.
68. Canavan PK: Designing a rehabilitation program related to strength and conditioning, in Wilmarth MA (ed): Orthopaedic Physical Therapy: Topic—Strength and Conditioning—Independent Study Course 15.3. La Crosse, Wisc, Orthopaedic Section, APTA, Inc, 2005.
69. Pearson D, Faigenbaum A, Conley M, et al: The National Strength and Conditioning Association's basic guidelines for resistance training of athletes. Strength Cond 22:14-27, 2000.
70. Joynt RL: Therapeutic exercise, in DeLisa JA (ed): Rehabilitation Medicine: Principles and Practice. Philadelphia, JB Lippincott, 1988, pp 346-371.
71. Yoder E: Physical therapy management of nonsurgical hip problems in adults, in Echternach JL (ed): Physical Therapy of the Hip. New York, Churchill Livingstone, 1990, pp 103-137.
72. Travell JG, Simons DG: Myofascial Pain and Dysfunction—The Trigger Point Manual. Baltimore, Williams & Wilkins, 1983.
73. Swezey RL: Arthrosis, in Basmajian JV, Kirby RL (eds): Medical Rehabilitation. Baltimore, Williams & Wilkins, 1984, pp 216-218.
74. Kottke FJ: Therapeutic exercise to maintain mobility, in Kottke FJ, Stillwell GK, Lehman JF (eds): Krusen's Handbook of Physical Medicine and Rehabilitation. Baltimore, WB Saunders, 1982, pp 389-402.
75. Wallman HW: Stretching and flexibility, in Wilmarth MA (ed): Orthopaedic Physical Therapy: Topic—Strength and Conditioning—Independent Study Course 15.3. La Crosse, Wisc, Orthopaedic Section, APTA, Inc, 2005.
76. Nelson RT: A comparison of the immediate effects of eccentric training vs. static stretch on hamstring flexibility in high school and college athletes. North Am J Sports Phys Ther 1:56-61, 2006.
77. Thacker SB, Gilchrist J, Stroup DF, et al: The impact of stretching on sports injury risk: a systematic review of the literature. Med Sci Sports Exerc 36:371-378, 2004.

78. Herbert RD, Gabriel M: Effects of stretching before and after exercising on muscle soreness and risk of injury: systematic review. BMJ 325:468, 2002.

79. Shrier I: Does stretching improve performance? A systematic and critical review of the literature. Clin J Sport Med 14:267-273, 2004.

80. Murphy DR: A critical look at static stretching: Are we doing our patient harm? Chiropractic Sports Med 5:67-70, 1991.

81. Prentice WE: Impaired mobility: Restoring range of motion and improving flexibility, in Voight ML, Hoogenboom BJ, Prentice WE (eds): Musculoskeletal Interventions: Techniques for Therapeutic Exercise. New York, McGraw-Hill, 2007, pp 165-180.

82. Markos PD: Ipsilateral and contralateral effects of proprioceptive neuromuscular facilitation techniques on hip motion and electromyographic activity. Phys Ther 59:1366, 1979.

83. Holt LE, Travis TM, Okita T: Comparative study of three stretching techniques. Percep Motor Skills 31:611-616, 1970.

84. Tanigawa MC: Comparison of hold-relax procedure and passive mobilization on increasing muscle length. Phys Ther 52:725-735, 1972.

85. Sady SP, Wortman MA, Blanke D: Flexibility training: Ballistic, static or proprioceptive neuromuscular facilitation? Arch Phys Med Rehabil 63:261-263, 1982.

86. Prentice WE: A comparison of static stretching and PNF stretching for improving hip joint flexibility. Athl Train 18:56-59, 1983.

87. Hartley-O'Brien SJ: Six mobilization exercises for active range of hip flexion. Res Q 51:625-635, 1980.

88. Muir IW, Chesworth BM, Vandervoort AA: Effect of a static calf-stretching exercise on the resistive torque during passive ankle dorsiflexion in healthy subjects. J Orthop Sports Phys Ther 29:106-113; discussion 114-115, 1999.

89. DeVries HA: Evaluation of static stretching procedures for improvement of flexibility. Res Q 33:222-229, 1962.

90. Logan GA, Egstrom GH: Effects of slow and fast stretching on sacrofemoral angle. J Assoc Phys Ment Rehabil 15:85-89, 1961.

91. Davies CT, White MJ: Muscle weakness following eccentric work in man. Pflugers Arch 392:168-171, 1981.

92. Friden J, Sjostrom M, Ekblom B: A morphological study of delayed muscle soreness. Experientia 37:506-507, 1981.

93. Hardy L: Improving active range of hip flexion. Res Q Exerc Sport 56:111-114, 1985.

94. Starring DT, Gossman MR, Nicholson GG, Jr., et al: Comparison of cyclic and sustained passive stretching using a mechanical device to increase resting length of hamstring muscles. Phys Ther 68:314-20., 1988.

95. Depino GM, Webright WG, Arnold BL: Duration of maintained hamstring flexibility after cessation of an acute static stretching protocol. J Athl Train 35:56-59, 2000.

96. Spernoga SG, Uhl TL, Arnold BL, et al: Duration of maintained hamstring flexibility after a one-time, modified hold-relax stretching protocol. J Athl Train 36:44-48, 2001.

97. Bandy WD, Irion JM, Briggler M: The effect of time and frequency of static stretching on flexibility of the hamstring muscles. Phys Ther 77:1090-1096, 1997.

98. Roberts JM, Wilson K: Effect of stretching duration on active and passive range of motion in the lower extremity. Br J Sports Med. 33:259-263, 1999.

99. Taylor DC, Dalton JD, Jr., Seaber AV, et al: Viscoelastic properties of muscle-tendon units. The biomechanical effects of stretching. Am J Sports Med 18:300-309, 1990.

100. American College of Sports Medicine Position Stand. The recommended quantity and quality of exercise for developing and maintaining cardiorespiratory and muscular fitness, and flexibility in healthy adults. Med Sci Sports Exerc 30:975-991, 1998.

101. Fulk GD: Traumatic brain injury, in O'Sullivan SB, Schmitz TJ (eds): Physical Rehabilitation (ed 5). Philadelphia, FA Davis, 2007, pp 895-935.

102. de Jong LD, Nieuwboer A, Aufdemkampe G: Contracture preventive positioning of the hemiplegic arm in subacute stroke patients: a pilot randomized controlled trial. Clin Rehabil 20:656-667, 2006.

103. Chatterton HJ, Pomeroy VM, Gratton J: Positioning for stroke patients: a survey of physiotherapists' aims and practices. Disabil Rehabil 23:413-421, 2001.

104. Risberg MA, Mork M, Krogstad-Jenssen H, et al: Design and implementation of a neuromuscular training program following anterior cruciate ligament reconstruction. J Orthop Sports Phys Ther 31:620-631, 2001.

105. Chmielewski TL, Hewett TE, Hurd WJ, et al: Principles of neuromuscular control for injury prevention and rehabilitation, in Magee D, Zachazewski JE, Quillen WS (eds): Scientific Foundations and Principles of Practice in Musculoskeletal Rehabilitation. St Louis, WB Saunders, 2007, pp 375-387.

106. Voight ML, Cook G, Blackburn TA: Functional lower quarter exercises through reactive neuromuscular training, in Bandy WD (ed): Current Trends for the Rehabilitation of the Athlete—Home Study Course. La Crosse, Wisc, Sports Physical Therapy Section, APTA, Inc, 1997.

107. Fitts PM, Posner MI: Human Performance. Belmont, CA, Brooks/Cole, 1967.

108. Litzinger ME, Osif B: Accommodating diverse learning styles: Designing instruction for electronic information sources, in Shirato L (ed): What Is Good Instruction Now? Library Instruction for the 90s. Ann Arbor, Mich, Pierian Press, 1993, pp 26-50.

109. Schmidt R, Lee T: Motor Control and Learning (ed 4). Champaign, Ill, Human Kinetics, 2005.

110. Kisner C, Colby LA: Therapeutic exercise: Foundational concepts, in Kisner C, Colby LA (eds): Therapeutic Exercise. Foundations and Techniques (ed 5). Philadelphia, FA Davis, 2002, pp 1-36.

111. Gentile AM: Skill acquisition: action, movement, and neuromotor processes, in Carr J, Shepherd R (eds): Movement Science: Foundations for Physical Therapy in Rehabilitation. Gaithersburg, Md, Aspen, 2000, pp 111-187.

112. Magill RA: Motor learning and control: Concepts and applications (ed 8). New York, NY, McGraw-Hill, 2007.

113. Zwicker JG, Harris SR: A reflection on motor learning theory in pediatric occupational therapy practice. Can J Occup Ther 76:29-37, 2009.

114. Peck AC, Detweiler MC: Training concurrent multistep procedural tasks. Human Factors 42:379-389, 2000.

115. Ma HI, Trombly CA: The comparison of motor performance between part and whole tasks in elderly persons. Am J Occup Ther 55:62-67, 2001.

116. Mathiowetz V, Bass-Haugen J: Assessing abilities and capacities: Motor behavior, in Radomski MV, Trombly-Latham CA (eds): Occupational Therapy for Physical Dysfunction (ed 6). Baltimore, Md, Williams & Wilkins, 2008, pp 186-211.

117. Salive ME, Mayfield JA, Weissman NW: Patient outcomes research teams and the agency for health care policy and research. Health Serv Res 25:697-708, 1990.

118. Jette AM, Keysor JJ: Uses of evidence in disability outcomes and effectiveness research. Milbank Q 80:325-345, 2002.

119. Blair SJ, McCormick E, Bear-Lehman J, et al: Evaluation of impairment of the upper extremity. Clin Orthop 221:42-58, 1987.

120. Van der Wurff P, Meyne W, Hagmeijer RHM: Clinical tests of the sacroiliac joint, a systematic methodological review. part 2: validity. Man Ther 5:89-96, 2000.

121. Resnik L, Dobrzykowski E: Guide to outcome measurement for patients with low back pain syndromes. J Orthop Sports Phys Ther 33:307-318, 2003.

122. Hebert R, Spiegelhalter DJ, Brayne C: Setting the minimal metrically detectable change on disability rating scales. Arch Phys Med Rehabil 78:1305-1308, 1997.

123. Fritz JM, Irrgang JJ: A comparison of a modified Oswestry Low Back Pain Disability Questionnaire and the Quebec Back Pain Disability Scale. Phys Ther 81:776-788, 2001.

124. Stratford PW: Invited commentary: Guide to outcome measurement for patients with low back pain syndromes. J Orthop Sports Phys Ther 33:317-318, 2003.

125. Grimmer K, Sheppard L, Pitt M, et al: Differences in stakeholder expectations in the outcome of physiotherapy management of acute low back pain. Int J Qual Health Care 11:155-162, 1999.

126. Reuben DB, Siu AL: Measuring physical function in community dwelling older persons: a comparison of self administered, interviewer administered, and performance-based measures. J Am Geriatr Soc 43: 17-23, 1995.

127. Tager IB, Swanson A, Satariano WA: Reliability of physical performance and self-reported functional measures in an older population. J Gerontol 53:M295-M300, 1998.

128. de Bruin AF, de Witte LP, Stevens F, et al: Sickness Impact Profile: The state of the art of a generic functional status measure. Soc Sci Med 35:1003-1014, 1992.

129. Bergner M, Bobbitt RA, Carter WB, et al: The Sickness Impact Profile: Development and final revision of a health status measure. Med Care 19:787, 1981.

130. Feise RJ, Michael Menke J: Functional rating index: a new valid and reliable instrument to measure the magnitude of clinical change in spinal conditions. Spine 26:78-86; discussion 87, 2001.

131. Stratford P, Gill C, Westaway M, et al: Assessing disability and change on individual patients: a report of a patient specific measure. Physiother Can 47:258-263, 1995.

132. Cleland JA, Fritz JM, Whitman JM, et al: The reliability and construct validity of the Neck Disability Index and patient specific functional scale in patients with cervical radiculopathy. Spine 31:598-602, 2006.

133. Chatman AB, Hyams SP, Neel JM, et al: The Patient-Specific Functional Scale: measurement properties in patients with knee dysfunction. Phys Ther 77:820-829, 1997.

134. Westaway MD, Stratford PW, Binkley JM: The patient-specific functional scale: validation of its use in persons with neck dysfunction. J Orthop Sports Phys Ther 27:331-338, 1998.

135. Swiontkowski MF, Engelberg R, Martin DP, et al: Short musculo-skeletal function assessment questionnaire: validity, reliability, and responsiveness. J Bone Joint Surg 81A:1256-1258, 1999.

136. Patrick DL: Rethinking prevention for people with disabilities. Part I: A conceptual model for promoting health. Am J Health Promot 11:257-260, 1997.

137. Barnett D: Assessment of quality of life. Am J Cardiol 67:41c-44c, 1991

138. Carr A, Thompson P, Kirwan J: Quality of life measures. Br J Rheum 35:275-281, 1996.

139. Felce D, Perry J: Quality of life: its definition and measurement. Res Dev Disabil 16:51-74, 1995.

140. Krause JS, Bell. RB: Measuring quality of life and secondary conditions: Experiences with spinal cord injury, in Simeonsson RJ, McDevitt LN (eds): Issues in Disability and Health: The Role of Secondary Conditions and Quality of Life. Chapel Hill, University of North Carolina Press, 1999, pp 129-143.

141. Patrick DL, Deyo RA: Generic and disease-specific measures in assessing health status and quality of life. Med Care 27(suppl 3):217-232, 1989.

142. Simeonsson RJ, Leskinen M: Disability, secondary conditions and quality of life: Conceptual issues, in Simeonsson RJ, McDevitt LN (eds): Issues in Disability and Health: The Role of Secondary Conditions and Quality of Life. Chapel Hill, University of North Carolina Press, 1999, pp 51-72.

143. Fisher C, Dvorak M: Orthopaedic research: What an orthopaedic surgeon needs to know, Orthopaedic Knowledge Update: Home Study Syllabus. Rosemont, Ill, American Academy of Orthopaedic Surgeons, 2005, pp 3-13.

144. Ware JE, Jr., Snow KK, Kosinski M, et al: SF-36 Health Survey: Manual and Interpretation Guide. Boston, The Health Institute, 1993.

145. Beaton DE, Richards RR: Measuring function of the shoulder. A cross-sectional comparison of five questionnaires. J Bone Joint Surg 78A:882-890, 1996.

146. Mastos M, Miller K, Eliasson AC, et al: Goal-directed training: linking theories of treatment to clinical practice for improved functional activities in daily life. Clin Rehabil 21:47-55, 2007.

Preparation for Patient Care

CHAPTER 8

CHAPTER OBJECTIVES

*At the completion of this chapter,
the reader will be able to:*

1. Discuss the differences between values and beliefs

2. List some of the most common negative biases of healthcare workers

3. Provide some examples of nonverbal communication

4. Define *empathy*

5. Discuss the importance of health equity and cultural competency among healthcare providers

6. Describe what health disparity is

7. List the five steps to achieving cultural competence

8. Discuss the importance of infection control in healthcare

9. Describe some of the microorganisms that can be encountered in healthcare and their various modes of transmission

10. List some of the precautions that must be used with special populations

OVERVIEW

Patient care is a partnership between a patient and the clinician—it is something a clinician does *with* a patient, not *to* a patient. The primary focus of patient care is to enhance a patient's function through positive interactions, with each interaction having an objective. In some cases, this involves helping a patient to regain former skills, whereas in other cases, it may involve teaching a patient ways to compensate for the loss of a physical or mental attribute. Generally speaking, most interventions involve increasing either a patient's mobility or a patient's stability. Determining what the focus or objective will be requires clinical decision making and preparation.

CLINICAL PEARL

Essential for the preparation for patient care is the knowledge of a number of general principles so that patient and clinician safety is ensured. For example, having to leave a patient unguarded to retrieve a piece of equipment must be avoided at all times. All equipment is required to be inspected before use. In the event that a piece of equipment is found to be malfunctioning, correct procedures must be followed. This typically involves labeling the piece of equipment as defective and reporting the defect to the appropriate personnel, such as the clinical engineering department.

THE HEALTHCARE TEAM

In many physical therapy settings, a physical therapist does not work in isolation. Often, a healthcare team made up of many different professions plays a role in reviewing a patient's condition and making decisions (see Chapter 1). This patient-centered interprofessional collaboration, which is more common outside the outpatient work areas, serves to enhance problem solving and the coordination of care. In most cases, team conferences involving members from each of the disciplines (nursing, social services, etc.) are held on the patient's behalf. In addition to these discussion meetings, it is not unusual for fellow professionals to co-treat a patient. For example, a patient who has undergone hip replacement is often co-treated by a physical therapist and an occupational therapist. The advantage of co-treatment is that it reduces duplication of treatments, enhances input from different professionals, and often results in interventions for complex problems that exceed what an individual could accomplish. Another example of co-treatment occurs when a physical therapist and a physical therapist assistant work together with the same patient. The physical therapist evaluates the patient, provides a plan of care, establishes the goals or desired outcomes, and determines the therapeutic interventions to be used. The physical therapist assistant performs the treatment activities for which he or she is qualified and communicates frequently, both orally and in writing, with the physical therapist, who evaluates the results of the treatment and the patient's responses to it so that alterations or adjustments to the plan of care can be made as necessary.

INITIAL PREPARATION

A significant component of the clinician-patient interaction takes place before the clinician ever comes into contact with the patient. Before the start of any procedure, the clinician must prepare for the steps ahead, both mentally and physically. For example, the treatment area must be organized with safety in mind, as well as for efficient use. This may include the removal of any obstacles, adjusting the height of the treatment table, or checking the availability of a particular piece of equipment. Enough room must be allowed for unimpeded movement. Before meeting the patient, the clinician should perform a comprehensive review of the patient's medical record or chart, including all of the following:

► Diagnosis or reason for admittance
► Past medical history
► Past surgical history
► Current history and physical findings
► Imaging test results, as appropriate
► Laboratory test results, as appropriate
► Prescribed medications
► Other consultations prescribed
► Confirmation that orders for physical therapy exist

After the chart review, the clinician enters the patient's room, performs a personal introduction, and then informs the patient about the reason that physical therapy has been ordered. This can include the treatment goals and the desired outcomes, as well as a review of any pertinent precautions (e.g., physician-ordered restrictions of motion). The patient should be asked if he or she has any questions before the clinician proceeds with the more formal part of the examination (see Chapter 5).

COMMUNICATION

Patient-clinician interactions can take place in a number of environments, including hospital rooms, outpatient clinics, and the home. Much about becoming a clinician relates to an ability to communicate with the patient, the patient's family, and the other members of the healthcare team. It is important to remember that listening is often more critical than speaking. Nonverbal cues are especially significant, because they often are performed subconsciously. Even when performing a dependent mobility task, the clinician can engage the patient both physically and cognitively to some degree. Special attention needs to be paid to cultural diversity and to nonverbal communication such as:

► *Facial expression.* The facial expression should be one of interest and concern.
► *Voice volume.* The voice volume should be at a level that is sufficient for the patient to hear. Avoid speaking

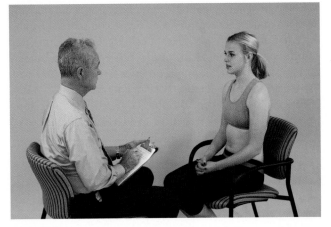

FIGURE 8-1 Clinician-patient interaction

loudly when possible, especially to those who are hard of hearing.
► *Posture.* An upright and attentive posture is preferable (Figure 8-1).
► *Touch.* Any touch, based on respect of the patient's cultural preferences and personal boundaries, should be confident and firm.
► *Gestures.* Gestures should be limited to those describing a particular activity.
► *Physical closeness.* Comfort with physical closeness varies according to culture. In the United States a distance of 18 inches to 4 feet is considered normal for a professional distance.
► *Eye contact.* Maintaining eye contact enhances trust and demonstrates attentiveness (see Figure 8-1).
► *Eye level.* Whenever possible, the clinician should alter his or her position so that the eye level between patient and clinician is the same. For example, if the patient is sitting, the clinician should assume a sitting position (see Figure 8-1).

The appearance of the clinician should convey an air of professionalism (see Figure 8-1). Most institutions have a dress code that should be adhered to.

CLINICAL PEARL

Learn to be a good listener by:

► Looking at the person who is talking and give him or her your full attention
► Making appropriate eye contact
► Showing understanding by summarizing and asking for confirmation
► Letting the speaker finish the point they were making
► Showing interest
► Being respectful

Communication between the clinician and the patient begins when the clinician first meets the patient and continues throughout any future sessions. Communication involves interacting with the patient using terms he or she can understand. The introduction to the patient should be handled in a professional yet empathetic tone. Listening with empathy involves understanding the ideas being communicated and the emotion behind the ideas. In essence, empathy is seeing another person's viewpoint, so that a deep and true understanding of what the person is experiencing can be obtained. Particularly important aspects of empathy are the recognition of patients' rights, potential cultural differences (see Cultural Competence), typical responses to loss, and the perceived role of spirituality in health and wellness to the patient.

CLINICAL PEARL

A patient's privacy and dignity should be maintained at all times. Privacy includes the patient's personal space. Whenever appropriate, the clinician should ask permission from the patient before carrying out an action (moving the patient's belongings off the bedside table, sitting down, etc.).

Given the nature of the physical therapy profession, physical therapists interact frequently with people with disabilities. When writing or speaking about people with disabilities, it is important to put the person first. Group designations such as "the blind" or "the disabled" are inappropriate because they do not reflect the individuality, equality, or dignity of people with disabilities. Similarly, words such as "normal person" imply that the person with a disability is not normal, whereas "person without a disability" is descriptive but not negative. Etiquette considered appropriate when interacting with people with disabilities is based primarily on respect and courtesy. Outlined next are tips to help when communicating with persons with disabilities, provided by the Office of Disability Employment Policy; the Media Project, Research and Training Center on Independent Living, University of Kansas, Lawrence, KS; and the National Center for Access Unlimited, Chicago, IL.

General Tips. When introduced to a person with a disability, it is appropriate to offer to shake hands. People with limited hand use or who wear an artificial limb can usually shake hands (shaking hands with the left hand is an acceptable greeting). If you offer assistance to a person with a disability, wait until the offer is accepted, then listen to or ask for instructions. Address people who have disabilities by their first names only when extending the same familiarity to all others.

Communicating with Individuals Who Are Blind, or Visually Impaired. The clinician should speak to the individual when approaching him or her, and should speak in a normal tone of voice. When conversing in a group, remember to identify yourself and the person to whom you are speaking. The clinician should not attempt to lead the individual without first asking; allow the person to hold your arm and control her or his own movements. Direct action should be given using descriptive words giving the person verbal information that is visually obvious to individuals who can see. For example, if you are approaching a series of steps, mention how many steps. If you are offering a seat, gently place the individual's hand on the back or arm of the chair so that the person can locate the seat. At the end of the session, the clinician should tell the individual that he or she is leaving.

Communicating with Individuals Who Are Deaf or Hard of Hearing. The clinician should gain the patient's attention before starting a conversation (e.g., tap the person gently on the shoulder or arm), and then look directly at the individual, face the light, speak clearly, in a normal tone of voice, and keep the hands from obstructing the mouth. Short, simple sentences should be used. If the patient uses a sign language interpreter, the clinician should speak directly to the person, not the interpreter. If the clinician places a phone call, he or she should let the phone ring longer than usual. If a Text Telephone (TTY) is not available, the clinician should dial 711 to reach the national telecommunications relay service, which will facilitate the call.

Communicating with Individuals with Mobility Impairments. Whenever possible, the clinician should position himself or herself at the wheelchair user's eye level without leaning on the wheelchair or any other assistive device. Never patronize people who use wheelchairs by patting them on the head or shoulder. Do not assume that an individual wants to be pushed—ask first.

Communicating with Individuals with Speech Impairments. If the clinician does not understand something the patient said, he or she should not pretend that they did but should ask the individual to repeat what was said and then repeat it back. To help the patient, the clinician should try to ask questions that require only short answers or a nod of the head. The clinician should not speak for the individual or attempt to finish her or his sentences. If the clinician is having difficulty understanding the individual, writing should be considered as an alternative means of communicating, but only after asking the individual if this is acceptable.

Communicating with Individuals with Cognitive Disabilities. Whenever possible, the clinician and patient should communicate in a quiet or private location and should be prepared to repeat what is said, orally or in writing. It is important that the clinician be patient, flexible, and supportive. The clinician should wait for the individual to accept an offer of assistance; do not "overassist" or be patronizing.

At the end of the first visit and at subsequent visits, the clinician should ask if there are any questions. Each session should have closure, which may include a handshake, if appropriate.

VALUES AND BELIEFS

Every individual has an internalized system of values and beliefs that have developed throughout life. Consciously or otherwise, a clinician brings a set of values and beliefs to every patient interaction. These values and beliefs have been honed by prior experiences. Values and beliefs not only guide actions and behavior but also help to form attitudes toward different things and situations.

▶ *Values.* Values are characteristics that are deemed important. Examples include honesty, effort, perseverance, and loyalty. Numerous studies have demonstrated that both conscious and unconscious values can have an impact on interactions with others.

▶ *Beliefs.* Beliefs are assumptions that are made based on life's experiences. Examples include religion, gender bias, and racial equality. Belief bias occurs when someone's evaluation of the logical strength of an argument is biased by their belief in the truth or falsity of the conclusion. People tend to accept any and all conclusions that fit in with their systems of belief. A bias can be negative or positive. The most common negative biases of healthcare workers involve:

- *Race/ethnicity.* In the United States, patients of racial and ethnic minorities tend to receive healthcare interventions that are inferior to those received by White patients even when income and insurance levels are similar.

- *Gender.* Research is commonly conducted on male subjects, and the conclusions from this research have been generalized and applied to women without consideration of structural or biochemical differences.

- *Ageism.* Older patients are often considered to be senile, hard of hearing, frail, lonely, and incapable of learning new things.

- *Obesity.* Assumptions are made that this population is lazy, lacking in self-discipline and motivation, and ugly, and that they have brought their weight problems on themselves.

- *Disability.* Although patients with disabilities are often viewed positively, they are often treated with pity.

- *Substance abuse.* It is a generally held belief that substance abuse is the fault of the individual because of a lack of willpower.

As clinicians, we are likely to interact frequently with individuals whose values and cultural practices differ from our own. These differences can result in a judgmental response that will either validate or invalidate those values and cultural practices. It is important that the judgmental response not be critical, biased, or one of disapproval, but that every conscious effort be made to accept differences as long as those differences serve the well-being of the patients.

CLINICAL PEARL

The following behaviors are associated with negative beliefs:

▶ Avoiding or minimizing patient interactions

▶ Using derogatory terms or nicknames when describing a patient

▶ Ignoring patient requests or needs

▶ Treating a patient without compassion, commitment, or respect

▶ Referring to the patient as a number and not using his or her name

CULTURAL COMPETENCE

In today's healthcare, a clinician will encounter people of racial, ethnic and cultural minorities, immigrant and refugee communities, those with disabilities, and lesbian, gay, bisexual, and transgender populations. In addition, within these populations can be economically and socially disadvantaged groups. One of the goals of the U.S. government is to create health equity and to promote cultural competency among healthcare providers so as to increase positive outcomes for all people.

CLINICAL PEARL

A health disparity is a difference in rates of illness, disease, or conditions among different populations and a difference in the health outcomes for these populations. Some of these health disparities are the result of poverty, acculturation, behavior and lifestyle, nutrition, access to healthcare services, genetic predisposition, education level, discrimination, differing levels of insurance coverage, and differing access to high-quality networks of preventive and primary care.

In 2010, according to the U.S. Census Bureau, about 30% of the nation's population identified themselves as members of racial or ethnic minority groups. By 2050, these groups are expected to account for almost half of the country's population. It is widely accepted that racial and ethnic minority populations on average receive lower levels of care and have higher rates of certain conditions and diseases than Whites. It has also become clear that economic and social conditions under which people live can affect a person's health and well-being. The World Health Organization recently published a final report and recommendations for creating health equity through action on the social determinants of health (http://www.who.int/social_determinants/en).

A precise definition of "culture" has been widely debated and broadly described, with certain common characteristics including an integrated pattern of learned beliefs and behaviors that can be shared among groups. Included in the pattern are thoughts, styles of communicating, ways of interacting, views on roles and relationships, values, practices, and customs. In essence, culture serves to help individuals to shape and explain their values and to provide meaning. Too often, a different culture is considered to be "exotic" or about "other people" and has been associated with socioeconomic status, religion, gender, and sexual orientation.

Cultural competence can be viewed as a set of congruent behaviors, attitudes, and policies that blend together to form effective interactions within a cross-cultural framework. To be culturally competent, an individual must be aware of, respect, and accept different cultures and must resist the temptation to make assumptions about people and situations.

CLINICAL PEARL

The five steps to achieving cultural competence include:

▶ Awareness

▶ Acknowledgment

▶ Validation

▶ Negotiation

▶ Accomplishment

Examples of how culture can affect healthcare include differences in languages and nonverbal communication patterns, cultural differences in the perception of illness, disease, medical roles and responsibilities, and cultural preferences for treatment of illnesses. Overcoming these barriers requires the cooperation of the patient, the organization, and the clinician.

CLINICAL PEARL

Ways to improve interpersonal communication with culturally diverse patients or those with limited English proficiency or low health literacy include:

1. Slowing down the rate of speaking, rather than speaking loudly
2. Using or drawing pictures
3. Limiting the amount of information provided and using simple, nonmedical language
4. Using the "teach-back" or "show-me" technique

Wherever possible, questions should be asked to help with patients and families from culturally diverse backgrounds. Such questions can include:

▶ Can you tell me the languages that you understand and speak?

▶ Do you use any traditional health remedies to improve your health?

▶ Is there someone, in addition to yourself, with whom you want us to discuss your medical condition?

▶ Are there certain healthcare procedures and tests that your culture prohibits?

▶ Are there any situations where you would prefer to be treated by a clinician of a specific gender?

To minimize the level of difficulty encountered by patients with limited or no English proficiency, system-wide procedures or resources can be put in place. Resources to support this capacity may include:

▶ Trained interpreters

▶ Bilingual/bicultural or multilingual/multicultural staff

▶ Materials developed for specific cultural, ethnic and linguistic groups, including culturally and linguistically appropriate signage

The National Standards on Culturally and Linguistically Appropriate Services (CLAS) (http://clas.uiuc.edu/) are directed at healthcare organizations. The 14 CLAS standards are organized by themes: culturally competent care, language access services, and organizational supports for cultural competency.

PATIENT COMFORT AND SAFETY

The patient's well-being is always the central focus of any interaction or procedure. Treatment tables, mats, or beds should be prepared with linens and pillows before the patient arrives in the treatment area. Additional sheets may be required as

pull sheets for transfers or for draping. Pillows can be used for patient positioning and/or comfort. Call bells must be within reach of patients in areas where patients will be left unattended. Finally, the clinician should always emphasize cleanliness, particularly hand hygiene (see Infection Control).

INFECTION CONTROL

A major focus of healthcare is the prevention of the spread of infection by fostering a clean environment. The degree of cleanliness required depends on the level of the contamination threat. A pathogen, commonly referred to as a germ, is a microorganism that causes disease in (infects) its host. Some healthcare environments and situations can increase the potential for infection. Nosocomial infections are those that originate or occur in a hospital or hospital-like setting. These infections are responsible for about 20,000 deaths per year in the United States.[1]

CLINICAL PEARL

Nosocomial infections are those that originate or occur in a hospital or hospital-like setting. A healthcare-associated infection (HAI) refers to an infection acquired in any healthcare setting.

Approximately 10% of American hospital patients (about 2 million every year) acquire a clinically significant nosocomial infection.[1] Nosocomial infections are due to a number of factors occurring in tandem:

▶ A high prevalence of pathogens

▶ A high prevalence of immunocompromised hosts

▶ High potential of the chains of transmission from patient to patient

Although the purpose of hospitals is to corral the sick and injured into one place in order to efficiently treat them, this environment increases the potential for the movement of pathogens from individual to individual via various routes. In addition to the higher likelihood of pathogen transmission, the high prevalence of pathogens provides an environment for the potential evolution of new microorganisms that are resistant to conventional methods of treatment. Hospitals or hospital-like settings are hosts to a number of opportunistic microorganisms. An opportunistic microorganism is one that takes advantage of certain opportunities (e.g., compromised host) to cause disease. Compromised hosts include:

▶ Those with broken skin or mucous membranes (wounds)

▶ The immunocompromised

The most common sites of nosocomial infections are as follows:

▶ Urinary tract

▶ Surgical wounds

▶ Respiratory tract

▶ Skin (especially after a serious burn)

▶ Blood (bacteremia)

- Gastrointestinal (GI) tract
- Central nervous system

CLINICAL PEARL

The transmission of microorganisms in a healthcare setting is generally a consequence of either accidental or deliberate disregard of established protocols designed to minimize transmission between patients or from hospital workers to patients.

Infection is the process by which this microorganism establishes a parasitic relationship with its host. This invasion and multiplication of microorganisms produces an immune response and subsequent signs and symptoms.[2]

CLINICAL PEARL

- *Apparent infection:* An infection that produces symptoms.
- *Unapparent or subclinical infection:* An infection that is active, but does not produce noticeable symptoms.
- *Latent infection:* An infection that is inactive or dormant.
- A short-term infection is an acute infection.
- A long-term infection is a chronic infection.

For an infection to occur a chain of events that involves several steps must occur in a chronological order (Table 8-1). These steps include the infectious agent encountering a reservoir (host), entering a susceptible reservoir, exiting the reservoir, and then being transmitted (by a vehicle) to new hosts. Examples of how the infectious agent can exit the reservoir include:

- The nose
- The mouth and throat
- The eyes
- The intestinal tract
- The urinary tract
- Multiple body fluids

Examples of the vehicle of transmission include the following:

- *Air:* droplets of body fluid from a cough or sneeze
- *Indirect contact:* occurs when an uninfected person comes into contact with pathogens on a person or object (e.g., clothing, equipment, patient care items, toys)
- *Direct contact:* with another person's skin, body fluids such as blood, semen, and saliva, and eating utensils

Without this transmission, the infection cannot take place. Once the infectious agent has left the host, it must be able to enter another host in order for the infection to spread. An infectious agent can enter a host through a break in a person's skin barrier, mucous membranes, eyes, mouth, nose, or genitourinary tract.

CLINICAL PEARL

The body has a number of natural defense mechanisms to prevent the entry of an infectious agent:

- An intact skin is the primary barrier to infection, as it is relatively resistant to the absorption of microorganisms and to the loss of many body fluids.
- The respiratory tract is lined with cilia, minute hair-like organelles that function to filter and trap microorganisms and prevent them from entering other areas of the lungs.

TABLE 8-1	The Chain of Infection
Element	**Description**
Pathogen reservoir	A pathogen can be found in food, water, people, and inanimate objects. An individual may carry a pathogen without showing any signs or symptoms of disease. In addition, healthcare workers who are sick can put both co-workers and patients at risk and so may be required to wear a face mask. A common pathogen reservoir is the nails of the hand, including artificial nails. The CDC recommends keeping natural nail length to less than one quarter of an inch. Visitors can be significant pathogen reservoirs. Good hand hygiene is encouraged and, on occasion, the use of face masks.
Portal of exit	Pathogens can exit their host through bodily excretions and secretions through openings in the skin.
Means of transmission	Pathogens are transmitted primarily by three modes: - *Contact* (direct and indirect). Direct-contact transmission involves physical transfer of pathogens directly from one person to another through physical contact. An indirect transmission occurs when an uninfected person comes into contact with pathogens on a person or object, and then passes those pathogens on to another person through physical contact. - *Droplet.* This involves large pathogenic particle droplets coming into contact with either the host's conjunctivae or the mucous membranes of the nose or mouth, usually through coughing or sneezing. - *Airborne.* This involves small pathogenic particle droplets being either inhaled or deposited on a susceptible host.
Mode of entry	The most common modes of entry are the mucous membranes of the nose, the eyes, and openings in the skin.
Susceptibility	The risk of infection increases based on both the virulence of the pathogen and the susceptibility of the host.

Entry into a host does not guarantee that the infection will spread. For that to occur, the host must be susceptible or the organism must be difficult to destroy. Multidrug-resistant organisms (MDROs) are organisms that have developed resistance to one or more antibiotics. Most healthy individuals are not susceptible to the majority of infections, but those who are sick, at either end of the life span, malnourished, or immunocompromised are at a greater risk.

CLINICAL PEARL

▶ The majority of microorganisms proliferate best in a dark, warm, moist environment.

▶ The majority of microorganisms cannot proliferate in a cool, dry, light, or extremely cold environment.

A great variety of microorganisms are responsible for infectious diseases, including fungi (yeast and molds); helminths (e.g., tapeworms); viruses; bacteria, protozoa; and prions.

▶ *Fungi.* Certain types of fungi (such as *Candida*) are commonly present on body surfaces or in the intestines. Although generally innocuous, these fungi sometimes cause local infections of the skin and nails, vagina, mouth, or sinuses in immunocompromised individuals. In these individuals, fungal infections can be aggressive—spreading quickly to other organs and often proving fatal. Some fungi reproduce by spreading microscopic spores. These spores are often present in the air, where they can be inhaled or contact the body surfaces. Of the wide variety of spores that land on the skin or end in the lungs, most do not cause infection.

CLINICAL PEARL

Fungal diseases in humans are called mycoses.

Even in otherwise healthy people, some fungal infections (for example, blastomycosis and coccidioidomycosis) can have serious outcomes.

▶ *Bacteria.* Bacteria are microscopic, single-celled organisms, which are encountered in the environment, on the skin, in the airways, in the mouth, and in the digestive and genitourinary tracts of people and animals.

Bacteria can be classified according to shape (cocci [spherical], bacilli [rod-like], and spirochetes [spiral or helical]), their use of oxygen (aerobes, those that can live and grow in the presence of oxygen, and anaerobes, those that can tolerate only low levels of oxygen such as those found in the intestine or in decaying tissue), or by color after a particular chemical (Gram) stain is applied (the bacteria that stain blue are called gram-positive, whereas those that stain pink are called gram-negative). Gram-positive and gram-negative bacteria differ in the types of infections they produce and in the types of antibiotics that are required to manage them.

■ *Gram-negative bacteria.* These bacteria possess a unique outer membrane that is rich in molecules called lipopolysaccharides (endotoxins) that make them more resistant to antibiotics than gram-positive bacteria. The lipopolysaccharides can potentially cause high fever and a life-threatening drop in blood pressure. Gram-negative bacteria have a great facility for mutation—the capacity to exchange genetic material (DNA) with other strains of the same species and even with different species.

■ *Gram-positive bacteria.* These bacteria are usually slow to develop resistance to antibiotics but some (e.g., *Bacillus anthracis* and *Clostridium botulinum*) can produce toxins that cause serious illness. Disease-causing anaerobes include clostridia and peptococci and peptostreptococci, the latter two of which are part of the normal bacterial population (flora) of the mouth, upper respiratory tract, and large intestine.

CLINICAL PEARL

Bacteremia is the presence of viable bacteria in the circulating blood. Most bacteria that enter the bloodstream are rapidly removed by white blood cells. However, if the bacteria become viable, they may establish a focal infection, or the infection may progress to septicemia; the possible sequelae of septicemia include shock, disseminated intravascular coagulation, multiple organ failure, and death.[3]

■ *Mycoplasmas.* Mycoplasmas are unusual, self-replicating bacteria that have no cell wall component and very small genomes.[2] For this reason, antibiotics that are active against bacterial cell walls have no effect on mycoplasmas.[2]

■ *Clostridia.* Clostridia, which normally inhabit the human intestinal tract, soil, and decaying vegetation, are toxin-producing anaerobes that can cause tetanus, botulism, and tissue infections. Clostridia, particularly *Clostridium perfringens*, also infect wounds. Clostridial wound infections, including skin gangrene, muscle gangrene (clostridial myonecrosis), and tetanus, are rather uncommon but may be fatal.

■ *Rickettsiae.* Rickettsiae are small, gram-negative, obligate intracellular organisms that cause several diseases, including Rocky Mountain spotted fever and epidemic typhus. Like viruses, rickettsiae require a host for replication and cannot survive on their own in the environment. In humans, rickettsiae infect the cells lining small blood vessels, causing the blood vessels to become inflamed or choked or to bleed into the surrounding tissue. The various types of rickettsial infections produce similar symptoms, which include fever, severe headache, a characteristic skin rash, and a general feeling of malaise. As rickettsial disease progresses, a person typically experiences confusion and severe weakness—often with cough, dyspnea, and sometimes vomiting and diarrhea. In some people, the liver or spleen enlarges, the kidneys fail, and blood pressure falls dangerously low. Death can occur.

Because ticks, mites, fleas, and lice transmit rickettsiae, a report of a bite from one or more of these vectors is a helpful clue—particularly in geographic areas where rickettsial infection is common.

- *Ehrlichioses.* Ehrlichiae are similar to rickettsiae: they are microorganisms that can live only inside the cells of an animal or person. Unlike rickettsiae, however, ehrlichiae inhabit white blood cells (such as granulocytes and monocytes). Ehrlichioses occur in the United States and Europe, but are most common in the midwestern, southeastern, and south-central United States. Ehrlichioses are most likely to develop between spring and late fall, when ticks are most active.

▶ *Virus.* A virus is a subcellular organism made up only of a ribonucleic acid (RNA) or a deoxyribonucleic acid (DNA) nucleus covered with proteins.[2] Viruses are completely dependent on host cells and cannot replicate unless they invade a host cell and stimulate it to participate in the formation of additional virus particles.[2] The virus can either kill the cell it enters or alter its function. Some viruses leave their genetic material in the host cell, where it remains dormant for an extended time (latent infection; e.g., herpesviruses). Viruses are not susceptible to antibiotics and cannot be destroyed by pharmacologic means.[2] However, antiviral medications can mitigate the course of the viral illness.[2]

Probably the most common viral infections are upper respiratory infections. In small children, viruses also commonly cause croup, laryngitis, bronchiolitis, or bronchitis.

Some viruses (for example, rabies, West Nile virus, and several encephalitis viruses) infect the nervous system. Viral infections may also develop in the skin, sometimes resulting in warts or other blemishes.

▶ *Prions.* Prions are newly discovered proteinaceous, infectious particles consisting of proteins but without nucleic acids.[2] These particles are transmitted from animals to humans and are characterized by a long, latent interval in the host. Examples include Creutzfeldt-Jakob disease and bovine spongiform encephalopathy or "mad cow disease."[2]

▶ *Parasite.* A parasite is an organism that resides on or inside another organism (the host) and causes harm to the host. Parasitic infections are common in rural parts of Africa, Asia, and Latin America and less prevalent in industrialized countries.

Parasites enter the body through the mouth or skin. Parasites that enter through the mouth are swallowed and can remain in the intestine or burrow through the intestinal wall and invade other organs. Parasites that enter through the skin bore directly through the skin or are introduced through the bites of infected insects (the vector). Some parasites enter through the soles of the feet when a person walks barefoot or through the skin when a person swims or bathes in water where the parasites are present.

The diagnosis of a parasitic infection can be made from samples of blood, tissue, stool, or urine for laboratory analysis.

Some parasites, particularly those that are single-celled, reproduce inside the host. Other parasites have complex life cycles, producing larvae that spend time in the environment or as an insect vector before becoming infective. If egg-laying parasites live in the digestive tract, their eggs may be found in the person's stool when a sample is examined under a microscope. Antibiotics, laxatives, and antacids can substantially reduce the number of parasites, making their detection in a stool sample more difficult.

Food, drink, and water are often contaminated with parasites in areas of the world with poor sanitation and unhygienic practices.

CLINICAL PEARL

▶ *Sanitization:* the cleaning of pathogenic microorganisms from public eating utensils and objects.

▶ *Decontamination:* to remove, inactivate, or abolish blood-borne pathogens (BBP) on a surface or object to the point where the BBP are no longer capable of transmitting infectious particles and the surface or object is rendered safe for handling, use, or disposal.

▶ *Disinfection:* refers to a reduction in the number of viable microorganisms present in a sample. Not all disinfectants are capable of sterilizing. Many disinfectants are used alone or in combinations (e.g., hydrogen peroxide) in the healthcare setting. These include alcohols, chlorine and chlorine compounds, formaldehyde, glutaraldehyde, peracetic acid, and quaternary ammonium compounds.

▶ *Sterilization:* any process that abolishes all forms of microbial life, including transmissible agents (e.g., fungi, bacteria, or viruses) present on a surface, within a fluid, in medication, or in a biological culture medium. A surface or an object is either sterile or nonsterile; there are no gradations in sterility. Sterilization can be accomplished using a variety of methods, including heat, chemicals, physical cleaning, and forced air purification.

Infectious Diseases

Infectious agents are now suspected in the origins of chronic diseases such as sarcoidosis, various forms of inflammatory bowel disease, scleroderma, rheumatoid arthritis, systemic lupus erythematosus, diabetes mellitus, Kawasaki disease, Alzheimer's disease, and many forms of cancer. All healthcare professionals need to have an understanding of the infectious process, the sequence of transmission, and approaches to lessen the spread of infections.

Staphylococcal Infections

Most infections caused by staphylococci are because of *Staphylococcus aureus*. However, the prevalence of infections because of *Staphylococcus epidermidis* and other coagulase-negative staphylococci has been steadily increasing in recent years.

Staphylococcus aureus (S. aureus)

S. aureus is a gram-positive coccus that is catalase positive and coagulase positive. *S. aureus* produces a wide variety of toxins, including enterotoxins; Panton-Valentine leukocidin (PVL), associated with necrotic skin and lung infections; and toxic shock syndrome toxin–1 (TSST-1).

S. aureus occurs worldwide. Healthcare workers, anyone with diabetes, and patients on dialysis all have higher rates of colonization. The anterior nares are the chief site of colonization in adults; other potential sites of colonization include the axilla, rectum, and perineum.[4]

Common expressions of staphylococcal infections include skin, wound, and soft tissue infections (burns, surgical wounds, pyomyositis, septic bursitis), toxic shock syndrome, endocarditis, osteomyelitis, food poisoning, and infections related to prosthetic devices (prosthetic joints and heart valves and vascular shunts, grafts, and catheters).[4] The clinical manifestations vary enormously according to the site and type of infection.[2]

Many antibiotics are effective against *S. aureus*. Methicillin-resistant *S. aureus* (MRSA) are resistant to most agents other than vancomycin or non–beta-lactam antibiotics. Many coagulase-negative staphylococci are resistant to all antimicrobials other than vancomycin.

Streptococcal Infections

Streptococcus pyogenes (group A *Streptococcus*) is one of the most common pathogens faced in clinical practice. It causes many diseases in diverse organ systems, ranging from skin infections to infections of the upper respiratory tract.

Signs and symptoms of streptococcus contamination are varied. Classic acute disease involves the skin and oropharynx, but any organ system may be involved. Spread is by skin contact, not by the respiratory tract, although impetigo serotypes may colonize the throat. Respiratory droplet spread is the major route for transmission of strains associated with upper respiratory tract infection. Fingernails and the perianal region can harbor streptococci and play a role in spreading impetigo.

Diagnosis is by culture of streptococci from pharyngeal secretions, blood, cerebrospinal fluid, joint aspirate, skin biopsy specimen, sputum, bronchoalveolar lavage fluid, or thoracocentesis fluid. Types include:

- Group A (*S. pyogenes*)—responsible for pharyngitis, rheumatic fever, scarlet fever, impetigo, necrotizing fasciitis, cellulitis, myositis

- Group B (*S. agalactiae*)—responsible for neonatal and adult infections

- Group C (*S. pneumoniae*)—responsible for pneumonia, otitis media, meningitis, endocarditis

The interventions for streptococcal infections vary depending on the clinical syndrome. In general, penicillin therapy remains the intervention of choice in most situations (except in penicillin-allergic individuals). Remarkably, no penicillin-resistant strains of *S. pyogenes* have yet been encountered in clinical practice.

Hepatitis

Hepatitis is defined as an inflammation of the liver. Several different viruses cause viral hepatitis. They are named the hepatitis A, B, C, D, and E viruses. Some cases of viral hepatitis cannot be attributed to the hepatitis A, B, C, D, or E viruses. These types are called non–A-E hepatitis.

The hepatitis A, B, C, D, and E viruses cause acute, or short-term, viral hepatitis. The hepatitis B, C, and D viruses can also cause chronic hepatitis, in which the infection is prolonged, sometimes lifelong.

Signs and symptoms (some people do not have symptoms) include:

- Low-grade fever—usually an early sign (preicteric phase), with anorexia, nausea, headache, malaise, fatigue, vomiting, abdominal pain, loss of appetite

- Jaundice (yellowing of the skin and eyes)—usually a sign of the icteric phase, with an enlarged liver with tenderness and abatement of the earlier symptoms

- Elevated lab values (hepatic transaminases and bilirubin)

Hepatitis A (HAV, Acute Infectious Hepatitis)

Hepatitis A spreads mostly through food or water contaminated by feces from an infected person. Rarely, it spreads through contact with infected blood. People at risk include international travelers; people living in areas where hepatitis A outbreaks are common; people who live with or have sex with an infected person; and, during outbreaks, day-care children and employees, men who have sex with men, and injection drug users. The best methods of prevention are:

- The hepatitis A vaccine

- Avoiding tap water when traveling internationally

- Practicing good hygiene and sanitation—handwashing

Hepatitis A is usually self-limiting, lasting several weeks.

Hepatitis B (HBV, Serum Hepatitis)

Hepatitis B is spread through contact with infected blood, through sex with an infected person, or from mother to child during childbirth. People at risk are those who have sex with an infected person, gay men, injection drug users, children of immigrants from disease-endemic areas, infants born to infected mothers, people who live with an infected person, healthcare workers, hemodialysis patients, people who received a transfusion of blood or blood products before July 1992 or clotting factors made before 1987, and international travelers. The best method of prevention for this type is the hepatitis B vaccine.

Acute hepatitis B is usually self-limiting. The intervention for chronic hepatitis B includes drug treatment with alpha interferon, peginterferon, lamivudine, or adefovir dipivoxil.

Hepatitis C (HCV, non-A, non-B)

This type of hepatitis spreads mostly through contact with infected blood and, less commonly, through sexual contact and childbirth. People at risk include injection drug users, people who have sex with an infected person, people who have multiple sex partners, healthcare workers, infants born to infected women, hemodialysis patients, and people who received a transfusion of blood or blood products before July 1992 or clotting factors made before 1987. The best method for prevention is through a reduction in the risk of exposure to the virus (there is no vaccine for hepatitis C)—avoiding behaviors such as sharing drug needles or sharing personal items like toothbrushes, razors, and nail clippers with an infected person. The intervention for chronic hepatitis C is pharmacology: peginterferon alone, or combination treatment with peginterferon and the drug ribavirin.

Hepatitis D

Hepatitis D spreads through contact with infected blood. This disease occurs only in people who are already infected with hepatitis B. People at risk include anyone infected with hepatitis B—injection drug users who have hepatitis B have the highest risk. People who have hepatitis B are also at risk if they have sex with a person infected with hepatitis D or if they live with an infected person. Also at risk are people who received a transfusion of blood or blood products before July 1992 or clotting factors made before 1987. The best method of prevention for this type is:

▶ Immunization against hepatitis B for those not already infected

▶ Avoiding exposure to infected blood, contaminated needles, and an infected person's personal items (toothbrush, razor, nail clippers)

The intervention for chronic hepatitis D is alpha interferon.

Hepatitis E

This type of hepatitis spreads through contaminated food or water (by feces from an infected person). The disease is uncommon in the United States. People at risk include international travelers; people living in areas where hepatitis E outbreaks are common; and people who live with or have sex with an infected person. The best way to prevent hepatitis E is to reduce the risk of exposure to the virus (there is no vaccine for hepatitis E)—avoiding tap water when traveling internationally and practicing good hygiene and sanitation.

Hepatitis E is usually self-limiting, lasting several weeks to months.

Acquired Immunodeficiency Syndrome (AIDS)

In 1984, 3 years after the first reports of a disease that was to become known as AIDS, researchers discovered the primary causative viral agent, the human immunodeficiency virus type 1 (HIV-1).[5] In 1986, a second type of HIV, called HIV-2, was isolated from AIDS patients in West Africa, where it may have been present decades earlier.[5] Both HIV-1 and HIV-2 have the same modes of transmission and are associated with similar opportunistic infections and AIDS.[6] In persons infected with HIV-2, immunodeficiency seems to develop more slowly and to be milder. Compared with persons infected with HIV-1, those with HIV-2 are less infectious early in the course of infection.[6]

The primary cause of AIDS is through transmission of the HIV retrovirus by body fluid exchange (in particular blood and semen), which is associated with high-risk behaviors:

▶ Unprotected sexual contact

▶ *Contaminated needles:* sharing, frequent injection of Institute for Applied Biomedicine drugs, transfusions (although no longer a major risk)

▶ Maternal-fetal transmission in utero or at delivery or through contaminated breast milk

Low-risk behaviors for HIV transmission include:

▶ *Occupational transmission:* needle sticks

▶ *Casual contact:* kissing

The HIV retrovirus chiefly infects human T4 (helper) lymphocytes, the major regulators of the immune response, and destroys or inactivates them.[6] Once HIV enters the body, cells containing the CD4 antigen, including macrophages and T4 cells, serve as receptors for the HIV retrovirus.[6] After invading a cell, a virus particle (virion) injects the core proteins and the two strands of viral RNA into the cell. HIV contains reverse transcriptase, an enzyme that allows for successful replication of the virus in reverse fashion, transcribing the RNA code into DNA.[5]

HIV infection manifests itself in many different ways and differs between adult and pediatric populations. The clinical expressions of HIV infection are classified into three stages[5,6]:

▶ *Asymptomatic stage:* although positive for laboratory tests, a patient in the early stages remains asymptomatic. Some individuals can develop an acute, self-limiting infectious mononucleosis–like condition.

▶ *Early symptomatic stage:* AIDS-related complex (ARC), as the infection progresses and the immune system becomes increasingly compromised. This stage may last for weeks or months and is a forerunner to full-blown AIDS. Symptoms and conditions during this stage involve:

■ Generalized adenopathy, deconditioning, anxiety and depression.

■ Nonspecific symptoms, including weight loss, fatigue, night sweats, swollen lymph glands, loss of appetite, apathy and fevers.

■ Neurologic symptoms, including encephalopathy, headache, blurred vision, mild dementia, seizures, focal neurologic signs.

■ *Opportunistic infections:* the most common are *Pneumocystis jirovecii* pneumonia, oral and esophageal candidiasis, cytomegalovirus infection, *Cryptococcus*, herpes simplex, *Mycobacterium tuberculosis*.

▶ *HIV advanced disease:* this stage can include:

■ Neurologic manifestations of central, peripheral, and autonomic nervous systems, including:

● AIDS encephalopathy (HIV-associated dementia).

● *Peripheral neuropathy:* distal, symmetric, and mainly sensory.

● *Neuromusculoskeletal diseases:* osteomyelitis, bacterial myositis, non-Hodgkin's lymphoma, and infectious arthritis.

■ *HIV wasting syndrome:* characterized by a disproportionate loss of metabolically active tissue, specifically body cell mass secondary to weight loss, chronic diarrhea, unexplained weakness, and malnutrition.

■ Rheumatologic manifestations.

■ *HIV-associated myopathy:* a progressive painless weakness in the proximal limb muscles.

■ *Malignancies:* the most common are Kaposi's sarcoma, non-Hodgkin's lymphoma, and primary brain lymphoma.

The diagnosis is by clinical findings and systemic evidence of HIV infection and nonexistence of other known causes of immunodeficiency. Early identification is important so that early and preventive therapies may be introduced.

Controlling the Transmission of Infection

Contamination refers to any instance when an object, surface, or field comes into contact with anything that is not sterile. The most effective ways of preventing contamination and the spread of infection include effective personal and hand hygiene, and effective cleaning and handling techniques.

> ### CLINICAL PEARL
> A *fomite* is any inanimate object or substance such as clothing, book, or furniture that is capable of carrying an infectious organism.

The best way of preventing or controlling the transmission of infection is through the use of sterile techniques and an emphasis on cleanliness.

> ### CLINICAL PEARL
> Depending on the clinical setting, the physical therapist may be required to interact with patients who have open wounds, are immunocompromised, or require the use of medical or surgical aseptic techniques.
> - *Medical asepsis:* any practice that helps to reduce the number and spread of microorganisms. The practice of medical asepsis includes patient isolation in cases of tuberculosis or hepatitis.
> - *Surgical asepsis:* the complete removal of microorganisms and their spores from the surface of an object. The practice of surgical asepsis begins with cleaning the object in question using the principles of medical asepsis followed by a sterilization process.

In 1985, the Centers for Disease Control and Prevention (CDC) introduced the use of Universal Precautions to protect healthcare workers and to reduce the transmission of diseases.

The CDC has since revised its previous information and currently recommends the use of Standard Precautions by healthcare workers when they have contact with any patient's body fluid (secretions or excretions) or blood, and Transmission-Based Precautions when in contact with special patient populations that have highly transmissible pathogens.

> ### CLINICAL PEARL
> Universal Precautions applies to the following body fluids: blood, semen, and vaginal, tissue, cerebrospinal, synovial (joint cavity), pleural, peritoneal, pericardial, and amniotic fluids. The CDC has stated that Universal Precautions also apply to feces, nasal secretions, sputum, sweat, tears, urine, and vomitus.[7]

In addition to these recommendations, most institutions and agencies have enacted additional policies and procedures to control the transmission of infection and disease (Table 8-2). These policies and procedures emphasize good hand hygiene, good respiratory hygiene, a clean environment, the correct disposal of soiled articles (e.g., patient linens, wound dressings), and the safe disposal of needles and other sharps (Table 8-3).

Standard Precautions

Standard Precautions (Table 8-4) are required when working with all patients and clients in any healthcare setting, including the patient's home. Generally, the clinician should:

- Avoid direct contact with patients, fomites, or, especially, body fluids
- Wear barriers such as gloves when contact is necessary or expected
- Avoid puncturing himself or herself with anything and therefore should minimize exposure to sharp instruments, especially body fluid–contaminated sharp instruments
- Avoid exposing patients to any body fluids (or substances, e.g., "weeping dermatitis") of others, such as that of healthcare workers

The most basic standard precaution is hand hygiene. There are two primary methods of hand hygiene: hand rubbing and handwashing.

- *Hand rubbing.* This technique uses an alcohol-based (60% to 95% alcohol [isopropyl, ethanol, *n*-propanol]) and skin conditioner product (to prevent skin irritation and dryness) dispensed from a wall-mounted unit, or an antimicrobial/antiseptic hand wipe. Hand rubbing is used to decontaminate hands in lieu of handwashing. After performing several hand rubs, the hands may become sticky, and handwashing should be used to cleanse them.

> ### CLINICAL PEARL
> A typical hand rubbing procedure involves:
> - The removal of all jewelry from the hands and wrists.
> - The cleansing agent is applied from the dispenser to one palm, and the hands are rubbed vigorously together using friction or rubbing motions, covering all surfaces of both hands.
> - The rubbing is continued until the hands are dry, which can take 25 to 30 seconds depending on the product.

- *Handwashing.* Handwashing with soap and water is necessary when organic material such as blood or dirt is visible, when the pathogen is known to be *C. difficile,* in between patients, or after multiple applications of hand rubbing. It is important to avoid touching any potentially contaminated surface during or at the conclusion of the handwashing process. It is important to remember that the sink, soap dispenser, and towel container are considered to be contaminated.

TABLE 8-2 Basic Precautions

Hand hygiene	The single most effective way to protect the patient and the caregiver.
	Should be performed by every caregiver and hospital visitor before or after a treatment or contact with a patient.
	Hand rubbing: advantages include requires less time to use, is more effective than soap and water, is more accessible than sinks, significantly reduces bacterial counts on hand, and causes less damage to the skin than soap and water.
	Handwashing: not the most effective method to decontaminate the hands except when hands are visibly dirty, soiled, or considered to be contaminated. The soap typically includes an antimicrobial or germicidal agent. Many handwashing stations have knee- or foot-operated controls for the faucet. Warm water promotes lather and is less irritating than hot or cold water.
Respiratory hygiene	Often referred to as "cough etiquette." Includes:
	▶ Covering of the mouth and nose with a tissue during a cough or sneeze.
	▶ Coughing or sneezing into the upper sleeve or elbow rather than into the hands, if no tissue is available.
	▶ Hand hygiene after contact with respiratory secretions.
	▶ Maintaining a distance of more than 3 feet from persons with respiratory infections in common waiting areas.
	▶ Wearing a face mask on entering a healthcare facility if one has increased production of infectious respiratory secretions.
Clean environment	▶ Treatment tables or mat tables require regular cleaning, ideally between each use (except in the case where a linen covering or paper sheet is used).
	▶ Linens, including sheets, pillowcases, and towels, should be changed after each use and should be properly laundered and stored.
	▶ Equipment that comes into contact with a patient or with a contaminated area, including such things as goniometers, ambulation devices, ankle weights, and exercise machines, must be cleaned regularly.
	▶ Toys are common clinical items that can serve as pathogen reservoirs; therefore, only toys that can be easily cleaned and disinfected should be provided (avoid the use of stuffed or furry toys). Containers should be designated for toys that have been cleaned and for those that require cleaning.
Disposal of soiled items	All items that have been used by or with a patient are considered soiled, even if no contamination is visible. Linens should be placed in an appropriate laundry container, and gloves should be worn when handling soiled items. Soiled items that have come in contact with the patient's blood or suspected infectious material require special handling and should be disposed of in specially labeled biohazard containers. Hand hygiene should always be performed after disposing of used and soiled items.
Sharps containers	Any instrument capable of puncturing the skin, such as needles and scalpels, must be discarded in a specific container, typically referred to as a "sharps container."

TABLE 8-3 Correct Disposal of Clinical Items

Item	Disposal Method
Instruments and equipment	Cleaned or disposed of according to institutional or agency policies and procedures.
	▶ Contaminated reusable equipment should be placed carefully in a container, labeled, and returned to the appropriate department for sterilization.
	▶ Contaminated disposable items should be placed carefully in a container, labeled, and discarded.
	Staff members who handle contaminated instruments or equipment should wear gloves and wash or rub the hands before and after the gloves have been applied and removed.
Needles, scalpels, and other sharp instruments	Should be placed in puncture-proof containers.
	No attempt should be made to bend, or break the needle before it is discarded according to institutional or agency policies and procedures.
Departmental stethoscope	The ear tips should be wiped with alcohol before and after each use.
Contaminated or soiled linen	Should be disposed of with minimal handling, sorting, and movement according to institutional or agency policies and procedures.
Contaminated dressings, bandages, and other disposable materials	Should be properly placed in a nonporous container or bag, labeled, and discarded according to institutional or agency policies and procedures.

TABLE 8-4   Standard Precautions

Handwashing

1. Wash hands after touching blood, body fluids, secretions, excretions, and contaminated items, whether or not gloves were worn.
2. Wash hands immediately after removing gloves, between patient contacts, and when otherwise indicated to reduce transmission of microorganisms.
3. Wash hands between tasks and procedures on the same patient to prevent cross-contamination of different body sites.
4. Use plain (non-antimicrobial) soap for routine handwashing.
5. An antimicrobial agent or a waterless antiseptic agent may be used for specific circumstances (hyperendemic infections) as defined by infection control.

Gloves

1. Wear gloves (clean, unsterile gloves are adequate) when touching blood, body fluids, secretions, excretions, and contaminated items; put on clean gloves just before touching mucous membranes and nonintact skin.
2. Change gloves between tasks and procedures on the same patient after contact with materials that may contain high concentrations of microorganisms.
3. Remove gloves promptly after use, before touching uncontaminated items and environmental surfaces, and before going on to another patient; wash hands immediately after glove removal to avoid transfer of microorganisms to other patients or environments.

Mask and Eye Protection or Face Shield

1. Wear a mask and eye protection or a spray shield to protect mucous membranes of the eyes, nose, and mouth during procedures and patient care activities that are likely to generate splashes or sprays of blood, body fluids, secretions, and excretions.

Gown

1. Wear a gown (a clean, unsterile gown is adequate) to protect skin and prevent soiling of clothing during procedures and patient care activities that are likely to generate splashes or sprays of blood, body fluids, secretions, and excretions.
2. Select a gown that is appropriate for the activity and the amount of fluid likely to be encountered.
3. Remove a soiled gown as soon as possible and wash hands to avoid transfer of microorganisms to other patients or environments.

Patient Care Equipment

1. Handle used patient care equipment soiled with blood, body fluids, secretions, and excretion in a manner that prevents skin and mucous membrane exposures, contamination of clothing, and transfer of microorganisms to other patients or environments.
2. Ensure that reusable equipment is not used for the care of another patient until it has been cleaned and reprocessed appropriately.
3. Ensure that single-use items are discarded properly.

Environmental Control

1. Follow hospital procedures for the routine care, cleaning, and disinfection of environmental surfaces, beds, bed rails, bedside equipment, and other frequently touched surfaces.

Linen

1. Handle, transport, and process used linen soiled with blood, body fluids, secretions, and excretion in a manner that prevents skin and mucous membrane exposures and contamination of clothing, and avoids transfer of microorganisms to other patients or environments.

Occupational Health and Blood-Borne Pathogens

1. Prevent injuries when using needles, scalpels, and other sharp instruments or devices; when handling sharp instruments and procedures; when cleaning used instruments; and when disposing of used needles.
2. Never recap used needles, or otherwise manipulate them using both hands, or use any other technique that involves directing the point of the needle toward any part of the body; rather, use either a one-handed "scoop" technique or mechanical device designed for holding the needle sheath.
3. Do not remove used needles from disposable syringes by hand, and do not bend, break, or otherwise manipulate used needles by hand.
4. Place used disposable syringes and needles, scalpel blades, or other sharp items in an appropriate puncture-resistant container for transport to the reprocessing area.
5. Use mouthpieces, resuscitation bags, or other ventilation devices as an alternative to mouth-to-mouth resuscitation.

Patient Placement

1. Use a private room for a patient who contaminates the environment or who does not (or cannot be expected to) assist in maintaining appropriate hygiene or environmental control.
2. Consult Infection Control if a private room is not available.

From Centers for Disease Control, Hospital Infection Control Practices Advisory Committee. Part II. Recommendations for Isolation Precautions in Hospitals. February 2007.

CLINICAL PEARL

Handwashing procedure:

▶ All jewelry is removed from the hands and wrists.

▶ The faucet is adjusted (Figure 8-2) until the water is warm and then the wrists and hands are immersed.

▶ Soap is applied (Figure 8-3), water is applied (Figure 8-4), and the hands are washed vigorously using rubbing (Figure 8-5) or friction (Figure 8-6) motions for approximately 15 seconds (or approximately 60 seconds if the hands have contacted body fluids, an infectious wound, or a contaminated surface), making sure that all areas of

the hands and wrists (between the fingers [Figure 8-7], the dorsum of the hands, and the thumbs) are included.

▶ The hands and then wrists are rinsed thoroughly while the hands are directed downward and maintaining no contact with the sink rim or basin (Figures 8-8 and 8-9).

▶ Once the soap lather has been completely removed from all surfaces, the hands are dried with a disposable paper towel while the water continues to flow (Figures 8-10 through 8-12).

▶ The towels used to dry the hands are discarded, and a clean, dry towel is used to turn off the faucet (Figures 8-13 and 8-14) before also being discarded.

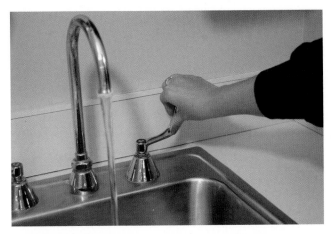

FIGURE 8-2 Handwashing procedure—adjusting the faucet to correct temperature

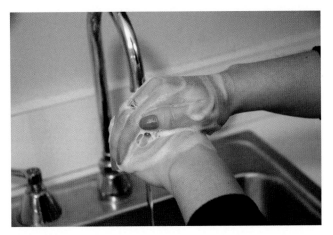

FIGURE 8-5 Handwashing procedure—rubbing motions

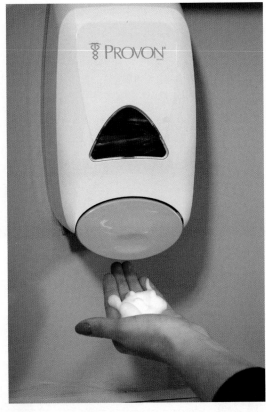

FIGURE 8-3 Handwashing procedure—applying the soap

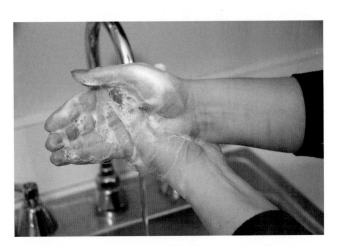

FIGURE 8-6 Handwashing procedure—friction motions

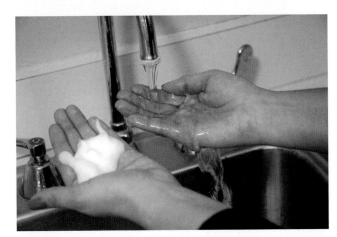

FIGURE 8-4 Handwashing procedure—adding water

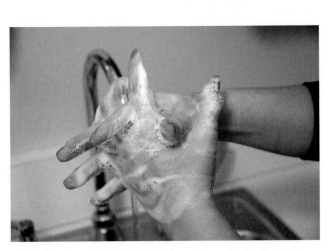

FIGURE 8-7 Handwashing procedure—between the fingers

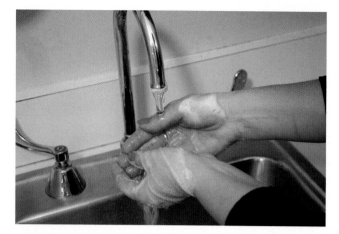

FIGURE 8-8 Hand rinsing procedure—hands are directed downward

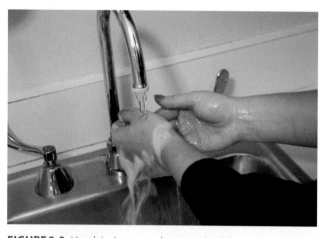

FIGURE 8-9 Hand rinsing procedure—maintaining no contact with the sink rim or basin

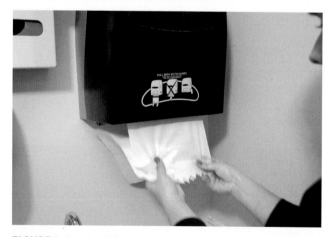

FIGURE 8-10 Hand drying

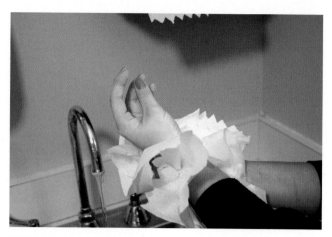

FIGURE 8-11 Hand drying

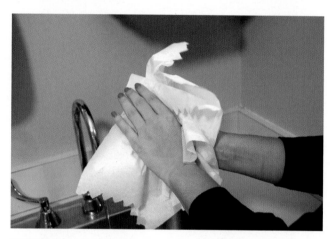

FIGURE 8-12 Hand drying

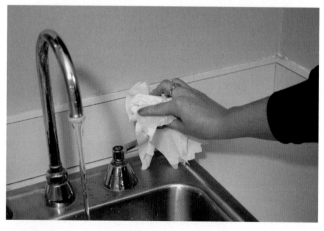

FIGURE 8-13 Turning off the faucet

Transmission-Based Precautions

Transmission-based precautions (Table 8-5) are required for patients known to be at risk for the presence of pathogens. Transmission-based precautions are standard precaution procedures that include additional practices specific to the infectious microorganism's mode of transmission.

Personal Protective Equipment

The use of personal protective equipment (PPE) may be necessary to protect the clinician from the patient, although in some cases PPE can be worn by patients. The amount and type of PPE worn is determined by the likelihood of encountering body fluids and contaminated areas and by the modes

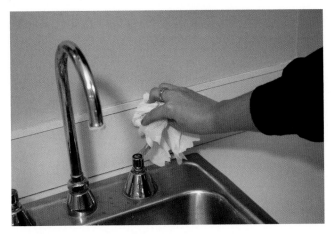

FIGURE 8-14 Turning off the faucet

in which known or suspected pathogens are transmitted. The various types of PPE are described in Table 8-6. Special procedures must be followed when donning and doffing PPE so that the items are donned and doffed in a particular order to avoid contamination.

CLINICAL PEARL

A common axiom used when donning and doffing PPE is "clean to clean and dirty to dirty." When a patient is in protective isolation, the sequence of donning garments is

extremely critical, whereas the garment doffing sequence is less critical. Conversely, when the clinician is to be protected from the patient, the common donning sequence is less critical, whereas the garment doffing sequence is extremely critical. In either scenario, the clinician should perform hand hygiene after removing the gloves and clothing and avoid contact until this has been performed thoroughly.

Hand hygiene should be performed before donning PPE and immediately after removal of PPE. Although each facility has its own specific protocols related to donning and doffing of PPE, an example of such a method follows.

▶ *Donning and doffing gloves.* If exam gloves are donned, no specific techniques are required (Figures 8-15 through 8-17). However, if sterile gloves are being used, a specific (clean) technique must be used (see Clinical Pearl). In either situation, if a tear develops while donning a glove, it should be disposed of and replaced with a new one. Depending on the procedure, the clinician may go through several pairs of sterile gloves in one session. For example, one pair must be used for the removal of the soiled dressings, then a new set is needed to examine and treat the wound, and then a further pair is used to apply a new dressing. Each separate wound is treated as a separate treatment site to prevent cross contamination.

TABLE 8-5	Transmission-Based Isolation Precautions

Airborne Precautions

In addition to Standard Precautions, use Airborne Precautions, or the equivalent, with all patients known or suspected to be infected with serious illness transmitted by airborne droplet nuclei (small-particle residue) that remain suspended in the air and that can be dispersed widely by air currents within a room or over long distance (for example, *Mycobacterium tuberculosis*, measles virus, chickenpox virus).

1. Respiratory isolation room.
2. Wear respiratory protection (mask) when entering room.
3. Limit movement and transport of patient to essential purposes only. Mask patient when transporting out of area.

Droplet Precautions

In addition to Standard Precautions, use Droplet Precautions, or the equivalent, for patients known or suspected to be infected with serious illness due to microorganisms transmitted by large-particle droplets that can be generated by the patient during coughing, sneezing, talking, or the performance of procedures (for example, mumps, rubella, pertussis, influenza).

1. Isolation room.
2. Wear respiratory protection (mask) when entering room.
3. Limit movement and transport of patient to essential purposes only. Mask patient when transporting out of area.

Contact Precautions

In addition to Standard Precautions, use Contact Precautions, or the equivalent, for specified patients known or suspected to be infected or colonized with serious illness transmitted by direct patient contact (and or skin-to-skin contact) or contact with items in patient environment.

1. Isolation room. Complete isolation precaution policies can be found in a healthcare facility's infection control manual.
2. Wear gloves when entering room; change gloves after having contact with infective material; remove gloves before leaving patient's room; wash hands immediately with an antimicrobial agent or waterless antiseptic agent. After glove removal and handwashing, ensure that hands do not touch contaminated environmental items.
3. Wear a gown when entering room if you anticipate your clothing will have substantial contact with the patient, environmental surfaces, or items in the patient's room, or if the patient is incontinent or has diarrhea, ileostomy, colostomy, or wound drainage not contained by dressing. Remove gown before leaving patient's room; after gown removal, ensure that clothing does not contact potentially contaminated environmental surfaces.
4. Single patient use equipment.
5. Limit movement and transport of patient to essential purposes only. Use precautions when transporting patient to minimize risk of transmission of microorganisms to other patients and contamination of environmental surfaces or equipment.

Data from Guideline for isolation precautions in hospitals. Part II. Recommendations for isolation precautions in hospitals. Hospital Infection Control Practices Advisory Committee 2008.

TABLE 8-6	Personal Protective Equipment	
Equipment	**Description of Use**	**Purpose and Precautions**
Gloves	Two types: ▶ Exam—the gloves are clean but have not undergone sterilization. Dispensed singly from a box. ▶ Sterile—have been treated to remove microorganisms. Packaged in pairs and sealed to prevent contamination. Used when there is a potential for coming in contact with a patient's body fluids, direct contact with someone who has an infection, handling equipment or touching surfaces that may be contaminated, or when there is a cut, wound, or break in the skin.	To prevent pathogens entering small cuts, wound, or breaks in the skin. Latex sensitivity is common in healthcare workers. Nonlatex and nonvinyl gloves are available for those who have latex sensitivity.
Gowns	Disposable gowns that are designed to cover the arms and the front of the clinician's body to at least the mid-thigh.	Used to protect the clinician skin and clothing from possible contact with pathogens.
Face protectors	These come in a variety of designs: ▶ Facemask: fits over the clinician's nose and mouth. ▶ Goggles: often worn with facemasks. ▶ Face shield: a combination of a face mask and goggles.	Face masks help protect against the spray of body fluids and secretions but also to prevent the dispersal of potentially infectious respiratory particles. Goggles protect the eyes against splashes from body fluids or chemicals.
Particulate respirators	Fully disposable or reusable face masks designed to filter particulate matter in the air at a higher level than standard surgical masks. The CDC recommends N95 (95% filter with no resistance to oils).	Typically used in the presence of tuberculosis (TB), and severe acute respiratory syndrome (SARS).

CLINICAL PEARL

To don a sterile pair of gloves, the clinician creates a clean field by clearing a surface that is at least 1 to 2 feet away from other objects. The clear surface is then covered with a clean item such as a towel or disposable patient protective barrier, and all items to be used are placed on the clean area. If a sterile field is required, a sterile covering is placed on the work surface by holding only the tips of the edges. Any tape that may be needed to secure dressings is prepared ahead of time by ripping the strips and hanging them from the edge of the work surface, before cleaning the hands again and donning new gloves before proceeding. Once the area has been prepared, the clinician, while taking care not to touch the sterile surface with the hands, opens the inner packet containing the gloves, like a book, with the flaps facing the clinician and without touching the outside of the gloves with the bare hands. Each glove has

a cuff rolled back about 2 inches. The clinician picks up one glove, by the inside of the glove, using one hand, which either is still inside the gown cuff (see above) or is bare. The glove is placed palm down on its proper hand so that the thumb of the glove rests on the thumb of the hand and the fingers of the glove are directed toward the elbow. Grasping the cuff of the glove by the hand or through the cuff of the gown, the clinician covers the cuff over the hand to seal or enclose the hand within the glove cuff, and then gently maneuvers the fingers and hand into the glove, while the other hand remains within the gown sleeve. The other glove is donned in the same manner. Once both gloves have been donned completely, they are held above waist level and should not be allowed to touch the gown or other objects to maintain sterility. If necessary, a sterile towel can be wrapped over the gloved hands to protect them until it is time to treat the patient.

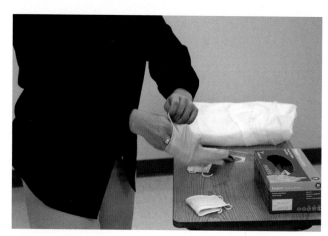

FIGURE 8-15 Donning nonsterile gloves

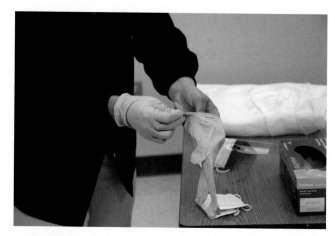

FIGURE 8-16 Donning nonsterile gloves

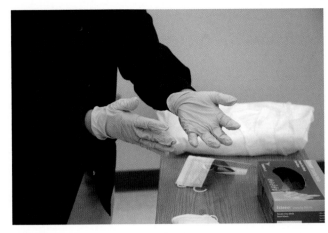

FIGURE 8-17 Donning nonsterile gloves

After treating the patient, the gloves can be removed in any sequence, after which good hand hygiene is performed. The most common method to remove gloves is as follows (Figures 8-18 through 8-21): using one gloved hand to pull the opposite glove away from the hand, then placing the fingers of the bare hand under the remaining glove and using them to remove the glove without touching the outside of the gloves with the bare hands. The gloves are then disposed in the appropriate receptacle (Figure 8-22).

CLINICAL PEARL

Never leave a patient's room while still wearing gloves. Gloves should be removed before leaving the patient's room and washing the hands.

▶ *Donning and doffing a face mask or respirator.* If a face mask or respirator is to be used, the clinician applies it while holding it by its ties or edges (Figure 8-23). The mask or respirator should be positioned on the face so that it fits

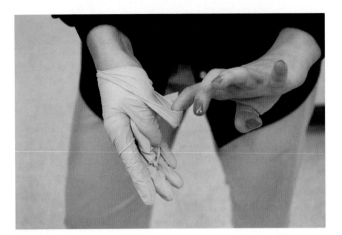

FIGURE 8-20 Doffing nonsterile gloves

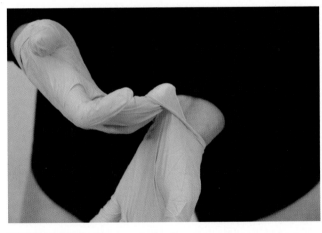

FIGURE 8-18 Doffing nonsterile gloves

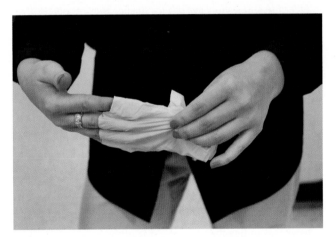

FIGURE 8-21 Doffing nonsterile gloves

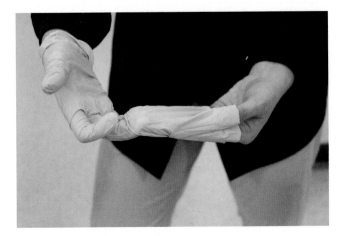

FIGURE 8-19 Doffing nonsterile gloves

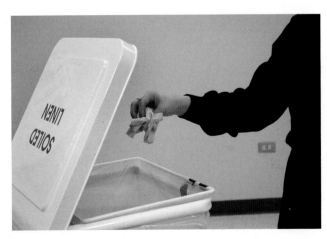

FIGURE 8-22 Disposing of gloves

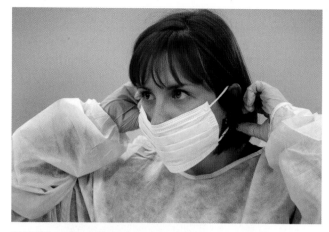

FIGURE 8-23 Applying a face mask

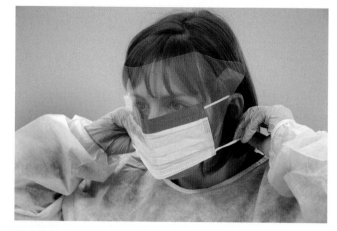

FIGURE 8-25 Donning a face shield

over the nose and under the chin. The upper ties are tied at the middle of the back of the head. The lower ties are tied at the neck while ensuring that the neck or cap is not touched as the mask is being tied. If the mask has a flexible piece designed to fit on the bridge of the nose, the clinician can gently press on the nose piece to contour it for a better fit once the face mask has been donned (Figure 8-24). A mask or respirator can be removed by carefully untying each of the ties and then handling it by the ties while avoiding touching the center of the mask with the hands before being disposed of in an appropriate receptacle.

▶ *Donning and doffing eye or face shields.* If eye protection is necessary, the clinician can apply goggles or a face shield (Figure 8-25). Modern goggles are similar to glasses and are worn accordingly, but some goggles have elastic straps that fit snugly around the head. It is important that the goggles be comfortable, provide good peripheral vision, and ensure a secure fit. In place of a face mask and goggles, a chin-length face shield may be used, although it is important to remember that face shields do not protect against airborne transmission and, therefore, often have to be used in conjunction with a surgical mask, or respirator. Goggles are removed by handling the earpieces or headbands, and not the front of the goggles. Face shields are removed in a similar fashion by touching only the earpieces or headbands at the side of the head before they are disposed of in an appropriate receptacle (Figure 8-26).

▶ *Donning and doffing a disposable gown.* If a gown is required, once the inside of the gown comes into contact with the clinician's clothing it is considered contaminated. The clinician picks up the gown with one hand by grasping the center or neck of the gown and allows it to unfold without letting it touch the body (Figure 8-27). The clinician may need to gently shake the gown, which is folded inside out, so that it opens fully. Once opened fully, the clinician inserts one hand and arm through one sleeve inside the gown (Figure 8-28), maintaining gown-to-gown contact, but not allowing the hand to extend through the gown cuff (if a closed glove technique is to be used) (Figure 8-29). The clinician then places the other arm through the other sleeve in the gown (Figure 8-30), again maintaining gown-to-gown contact and keeping that hand inside the cuff (if a closed glove technique is to be used). Once the clinician has checked to be sure that the gown covers the arms on the front of the body to at least mid-thigh level (Figure 8-31), the straps are tied behind the clinician at the neck (Figures 8-32 through 8-35) and waist (Figures 8-36 and 8-37). After treating the patient, the gown can usually be removed in any sequence such as the one outlined in Figures 8-38 through 8-46, and then good hand hygiene is performed. To remove a gown following isolation precautions, the clinician unties the waist tie of the gown and then carefully unties the neck tie while avoiding touching the neck, cap, or outer

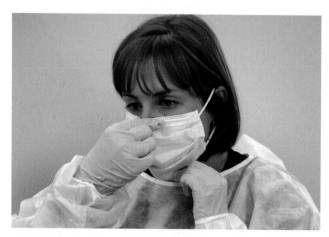

224   **FIGURE 8-24** Pressing on the nose piece to contour it for a better fit

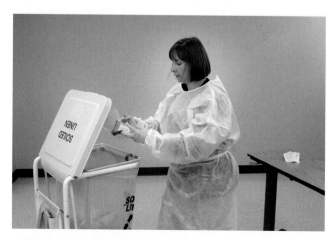

FIGURE 8-26 Disposing of a face shield

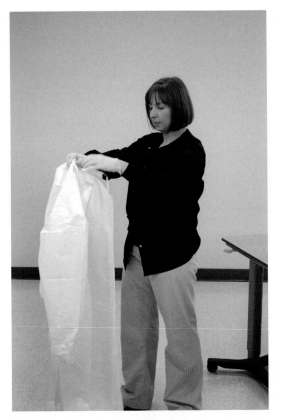

FIGURE 8-27 Allowing the gown to unfold without letting it touch the body

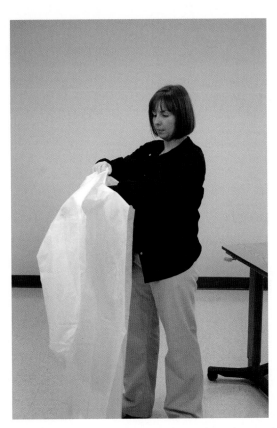

FIGURE 8-28 Inserting one hand and arm through one sleeve inside the gown

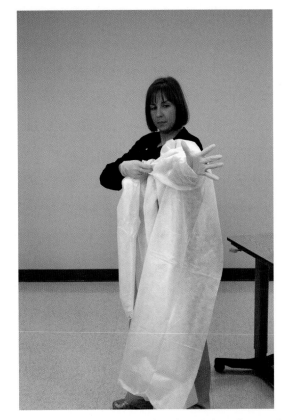

FIGURE 8-29 Inserting one hand and arm through one sleeve inside the gown

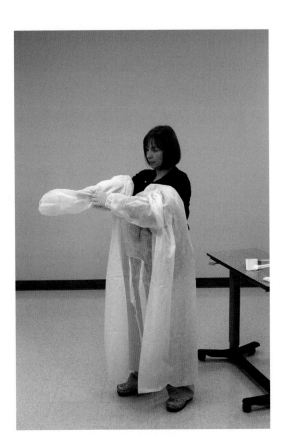

FIGURE 8-30 Placing the other arm through the other sleeve in the gown

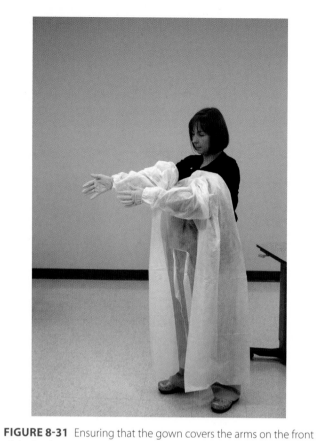

FIGURE 8-31 Ensuring that the gown covers the arms on the front of the body

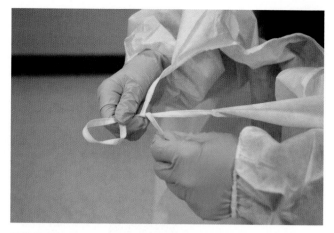

FIGURE 8-33 Sequence of applying and tying the straps behind the clinician at the neck

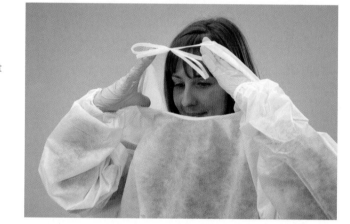

FIGURE 8-34 Sequence of applying and tying the straps behind the clinician at the neck

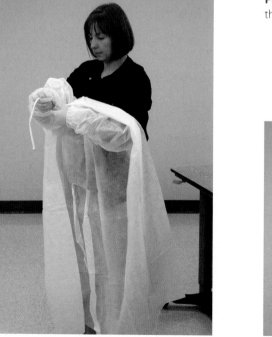

FIGURE 8-32 Sequence of applying and tying the straps behind the clinician at the neck

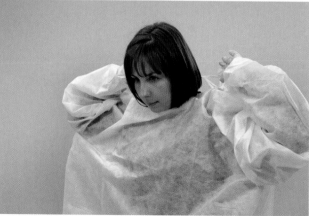

FIGURE 8-35 Sequence of applying and tying the straps behind the clinician at the neck

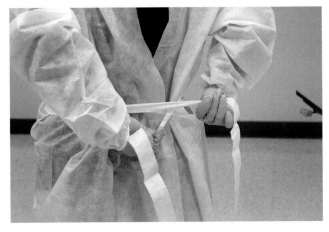

FIGURE 8-36 Tying the straps at the waist

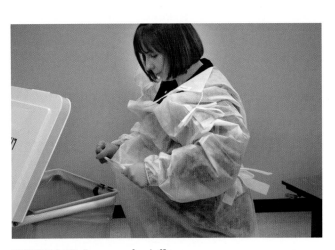

FIGURE 8-39 Sequence for doffing gown

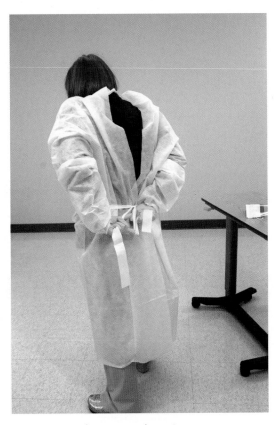

FIGURE 8-37 Tying the straps at the waist

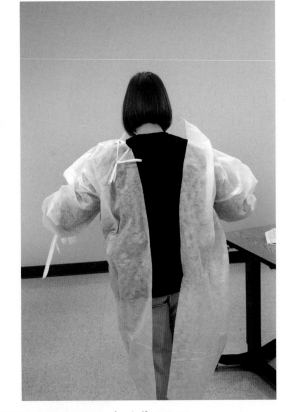

FIGURE 8-40 Sequence for doffing gown

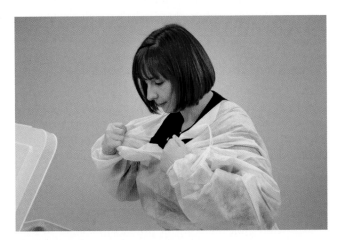

FIGURE 8-38 Sequence for doffing gown

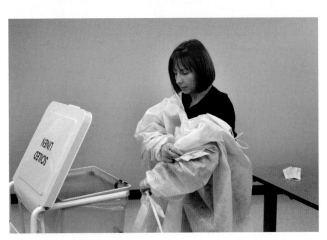

FIGURE 8-41 Sequence for doffing gown

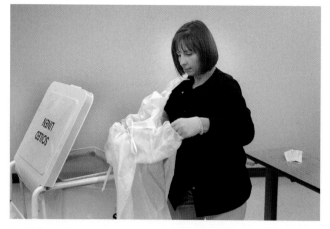

FIGURE 8-42 Sequence for doffing gown

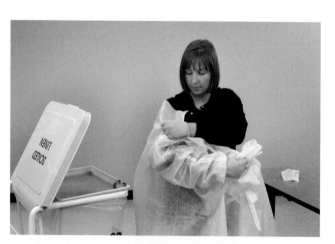

FIGURE 8-43 Sequence for doffing gown

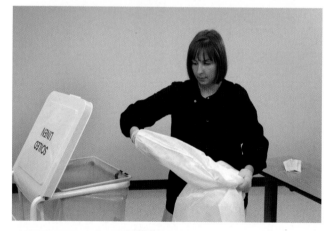

FIGURE 8-44 Sequence for doffing gown

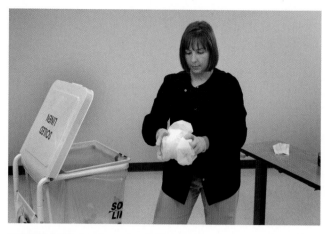

FIGURE 8-45 Sequence for doffing gown

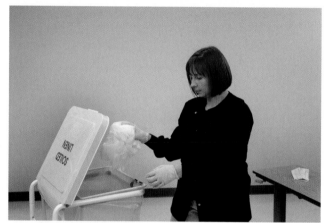

FIGURE 8-46 Sequence for doffing gown

CLINICAL PEARL

The order of gown and glove removal depends on how the gown was used and how contaminated it became. Most often, the gown is removed first.

▶ *Donning and doffing a cap.* If a cap is to be used, the clinician should apply it before donning the gown. The cap should be applied while avoiding touching the head as much as possible, and including all of the head and ears in the cap. To remove a cap, the clinician handles it by its ties or gently grasps the center at the top and lifts it from the head.

Precautions for Special Populations

Certain populations with impaired resistance to infection require extra precautions to protect the patient. These populations include patients who are transplant recipients, including bone marrow transplants, and those undergoing chemotherapy. These precautions include, but are not limited to[8]:

▶ Placing a patient in a private room with the air pressure positive in relation to the corridor outside.

▶ Performing good hand hygiene using an antimicrobial soap before either entering the patient's room or before providing direct patient care.

side of the gown. The clinician then slips both hands under the gown at the neck and shoulders and peels the gown away from the body, turning the sleeves inside out. Grasping the cuffs one of the time by slipping the fingers underneath each of them, each arm is then pulled out of the gown. Then, while holding the inside surface of the gown at the shoulders, the clinician folds or rolls the gown in on itself so that the inner surface of the gown is exposed and the contaminated surfaces are contained within. The gown is then discarded into an appropriate receptacle.

- Permitting only essential personnel and visitors to enter the patient's room and preventing anyone who is ill, or feels like they may be getting sick, from entering.

- Permitting no live plants, fresh fruits, or uncooked vegetables without the approval of the attending physician.

- Allowing the patient to leave his or her room only for essential purposes with the attending physician's permission. If allowed to leave, the patient must wear a surgical mask.

In addition to those populations already mentioned, pediatric and geriatric patients bring their own set of challenges. This is because these populations tend to be at higher risk of infection than other patients, especially when potentially having weakened immune systems as a result of an acquired or congenital health problem. Key precautions with these populations in addition to standard precautions include the implementation of respiratory hygiene and cough-etiquette strategies for patients with suspected influenza or infection with another respiratory-tract pathogen to the extent feasible; separation of infected, contagious children from uninfected children when feasible; and appropriate sterilization, disinfection, and antisepsis.

CLINICAL PEARL

To help prevent a nosocomial infection, and to break the chain of transmission, the clinician should:

- Observe aseptic technique
- Frequently perform handwashing especially between patients
- Perform careful handling, cleaning, and disinfection of fomites
- Where possible, use single-use disposable items
- Enforce patient isolation
- Avoid, where possible, any medical procedures that can lead with high probability to nosocomial infection

THE CRITICAL CARE ENVIRONMENT

Critical care environments have different names depending on the area of specialization:

- ICU—intensive care unit or intermediate care unit
- CCU—coronary care unit or critical care unit
- MICU—medical intensive care unit
- SICU—surgical intensive care unit
- NICU—neurologic intensive care unit or neonatal intensive care unit
- PACU—Postanesthesia care unit

Physical therapists who practice in these critical care settings face a variety of complex challenges. The amount of preparation required to treat patients in this environment requires is more than for a typical hospital setting. Critically ill patients have limited mobility because of tenuous hemodynamic status, multiple central catheters, life-support monitors, artificial airways,

sedative medication, impaired levels of alertness, electrolyte imbalances, multiple medical problems, deconditioning, sleep disturbances, and muscle weakness. The benefits of early mobilization of this population include weaning from mechanical ventilation, improving tissue perfusion, promoting better rest periods, improving emotional state, decreasing the incidence of acquired pressure ulcers, restoring function and mobility, relieving pain, and decreasing the length of stay (thereby reducing healthcare costs). However, mobilizing patients in this environment is not without risk. Catheters and supportive equipment attached to patients can become dislodged and cause injury, and reinsertion of catheters can increase infection risk and cause unwanted stress and pain for patients and families.[9] The treating clinician may find the highly technical environment somewhat daunting, especially as the stakes are high. However, provided that the clinician approaches these situations in a logical and organized manner, a degree of comfort level will be reached fairly quickly. In most cases, orientation is provided to new clinicians, which includes a formal introduction to the nursing staff and other key members of the healthcare team as well as information regarding the equipment and the various treatment protocols. Most critical care environments consist of a series of individualized cubicles, with one patient to each cubicle. Typically, before entering an intensive care unit, the clinician reviews the patient's medical record for any changes in the patient status, any procedures that are scheduled, any special precautions that need to be taken (e.g., respiratory isolation), or any changes in the orders for the patient.

Contained within the medical chart are laboratory values, which provide information about the patient's blood chemistry, blood gases, and urinalysis depending on the patient's diagnosis. Reference laboratory values are provided in Table 8-7.

It is also worth noting whether the patient has a do not resuscitate (DNR) directive in the medical record.

CLINICAL PEARL

In general, if a patient has a DNR status, no attempt is made to administer chest compressions, insert an artificial airway, administer resuscitative drugs, defibrillate, provide respiratory assistance (other than suctioning the airway and administering oxygen), initiate resuscitative IV, or initiate cardiac monitoring. However, the following procedures are generally accepted as part of the DNR status: suctioning of the airway, administering oxygen, positioning the patient for comfort, splinting or immobilization, controlling bleeding, providing pain medication, providing emotional support, and contacting other appropriate healthcare providers. Recently, varying degrees of DNR have been introduced:

- *DNR Comfort Care:* permit comfort care only both before and during a cardiac or respiratory arrest. Resuscitative therapies are not administered before an arrest. This order is generally regarded as appropriate for patients who have a terminal illness, short life expectancy, little chance of surviving CPR, and a desire to let nature take its course in the face of an impending arrest.

- *DNR Comfort Care–Arrest:* Resuscitative therapies will be administered before an arrest but not during an arrest.

TABLE 8-7   Reference Laboratory Values

Profile	Component	Related Physiology	Reference Value	Significance
Arterial blood gases (ABGs)	Arterial PaO$_2$	Reflects the dissolved oxygen level based on the pressure it exerts on the bloodstream.	80–100 mm Hg	A decrease indicates pulmonary dysfunction, e.g. hypoventilation.
	Arterial PaCO$_2$	Reflect the dissolved carbon dioxide level based on the pressure it exerts on the bloodstream.	35–45 mm Hg	Indicates pulmonary dysfunction—hypoventilation leads to an elevation.
	Arterial pH	Reflects the free hydrogen ion concentration.	7.35–7.45	<7.35 = acidosis >7.45 = alkalosis Collectively this test and the arterial PO$_2$ and arterial PCO$_2$ tests help reveal the acid-based status and how well oxygen is being delivered to the body.
	Oxygen saturation (SAO$_2$)	Usually a bedside technique (pulse oximetry) is used to indicate the level of oxygen transport.	95%–98%	During exercise or physical activity, a minimum of 90% saturation should be maintained to avoid hypoxemia.
Fluids and electrolytes	Sodium (Na)	Major extracellular cation that serves to regulate serum osmolality, fluid, and acid-base balance; maintains transmembrane electric potential for neuromuscular functioning.	135–145 mEq/L	*Increased* values found with excessive sweating, hypothalamus disease, diabetes insipidus, hypoadrenalism, excess sodium intake. *Decreased* values found with diuretic medication, kidney disease, congestive heart failure, diabetic ketoacidosis, sweating, severe vomiting and diarrhea.
	Potassium (K)	Major intracellular cation: maintains normal hydration and osmotic pressure.	3.5–5.0 mEq/L	*Increased* values with tissue damage, urinary obstruction, primary adrenal insufficiency, diabetes mellitus. *Decreased* values with prolonged vomiting and diarrhea, diuretic medication, corticosteroid excess.
	Calcium (Ca)	Transmission of nerve impulses, muscle contractility; cofactor in enzyme reactions and blood coagulation.	8.5–10.8 mg/dL; inversely related to phosphorus level	*Increased* values with hyperparathyroidism, carcinoma metastatic to bone, multiple myeloma; loss of neuromuscular excitability and muscle weakness may be seen. *Decreased* values with vitamin D deficiency, malabsorption, kidney disease, hypoparathyroidism; muscle tetany may be observed.
	Phosphorus (PO$_4$)	Integral to structure of nucleic acids, in adenosine triphosphate energy transfer, and in phospholipid function. Phosphate helps to regulate calcium levels, metabolism, base balance, and bone metabolism.	2.6–4.5 mg/dL; inversely related to calcium level	*Increased* values with renal disease, hypoparathyroidism, hyperthyroidism. *Decreased* values with malabsorption, hyperparathyroidism.
Blood Enzymes	Creatine kinase (CK)	An enzyme found predominantly in the heart, brain, and skeletal muscle. Aids in protein catabolism. Can be separated into subunits or isoenzymes, each derived from a specific tissue; CPK-MB = cardiac CPK-MM = skeletal muscle. Blood levels of CPK-MB typically rise within 2 to 6 hours after a heart attack, reach their highest levels within 12 to 24 hours, and fall to normal levels within 3 days.	CK-Total = 25–255 µL/L CK-MB = 0–5.9 mL/L CK-MM = 5–70 µL/L	CK-Total: severe hypokalemia, carbon monoxide poisoning, seizures, pulmonary and cerebral infarctions. CPK-MB: myocardial infarction (an ongoing high level of CPK-MB levels after 3 days may mean that an MI is progressing and more heart muscle is being damaged), post cardiac surgery, muscular dystrophies, polymyositis. CPK-MM: trauma, muscular dystrophy, dermatomyositis, hypothyroidism, seizures.

		Description	Normal values	Clinical significance
	Lactate dehydrogenase (LDH)	Present in all body tissues and is abundant in red blood cells. Acts as a marker for hemolysis. Isoenzymes are LDH 1–5.	105–333 IU/L	LDH 1–2: myocardial infarction, myocarditis, shock, hemolytic and sickle cell anemia. LDH 3: shock, pulmonary infarction. LDH 4: shock. LDH 5: congestive heart failure, shock, hepatitis, cirrhosis, liver congestion.
	Alkaline phosphatase	An enzyme most effective in an alkaline environment. Associated with bone metabolism/calcification and lipid transport.	Adults: 20–140 IU/L Infants to adolescents: Up to 104 IU/L	*Increased* = severe biliary obstruction, cirrhosis, hepatitis. Indicates increased osteoblastic activity: 150–250 IU/L indicates a fracture. 350–700 IU/L indicates active heterotrophic ossification. Used as an indicator for Paget's disease, bone metastasis, osteomalacia, and hyper-parathyroidism. *Decreased* = the healing of bone has ceased (nonunion fracture), or normal finding indicating bone growth has stopped with skeletal maturity.
Cellular blood elements	White blood cells (WBCs)	Produced in bone marrow; provide defense against foreign agents/organisms.	$4.3–10.8 \times 10^9$/L	*Increased* values with infection (bacterial), most illnesses, inflammation, allergic reactions, parasitic infections, leukemias, stress, overall stimulation of bone marrow. *Decreased* values with chemotherapy, bone marrow failure, viral infections, alcoholism, AIDS.
	Red blood cells (RBCs)	Produced in bone marrow, carry oxygen to tissues.	$4.6–6.2 \times 10^{12}$/L (male) $4.2–5.4 \times 10^{12}$/L (female)	*Increased* values with lack of oxygen, smoking, exposure to carbon monoxide, long-term lung disease, diseases of kidney, heart, bone marrow; dehydration, vomiting, diarrhea, sweating, severe burns, diuretics. *Decreased* values with anemia from blood loss (colon cancer), decreased in RBC production (tumor, medication, lack of nutrients), increased RBC destruction (sickle cell disease).
	Hemoglobin (Hgb)	Reflects oxygen-carrying capacity.	14–18 g/dL (male) 13–16 g/dL (female)	Values of 8–10 g/dL typically result in decreased exercise tolerance, increased fatigue, and tachycardia, conditions that may contraindicate aggressive therapeutic measures, including strength and endurance training.
	Hematocrit	Measure of the ratio of packed red blood cells to whole blood.	40–54 mL/dL (male) 37–48 mL/dL (female)	By dividing the hematocrit level by 3, one can approximate the hemoglobin level.
	Platelet count	Reflects potential to address injury to vessel walls, thus regulating homeostasis.		*Increased* values with severe bleeding, infection, strenuous exercise, pregnancy, splenectomy, iron deficiency, rheumatoid arthritis, leukemia. *Decreased* values with infection, vitamin B_{12} or folic acid deficiency, severe internal bleeding, cancer, and autoimmune conditions.

Once the medical record has been reviewed, the clinician then communicates with the nursing staff to get the most recent update on the patient and to inform the nurse responsible for the patient about the activities planned for the patient.

On entering the patient's cubicle, the clinician should begin to systematically observe the equipment on the bed, on the wall, and on the floor. In addition, the clinician should observe the patient and determine the patient's level of arousal and overall condition before proceeding. In most cases, the patient's vital signs will be displayed on a monitor.

If the patient is conscious, the clinician should introduce himself or herself, explain the purpose of the visit, and describe what the patient can expect.

The following sections provide a description of the most common types of equipment and devices that are found in the critical care environment.

Bed Type

Standard Adjustable. The standard hospital bed has two motors: one for the legs and one for the back. These beds can also have a third motor as an option that allows the whole bed to go up and down. The lower portion of the bed is typically hinged so it can be adjusted to provide knee flexion/hip flexion (Fowler's position). The average size for this type of bed is 36 inches wide × 80 inches long. In the interest of safety, these beds are fitted with side rails that can be lifted until a locking mechanism is engaged, and lowered to allow the patient to get out of bed. If a side rail is to be lifted or lowered, the clinician must check that such a movement will not compress or stretch any line, lead, or tube that is connected to the patient, and whenever the patient is returned to the bed, the clinician should ensure that the side rail is in its correct position. The majority of these beds have a device (call button) attached to the side rail that can be used to contact nursing personnel, or a similar device, attached to an electrical cord, is provided for the patient. These beds come with a standard vinyl-covered innerspring or foam mattress, but designs are available for skin shear, reinforced borders to help a patient get in and out of bed, and several layers of foam for circulation, cushioning, pressure relief, and comfort. These beds are typically used with patients who do not require specialized equipment such as those in the late stages of dementia (bed rails can be used as a restraint method for short periods) and postsurgery patients. The benefits of this type of bed are that they ease caregiving, enhance patient comfort, are adjustable, and can help relieve various conditions including:

- Respiratory difficulties
- Patients susceptible to aspiration
- Patients with digestive problems such as reflux
- Cardiac patients

The ability to raise the upper part of the bed aids with activities of daily living such as:

- *Sitting up in bed.* A person is more likely to slip down when in a sitting position in bed if a pillow or wedge is not under his/her knees.
- Eating/drinking using a bed tray.
- Brushing teeth.

If the patient frequently sits up in bed, the clinician should make sure that the patient is educated on correct body alignment and posture. If the patient is unable to self-support good body alignment, the clinician can use pillows to help prop him/her up. A small pillow placed under the head can also increase comfort.

Bariatric. These hospital beds are electrically operated beds with reinforced frames and decks that are designed for people from 600 to 1000 lb depending on the design. The dimensions can be 42 inches wide (600 lb), 48 inches wide (750 lb), and 54 inches wide (1000 lb).

Air Fluidized (Clinitron). These beds contain 1600 lb of silicone-coated glass beads called microspheres through which heated and pressurized air flows through to suspend a polyester cover that supports the patient. The airflow combined with the microspheres develop the properties associated with fluids and provide a contact pressure to the patient's body of only 11 to 15 mm Hg. The indications for this type of bed include patients who have several infected lesions, obese patients with risk of skin deterioration, patients who require skin protection, and patients whose position cannot be altered easily (those with extensive skin grafts and those who require prolonged immobilization). The advantages of using this type of bed include:

▶ Reduced need for topical medication and dressings because the microclimate is favorable for the healing process

▶ Ability to control the temperature of the bed

▶ Reduction in overall skin pressure

When the unit is turned off, the polyester cover becomes a firm surface, which may be beneficial for certain nursing procedures (turning a patient during dressing changes).

In addition to being very expensive, the disadvantages of using this type of bed include:

▶ The polyester cover can be easily punctured.

▶ The air flowing across the patient's skin may cause dehydration.

▶ Tall or obese persons may be uncomfortable in this bed.

▶ The height of the bed surface from the floor is fixed.

▶ These beds tend to be very noisy.

Circular Turning Frame (Circ-O-Lectric Bed or Stryker Wedge). This type of bed has an anterior/posterior frame that is attached to two circular supports, which can move a patient vertically from supine to prone as the circular supports rotate through 180° around a short axis. At any point within their half-circle range during the rotation, the circular supports can be stopped. This type of bed is indicated when skeletal stability and alignment are required. The advantages of using this type of bed include:

▶ One person can safely and easily turn or position a patient.

▶ It provides easy access for a variety of therapeutic interventions.

▶ Attachments can be added to provide traction (cervical) or immobilization.

▶ The unit can be elevated to several heights.

▶ Various patient positioning options are available (e.g., hip and knee flexion, and semirecumbent). In addition, it is possible to position a patient in the fully upright position to allow him or her to step off the bed onto the floor.

The disadvantages of using this type of bed include:

▶ The amount of space required to allow the frames to rotate.

▶ A doorway must be over 7 feet high to allow the bed to pass through.

▶ Increased axial compressive pressure through the patient as he or she is moved into the vertical position during transition.

The use of this bed is contraindicated for unhealed, unstable vertebral fractures, any patient whose skin is susceptible to shearing and pressure, and any patient who suffers from motion sickness, vertigo, nausea, or orthostatic hypotension.

Posttrauma Mobility (Keane, Roto-rest). This type of bed is designed to maintain a seriously injured patient in a stable position and to maintain proper postural alignment through the use of adjustable bolsters. The bed, which is designed to oscillate from side to side in a cradle-like motion to reduce the amount of prolonged pressure on the patient's skin, is indicated for patients with restricted respiratory function, advanced or multiple pressure sores, severe neurologic deficits, and those who require stabilization and skeletal alignment after extensive trauma (spinal injuries, with or without the complication of paraplegia or quadriplegia, and also for head injuries and certain orthopedic cases to help manage patients at risk for pulmonary complications as a result of immobility).

The side-to-side motion provided by the bed improves upper respiratory function, reduces the need to turn the patient, provides environmental stimulation for the neurologically impaired patient, reduces urinary stasis, and improves bowel function. However, there are a number of disadvantages associated with this type of bed, including:

▶ The constant motion of the bed may induce motion sickness.

▶ Exercising may be restricted by bolsters and alignment supports.

▶ The bed requires a lot of room to oscillate.

Low Air Loss (Alternating Pressure) Therapy. These mattresses feature air flow throughout the sacral and torso areas to help minimize skin maceration by reducing excess moisture under patient. These mattress systems are available to fit all standard hospital beds including pediatric, geriatric, and bariatric configurations and are a proven way to help prevent and treat pressure ulcers by suspending the patient on several segmental air-filled cells while circulating air across the skin to reduce moisture and help maintain a constant skin interface pressure. The user has the ability to electronically adjust the amount of air pressure in each cell and to electronically adjust the bed to several different positions, including hip and knee flexion, sitting, or a semirecumbent position. This type of bed is indicated for patients who require prolonged immobilization, patients who are high risk of developing pressure ulcers or who have existing ulcers, patients who are obese, and those patients whose condition requires frequent elevation of the trunk. The advantages of this type of bed are that the patient's weight is measured by the sensors in the bed and the air bladders are inflated or deflated automatically to correctly distribute the patient's weight. The disadvantages of this type of bed include:

▶ The air cells can be punctured or torn by sharp objects.

▶ The patient's position must be frequently altered to prevent pressure ulcers.

Lines, Leads, and Tubes

Intravenous (IV) Line. IV lines are used for a number of purposes:

- To infuse fluids, nutrients, electrolytes, and medications via a plastic bag that measures the number of drops of fluid administered per minute

- To obtain venous blood samples

- To insert catheters into the central circulatory system

IVs are most commonly placed in the forearm or back of the hand. Complications associated with IV administration include cellulitis, phlebitis, thrombosis, sepsis, air embolus, and pulmonary thromboembolism.

Hickman Line. A central venous line/catheter most often used for the administration of chemotherapy or other medications, measurement of central venous pressure, or for the withdrawal of blood. Unlike the single entry point of an IV line, the Hickman has both an entry and exit point. The entry is usually through the jugular vein in the neck, and the catheter is then run through part of the body until it reaches the tip of the right atrium. It emerges from there and is attached to two or three tubes that are exterior to the chest. As with most permanent IV lines or catheters, the Hickman can be prone to infection. Because the line is inserted into the major veins, this can be very serious.

Nasogastric (NG) Tube. A flexible tube connected to an electric pump is passed through the nose and down through the nasopharynx and esophagus into the stomach, which provides access to the stomach for diagnostic and therapeutic purposes (feeding and administering drugs and other oral agents directly into the GI tract). Before treating a patient who is on an NG tube, the pump must be stopped and the patient positioned in an upright or semiupright position for at least 30 minutes (1 hour for pediatric patients) before supine activities.

Enterostomy Feeding Tube. A flexible feeding tube (percutaneous endoscopic gastrostomy/jejunostomy [PEG/PEJ]) that is inserted by endoscopic or a small surgical opening in the abdomen so that nutritional solutions can be conveyed directly into the stomach or jejunum through a tube. The main difference between a PEG and a PEJ is that the physician inserts the PEG tube percutaneously into the stomach with an endoscope, whereas the PEJ tube is inserted into the intestine to the jejunum.

Endotracheal Tube. An endotracheal tube is a specific type of artificial airway for a patient who is unable to oxygenate/ventilate independently. A large-diameter flexible tube can be inserted through the mouth (orotracheal) or nose (nasotracheal). Verification of correct placement is done by x-ray. Once correctly placed, the tube must not be moved unless there is a written order from the physician.

Chest Tube (Pleur-Evac). This is a flexible plastic tube that is surgically inserted through an incision on the side of a patient's chest and into the pleural space. It is used to remove air (pneumothorax) if placed in the anterior or lateral chest wall, fluid (pleural effusion, blood, chyle) if placed inferiorly and posteriorly, or pus (empyema) from the intrathoracic space, using mediastinal tubes. The chest tube is connected to one to three large bottles, which are responsible for collecting air/fluid without permitting the lung to collapse. The clinician should avoid activities that pull on these tubes because if they are accidentally dislodged or disconnected from the bottle, the patient's lung will collapse completely.

Jackson-Pratt Drain. A drainage device, which consists of a surgical tube connected to a suction bulb, that is used to pull excess fluid from the body by constant suction.

Autofusion Surgical Drain (Hemovac or Autovac). A disposable, self-contained postsurgical drain that is used to remove pus, blood, or other fluids from a wound. Before a treatment session, the clinician should ask the nursing staff to empty any drain that is more than half full.

Patient-controlled Analgesia (PCA). PCA is commonly assumed to imply on-demand, intermittent, IV administration of opioids under patient control—a sophisticated microprocessor-controlled infusion pump delivers a preprogrammed dose of opioid when the patient pushes a demand button.

Catheters

Indwelling Urinary (Foley) Catheter. This type of catheter is inserted into the bladder via the urethra. Urinary catheters are used to drain the bladder in cases of:

- Urinary incontinence (leaking urine or being unable to control urination)

- Urinary retention (being unable to empty the bladder on demand)

- Surgery on the prostate or genitals

- Other medical conditions such as multiple sclerosis, spinal cord injury, or dementia

An indwelling urinary catheter is one that is left in the bladder. It is held in place in the bladder by a small balloon. The urine drains through plastic tubing into a collection bag, bottle, or urinal. Complications associated with urinary catheters include infection of the urinary tract or bladder, development of a urethral fistula, and kidney failure. Before starting a treatment session, the clinician should drain urine from the catheter tubing. During treatment sessions, the clinician should ensure that the collection bag is always placed below the level of the bladder. Any signs of foul-smelling urine, cloudy dark urine, or urine with blood in it should be reported to the patient's physician or nurse.

Suprapubic Catheter. This type of catheter is inserted directly into the bladder through a small incision in the stomach and the bladder. Indications for a suprapubic catheter include:

- Failed trial using a urethral catheter

- Long-term use (if left in for long periods, urethral catheters can lead to acquired hypospadias and recurrent/chronic urinary tract infections [UTIs])

Contraindications include:

- Lower abdominal incisions, which can lead to adhesions
- Pelvic fracture

Complications associated with this type of catheter include:

- UTIs
- Blockages
- Bladder stones
- Bladder cancer

The clinician should use caution to avoid placing a gait or transfer belt directly over the insertion site.

Colostomy Bag. A colostomy is a surgical procedure in which a stoma is formed by drawing the healthy end of the large intestine or colon through an incision in the anterior abdominal wall and suturing it into place via an ostomy. This opening, in conjunction with the attached stoma appliance, provides an alternative channel for feces to leave the body. People with colostomies must wear an ostomy pouching system to collect intestinal waste. Ordinarily the pouch must be emptied or changed a couple of times a day depending on the frequency of activity; in general the further from the anus (i.e., the further "up" the intestinal tract) the ostomy is located, the greater the output and more frequent the need to empty or change the pouch.

Rectal Tube. The purpose of a rectal tube is to remove gas from the lower intestines or to remove or contain fecal matter. The collection bag should be kept below the level of the tube.

Life-Support Equipment

Mechanical Ventilator. A machine that generates a controlled flow of gas into a patient's airways using positive pressure from oxygen and air received from cylinders or wall outlets. The incoming gas is pressure reduced and blended according to the prescribed inspired oxygen tension (FiO_2), accumulated in a receptacle within the machine, and then delivered to the patient using one of many available modes of ventilation. Flow is either volume targeted and pressure variable, or pressure limited and volume variable. There are two phases in the respiratory cycle, high lung volume and lower lung volume (inhalation and exhalation). Gas exchange occurs in both phases. Inhalation serves to replenish alveolar gas. Prolonging the duration of the higher volume cycle enhances oxygen uptake, while increasing intrathoracic pressure and reducing time available for CO_2 removal. A variety of mechanical ventilators exist including:

▸ *Positive pressure.* These ventilators require an artificial airway (endotracheal or tracheostomy tube) and use positive pressure to force gas into a patient's lungs. Inspiration can be triggered either by the patient or the machine. There are four types of positive-pressure ventilators:

  ■ *Volume-cycled.* This type, which is the most commonly used in critical care environments, delivers a preset tidal volume then allows passive expiration. This is ideal for patients with acute respiratory distress syndrome (ARDS) or bronchospasm, since the same tidal volume is delivered regardless of the amount of airway resistance.

  ■ *Pressure-cycled.* These ventilators, which are also commonly used in the critical care environment, deliver gases at a preset pressure, then allow passive expiration. The benefit of this type is a decreased risk of lung damage from high inspiratory pressures, which is particularly beneficial for neonates who have a small lung capacity. The disadvantage is that the tidal volume delivered can decrease if the patient has poor lung compliance and increased airway resistance.

This type of ventilation is usually used for short-term therapy (less than 24 hours). Some ventilators have the capability to provide both volume-cycled and pressure-cycled ventilation.

  ■ *Flow-cycled.* This type delivers oxygenation until a preset flow rate is achieved during inspiration.

  ■ *Time-cycled.* This type delivers oxygenation over a preset time period. These types of ventilators are not used as frequently as the volume-cycled and pressure-cycled ventilators.

▸ *Negative pressure.* Negative-pressure ventilation is typically only used in a few situations. These units allow negative pressure to be applied only to the patient's chest by using a combination of a form-fitted shell and a soft bladder. Rather than connecting to an artificial airway as with the more modern ventilators, these ventilators were designed to enclose the body from the outside so that when the gas is pulled out of the ventilator chamber, the resulting negative pressure causes the chest wall to expand, which pulls air into the lungs. For exhalation to occur, cessation of the negative pressure causes the chest wall to fall. These devices can be used for patients with neuromuscular disorders, especially those with some residual muscular function, because they do not require a tracheostomy with its inherent problems.

Modes of Ventilation

The mode of ventilation refers to how a machine ventilates the patient in relation to the patient's own respiratory efforts (http://www.enotes.com/ventilators-reference/ventilators).

Control Ventilation (CV). CV, which delivers the preset volume or pressure regardless of the patient's own inspiratory efforts, is used for patients who are unable to initiate their own breath. If it is used with spontaneously breathing patients, they must be sedated and/or pharmacologically paralyzed so they do not breathe out of synchrony with the ventilator.

Assist-control Ventilation (AC) or Continuous Mandatory Ventilation (CMV). AC or CMV, which delivers a preset volume or pressure in response to the patient's inspiratory effort, initiates the breath if the patient does not do so within a preset amount of time. This mode is used for patients who can initiate a breath but who have weakened respiratory muscles. The patient may need to be sedated to limit the number of spontaneous breaths, as hyperventilation can occur in patients with high respiratory rates.

Synchronous Intermittent Mandatory Ventilation (SIMV). SIMV, which delivers a preset volume or pressure and a preset respiratory rate while allowing the patient to breathe spontaneously, initiates each breath in synchrony with the patient's breaths. SIMV is used as a primary mode of ventilation as well as a weaning mode. (During weaning, the preset rate is gradually reduced, allowing the patient to slowly return to breathing independently.) The disadvantage of this mode is that it may increase the effort of breathing and cause respiratory muscle fatigue. (Breathing spontaneously through ventilator tubing has been compared to breathing through a straw.)

Positive-end Expiratory Pressure (PEEP). PEEP, which is positive pressure that is applied by the ventilator at the end of expiration, does not deliver breaths but is used as an adjunct to CV, AC, and SIMV to improve oxygenation by opening collapsed alveoli at the end of expiration. Complications from the increased pressure can include decreased cardiac output, lung rupture, and increased intracranial pressure.

Constant Positive Airway Pressure (CPAP). CPAP is similar to PEEP, except that it works only for patients who are breathing spontaneously. The effect of CPAP (and PEEP) is compared to inflating a balloon but not letting it completely deflate before inflating it again. The second inflation is easier to perform because resistance is decreased. CPAP can also be administered using a mask and CPAP machine for patients who do not require mechanical ventilation but who need respiratory support (for example, patients with sleep apnea).

Pressure Support Ventilation (PSV). PS is preset pressure that augments the patient's spontaneous inspiration effort and decreases the work of breathing. The patient completely controls the respiratory rate and tidal volume. PS is used for patients with a stable respiratory status and is often used with SIMV during weaning.

Independent Lung Ventilation (ILV). This method is used to ventilate each lung separately in patients with unilateral lung disease or a different disease process in each lung. It requires a double-lumen endotracheal tube and two ventilators. Sedation and pharmacologic paralysis are used to facilitate optimal ventilation and increase comfort for the patient in whom this method is used.

High-frequency Ventilation (HFV). HFV delivers a small amount of gas at a rapid rate (as many as 60 to 100 breaths per minute). It is used when conventional mechanical ventilation would compromise hemodynamic stability, during short-term procedures, or for patients who are at high risk for lung rupture. Sedation and/or pharmacologic paralysis are required.

Inverse Ratio Ventilation (IRV). The normal inspiratory: expiratory ratio is 1:2, but this is reversed during IRV to 2:1 or greater (a maximum of 4:1). This method is used for patients who are still hypoxic, even with the use of PEEP. Longer inspiratory time increases the amount of air in the lungs at the end of expiration (the functional residual capacity) and improves oxygenation by reexpanding any collapsed alveoli. The shorter expiratory time prevents the alveoli from collapsing again. This method requires sedation and therapeutic paralysis because it is very uncomfortable for the patient.

Monitoring Equipment

Arterial Line. The arterial line (A-line) is connected to a pressure transducer that provides a way to constantly measure a patient's blood pressure and also provides access for frequent blood sampling, thereby avoiding repeated needle punctures. An A-line is typically inserted into one of four arteries: radial, femoral, dorsal pedal, or axillary. Arterial lines are usually changed every 4 to 5 days to decrease the risk of infection. Accidental displacement of an A-line is a life-threatening emergency, as significant blood loss can occur very quickly unless direct pressure is promptly applied to the insertion site.

Cardiac Leads. A series of 12 leads that are connected to the anterior chest to monitor electrical activity of the heart.

Pulse Oximeter. A noninvasive method allowing the monitoring of the saturation of a patient's hemoglobin levels in the blood. Usually, an external clip is attached to the patient's fingertip or earlobe.

Pulmonary Artery Catheterization (Swan-Ganz). Initially developed for the management of acute myocardial infarction, this catheter has gained widespread use in the management of a variety of critical illnesses and surgical procedures such as the diagnosis of idiopathic pulmonary hypertension, valvular disease, intracardiac shunts, cardiac tamponade, and pulmonary embolus (PE). The catheter is inserted into the internal jugular or the femoral vein and is then glided into the basilic or subclavian vein, before being passed into the pulmonary artery. The catheter is designed to provide accurate and continuous measurements of pulmonary artery pressure, which can detect even subtle changes in a patient's cardiovascular system. Accidental displacement of this device creates a life-threatening emergency for the patient, as significant blood loss can occur very quickly unless direct pressure is promptly applied to the insertion site.

Intracranial Pressure (ICP) Monitor. Cerebrospinal fluid (CSF) is a colorless, clear fluid produced by the highly vascular choroid plexus in the lateral third and fourth ventricles that functions as a cushion for the brain and spinal cord. ICP monitoring, which calculates the pressure exerted against the skull by brain tissue, blood, or CSF, is a common practice when treating intracranial pathology with risk for elevated ICP, including patients who have sustained a closed head injury, a cerebral hemorrhage, or an overproduction of CSF. When the brain suffers an insult or injury, changes occur that affect cerebral hemodynamics, including changes in ICP, cerebral blood flow, and oxygen delivery. ICP data are very useful to help predict outcomes and worsening intracranial pathology, such as cerebral edema or hemorrhage. Intraventricular catheters, which are antibiotic-impregnated and coated ventricular catheters to prevent infections, are considered the gold standard for measuring ICP because they are placed directly into the ventricle and are attached to a pressure transducer. An external ventricular device can assist with controlling increased ICP by allowing for therapeutic CSF drainage.

CLINICAL PEARL

Extreme care must be taken with patients who have an ICP inserted when raising the head of the bed (increases the drainage, thereby lowering the ICP) or lowering the head of the bed (increases the ICP). In addition, activities such as isometric exercises and the Valsalva maneuver have been shown to increase ICP and should therefore be avoided. Other precautions include:

▶ Avoiding hip flexion greater than 90°

▶ Avoiding neck flexion

▶ Avoiding placing the patient in the prone position

▶ Avoid lowering the patient's head more than 15° below horizontal

Oxygen Delivery Systems

Nasal Cannula. A device with two plastic prongs, which are inserted into each of the patient's nostrils, to deliver supplemental oxygen or airflow to a patient who requires low to moderate concentrations of oxygen.

Oronasal Mask. A triangular plastic device covered with small vent holes that covers the patient's nose and mouth and allows exhaled air to be expelled.

Tracheotomy/Tracheostomy. This is a method to provide a semipermanent, or permanent, oxygen delivery system to a patient via an incision on the anterior aspect of the neck to form a direct connection with the trachea and to allow a patient to breathe without the use of his or her mouth or nose. The tracheostomy tube is a 2- to 3-inch-long (51- to 76-mm) curved metal or plastic tube that is connected to a wall unit via a long plastic tube that is inserted into a tracheostomy stoma to maintain a patent lumen. This type of procedure is usually not used unless the patient has had an endotracheal tube in for an extended period of time and is unable to be weaned from the ventilator. Indications in the acute setting include severe facial trauma, head and neck cancers, and large congenital tumors of the head and neck. Indications in the chronic setting include the need for long-term mechanical ventilation and tracheal hygiene.

THE GRIEVING PROCESS

It is not uncommon for a healthcare provider to encounter a patient who has suffered the loss of someone or something close to them (loved one, pet, a job, or possibly a role—entering retirement). Grief, itself, is a normal and natural response to a loss, so it is important to realize that acknowledging the grief promotes the healing process. There are a variety of ways in which individuals respond to loss, some healthy and some that may hinder the grieving process.

CLINICAL PEARL

Factors that can hinder the grieving process include:

▶ Avoidance or minimization of one's emotions

▶ Use of alcohol or drugs to self-medicate

▶ Use of work (overfunction at workplace) to avoid feelings

Healthy responses to grief include:

▶ Allowing sufficient time to experience thoughts and feelings openly to self.

▶ Acknowledging and accepting all feelings, both positive and negative.

▶ Using a journal to document the healing process.

▶ Confiding in a trusted individual.

▶ Expressing feelings openly. Crying offers a release.

▶ Identifying any unfinished business and attempting to come to a resolution.

▶ Attending bereavement groups—this can provide an opportunity to share grief with others who have experienced similar loss.

Invariably an individual passes through a series of stages during the grieving process. These stages reflect a variety of reactions that may surface as an individual makes sense of how a loss affects them. Experiencing and accepting all feelings remains an important part of the healing process. Elizabeth Kübler-Ross[10] identified a number of stages that occur during the grieving process:

▶ *Stage 1:* Shock, numbness, and denial.

  ■ Shock usually occurs as the initial reaction to a psychological trauma or severe and sudden physical injury.[11] During stressful situations, individuals express themselves through physiologic and emotional responses. These reactions serve to protect the individual from an overwhelming experience.

  ■ Numbness is a normal reaction to an immediate loss and should not be confused with "lack of caring."

  ■ Denial is often used as a defense mechanism to alleviate anxiety and pain associated with a disability or illness.[11] Denial, and feelings of disbelief, occur as a specific phase early in the adaptation process and serve to protect the person from having to confront the overwhelming implications of illness or injury at once.[11] Denial and disbelief will diminish as the individual slowly acknowledges the impact of this loss and accompanying feelings.

It is common for people to avoid making decisions or taking action at this point.

▶ *Stage 2:* Anger. This reaction usually occurs when an individual feels helpless and powerless. Anger may result from feeling abandoned, occurring in cases of loss through death. Feelings of resentment may occur toward one's higher power or toward life in general for the injustice of this loss. After an individual acknowledges anger, guilt may surface because of expressing these negative feelings.

Making decisions at this point is difficult because an individual's energy is focused on the emotion rather than on problem solving.

▶ *Stage 3:* Depression and detachment. After recognizing the true extent of the loss, some individuals may experience depressive symptoms. Sleep and appetite disturbance, lack of energy and concentration, and crying spells are some typical symptoms. Feelings of loneliness, emptiness, isolation, and self-pity can also surface during this phase, contributing to this reactive depression. For many, this phase must be experienced in order to begin reorganizing one's life.

▶ *Stage 4:* Dialogue and bargaining. People become more willing to explore alternatives after expressing their feelings. At times, individuals may ruminate about what could have been done to prevent the loss. Individuals can become preoccupied with ways that things could have been better, imagining all the things that will never be. This reaction can provide insight into the impact of the loss; however, if not properly resolved, intense feelings of remorse or guilt may hinder the healing process. This phase may be marked by externalized hostility toward other people or objects in the environment.

► *Stage 5:* Acceptance. Time allows the individual an opportunity to resolve the range of feelings that surface. Acknowledgment is the first sign that the patient has accepted or recognized the permanency of the condition and its future implications.[11] Decisions are much easier to make because people have found new purpose and meaning as they have begun to accept the loss. Adjustment is the final phase in adaptation and involves the development of new ways of interacting successfully with others and one's environment.[11]

Physical Therapy Approach During the Grieving Process

► Discuss quality-of-life issues with patient/family.

► Make time for grief work.

► Focus on the positive: realize and maximize all clinical opportunities.

► Learn to deal with the patient's or family's anger during the discharge crisis.

► Realize the importance of comfort measures and pain management to patient/family.

► Work with appropriate pastoral supports.

► Try to engage the patient's interest in things.

► Respect the needs of privacy, independence, and decathexis (the gradual weakening and separating of emotional ties) on the part of the patient.

REFERENCES

1. Decoster A, Grandbastien B, Demory MF, et al: A prospective study of nosocomial-infection-related mortality assessed through mortality reviews in 14 hospitals in Northern France. J Hosp Infect 80:310-315, 2012.
2. Goodman CC, Kelly Snyder TE: Infectious disease, in Goodman CC, Boissonnault WG, Fuller KS (eds): Pathology: Implications for the Physical Therapist (ed 2). Philadelphia, Saunders, 2003, pp 194-235.
3. Bass JW, Wittler RR, Weisse ME: Social smile and occult bacteremia. Pediatr Infect Dis J 15:541, 1996.
4. Eady EA, Cove JH: Staphylococcal resistance revisited: community-acquired methicillin resistant *Staphylococcus aureus*—an emerging problem for the management of skin and soft tissue infections. Curr Opin Infect Dis 16:103-124, 2003.
5. Wong KH, Lee SS, Chan KC: Twenty years of clinical human immunodeficiency virus (HIV) and acquired immunodeficiency syndrome (AIDS) in Hong Kong. Hong Kong Med J 12:133-140, 2006.
6. Goodman CC: The immune system, in Goodman CC, Boissonnault WG, Fuller KS (eds): Pathology: Implications for the Physical Therapist (ed 2). Philadelphia, Saunders, 2003, pp 153-193.
7. Black JG: Epidemiology and nosocomial infections, in Microbiology: Principles and Applications (ed 7). Upper Saddle River, NJ, Prentice Hall, 2008, pp 426-462.
8. University of North Carolina Hospitals: Understanding isolation precautions: http://www.unc.edu/~rlensley/tb2.htm#PROTECTIVE, UNC Hospitals' Precautions for the Prevention of Disease Transmission: Protective Precautions.
9. Adler J, Malone D: Early mobilization in the intensive care unit: a systematic review. Cardiopulm Phys Ther J 23:5-13, 2012.
10. Kübler-Ross E: On Death and Dying. New York, Macmillan, 1969.
11. Precin P: Influence of psychosocial factors on rehabilitation, in O'Sullivan SB, Schmitz TJ (eds): Physical Rehabilitation (ed 5). Philadelphia, FA Davis, 2007, pp 27-63.

CHAPTER 9

Monitoring Vital Signs

CHAPTER OBJECTIVES

At the completion of this chapter,
the reader will be able to:

1. List the vital signs that are used to help determine a patient's status

2. Explain the importance of monitoring each of the vital signs

3. Describe the signs and symptoms that would warrant an assessment of the vital signs

4. List some of the variables that can affect the accuracy of the vital signs

5. Describe the correct techniques to assess heart rate

6. Describe the correct techniques to assess respiration rate

7. Describe the correct techniques to assess blood pressure

8. Describe the correct techniques to assess temperature

9. List the various tools that are available for the assessment of pain

10. Describe how to respond to an emergency situation

OVERVIEW

The triad of pulse, respiration rate, and blood pressure is often considered as a baseline indicator of a patient's health status, which is why each is called a vital or cardinal sign. All four practice patterns in the *Guide to Physical Therapist Practice*[1] include the measurement of pulse, blood pressure, and respiration as a routine part of any physiologic examination. Temperature is not included in the practice patterns because it is not routinely assessed by physical therapists. However, as temperature can often provide an important clue to the severity of the patient's illness, particularly the presence of infection, it is discussed in this chapter. Additional measurements of physiologic status, which are not universally considered vital signs, include the assessment of perceived exertion ratings, pain, and pulse oximetry.

Depending on the health history and familiarity with a patient, the taking of vital signs should be a standard procedure for all patients. Clinical indicators that highlight the need for an assessment of vital signs include dyspnea, hypertension, fatigue, syncope, chest pain, irregular heart rate, cyanosis, intermittent claudication, nausea, diaphoresis, and pedal edema. Certain patient populations also warrant a vital sign assessment, including elderly patients (older than 65 years), very young patients (younger than two years), debilitated patients, patients with a history of physical inactivity, and patients recovering from recent trauma. The measurement of vital signs can be used to establish goals and to assess a patient's response to activity.

CLINICAL PEARL

The taking of vital signs can be delegated to a physical therapist assistant (PTA).

It is worth remembering that a number of variables can influence the results of the vital signs measurements. These include caffeine consumption, alcohol consumption, tobacco use, physical activity level, medications, and the use of illegal drugs.[2] The other variables that can influence the results are outlined in Table 9-1.

CLINICAL PEARL

▶ Pulse oximetry (Figure 9-1) is an important related measure, as it provides information on arterial blood oxygen saturation levels.

▶ Pain is considered by many to be a vital symptom.[3–12]

HEART RATE

When the heart muscle of the left ventricle contracts, blood is ejected into the aorta, and the aorta stretches (see Chapter 4). At this point, the wave of distention (pulse wave) is most pronounced and can be detected as a pulse at certain points around the body. The pulse rate (or frequency) is the number of pulsations (peripheral pulse waves) per minute.

TABLE 9-1	Variables That Can Influence Vital Signs Data
Hormonal status	
Age	
Stress	
Obesity	
Diet	
Gender	
Family history	
Time of day	
Menstruation	
General health status	
Pain	

CLINICAL PEARL

In most people, the pulse is an accurate measure of heart rate. However, in certain cases, including arrhythmias, the heart rate can be (much) higher than the pulse rate. In these cases, the heart rate should be determined by auscultation of the central pulse at the heart apex (fifth interspace, midclavicular vertical line, also known as the apical pulse or point of maximal impulse [PMI]). The pulse deficit (difference between heart beats and pulsations at the periphery) is determined by simultaneous palpation at the radial artery and auscultation at the heart apex. Except in the case of cardiac disease or peripheral arterial disease, the apical and radial pulse rates will be equal. If there is a difference between the apical and radial pulse rates, only the apical pulse should be used to assess the patient, and the differences should be noted in the patient's medical record.

The pulse, measured in beats per minute (bpm), is taken to obtain information about the resting state of the cardiovascular system and the system's response to activity or exercise and recovery.[13] Such information includes the resting heart rate, the pulse quality, the pulse amplitude, and the presence of any irregularities in the rhythm.[13]

▶ *Resting heart rate:* The normal adult heart rate is 70 bpm, with a range of 60 to 80 bpm. A rate of greater than 100 bpm is referred to as tachycardia. Normal causes of tachycardia include anxiety, stress, pain, caffeine, dehydration, or exercise. A rate of less than 60 bpm is referred to as

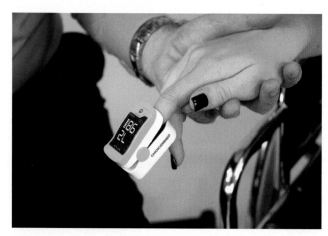

FIGURE 9-1 Pulse oximeter

bradycardia. Athletes may normally have a resting heart rate lower than 60 bpm. The normal range of resting heart rate in children is between 80 and 120 bpm. The rate for a newborn is 120 bpm (normal range 70 to 170 bpm).

▶ *Pulse quality:* The quality of the pulse refers to the amount of force created by the ejected blood against the arterial wall during each ventricular contraction.[14]

▶ *Pulse amplitude:* The pulse amplitude is an indication of the heart's efficiency in pushing blood into the arteries and the pressure being placed on the vessel's walls. A high volume may result in a bounding pulse, whereas a low volume may present as a weak or thready pulse.

▶ *Rhythm irregularities:* The pulse rhythm is the pattern of pulsations and the intervals between them.[14] In a healthy individual, the rhythm is regular and indicates that the time intervals between pulse beats are essentially equal. Arrhythmia or dysrhythmia refers to an irregular rhythm in which pulses are not evenly spaced.[14]

As the pulse travels toward the peripheral blood vessels, it gradually diminishes and becomes faster. In the large arterial branches, its velocity is 7 to 10 m/s; in the small arteries, it is 15 to 35 m/s.

The pulse can be taken at a number of points including the temporal (Figure 9-2), carotid (Figure 9-3), brachial (Figure 9-4), radial (Figure 9-5), femoral (within the femoral triangle), popliteal (Figure 9-6), dorsal pedal (Figure 9-7), and posterior tibial artery (Table 9-2).

CLINICAL PEARL

The most accessible pulse points are usually the radial or carotid pulse. The radial pulse is normally used when the patient is alert and active, whereas the carotid pulse is used when the detection of the pulse is critical.

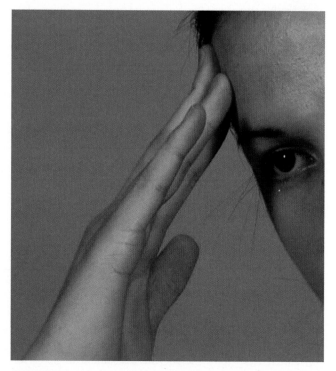

FIGURE 9-2 Pulse point—temporal

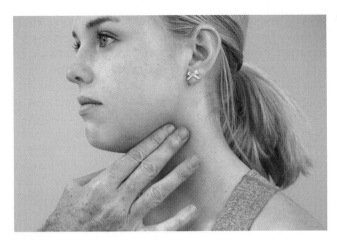

FIGURE 9-3 Pulse point—carotid

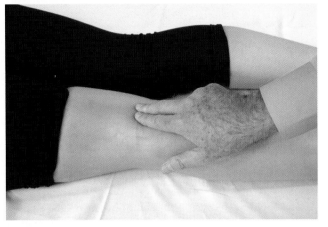

FIGURE 9-6 Pulse point—popliteal

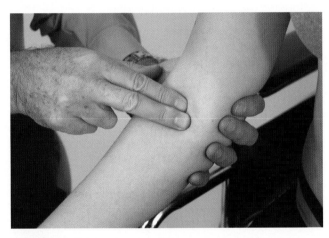

FIGURE 9-4 Pulse point—brachial

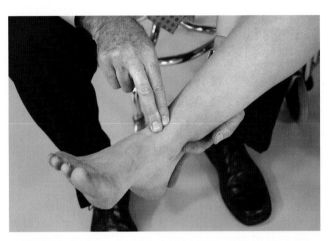

FIGURE 9-7 Pulse point—dorsal pedal

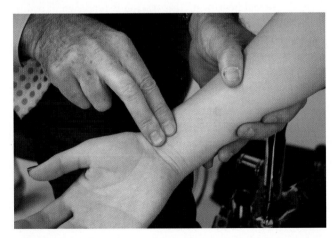

FIGURE 9-5 Pulse point—radial

On occasion, a specific pulse point site is chosen based on the patient's condition. For example, points in the lower extremity may be used if the clinician is assessing for peripheral vascular disease—if there is an arterial occlusion of the knee, the pulse of the groin will be stronger than the pulse palpated on the foot. A more specific diagnosis can then be made using Doppler technology.

TABLE 9-2	Palpation Sites for Pulse Reading
Pulse	**Location**
Radial	The distal radial artery is located on the lateral (thumb) side of the anterior surface of the wrist.
Carotid	The carotid artery is located to the side of the larynx and medial to the sternocleidomastoid muscle.
Brachial	In an adult, the brachial artery is located in the antibrachial fossa, just medial to the biceps brachii tendon. In an infant, the brachial artery can be located at the middle of the upper arm.
Temporal	At a point anterior and adjacent to the ear.
Femoral	At the femoral triangle, slightly lateral and anterior to the inguinal crease.
Popliteal	At the midline of the posterior knee crease between the tendons of the hamstring muscles.
Dorsal pedal	Along the midline or slightly medial on the dorsum of the foot.
Posterior tibial	On the medial aspect of the foot inferior to the medial malleolus.

One should avoid using the thumb when taking a pulse, as it has its own pulse that can interfere with detection of the patient's pulse. When taking a pulse, the fingers must be placed near the artery and pressed gently against a firm structure, usually a bone.

The main objective in assessing a patient's pulse rate is to determine if any physiologic response occurs during activity. The activity in question varies greatly depending on the patient's condition and functional demands. In addition to activity, there are a number of factors that can affect the pulse rate. These include:

▸ *Medications.* Medications can cause the pulse rate to either increase or decrease.

▸ *Emotional status.* The pulse rate typically increases during episodes of high stress, anxiety, and fear.

▸ *Age.* Adolescents persons and younger typically exhibit an increased rate, whereas persons older than 65 years may exhibit a decreased rate.

▸ *Gender.* Male pulse rates are usually slightly lower than female rates.

▸ *Temperature of the environment.* A pulse rate tends to increase with high temperature and decrease with low temperature.

▸ *Physical conditioning.* Individuals who perform frequent, sustained, and vigorous aerobic exercise exhibit a lower than normal pulse rate.

Abnormal responses to an increase in activity include the following:

▸ The pulse rate does not increase, or only increases slowly.

▸ The pulse rate declines before the intensity of the activity declines.

▸ The rate of the pulse increase exceeds the level expected for a particular activity.

▸ The pulse rate demonstrates an abnormal rhythm.

Procedure. The clinician washes his or her hands, obtains a timepiece that measures seconds, and explains the procedure to the patient. The patient is typically positioned in sitting but may also be recumbent or standing. The clinician selects an arterial site and gently places two or three fingertips over the artery. Gentle pressure is applied to the point when the patient's pulse can be detected. The count typically begins with the first beat that occurs after a time interval. For example, if the interval begins when a digital counter is at 0 seconds, "1" is the first beat felt after the 0 starting point. Alternatively, the clinician starts the time frame when the first beat is felt. The length of time for taking the pulse depends on the patient's situation. For example, the clinician can palpate for 15 seconds and multiply by 4 (or 30 seconds and multiply by 2) with a regular rhythm (evenly spaced beats), or 60 seconds for a baseline measurement, or in the presence of a regularly irregular rhythm (regular pattern overall with "skipped" beats) or irregularly irregular rhythm (chaotic, no real pattern) rhythm. The clinician documents the findings in terms of beats per minute, any variation in rhythm or volume, the location used, and the patient position.

Although the simplest way to assess the heart rate is by measuring the pulse, the most accurate way to examine heart rhythm is to use an electrocardiogram (ECG or EKG).[15] By placing 4 to 12 electrodes on the skin near the patient's heart, a typical ECG can provide information about the electrical activity of the heart by tracing the rate, rhythm, and waveform of normal heartbeat. This tracing is represented by a P wave, QRS complex, and T wave. The heart rate can also be monitored during a patient's activities of daily living (ADLs) through the use of a Holter monitor, a small device attached to the patient's belt that monitors the patient's heart rate through a series of electrodes placed on the patient's chest.

RESPIRATION RATE

The pulmonary or respiratory system is contained within a cagelike structure, which consists of the sternum, 12 pairs of ribs, the clavicle, and the vertebrae of the thoracic spine (see Chapter 4 and Chapter 6). The normal chest expansion difference between the resting position and the fully inhaled position is 2 to 4 cm (females > males).

The primary function of the respiratory system is to exchange gases between tissue, the blood, and the environment so that arterial blood oxygen, carbon dioxide, and pH levels remain within specific limits throughout many different physiologic limits.[18] The pulmonary system also plays a number of other roles, including contributing to temperature homeostasis via evaporative heat loss from the lungs and filtering, humidifying, and warming or cooling the air to body temperature.[18] This process protects the remainder of the respiratory system from damage caused by dry gases or harmful debris.[18]

In order for inspiration to occur, the lungs must be able to expand when stretched—they must have high compliance. In order for expiration to occur, the lungs must get smaller when this tension is released—they must have elasticity.

The diaphragm, innervated by the phrenic nerve, is the primary muscle of inspiration, with the ribs serving as levers. In addition, the 11 internal and external intercostals, which connect one rib to the next, serve to elevate the ribs and increase thoracic volume.[19]

▶ The external intercostals function to elevate the ribs and to increase thoracic volume.

▶ The internal intercostals function to lower the ribs, thereby decreasing thoracic volume.[19]

In order to inflate the lungs, the inspiratory muscles must perform two types of work: they must overcome the tendency of the lung to recoil inward; and they must overcome the resistance to flow offered by the airways.[20] Therefore, any factor that affects the efficiency of the respiratory muscles will also affect the quality and quantity of respiration.

When the diaphragm contracts, it descends over the abdominal contents, flattening the dome, which causes the lower ribs to move outward, resulting in protrusion of the abdominal wall. In addition, the contracting diaphragm causes a decrease in intrathoracic pressure, which pulls air into the lungs.[19]

Normal inspiration results from muscle contraction of the inspiratory muscles, which expand the chest wall and lower the diaphragm. During relaxed breathing, expiration is essentially a passive process.[14] The structure of the rib cage and associated cartilages provides continuous inelastic tension, so that when stretched by muscle contraction during inspiration, the rib cage can return passively to its resting dimensions when the muscles relax.[20]

Respiratory muscle activity involves multiple components of the neural, mechanical, and chemical control and is closely integrated with the cardiovascular system.[14] The spontaneous neuronal activity that produces cyclic breathing originates in the respiratory centers in the dorsal region of the medulla, which is influenced by control centers in the pons. In addition to the neural influences, the automatic control of breathing is also influenced by chemoreceptors.[18]

Other factors that influence respiration include[14]:

▶ *Age:* the resting rate of the newborn is between 25 and 50 breaths per minute, a rate which gradually slows until adulthood, when it ranges between 12 and 20 breaths per minute.

▶ *Body size and stature:* men generally have a larger vital capacity than women, and adults larger than adolescents and children. Tall, thin individuals generally have a larger vital capacity than stout or obese individuals.

▶ *Exercise:* resting rate and debt increase with exercise as a result of increased oxygen demand and carbon dioxide production.

- *Body position:* the recumbent position can significantly affect respiration through compression of the chest against the supporting surface and pressure from abdominal organs against the diaphragm.
- *Environment:* exposure to pollutants such as gas and particle emissions, asbestos, chemical waste products, or coal dust can diminish the ability to transport oxygen.
- *Emotional stress:* can result in an increased rate and depth of respirations.
- *Pharmacologic agents:* any drug that depresses central nervous system (CNS) function will result in respiratory depression. Examples include narcotic agents and barbiturates. Conversely, bronchodilators decrease airway resistance and residual volume with a resultant increase in vital capacity and air flow.

Assessment of the respiratory system involves measurement of the rate, rhythm, depth, and character of the patient's breathing using observation and palpation.

- *Rate:* the rate of breathing refers to the number of breaths per minute. Normal respiration rates for an adult person at rest range from 12 to 20 breaths per minute (the normal rate for a newborn is between 25 and 50 breaths per minute). Respiration rates over 25 breaths per minute or under 10 breaths per minute (when at rest) may be considered abnormal. The expirations are normally approximately twice as long as the inspirations. The opposite occurs in conditions such as chronic obstructive pulmonary disease (COPD).
- *Rhythm:* the rhythm of breathing refers to the regularity of the breathing pattern and the interval between each breath.

CLINICAL PEARL

The following breathing patterns are characteristic of disease[21]:

- Cheyne–Stokes respiration, characterized by a periodic, regular, sequentially increasing depth of respiration, occurs with serious cardiopulmonary or cerebral disorders.
- Biot's respiration, characterized by irregular spasmodic breathing and periods of apnea, is almost always associated with hypoventilation due to CNS disease.
- Kussmaul's respiration, characterized by deep, slow breathing, indicates acidosis, as the body attempts to blow off carbon dioxide.
- Apneustic breathing is an abnormal pattern of breathing characterized by a postinspiratory pause. The usual cause of apneustic breathing is a pontine lesion.
- Paradoxical respiration is an abnormal pattern of breathing, in which the abdominal wall is sucked in during inspiration (it is usually pushed out). Paradoxical respiration is due to paralysis of the diaphragm.

- *Depth:* the depth of breathing refers to the amount of air exchange (volume of air that is being exchanged in the lungs) with each respiration. Deep breathing is associated with greater thoracic expansion, whereas shallow breathing is associated with minimal chest expansion.

TABLE 9-3	Rating of Perceived Exertion	
Traditional Scale	Verbal Rating	Revised 10-Grade Scale
6	No exertion at all	0
7	Very, very light	0.5
8		
9	Very light	1.0
10		
11	Light	
12	Fairly light	2.0
13	Moderate	3.0
14	Somewhat hard	4.0
15	Hard (heavy)	5.0
16		6.0
17	Very hard	7.0
18		8.0
19	Very, very (extremely) hard	9.0
20	Maximal (exhaustion)	10.0

Data from Borg GAV: Psychophysical basis of perceived exertion. Med Sci Sports Exerc 14:377–381, 1992; Borg's Perceived Exertion and Pain Scales. Champaign, IL: Human Kinetics; 1998.

The clinician should compare measurements of both the anterior–posterior diameter and the transverse diameter during rest and at full inhalation.

- *Character:* the character of breathing refers to a deviation from normal, resting, or quiet respiration. A normal breathing response would be an increase in the respiratory rate and depth with exercise. The Borg scale of Rate of Perceived Exertion (RPE) is commonly used to assess breathing intensity based on activity (Table 9-3). An abnormal breathing response would be difficulty with breathing (dyspnea) in a patient at rest. In addition, normal breathing is barely audible. Abnormal breathing can be associated with some distinguishing characteristics (Tables 9-4 and 9-5).

A number of pieces of equipment are required to assess the respiration rate, including a timing device and a tape measure. A full assessment of a patient's respiration rate includes all of the following:

- Observation for signs or symptoms of abnormal respiration, including the quality of the breathing in relation to the patient's activity level.
- Palpation of the patient's radial pulse and a recording of the pulse rate.
- Observation of the patient's rate of breathing. The rate is usually measured when a person is at rest and simply involves counting the number of breaths for 30 seconds and multiplying the total by 2. If the total appears abnormal, the clinician should count the breaths for one minute.
- A measurement of chest expansion with inspiration compared to the relaxed state.

CLINICAL PEARL

Pulse oximetry provides an easy way of partly assessing a patient's breathing by measuring the oxygen saturation of arterial blood. A two-sided sensor, which monitors the

TABLE 9-4	Abnormal Breathing Patterns
Pattern	Description
Cheyne-Stokes	A common and bizarre breathing pattern characterized by alternating periods of apnea and hyperpnea. Typically, over a period of 1 minute, a 10- to 20-second episode of apnea or hypopnea is observed, followed by respirations of increasing depth and frequency. The cycle then repeats itself. Despite periods of apnea, significant hypoxia rarely occurs. Occurs in congestive heart failure, encephalitis, cerebral circulatory disturbances, and drug overdose, manifesting as a lesion of the bulbar center of respiration. The condition may also, however, be present as a normal finding in children, and in healthy adults following fast ascension to great altitudes, or in sleep.
Kussmaul's breathing	Rhythmic, gasping, and very deep type of respiration with normal or reduced frequency, associated with severe diabetic or renal acidosis or coma. Also known as air hunger syndrome.
Hyperventilation	Rapid breathing, often due to anxiety.
Biot (ataxic) breathing	Breathing that is irregular in timing and depth. It is indicative of meningitis or medullary lesions.
Apneustic breathing	This is an abnormal pattern of breathing characterized by a postinspiratory pause. The usual cause of apneustic breathing is a pontine lesion.
Paradoxical respiration	This is an abnormal pattern of breathing in which the abdominal wall is sucked in during inspiration (it is usually pushed out). Paradoxical respiration is due to paralysis of the diaphragm.
Sleep apnea	Sleep apnea is defined as the cessation of breathing during sleep. There are three different types of sleep apnea: ▶ *Obstructive:* the most common. Characterized by repetitive pauses in breathing during sleep due to the obstruction and/or collapse of the upper airway (throat), usually accompanied by a reduction in blood oxygen saturation, and followed by an awakening to breathe. This is called an apnea event. Respiratory effort continues during the episodes of apnea. ▶ *Central:* a neurologic condition causing cessation of all respiratory effort during sleep, usually with decreases in blood oxygen saturation. The person is aroused from sleep by an automatic breathing reflex, so may end up getting very little sleep at all. ▶ *Mixed:* a combination of the previous two. An episode of mixed sleep apnea usually starts with a central component and then becomes obstructive. Generally the central component of the apnea becomes less troublesome once the obstructive apnea is treated.

oxygenation of the patient's hemoglobin, is placed on a thin part of the patient's body, usually a fingertip (see Figure 9-1) or earlobe. Light consisting of two different wavelengths is passed between one sensor and the other. Depending on the color of the blood, these two wavelengths are absorbed differently, and a ratio of the two wavelengths is represented on the digital display as a percentage of oxygen saturation. Acceptable normal ranges for patients are from 95% to 99%, whereas saturation levels between 88% and 94% indicate hypoxia.

BLOOD PRESSURE

Every single beat of the heart involves a sequence of interrelated events known as the cardiac cycle. The cardiac cycle consists of three major stages: atrial systole, ventricular systole, and complete cardiac diastole.

▶ The atrial systole consists of the contraction of the atria. This contraction occurs during the last third of diastole and complete ventricular filling.

▶ The ventricular systole consists of the contraction of the ventricles and flow of blood into the circulatory system. Once all the blood empties from the ventricles, the pulmonary and aortic semilunar valves close.

▶ The complete cardiac diastole involves relaxation of the atria (atrial diastole) and ventricles (ventricular diastole) in preparation for refilling with circulating blood. End diastolic volume is the amount of blood in the ventricles after diastole, about 120 mL.

CLINICAL PEARL

▶ The heart has a two-step pumping action. One action is involved in the pumping of blood from the right half of the heart through the lungs and back to the left half of the heart (pulmonary circulation); the other action is involved with pumping blood from the left half of the heart through all the tissues of the body (except, of course, the lungs) and back to the right half of the heart (systemic circulation).

▶ The ventricles are the pumps that produce the pressures which drive the blood through the entire pulmonary and systemic vascular systems and back to the heart by contracting and relaxing.

Blood pressure (BP), a product of cardiac output and peripheral vascular resistance, is defined as the pressure exerted by the blood on the walls of the blood vessels, specifically *arterial blood pressure* (the pressure in the large arteries).

245

TABLE 9-5	Abnormal Breath Sounds
Sound	**Description**
Crackles	Crackles are discontinuous, explosive, "popping" sounds that originate within the airways. They are heard when an obstructed airway suddenly opens and the pressures on either side of the obstruction suddenly equilibrate, resulting in transient, distinct vibrations in the airway wall. The dynamic airway obstruction can be caused either by accumulation of secretions within the airway lumen or by airway collapse caused by pressure from inflammation or edema in surrounding pulmonary tissue. Crackles can be heard during inspiration when intrathoracic negative pressure results in opening of the airways or on expiration when thoracic positive pressure forces collapsed or blocked airways open. Crackles are heard more commonly during inspiration than expiration. They are significant as they imply either accumulation of fluid secretions or exudate within airways or inflammation and edema in the pulmonary tissue.
Wheezes	Continuous musical tones that are most commonly heard at end inspiration or early expiration. Result when a collapsed airway lumen gradually opens during inspiration or gradually closes during expiration. As the airway lumen becomes smaller, the air flow velocity increases, resulting in harmonic vibration of the airway wall and thus the musical tonal quality. Can be classified as either high-pitched or low-pitched wheezes. May be monophonic (a single pitch and tonal quality heard over an isolated area) or polyphonic (multiple pitches and tones heard over a variable area of the lung). Wheezes are significant because they imply decreased airway lumen diameter caused either by thickening of reactive airway walls or by collapse of airways due to pressure from surrounding pulmonary disease.
Stridor	Intense continuous monophonic wheezes heard loudest over extrathoracic airways that can often be heard without the aid of a stethoscope. These extrathoracic sounds are often referred down the airways and can often be heard over the thorax. They are often mistaken as pulmonary wheezes. Tend to be accentuated during inspiration when extrathoracic airways collapse due to lower internal lumen pressure. Stridor is significant and indicates upper airway obstruction.
Stertor	A poorly defined and inconsistently used term to describe harsh discontinuous crackling sounds heard over the larynx or trachea. Also described as a sonorous snoring sound heard over extrathoracic airways. Stertor is significant because it is suggestive of accumulation of secretions within extrathoracic airways.
Rhonchi	Abnormal dry, leathery sounds heard in the lungs, which indicate inflammation of the bronchial tubes.

▶ Peak pressure in the arteries occurs during contraction of the left ventricle (systole) and provides the clinician with a measurement called the systolic pressure.

▶ The lowest pressure in the arteries occurs during cardiac relaxation when the heart is filling (diastole) and provides the clinician with a measurement called the diastolic pressure.

The difference between systolic and diastolic pressure is called the pulse pressure. To withstand and adapt to the pressures within, arteries are surrounded by varying thicknesses of smooth muscle that have extensive elastic and inelastic connective tissues.[13]

The assessment of BP provides information about the effectiveness of the heart as a pump and the resistance to blood flow. It is measured in mm Hg and is recorded in two numbers. The systolic pressure is the pressure that is exerted on the brachial artery when the heart is contracting, and the diastolic pressure is the pressure exerted on the artery during the relaxation phase of the cardiac cycle.[13] BP is recorded as the systolic pressure over the diastolic pressure.

CLINICAL PEARL

The mean arterial pressure (MAP), which is an important clinical measure in critical care, is determined by the cardiac output (CO), systemic vascular resistance (SVR),

and central venous pressure (CVP) and is based on the relationship between flow, pressure, and resistance. The following equation is used: $MAP = CO \times SVR$. A MAP of 60 or greater is necessary to diffuse oxygen to the body's major organs and vessels to maintain them. Typically physical therapy treatment is not permitted with a patient whose MAP is less than 60.

CLINICAL PEARL

A useful tool in assessing a patient with claudication is the ankle-brachial index (ABI), which is calculated as the ratio of systolic blood pressure at the ankle to the arm. A normal ABI is 0.9 to 1.1. However, any patient with an ABI less than 0.9, by definition, has some degree of arterial disease.

A category of prehypertension has established more aggressive guidelines for medical intervention of hypertension. The normal values for resting BP in adults are:

▶ *Normal:* systolic blood pressure <120 mm Hg and diastolic blood pressure <80 mm Hg

▶ *Prehypertension:* systolic blood pressure 120 to 139 mm Hg or diastolic blood pressure 80 to 90 mm Hg

▶ *Stage 1 hypertension:* systolic blood pressure 140 to 159 mm Hg or diastolic blood pressure 90 to 99 mm Hg

▶ *Stage 2 hypertension:* systolic blood pressure ≥160 mm Hg or diastolic blood pressure ≥100 mm Hg

The normal values for resting blood pressure in children are:

▶ *Systolic:* birth to 1 month, 60 to 90 mm Hg; up to 3 years of age, 75 to 130 mm Hg; and over 3 years of age, 90 to 140 mm Hg;

▶ *Diastolic:* birth to 1 month, 30 to 60 mm Hg; up to 3 years of age, 45 to 90 mm Hg; and over 3 years of age, 50 to 80 mm Hg.

CLINICAL PEARL

Ideally, BP should be determined in both arms. Causes of marked asymmetry in blood pressure of the arms include the following: errors in measurements, marked difference in arm size, thoracic outlet syndromes, embolic occlusion of an artery, dissection of an aorta, external arterial occlusion, coarctation of the aorta, and atheromatous occlusion.[21]

Hypertension is one of the most common worldwide diseases afflicting humans and is an important public health challenge. Regulation of normal blood pressure is a complex process. Persistent hypertension can result in organ damage to the aorta and small arteries, heart, kidneys, retina, and CNS.

There are many physical factors that influence blood pressure:

▶ *Age:* The normal systolic range generally increases with age. BP normally rises gradually after birth and reaches a peak during puberty. By late adolescence (18 to 19 years), adult BP is reached.[14] In older adults, the rise in blood pressure is primarily because of the degenerative effects of arteriosclerosis.[14]

▶ *Rate of pumping (heart rate):* the rate at which blood is pumped by the heart—the higher the heart rate, the higher (assuming no change in stroke volume) the blood pressure.

▶ *Volume of blood:* the amount of blood present in the body. The more blood present in the body, the higher the rate of blood returned to the heart and the resulting cardiac output.

▶ *Dehydration:* a significant decrease of body fluids may cause low blood pressure.

▶ *Cardiac output:* the rate and volume of flow—product of the heart rate, or the rate of contraction, multiplied by the stroke volume, the amount of blood pumped out from the heart with each contraction—the efficiency with which the heart circulates the blood throughout the body.

▶ *Resistance of the blood vessel walls (peripheral vascular resistance):* the higher the resistance, the higher the blood pressure; the larger the blood vessel, the lower the resistance. Factors that influence peripheral vascular resistance include arteriolar tone, vasoconstriction, and to a lesser extent, blood viscosity.

▶ *Viscosity, or thickness, of the blood:* if the blood gets thicker, the result is an increase in blood pressure. Certain

medical conditions can change the viscosity of the blood. For instance, low red blood cell concentration, anemia, reduces viscosity, whereas increased red blood cell concentration increases viscosity.

CLINICAL PEARL

The so-called blood thinners (e.g., Coumadin) do not affect the viscosity of the blood, but rather the ability of the blood to clot.

▶ *Body temperature:* an increase in body temperature causes the heart rate to increase. Conversely a decrease in body temperature causes the heart rate to decrease.

▶ *Arm position:* BP may vary as much as 20 mm Hg by altering arm position.[14] The pressure should be determined in both arms (see later).

▶ *Exercise:* physical activity will increase cardiac output, with a consequent linear increase in blood pressure. Greater increases are noted in systolic pressure owing to proportional changes in the pressure gradient of peripheral vessels.[14] Systolic readings greater than 250 mm Hg or diastolic readings greater than 115 mm Hg during exercise or other high-level activity should serve as serious warnings. Similarly, a drop in the systolic pressure more than 10 mm Hg from baseline or failure of the systolic pressure to increase with an increasing workload should also give cause for concern.

▶ *Valsalva maneuver:* An attempt to exhale forcibly with the glottis, nose, and mouth closed.[14] This results in:

  ■ An increase in intrathoracic pressure with an accompanying collapse of the veins of the chest wall

  ■ A decrease in blood flow to the heart, and a decreased venous return

  ■ A drop in arterial blood pressure

When the breath is released, the intrathoracic pressure decreases, and venous return is suddenly reestablished as an *overshoot* mechanism to compensate for the drop in blood pressure. This causes a marked increase in heart rate and arterial blood pressure.[14]

▶ *Orthostatic hypotension:* defined as a drop in systolic blood pressure within three minutes of assuming an upright position—a decrease in BP below normal (a systolic blood pressure decrease of at least 20 mm Hg or a diastolic blood pressure decrease of at least 10 mm Hg) to the point where the pressure is not adequate for normal oxygenation of the tissues.[13] Orthostatic hypotension can occur as a side effect of antihypertensive medications, in cases of low blood volume in patients who are postoperative or dehydrated, and in those with dysfunction of the autonomic nervous system, such as that which occurs with a spinal cord injury or post–cerebrovascular accident.[13] Activities that may increase the chance of orthostatic hypotension, such as application of heat modalities, hydrotherapy, pool therapy, moderate-to-vigorous exercise using the large muscles, sudden changes of position, and stationary standing, should be avoided in susceptible patients.[13]

There are a number of ways that BP can be measured. The most accurate method involves placing a cannula into a blood vessel and connecting it to an electronic pressure transducer. The less accurate, but less invasive, method is the auscultation method, which uses manual measurement using a sphygmomanometer, an inflatable (Riva Rocci) cuff (Figure 9-8) placed around the upper arm, at roughly the same vertical height as the heart in a sitting person, using the brachial artery. BP measurements are usually taken on the left arm because it is physically located nearer the aorta, but the right arm can also be used (Figure 9-8).

The chosen cuff must be the proper size to obtain an accurate measurement to prevent erroneous readings. The ideal cuff has a bladder length that is 80% of the arm circumference, and the width of the bladder should be 40% of the circumference of the midpoint of the limb.

The patient should be allowed to sit quietly for 1 to 2 minutes before the measurements are taken and should not have been exercising for 15 to 30 minutes. The clinician washes his or her hands and obtains a clean stethoscope and a sphygmomanometer. The procedure is explained to the patient while the patient is positioned in sitting with the forearm supported approximately at the level of the heart, and the feet are on the floor with the legs uncrossed. The clinician exposes the antecubital space of the patient's arm while making sure that any clothing that is rolled up does not create additional constriction, and palpates the brachial pulse (see Figure 9-4) for future placement of the cuff and stethoscope diaphragm. The deflated cuff is applied to the arm with the center of the bladder over the medial aspect of the arm (approximately 2 to

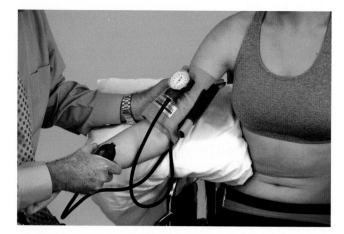

FIGURE 9-9 Placement of cuff

3 cm or 1½ fingerbreadths above the antecubital space) so that it will occlude the artery when it is inflated (Figure 9-9). The clinician applies the stethoscope to his or her ears with the earpieces directed forward and places the diaphragm on the skin where the brachial artery was palpated. Firm but gentle pressure is applied on the diaphragm (Figure 9-10). The clinician ensures that all of the air is out of the cuff bladder, the valve on the pump is closed, and the pressure gauge reading is zero. While listening with a stethoscope placed over the brachial artery at the elbow, the clinician uses the same hand to slowly inflate the blood pressure cuff by squeezing the bladder (Figure 9-11). The clinician uses the other hand to palpate the patient's radial pulse, and the cuff is slowly inflated until when the pressure level reaches either 20 to 30 mm Hg above the first Korotkoff sound (see Clinical Pearl) or 30 mm Hg above the point at which the radial pulse disappears. Some consider 200 mm Hg as the upper limit of inflation, but this can lead to a measurement error in patients with hypertension. At this point, the clinician uses the thumb and index finger of the hand used to squeeze the pump to slowly open the valve and release the pressure in the cuff (Figure 9-12). At the point when the clinician begins to hear a "whooshing" or pounding sound (first Korotkoff sound) the pressure reading (systolic) is noted. The cuff pressure is further released until a muffling sound can be heard (fourth Korotkoff sound). This is the diastolic blood pressure.

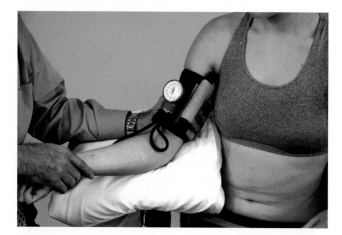

FIGURE 9-8 Sphygmomanometer

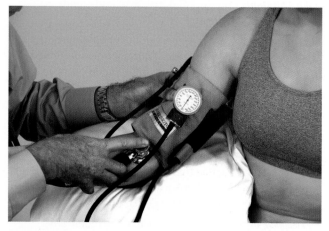

FIGURE 9-10 Diaphragm over the brachial pulse

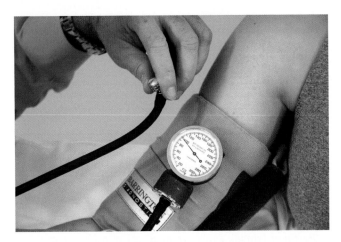

FIGURE 9-11 Inflation of cuff

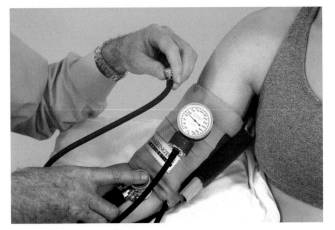

FIGURE 9-12 Controlled deflation of cuff

CLINICAL PEARL

Korotkoff sounds are the sounds that medical personnel listen for when they are taking blood pressure. Korotkoff actually described five phases of sounds:

1. The first clear, rhythmic tapping sound that gradually increases in intensity. This represents the highest pressure in the arterial system during ventricular contraction and is recorded as the systolic pressure. The clinician should be alert for the presence of an auscultatory gap, especially in patients with hypertension. An auscultatory gap is the temporary disappearance of sound normally heard over the brachial artery between phase 1 and phase 2 and may cover a range of as much as 40 mm Hg.[14] Not identifying this gap may lead to an underestimation of systolic pressure and overestimation of diastolic pressure.[14]

2. A murmur or swishing sound heard as the artery widens and more blood flows through the artery. This sound is heard for most of the time between the systolic and diastolic pressures.

3. Sounds become crisp, more intense, and louder.

4. The sound is distinct, abrupt muffling; soft blowing quality. At pressures within 10 mm Hg above the diastolic blood pressure (in children less than 13 years old, pregnant women, and in patients with high cardiac output or peripheral vasodilation), the muffling sound should be used to indicate diastolic pressure, but both muffling (phase 4) and disappearance (phase 5) should be recorded.

5. The last sound that is heard, which is traditionally recorded as diastolic blood pressure.

Although, the systolic blood pressure is commonly taken to be the pressure at which the first Korotkoff sound is first heard and the diastolic blood pressure reading is taken at the point at which the fourth Korotkoff sound is just barely audible, there has recently been a move toward the use of the fifth Korotkoff sound (i.e., silence) as the diastolic blood pressure, as this has been felt to be more reproducible.[25–30] In pregnancy a fifth phase may not be identifiable, in which case the fourth is used.[31–33]

CLINICAL PEARL

Any error that occurs during a blood pressure reading can result in highly inaccurate interpretations, especially in light of the fact that the cutoff levels for hypertension categories are close together, making the distinction between normal and hypotensive BP very slight. The most common errors include:

▶ The failure to accurately determine the first Korotkoff sound

▶ Use of inappropriate cuff size

▶ Incorrect patient positioning (unsupported tested arm, arm not level with the heart, legs crossed while sitting, and unsupported sitting)

▶ Incorrect placement of stethoscope

▶ Too rapid deflation of the cuff

The clinician records the BP readings, including the patient position and the upper extremity used. If it is necessary to repeat the measurements, the cuff is completely deflated and the patient is permitted to sit quietly for one to two minutes before proceeding again. Once the measurements are completed, the clinician cleans the equipment in preparation for future use.

CLINICAL PEARL

Many medical facilities currently use automated digital monitors to measure blood pressure. Similar units are also the most common devices used for at-home self-monitoring (Figure 9-13). The patient setup is the same as for the auscultation method. After the cuff is placed on the patient's upper arm, the cuff automatically inflates to a pressure higher than the systolic pressure using oscillometry. An electronically operated pump and valve then releases pressure gradually, and a transducer senses the periodic expansion and contraction of the wall of the brachial artery. The device uses this information to calculate the systolic and diastolic pressures, which are displayed digitally. Although these devices are less susceptible to human error, their accuracy varies widely based on manufacturer and model.

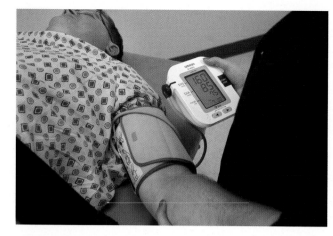

FIGURE 9-13 Automated digital blood pressure monitor

Recently, ultrasonic BP measuring devices have been introduced. These new devices work by using mathematically based software to measure blood flow and vein or artery wall distention as the heart beats, based on images generated by the ultrasound device. The patient setup is similar to that used by the auscultation method, but instead of using a stethoscope, ultrasonic waves are reflected off the brachial artery distal to the cuff.

TEMPERATURE

Body temperature, a balance between the heat that is produced and lost in the body, is one indication of the metabolic state of an individual. Temperature measurements provide information on basal metabolic state, possible presence or absence of infection, and metabolic response to exercise.[13] The "normal" core body temperature of an adult, found in the pulmonary artery, is generally considered to be 98.6°F (37°C). However, a temperature in the range of 96.5 to 99.4°F (35.8 to 37.4°C) is not at all uncommon. Fever or pyrexia is a temperature exceeding 100°F (37.7°C).[21] Hyperpyrexia refers to extreme elevation of temperature above 41.1°C (or 106°F).[13] Hypothermia refers to an abnormally low temperature (below 35°C or 95°F).

In most individuals, there is a diurnal (occurring every day) variation in body temperature of 0.5 to 2°F (1°C), with the low temperature occurring before waking and the high temperature occurring about 12 hours after waking. Menstruating women have a well-known temperature pattern that reflects the effects of ovulation, with the temperature increasing slightly (0.25 to 0.5°C measured in the morning) around ovulation.[21] In both aging and fit individuals, there is more temperature variation during the day. Finally, whereas ingestion of meals can slightly elevate or lower core temperature, alcohol ingestion slightly lowers core temperature.

CLINICAL PEARL

It is worth noting that in adults over 75 years of age and in those who are immunocompromised (e.g., transplant recipients, corticosteroid users, persons with chronic renal insufficiency, or anyone taking excessive antipyretic medications), the fever response may be blunted or absent.[13]

TABLE 9-6	Normal Temperatures Based on Site
Rectal	36.6°C to 38°C (97.9°F to 100.4°F)
Tympanic	35.8°C to 38°C (96.4°F to 100.4°F)
Oral	35.5°C to 37.5°C (95.9°F to 99.5°F)
Axillary	34.7°C to 37.3°C (94.5°F to 99.1°F)

The clinical measurement of temperature is merely an estimate of the true core temperature. A number of sites can be used, including the ear canal (tympanic), oral cavity, axilla, and rectum (Table 9-6).

▶ *Rectal or tympanic measurements:* commonly used with infants and unconscious patients because of the difficulty of maintaining the thermometer position at the other sites. Although there are concerns about the accuracy of tympanic measurements across all age groups,[34,35] a number of studies have shown them to be reliable.[36,37]

▶ *Axillary measurement:* only used when the other sites cannot be used because of its decreased accuracy.

CLINICAL PEARL

Rectal temperatures tend to be the highest and closest to the actual core temperature, whereas axillary temperatures tend to be the lowest and furthest from true core temperature.[34]

Oral Procedure. The oral temperature is generally taken by placing a probe thermometer under the patient's tongue. The thermometer can be a standard one (Figure 9-14) or a battery-operated electronic thermometer (Figure 9-15). After washing his or her hands, the clinician inserts a clean probe into the patient's mouth, positioned under the tongue, and held in place by the lips (not with the teeth). The patient is asked to breathe through the nose. Typically, the probe remains in place for 30 to 90 seconds. Electronic devices emit an audible alarm when the temperature reaches its final value. The clinician notes the value and then removes the probe from the patient's mouth, discards the probe cover, and turns

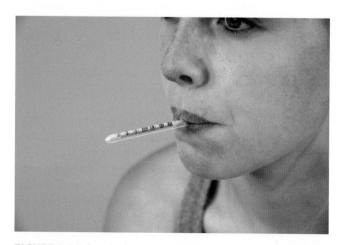

FIGURE 9-14 Standard thermometer

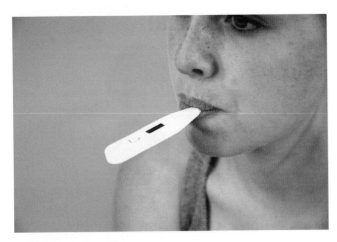

FIGURE 9-15 Battery operated electronic thermometer

the unit off. The clinician then washes his or her hands before recording the result.

Tympanic Procedure. The tympanic measurement involves placing a specially designed electronic monitor into the ear canal that reads the infrared energy emitted from the tympanic membrane (eardrum), detects when the maximum temperature has been reached, and then provides a liquid crystal display (LCD) of the temperature. The electronic monitor uses disposable, single-use probe covers. Newer designs of these monitors convert the tympanic temperature to an estimated core temperature. A number of precautions must be taken when using a tympanic device. Ideally, the clinician should[38,39]:

▶ Ensure that there is no excessive earwax present.

▶ Confirm that the patient's ear has not been resting against a pillow or similar object. If it has, the clinician should wait for 2 to 3 minutes before taking a reading.

▶ Take readings from both ears, as measurements can vary between sides. Alternatively, the clinician can take a reading from one ear and document which ear was used.

To take a tympanic temperature, the clinician washes his or her hands before applying a clean lens filter. As appropriate, the clinician selects the correct setting (some units have both an "oral" and a "rectal" setting) and then gently but firmly pulls on the patient's ear to straighten the ear canal. For an infant, the ear is pulled straight back, whereas for anyone who is older than one year, the ear is pulled up and back. The clinician then insert the thermometer lens cone, with its clean filter applied, into the ear opening, rocking it back and forth gently to insert it far enough to seal the ear canal. The clinician then depresses and holds the activation button for one second until the temperature reading appears in the display window, and mentally records the value. The lens cone is then removed from the patient's ear and discarded. Depending on the facility, the lens filter is also discarded or is thoroughly washed before being used again. The clinician washes his or her hands and records the temperature reading.

Rectal Procedure. Specifically designed rectal thermometers are used to record rectal temperatures. After washing his or her hands, the clinician applies a lubricant to the thermometer probe, and with the patient positioned in sidelying with the hips and knees flexed, the thermometer is inserted into the rectum far enough for the probe to be within the cavity but not so far as to push into tissue resistance. The thermometer remains in place for three minutes or until the electronic device indicates completion and the temperature reading is noted. The clinician then removes and cleans the probe, washes his or her hands, and then records the temperature.

> ## CLINICAL PEARL
>
> Ingestible telemetric body core temperature sensors, which measure approximately ¾ of an inch in length, have recently been introduced to measure and monitor the temperature of athletes. The "thermometer pill" has a silicone-coated exterior and microminiaturized circuitry on the interior, including a quartz crystal temperature sensor, and is powered by a miniature battery. As the pill is swallowed, the temperature sensor vibrates at a frequency relative to the body's temperature, transmitting a harmless and low-frequency signal through the body, which can be recorded by an external receiver. After 18 to 30 hours, the pill passes safely from the digestive system.

THE ASSESSMENT OF PAIN

Many clinical environments consider pain as the fifth vital sign, although strictly speaking pain is a symptom rather than a sign. Pain, always an abnormal finding, is felt by everyone at some point or other and is considered an emotional experience that is highly individualized and extremely difficult to evaluate. Pain is a broad and significant symptom that can be described in many ways. In addition, pain perception and the response to the painful experience can be influenced by a variety of cognitive processes, including anxiety, tension, depression, past pain experiences, and cultural influences.[40] As described in Chapter 5, pain is commonly described as *acute* or *chronic*.

Acute pain usually precipitates a visit to a physician, because it has not been experienced before, is severe and continuous, and is in a location that causes concern (chest, head).[41,42] In addition, there may be an autonomic component to acute pain.[43,44]

> ## CLINICAL PEARL
>
> ▶ Hyperalgesia is an increased sensitivity to pain.
>
> ▶ Allodynia is defined as a painful response to a previously innocuous stimulus.
>
> ▶ Referred pain is pain perceived at a site adjacent to or at a distance from the site of an injury's origin. For example, pain due to osteoarthritis of the hip is often felt in the anterior groin and thigh.

Pain that is not alleviated by rest, and that is not associated with acute trauma, may indicate the presence of a serious disorder such as a tumor, infection, or aneurysm. This pain is often described as deep, constant, and boring and is apt to be more noticeable and more intense at night.[45]

Chronic pain is much less intense than acute pain and can occur gradually over days or weeks.[42] In general, this type of pain has been experienced previously by the patient, is located at a site that does not cause as much concern, is usually of limited duration, and is more aggravating than debilitating.[46–49]

Typically chronic pain is aggravated by a specific movement or activity, and reduced with cessation of the specific movement or activity.

CLINICAL PEARL

Referred pain, which can be either acute or chronic, must be verified by the clinician by determining its cause and whether the cause is within the scope of practice.

The clinician should determine the location of the pain because this can indicate which areas need to be included in the physical examination. Information about how the location of the symptoms has changed since the onset can indicate whether a condition is worsening or improving. In general, as a condition worsens, the pain distribution becomes more widespread and distal (peripheralizes). As the condition improves, the symptoms tend to become more localized (centralized). A body chart may be used to record the location of symptoms (see Figure 9-16, later).

CLINICAL PEARL

It must be remembered that the location of symptoms for many musculoskeletal conditions is quite separate from the source, especially in those peripheral joints that are more proximal, such as the shoulder and the hip. For example, a cervical disk protrusion can produce symptoms throughout the upper extremity. The term *radiating pain* is used to describe symptoms that have their origin at a spinal nerve, but which is felt along the nerve's distribution into either the upper or lower extremity.

Although pain measurement does not provide a direct measure of a patient's physiologic status, it can provide important information to aid in diagnosis, prognosis, and intervention planning. Although largely subjective, pain assessment can be made more quantitative by using a variety of visual and verbal pain scales.

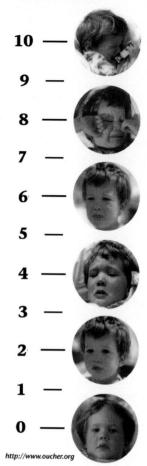

FIGURE 9-16 Caucasian ouchmeter to measure pain

CLINICAL PEARL

The Joint Commission requires appropriate assessment of the patient's pain as an element of standard care.

One of the simplest methods to quantify the intensity of pain is to use a 10-point visual analog scale (VAS). The VAS is a numerically continuous scale that requires the pain level be identified by making a mark on a 100-mm line, or by circling the appropriate number in a 1-to-10 series (Table 9-7).[50] The patient is asked to rate his or her present pain compared with the worst pain ever experienced, with 0 representing no pain, 1 representing minimally perceived pain, and 10 representing pain that requires immediate attention.[51] A modification of the VAS, which involves asking the patient to rate their pain from 0 to 10 with 0 corresponding to no pain and 10 indicating the maximum possible pain, is commonly used.

CLINICAL PEARL

It is important to remember that pain perception is highly subjective and is determined by a number of factors. The clinician must determine whether pain is the only symptom, or whether there are other symptoms that accompany the pain, such as bowel and bladder changes, tingling (paresthesia), radicular pain or numbness from a disk protrusion, associated weakness, or increased sweating.

TABLE 9-7   Patient Pain Evaluation Form

Name: _____

Date: _____   Signature: _____

Please use the diagram below to indicate where you feel symptoms right now. Use the following key to indicate different types of symptoms.

KEY: Pins and Needles = 000000   Stabbing = ///////   Burning = XXXXX   Deep Ache = ZZZZZZ

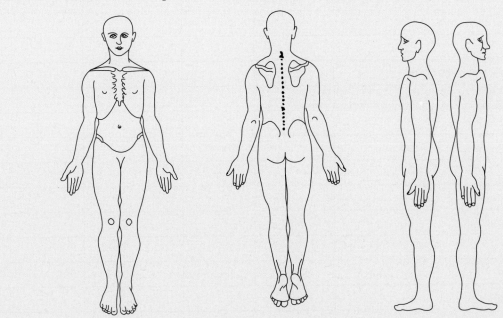

Please use the three scales below to rate your pain over the past 24 hours. Use the upper line to describe your pain level right now. Use the other scales to rate your pain at its worst and best over the past 24 hours.

RATE YOUR PAIN: 0 = NO PAIN, 10 = EXTREMELY INTENSE

1.	Right now	0	1	2	3	4	5	6	7	8	9	10
2.	At its worst	0	1	2	3	4	5	6	7	8	9	10
3.	At its best	0	1	2	3	4	5	6	7	8	9	10

Because pain is variable in its intensity and quality, describing pain is often difficult for the patient. The McGill Pain Questionnaire (MPQ),[52] designed in 1971 to use verbal descriptors to assess the intensity and quality of the patient's symptoms, is now widely used in pain research and practice (see Table 5-9). A patient first selects a single word from each group that best describes his or her pain, and then reviews the list to select three words from groups 1–10 that best reflect their pain, two words from groups 11–15, a single word from group 16, and then a single word from groups 17–20. Upon completion, the patient will have selected seven words that best describe his or her pain.[53] The implication is that each word chosen reflects a particular sensory quality of pain.

The patient is also asked to highlight on a body diagram.

A similar scale to the MPQ is the modified somatic perception questionnaire (MSPQ), a simple 13 item four-point self-report scale (Table 9-8), which is used to measure somatic and autonomic perception. The MSPQ has a minimum score of zero and a maximum score of 39. The higher the score the greater the somatic symptoms.

A number of pain rating scales exist for use with infants and children. The pain of infants can be assessed using a tool such as the FLACC (face, legs, activity, cry, and consolability), which is an observational scale assessing pain behaviors quantitatively with preverbal patients. Physiologic and behavioral responses to nociceptive or painful stimuli can also be used.[55] Physiologic manifestations of pain include increased heart rate, heart rate variability, blood pressure, and respirations, with evidence of decreased oxygenation (cyanosis).[55]

For the assessment of children, two common scales are currently used:

► *Faces Pain Rating Scale.*[56] This 0-to-5 scale consists of a series of six pictures of cartoonlike faces expressing various facial expressions from crying (Hurts worst—5) to smiling (No hurt—0). The child is asked to point to the face that best describes his or her pain.

► *The Oucher Scales.*[57] There are two ethnically based self-report Oucher scales; a (0 to 100) number scale for older children and a photographic scale for younger children (aged 3 to 5) (Figure 9-16). Children who are able to count to 100 by ones or tens and who understand, for example, that 72 is larger than 45 can use the numerical scale. Children who do not understand numbers should

TABLE 9-8	Modified Somatic Perceptions Questionnaire			

Please describe how you have felt during the PAST WEEK by marking a check mark (√) in the appropriate box. Please answer all questions. Do not think too long before answering.

	Not at All	A Little, Slightly	A Great Deal, Quite a Bit	Extremely, could not have been Worse
Heart rate increase				
Feeling hot all over				
Sweating all over				
Sweating in a particular part of the body				
Pulse in neck				
Pounding in head				
Dizziness				
Blurring of vision				
Feeling faint				
Everything appearing unreal				
Nausea				
Butterflies in stomach				
Pain or ache in stomach				
Stomach churning				
Desire to pass water				
Mouth becoming dry				
Difficulty swallowing				
Muscles in neck aching				
Legs feeling weak				
Muscles twitching or jumping				
Tense feeling across forehead				
Tense feeling in jaw muscles				

Source: Main C, Wood P, Hillis S, et al. The Distress and Risk Assessment Method. A simple patient classification to identify distress and evaluate the risk of poor outcome. *Spine* 1992;17: 42-52.

use the picture scale. The Oucher picture scale has three versions—Caucasian, African American, and Hispanic—that are suitable for children. Although this covers a wide variety of patients, females are not represented, nor are several other cultures. The scale uses six photographs of a child's face representing "no hurt" to "biggest hurt you can ever have" and includes a vertical scale with numbers from 0 to 10.

EMERGENCY FIRST AID

An emergency situation, whether characterized by unresponsiveness, an acute medical condition, drug intoxication, or trauma, demands a rapid response and management. A logical, sequential priority system must be implemented immediately. All healthcare employees who are involved in patient care should be aware of the emergency procedures of the facility in which they work and should be qualified to provide first aid in the case of an emergency. Most healthcare facilities have a series of emergency codes to indicate the occurrence of an emergency. For example:

▶ Code blue may represent a flood.

▶ Code amber may represent child abduction.

▶ Code red may represent a fire.

▶ Code black may represent a cardiac arrest.

At the very minimum, all healthcare employees should know how to contact and request emergency assistance (e.g., the use of 911 or the equivalent number to contact the police, fire, or emergency services).

It is not uncommon these days for patients to wear a medical alert bracelet or necklace, which inform others of any medical conditions, allergies, health history, medication needs, and so forth.

CLINICAL PEARL

A crash cart or code cart is a set of trays/drawers/shelves on wheels used in hospitals for transporting and dispensing emergency medication/equipment at the site of a medical/surgical emergency. The contents of a crash cart vary from institution to institution, but typically include the tools and drugs needed to treat a person in or near cardiac arrest. These include but are not limited to:

▶ Monitoring/defibrillators and suction devices

▶ Advanced Cardiac Life Support (ACLS) drugs

▶ First-line drugs for treatment of common problems (anaphylactic shock, deep venous thrombosis [DVT], etc.)

▶ Drugs for rapid sequence intubation, endotracheal tubes and other intubating equipment

▶ Drugs for peripheral and central venous access

▶ Pediatric equipment

▶ Other drugs and equipment as required by the facility

Physical therapists must be able to recognize the signs and symptoms that are associated with a medical emergency. Signs and symptoms of some common medical emergencies include:

▶ Difficulty breathing, shortness of breath.

▶ Chest or upper abdominal pain or pressure lasting two minutes or more.

▶ Loss of consciousness, fainting, unexplained nausea, sudden dizziness, or sudden weakness.

▶ *Seizure.* Any patient who convulses without a known cause should be evaluated and treated carefully.

▶ Incontinence of bowel or bladder without a known cause.

▶ Signs of a major burn.

▶ Reports of changes in vision.

▶ Difficulty speaking.

▶ Confusion or changes in mental status, unusual behavior, difficulty waking.

▶ Any sudden or severe pain.

▶ Head pain that lasts longer than five minutes.

▶ Uncontrolled bleeding.

▶ Shock symptoms, such as confusion, disorientation, and cool/clammy, pale skin.

▶ Severe or persistent vomiting or diarrhea.

▶ Coughing or vomiting blood.

▶ Unusual abdominal pain.

▶ Suicidal or homicidal feelings.

▶ Certain patient populations, such as the elderly, debilitated persons, and persons with cognitive deterioration, spinal cord injury, chronic respiratory condition, an acute/chronic cardiac condition, or acute/chronic diabetes.

CLINICAL PEARL

The "Good Samaritan" law provides certain protection from lawsuits to people who give first aid or other emergency care or treatment to someone suffering an injury or sudden illness. The care or treatment must be given at the scene of an emergency outside of a hospital, doctor's office, or other medical facility. The law protects volunteers who help when someone becomes ill or is injured in places such as on the street or highway, in parks, restaurants, businesses, even private residences. If someone is already at a hospital or other medical facility, the law does not apply.

Each physical therapy department has a number of policies and procedures regarding environmental, employee, and patient safety that are included in the unit's policy/procedure or safety manual. The typical contents of this manual are outlined in Table 9-9.

The initial response by the physical therapist should be an assessment of the patient's physiologic status performed in a sequence referred to as the ABCs (airway, breathing, circulation) for babies, and CAB (circulation, airway, breathing) for every other age group. The letters D (Disability—neurologic status) and E (Exposure—expose the sites of all injuries) follow (Table 9-10).

TABLE 9-9	Typical Contents of an Environmental, Employee, and Patient Safety Manual

Employee job duties, descriptions, and responsibilities

Supervisor relationships, organization table, and the chain of command

Plans for the evacuation and care of patients and the expected function of all personnel at the time of an emergency

Security measures for patient and employee valuables and procedures for items that are lost or found

The establishment of equipment inspection, repair, and maintenance records

The process and procedures for general infection control and handling of toxic materials

The application and use of personal protective equipment (PPE), the handling of body fluids, and the management of patients who are placed in isolation

TABLE 9-10	Situations That Require First Aid and Appropriate Action	
Situation	**Description**	**Appropriate Action**
Anaphylaxis	A life-threatening allergic reaction that can cause shock, a sudden drop in blood pressure and trouble breathing.	Immediately call 911 or facility's emergency number. Ask the person if he or she is carrying an epinephrine autoinjector to treat an allergic attack. Have the person lie still on his or her back and loosen tight clothing and cover the person with a blanket. Don't give the person anything to drink. If there's vomiting or bleeding from the mouth, turn the person on his or her side to prevent choking. If there are no signs of breathing, coughing, or movement, begin cardiopulmonary resuscitation (CPR).
Autonomic hyperreflexia	Occurs in individuals with a relatively recent complete injury to the cervical and upper thoracic portions of the spinal cord down to the T6 cord level. Signs and symptoms include severe hypertension, bradycardia, and profuse diaphoresis above the level of the cord lesion.	Immediately look for and remove any potential causes of any noxious stimuli below the level of the spinal cord lesion including bladder distention caused by urine retention, fecal impaction, tight straps from an orthosis or urine retention bag, localized pressure, open pressure ulcers, or exercise. The person should be placed in a sitting or semirecumbent position (not supine) and monitored.
Burn, including chemical burn	The severity of the burn depends on the extent of damage to body tissues.	For minor burns, including first-degree burns and second-degree burns limited to an area no larger than 3 inches (7.6 cm) in diameter, cool the burn by holding the burned area under cool (not cold) running water for 10 or 15 minutes or until the pain subsides. If this is impractical, immerse the burn in cool water or cool it with cold compresses. Cooling the burn reduces swelling by conducting heat away from the skin. Do not put ice on the burn. Next, cover the burn with a sterile gauze bandage. Wrap the gauze loosely to avoid putting pressure on burned skin. For major burns (third-degree), call 911 or the facility's emergency number. Until an emergency unit arrives, do not remove burned clothing, but make sure the victim is no longer in contact with smoldering materials or exposed to electricity, smoke, or heat. Do not immerse large, severe burns in cold water as this can cause a drop in body temperature (hypothermia) and deterioration of blood pressure and circulation (shock). Cover the area of the burn. Use a cool, moist, sterile bandage; clean, moist cloth; or moist towels. When possible, elevate the burned body part or parts above heart level. Check for signs of circulation (breathing, coughing or movement). If there is no breathing or other sign of circulation, begin CPR.
Cardiac arrest/heart attack	A cardiac arrest occurs as a result of cessation of normal circulation of the blood due to failure of the heart to contract effectively. A heart attack occurs when blood flow to the muscle of the heart is impaired.	All healthcare practitioners should be trained and certified to perform CPR and should be recertified every two years. The emergency services should be contacted as quickly as possible (before initiating CPR). If an automated external defibrillator (AED) is available, it should be applied after two cycles of CPR. CPR should be continued until medical assistance arrives or the person show signs of recovery.
Chemical splash in the eye	A number of chemicals used in the clinic can be very corrosive.	Immediately flush the eye with water. Use clean, lukewarm tap water for at least 20 minutes, and use whichever of these approaches is quicker: Get into a shower and, while holding the affected eye or eyes open, aim a gentle stream of lukewarm water on the forehead over the affected eye, or direct the stream on the bridge of the nose if both eyes are affected. Hold the affected eye or eyes open. Place the head down and turn it to the side. Or, ask the person to hold the affected eye open under a gently running faucet.

TABLE 9-10	Situations That Require First Aid and Appropriate Action (continued)	
Situation	**Description**	**Appropriate Action**
Choking	Occurs when a foreign object gets lodged in the throat or esophagus, blocking the flow of air.	To ensure that choking is occurring, determine whether the individual is demonstrating an inability to talk, difficulty breathing, and an inability to cough forcefully or whether the skin, lips, and nails are turning blue or dusky.
		If choking is occurring, first, deliver five back blows between the person's shoulder blades with the heel of your hand. Next, perform five abdominal thrusts (Heimlich maneuver). The Heimlich maneuver is performed by standing behind the person and wrapping your arms around their waist. The person is then tipped slightly forward. Making a fist with one hand, position it slightly above the person's navel and, while grasping the fist with the other hand, press hard into the abdomen with a quick, upward thrust (as if trying to lift the person up). Alternate between five back blows and five abdominal thrusts until the blockage is dislodged. If the person becomes unconscious, attempt to remove the blockage and perform CPR.
Convulsions/seizures	Occurs as a result of an electrical imbalance in the brain.	The person should be protected from injury as a result of violent or excessive movements of the extremities, and to protect the person's modesty of privacy.
Fainting	Occurs when the blood supply to the brain is momentarily inadequate, resulting in a temporary loss of consciousness.	Position the person on his or her back. If the person is breathing, restore blood flow to the brain by raising the person's legs above heart level—about 12 inches (30 cm)—if possible. Loosen belts, collars, or other constrictive clothing. If the person doesn't regain consciousness within one minute, call 911 or your local emergency number. In addition, check the person's airway to be sure it's clear. If vomiting occurs, turn the patient on his/her side. Check for signs of circulation (breathing, coughing, or movement). If absent, begin CPR. Call 911 or your local emergency number. Continue CPR until help arrives or the person responds and begins to breathe.
Fractures	Occurs when damage to the bone is sufficient to interrupt its continuity.	The objectives are to protect the fracture site and avoid further injury to it, prevent shock, and reduce pain, and prevent wound contamination if the bone ends have penetrated the skin. The clinician should apply support to the site to stabilize it, but should not attempt to align the bone ends. Any open fracture site should be covered with a sterile towel or dressing. If a spinal fracture is suspected, the clinician should use extreme caution and be sure to maintain the head and neck in a neutral position.
Cardiac arrest	Occurs when an artery supplying the heart with blood and oxygen becomes partially or completely blocked. A heart attack generally causes chest pain for more than 15 minutes, but it can also have no symptoms at all.	Call 911 or your local emergency medical assistance number. If possible, have the person chew and swallow an aspirin, unless he or she is allergic to aspirin. Begin CPR.
Heat illness	A number of heat illnesses exist including: ▶ Heat stroke—a body temperature of greater than 40.6°C (105.1°F) due to environmental heat exposure with lack of thermoregulation and inadequate fluid intake. Symptoms include dry skin, rapid, strong pulse and dizziness. ▶ Heat exhaustion—can be a precursor of heat stroke; the symptoms include heavy sweating, rapid breathing, and a fast, weak pulse.	Move the person out of the sun and into a shady or air-conditioned space. Call 911 or emergency medical help. Cool the person by covering him or her with damp sheets or by spraying with cool water. Direct air onto the person with a fan or newspaper. Have the person drink cool water or other nonalcoholic beverage without caffeine, if he or she is able.

(continued)

TABLE 9-10	Situations That Require First Aid and Appropriate Action (continued)	
Situation	**Description**	**Appropriate Action**
Heat illness (*Continued*)	▶ Heat syncope—fainting as a result of overheating. ▶ Heat edema—swelling of the digits. ▶ Heat cramps—muscle pains or spasms when exercising in hot weather. ▶ Heat rash—skin irritation from excessive sweating. ▶ Heat tetany—usually results from short periods of stress in intense heat. Symptoms may include hyperventilation, respiratory problems, numbness or tingling, or muscle spasms.	
Insulin-related illnesses	Hypoglycemia—occurs when the blood sugar level is too low. Hyperglycemia—occurs when the blood sugar level is too high.	The goal is to restore the person to a normal insulin glucose state and to remove, correct, or compensate for the cause of the condition. *Hypoglycemia:* if the person is conscious, provide some form of sugar (e.g., orange juice), and monitor the individual. *Hyperglycemia:* this is the more serious of the two as it can lead to a diabetic coma and death. Ideally, an injection of insulin should be given.

REFERENCES

1. Guide to Physical Therapist Practice. Second Edition. American Physical Therapy Association. Phys Ther 81:9-746, 2001.
2. Lewis PS: Cardiovascular assessment, in Ruppert SD, Dolan JT, Kernicki JG (eds): Dolan's Critical Care Nursing: Clinical Management Through the Nursing Process (ed 2). Philadelphia, FA Davis, 1996, pp 142-163.
3. Davis MP, Walsh D: Cancer pain: how to measure the fifth vital sign. Cleve Clin J Med 71:625-632, 2004.
4. Salcido RS: Is pain a vital sign? Adv Skin Wound Care 16:214, 2003.
5. Sousa FA: [Pain: the fifth vital sign]. Rev Lat Am Enfermagem 10:446-447, 2002.
6. Lynch M: Pain: the fifth vital sign. Comprehensive assessment leads to proper treatment. Adv Nurse Pract 9:28-36, 2001.
7. Lynch M: Pain as the fifth vital sign. J Intraven Nurs 24:85-94, 2001.
8. Merboth MK, Barnason S: Managing pain: the fifth vital sign. Nurs Clin North Am 35:375-383, 2000.
9. Torma L: Pain—the fifth vital sign. Pulse 36:16, 1999.
10. Pain as the fifth vital sign. J Am Optom Assoc 70:619-620, 1999.
11. Joel LA: The fifth vital sign: pain. Am J Nurs 99:9, 1999.
12. McCaffery M, Pasero CL: Pain ratings: the fifth vital sign. Am J Nurs 97:15-16, 1997.
13. Bailey MK: Physical examination procedures to screen for serious disorders of the low back and lower quarter, in Wilmarth MA (ed): Medical Screening for the Physical Therapist. Orthopaedic Section Independent Study Course 14.1.1 La Crosse, Wisc, Orthopaedic Section, APTA, Inc, 2003, pp 1-35.
14. Schmitz TJ: Vital signs, in O'Sullivan SB, Schmitz TJ (eds): Physical Rehabilitation (ed 5). Philadelphia, FA Davis, 2007, pp 81-120.
15. DeTurk WE, Cahalin LP: Electrocardiography, in DeTurk WE, Cahalin LP (eds): Cardiovascular and Pulmonary Physical Therapy: An Evidence-Based Approach. New York, McGraw-Hill, 2004, pp 325-359.
16. Boudet G, Chamoux A: Ability of new heart rate monitors to measure normal and abnormal heart rate. J Sports Med Phys Fitness 41:546-553, 2001.
17. Boudet G, Chamoux A: Heart rate monitors and abnormal heart rhythm detection. Arch Physiol Biochem 108:371-379, 2000.
18. Shaffer TH, Wolfson MR, Gault JH: Respiratory physiology, in Irwin S, Tecklin JS (eds): Cardiopulmonary Physical Therapy (ed 2). St Louis, Mosby, 1990, pp 217-244.
19. Collins SM, Cocanour B: Anatomy of the cardiopulmonary system, in DeTurk WE, Cahalin LP (eds): Cardiovascular and Pulmonary Physical Therapy: An Evidence-Based Approach. New York, McGraw-Hill, 2004, pp 73-94.
20. Van de Graaff KM, Fox SI: Respiratory system, in Van de Graaff KM, Fox SI (eds): Concepts of Human Anatomy and Physiology. New York, WCB/McGraw-Hill, 1999, pp 728-777.
21. Judge RD, Zuidema GD, Fitzgerald FT: Vital signs, in Judge RD, Zuidema GD, Fitzgerald FT (eds): Clinical Diagnosis (ed 4). Boston, Little, Brown and Company, 1982, pp 49-58.
22. Huber MA, Terezhalmy GT, Moore WS: White coat hypertension. Quintessence Int 35:678-679, 2004.
23. Chung I, Lip GY: White coat hypertension: not so benign after all? J Hum Hypertens 17:807-809, 2003.
24. Alves LM, Nogueira MS, Veiga EV, et al: White coat hypertension and nursing care. Can J Cardiovasc Nurs 13:29-34, 2003.
25. O'Sullivan J, Allen J, Murray A: The forgotten Korotkoff phases: how often are phases II and III present, and how do they relate to the other Korotkoff phases? Am J Hypertens 15:264-268, 2002.
26. Venet R, Miric D, Pavie A, et al: Korotkoff sound: the cavitation hypothesis. Med Hypotheses 55:141-146, 2000.
27. Weber F, Anlauf M, Hirche H, et al: Differences in blood pressure values by simultaneous auscultation of Korotkoff sounds inside the cuff and in the antecubital fossa. J Hum Hypertens 13:695-700, 1999.
28. Paskalev D, Kircheva A, Krivoshiev S: A centenary of auscultatory blood pressure measurement: a tribute to Nikolai Korotkoff. Kidney Blood Press Res 28:259-263, 2005.
29. Perloff D, Grim C, Flack J, et al: Human blood pressure determination by sphygmomanometry. Circulation 88:2460-2470, 1993.
30. Strugo V, Glew FJ, Davis J, et al: Update: Recommendations for human blood pressure determination by sphygmomanometers. Hypertension 16:594, 1990.
31. Higgins JR, Walker SP, Brennecke SP: Re: Which Korotkoff sound should be used for diastolic blood pressure in pregnancy? Aust N Z J Obstet Gynaecol 38:480-481, 1998.

32. Likeman RK: Re: Which Korotkoff sound should be used for diastolic blood pressure in pregnancy? Aust N Z J Obstet Gynaecol. 38:479-480, 1998.

33. Franx A, Evers IM, van der Pant KA, et al: The fourth sound of Korotkoff in pregnancy: a myth. Eur J Obstet Gynecol Reprod Biol 76:53-59, 1998.

34. Kelly G: Body temperature variability (Part 1): a review of the history of body temperature and its variability due to site selection, biological rhythms, fitness, and aging. Altern Med Rev 11:278-293, 2006.

35. Editors of Nursing: Take care with tympanic temperature readings. Nursing 37:52-53, 2007.

36. Sener S, Karcioglu O, Eken C, et al: Agreement between axillary, tympanic, and mid-forehead body temperature measurements in adult emergency department patients. Eur J Emerg Med 19:252–256, 2011.

37. Purssell E, While A, Coomber B: Tympanic thermometry—normal temperature and reliability. Paediatr Nurs 21:40-43, 2009.

38. Barton SJ, Gaffney R, Chase T, et al: Pediatric temperature measurement and child/parent/nurse preference using three temperature measurement instruments. J Pediatr Nurs 18:314-320, 2003.

39. Rush M, Wetherall A: Temperature measurement: practice guidelines. Paediatr Nurs 15:25-28, 2003.

40. Denegar CR, Donley PB: Impairment due to pain: Managing pain during the rehabilitation process, in Voight ML, Hoogenboom BJ, Prentice WE (eds): Musculoskeletal Interventions: Techniques for Therapeutic Exercise. New York, McGraw-Hill, 2007, pp 99-110.

41. Dray A: Inflammatory mediators of pain. Br J Anaesth 75:125-131, 1995.

42. Wiener SL: Differential Diagnosis of Acute Pain by Body Region. New York, McGraw-Hill, 1993, pp 1-4.

43. Adams RD, Victor M: Principles of Neurology (ed 5). New York, McGraw-Hill, Health Professions Division, 1993.

44. Chusid JG: Correlative Neuroanatomy & Functional Neurology (ed 19). Norwalk, Conn, Appleton-Century-Crofts, 1985, pp 144-148.

45. Judge RD, Zuidema GD, Fitzgerald FT: Musculoskeletal system, in Judge RD, Zuidema GD, Fitzgerald FT (eds): Clinical Diagnosis (ed 4). Boston, Little, Brown and Company, 1982, pp 365-403.

46. Bonica JJ: Neurophysiological and pathological aspects of acute and chronic pain. Arch Surg 112:750-761, 1977.

47. Burkhardt CS: The use of the McGill Pain Questionnaire in assessing arthritis pain. Pain 19:305, 1984.

48. Chaturvedi SK: Prevalence of chronic pain in psychiatric patients. Pain 29:231-237, 1987.

49. Dunn D: Chronic regional pain syndrome, type 1: Part I. AORN J 72:421-424, 426, 428-432, 435, 437-442, 444-449, 452-458, 2000.

50. Huskisson EC: Measurement of pain. Lancet 2:127, 1974.

51. Halle JS: Neuromusculoskeletal scan examination with selected related topics, in Flynn TW (ed): The Thoracic Spine and Rib Cage: Musculoskeletal Evaluation and Treatment. Boston, Butterworth-Heinemann, 1996, pp 121-146.

52. Melzack R: The McGill Pain Questionnaire: Major properties and scoring methods. Pain 1:277, 1975.

53. Melzack R, Torgerson WS: On the language of pain. Anaesthesiology 34:50, 1971.

54. Liebenson C: Pain and disability questionnaires in chiropractic rehabilitation, in Liebenson C (ed): Rehabilitation of the Spine: A Practitioner's Manual. Baltimore, Lippincott Williams & Wilkins, 1996, pp 57-71.

55. Kahn-D'Angel L, Unanue-Rose RA: The special care nursery, in Campbell SK, Vander Linden DW, Palisano RJ (eds): Physical Therapy for Children (ed 3). St Louis, Saunders, 2006, pp 1053-1097.

56. Hockenberry MJ, Wilson D, Winkelstein ML: Wong's Essentials of Pediatric Nursing (ed 7). St Louis, Mosby, 2004.

57. Beyer JE, Denyes MJ, Villarruel AM: The creation, validation, and continuing development of the Oucher: a measure of pain intensity in children. J Pediatr Nurs 7:335-346, 1992.

Bed Mobility, Patient Positioning, and Draping

CHAPTER 10

CHAPTER OBJECTIVES

At the completion of this chapter, the reader will be able to:

1. Understand the importance of bed mobility to prevent secondary complications

2. Describe some of the precautions when positioning a patient

3. Discuss the biomechanical principles behind correct body mechanics

4. Describe some of the challenges facing a clinician while moving a patient or heavy object

5. Describe some of the mechanical devices that can be used during bed mobility tasks

6. List the 12 principles of good body mechanics

7. Discuss the biomechanical principles and the integral elements of the motor control progression that can be implemented during a bed mobility tasks

8. Demonstrate how to provide bed mobility to a dependent patient

9. Demonstrate how to instruct a patient in bed mobility

10. Describe the importance and the principles behind patient positioning

11. Describe the importance and the principles behind patient draping

OVERVIEW

Bed mobility activities are designed to adjust the body position of a recumbent patient to prevent the development of joint contractures or skin breakdown. In contrast, depending on the patient's medical condition, such as after total joint replacement, there may be mobility restrictions or contraindications that affect bed mobility.

CLINICAL PEARL

A number of medical conditions can result in mobility and position restrictions or contraindications. These include:

▶ *Total hip arthroplasty (THA):* the restrictions and contraindications following this surgical technique depends on the approach the surgeon used:

■ For the posterolateral approach, this involves avoidance of hip flexion of the hip beyond 60–90°, 0° hip adduction and 0° of hip internal rotation.

■ Following a lateral or anterolateral approach, the patient should avoid hip extension, external rotation, and adduction across midline.

This patient population is prescribed a positioning device, a triangular foam cushion, which is strapped between the legs to keep the hip in an abducted position. It is important to remember that these range-of-motion restrictions apply in relation to both hip and trunk motion. For example, both lifting the knee while sitting or leaning forward at the waist result in hip flexion beyond 90°. From a clinical perspective, extra care must be taken when the patient is moving from supine to sitting to prevent both excessive hip flexion and excessive hip adduction.

▶ *Hemiplegia:* rolling from supine to sidelying on the hemiplegic side is relatively straightforward, but rolling to lie on the stronger side presents a greater challenge.

▶ *Spinal cord injury (SCI):* the functional ability of the patient who is post SCI depends on the level and degree of injury (Table 10-1). With respect to bed mobility, an injury at the level of the sixth cervical vertebra (C6) will typically allow a patient to achieve independent performance of bed mobility.

Bed mobility may be assisted by various types of equipment, with help from another individual or individuals, or performed independently by the patient. There are many occasions when a patient needs to be positioned by the clinician. Examples include when a patient has decreased sensation to pressure, or when the patient is unable to alter his or her position independently. Draping, or covering, a patient can be a natural consequence of positioning or can be performed to

TABLE 10-1	Functional Outcomes Related to Level of Spinal Cord Injury			
Level of Lesion	Function/Motion	Care Needs	ADLs	Equipment Needs

C1-C3	Limited head/neck movement
	Rotate/flex neck (sternocleidomastoid)
	Extend neck (cervical paraspinals)
	Speech and swallowing (neck accessories)
	Total paralysis of trunk, upper and lower extremity
		24 hr care needs
		Able to direct care needs
			Ventilator dependent
			Impaired communication
			Dependent for all care needs
			Mobility:
			  Power wheelchair
			  Hoyer lift
				Adapted computer
				Bedside/portable ventilator
				Suction machine
				Specialty bed
				Hoyer
				Reclining shower chair

C4	Head and neck control (cervical paraspinals)
	Shoulder shrug (upper traps)
	Inspiration (diaphragm)
	Lack of shoulder control (deltoids)
	Paralysis of trunk, UE and LE
	Inability to cough, low respiratory reserve
		24 hr care needs
		Able to direct care needs
			May or may not be vent dependent
			Improved communication
			Assisted cough
			Dependent for all care needs
			Mobility:
			  Power wheelchair
			  Hoyer lift
				Adapted computer
				Bedside/portable ventilator as needed
				Suction machine
				Specialty bed
				Hoyer
				Reclining shower chair

C5	Shoulder control (deltoids)
	Elbow flexion (biceps/elbow flexors)
	Supinate hands (brachialis and brachioradialis)
	Lack elbow extension and hand pronation
	Paralysis of trunk and LE
		10 hr personal care need
		6 hr homemaking assistance
			Setup/equipment: eating, drinking, face wash and teeth
			Assisted cough
			Dependent for bowel, bladder and lower body hygiene
			Dependent for bed mobility and transfers
			Mobility:
			  Hoyer or stand pivot
			  Power wheelchair w/ hand controls
			  Manual wheelchair
			  Drive motor vehicle w/ hand controls
				Power and manual wheelchairs
				Adaptive splints/braces
				Page turners/computer adaptations

C6	Wrist extension (extensor carpi ulnaris and extensor carpi radialis longus/brevis) Arm across chest (clavicular pectoralis) Lack elbow extension (triceps) Lack wrist flexion Lack hand control Paralysis of trunk and LE	6 hr personal care needs 4 hr homemaking assistance	Assisted cough Setup for feeding, bathing and dressing Independent bed mobility (if sufficient spinal rotation—approximately 66°—can be performed), pressure relief, turns and skin assessment. May be independent for bowel/bladder care	Independent slide board transfer Manual wheelchair Drive with adaptive equipment
C7	Elbow flexion and extension (biceps/triceps) Arm toward body (sternal pectoralis) Lack finger function Lack trunk stability	6 hr personal care needs 2 hr homemaking assistance	More effective cough Fewer adaptive aids Independent w/ all ADLs May need adaptive aids for bowel care	Manual wheelchair Transfers without adaptive equipment
C8-T1	Increased finger and hand strength Finger flexion (flexor digitorum) Finger extension (extensor communis) Thumb movement (pollicis longus and brevis) Separate fingers (interossei separates)	4 hr personal care needs 2 hr homemaking assistance	Independent w/ or w/o assistive devices Assist w/ complex meal prep and home management	Manual wheelchair

(continued)

TABLE 10-1   Functional Outcomes Related to Level of Spinal Cord Injury (continued)

Level of Lesion	Function/Motion	Care Needs	ADLs	Equipment Needs
T2-T6	Normal motor function of head, neck, shoulders, arms, hands and fingers Increased use of intercostals Increase trunk control (erector spinae)	3 hr personal care needs/ homemaking	Independent in personal care	Manual wheelchair May have limited walking with extensive bracing Drive with hand controls
T7-T12	Added motor function Increased abdominal control Increased trunk stability	2 hr personal care needs/ homemaking	Independent Improved cough Improved balance control	Manual wheelchair May have limited walking with bracing Driving with hand controls
L2-L5	Added motor function in hips and knees L2 Hip flexors (iliopsoas) L3 Knee extensors (quadriceps) L4 Ankle dorsiflexors (tibialis anterior) L5 Long toe extensors (ext hallucis longus)	May need 1 hr personal care/homemaking	Independent	Manual wheelchair May walk short distance with braces and assistive devices Driving with hand controls
S1-S5	Ankle plantar flexors (gastrocnemius) Various degrees of bowel, bladder, and sexual function Lower level equals greater function	No personal or homemaker needs	Independent	Increased ability to walk with less adaptive/ supportive devices Manual wheelchair for distance

expose a particular body part for examination or an intervention, such as a manual technique.

CLINICAL PEARL

As a patient becomes less dependent, less control from the clinician is needed.

BODY MECHANICS

Body mechanics refers to the way in which the clinician's body is positioned or aligned during tasks. Correct positioning and alignment places the center of mass (COM) of the clinician close to the patient (see Chapter 4), which increases the efficiency of movements and limits the stress and strain on musculoskeletal structures.

Healthcare workers often experience musculoskeletal disorders (MSDs), total lost workday injury and illness incidence at a rate exceeding that of workers in construction, mining, and manufacturing.[1] Most of these injuries are the result of lifting and transferring patients.[2] These injuries incur very high direct costs in workers' compensation, medical treatment and vocational rehabilitation as well as indirect costs due to lost production, retraining, and sick or administrative time, the latter of which can be at least four times the direct cost.[3,4]

CLINICAL PEARL

It is very important to remember that the greater the load, the greater the risk of injury.

The problem of lifting a patient is compounded by the increasing weight of patients to be lifted due to the obesity epidemic in the United States and the rapidly increasing number of older people who require assistance with their activities of daily living.[5]

The physical demands when working in healthcare involve variations of forceful exertion, repetition, and stressful positions or postures. Holding, pushing, or handling equipment can also involve these physical demands. A variety of individual factors also play an important role. Individuals who are not in good physical condition tend to have more injuries. Previous trauma or certain medical conditions involving bones, joints, muscles, tendons, nerves, and blood vessels may also predispose individuals to injuries. Finally, some psychological factors may influence the reporting of injuries, pain thresholds, and even the speed or degree of healing.

The amount of force involved can be determined as described in Chapter 4. An example is provided in Table 10-2.

Therefore, before any activities involving lifting, pushing, or pulling, the clinician must decide whether the transfer is to be performed by a team, a mechanical device, or a combination of both.

▶ *Team.* Choose the best body mechanics possible to accomplish the task with minimal effort and in a safe manner for everyone involved. The 12 principles of good body mechanics include:

1. Plan ahead by estimating the load and clearing the path of travel.

2. Stand as close to the load as is feasible. Being as close as possible to the person or object to be lifted or

TABLE 10-2	Calculating the Forces Involved When Preparing to Lift a Patient

Patient standing 0.5 m away from patient

Weight of clinician = 160 pounds (712 N)

Approximate weight of clinician's arms, trunk, and head (65% of the total weight of the body) = $712 \times 0.65 = 463$ N

The moment arm (MA) of the erector spinae (ES) muscles, which is the perpendicular distance between the line of action of the muscles and the axis about which they move, is approximately 0.05 m.

If the clinician keeps his or her knees straight, the approximate MA for the arms, trunk, and head of the clinician = 0.5 m.

If the clinician flexes his or her knees, the approximate MA for the arms, trunk, and head of the clinician = 0.25 m.

Therefore:

▶ The force applied to the ES with the clinician's knees straight = $(463 \text{ N} \times 0.5)/0.05 \text{ m} = 4630$ N (approx. 1041 lb).

▶ The force applied to the ES with the clinician's knees flexed = $(463 \text{ N} \times 0.25)/0.05 \text{ m} = 2315$ N (approx. 520 lb)

Note that the calculated forces do not include the patient's weight.

N, newtons.

carried allows the combined COM to be maintained within the base of support (BOS). When the COM is centered within the BOS and near the body's midline, both balance and good postural alignment are easier to maintain.

3. Use a BOS that is of the appropriate size and shape—stand with the feet apart, with one foot slightly in front of the other, and the toes pointing slightly outward.

4. Try to maintain normal spinal curvature. If the trunk is maintained in good alignment, the muscles only have to maintain this alignment, and do not have to work to extend the trunk during the lifting motion. Whenever possible the spine should be maintained in a neutral position. A simple method to determine pelvic neutral is to perform an anterior pelvic tilt and then a posterior pelvic tilt and to try and find the midpoint between the two [VIDEO 10-1]. Avoid twisting at the trunk, particularly when the trunk is flexed. Instead, pivot at the feet, or take several small steps to rotate the whole body.

5. Whenever possible, lifting should be initiated from a squatting position. The depth of the squat should be deep enough to permit the clinician to reach the person or object to be lifted, but not so deep that the leg muscles are moved out of their power position for lifting and lowering. This type of squat is achieved by flexing the hips and knees, rather than by trunk flexion. The other advantage of this position is that it maintains the COM of the body close to the center of the BOS—a shorter resistance lever arm requires less effort.

6. When possible, push rather than pull an object, as pushing permits a larger BOS and a lower COM as well as making it easier to use the larger muscles more efficiently.

7. Keep the combined COM of the clinician, equipment, and patient within the BOS by holding objects close.

8. If possible, elevate the surface to waist height. A load close to the height of the COM conserves energy and maintains stability during the lift.

9. Exhale during exertion to minimize any increase in intra-abdominal pressure, which in turn can elevate blood pressure.

10. Avoid rotation of the spine, particularly when the trunk is flexed, by moving the feet.

11. Before lifting, gently contract the abdominal muscles. Contracting the muscles of the trunk before lifting may reduce the potential for injury.

12. Know your own capabilities and do not attempt a task if there is any doubt about your ability to complete it safely.

▶ *Mechanical device.* A mechanically assisted or "zero-lift" transfer involves the transfer of an individual who is unable to provide minimal or any assistance.

When moving large pieces of equipment, the clinician should be positioned behind the equipment or patient, facing in the direction of movement. This allows the clinician to:

1. Determine a path free from obstruction

2. Use a lifting or pushing motion

3. Use larger muscles and body weight more efficiently during pushing or lifting

In all cases, plan movements and prepare the area to be used before starting. Use proper body mechanics and safety precautions.

CLINICAL PEARL

When in doubt about your ability to lift or carry a patient or object safely, always obtain additional assistance.

BED MOBILITY

Bed mobility activities are an important component of progressively improving a patient's independence and safety within his or her abilities. Regardless of the level of dependence of the patient, the clinician must always use proper body mechanics while also guarding the patient. If at all possible, the height of the bed or mat should be adjusted to enhance comfort and safety. As with all activities involving physical exertion, the clinician should first assess whether any physical or mechanical assistance is required before attempting the activity. Mechanical assistance can include use of the bed rails, a draw sheet, or an overhead bar or frame in cases where the patient is unable to safely perform the activity without equipment. Whenever possible, the patient should be encouraged to participate both mentally and physically in the bed mobility activity. Patient involvement fosters independence and boosts problem solving. The most common bed mobility activities include turning from a supine to a sidelying position and returning; moving from a supine to prone position and returning; moving from a lying to a sitting position and returning; and moving in a variety of horizontal directions (upward, downward, side to side) and returning to the center of the bed. More advanced activities include scooting in supine and sitting and scooting on the edge of the bed. The bed mobility progression should incorporate biomechanical principles and the integral elements of the motor control progression (see Chapter 4):

- Static stability
- Dynamic stability
- Controlled mobility
- Uncontrolled mobility

Closely associated with the motor control progression are the concepts of COM and BOS, which the clinician must consider with mobility activities. These concepts (see Chapter 4) include:

- The greater the mass, the greater the stability.
- The greater the friction, the greater the stability.
- The larger the BOS, the greater the stability.
- The lower the COM, the greater the stability.
- The more the BOS is widened in the direction of the line of force, the greater the stability.

From a clinical perspective, the concepts just listed can be applied when moving a patient. For example when pulling and sliding patient, the clinician places his or her COM as close to the patient's COM as possible, widens his or her feet to increase the BOS, and applies the force required to move the patient parallel to the surface of the bed, thereby reducing the energy required. Positioning the patient close to the clinician allows the muscles of the upper extremities to use short lever arms. Short lever arms can develop greater force than long lever arms, require less energy expenditure, and provide better patient control.

Assisted Mobility

Side-to-side Movement. With the patient positioned in supine, the clinician folds the patient's arm across the chest (Figure 10-1) and then positions one forearm under the

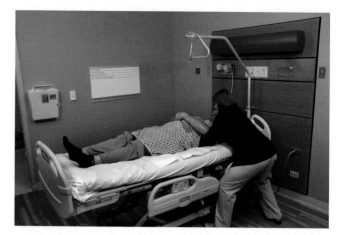

FIGURE 10-2 Clinician positions arms under the patient

patient's neck, supporting the patient's head, and one forearm under the middle of the patient's back (Figure 10-2). The clinician then gently slides the patient's upper body and head closer to where the clinician is standing (Figures 10-3 and 10-4). Next, the clinician can either place his or her forearms under the patient's lower trunk and just distal to the pelvis, or can use the bed mat (Figure 10-5) before gently sliding that body segment in the same direction as previous (Figure 10-6). Finally, the clinician places his or her forearms under the thighs and legs of the patient (Figure 10-7) and gently slides them toward him or her (Figure 10-8).

Upward Movement. This is one of the more difficult techniques and the one with the most potential for injury to the shoulders or lower back of the clinician. If the bed is adjustable, the portion that raises the head and trunk should be flat, and any pillows should be removed from under the patient's head and shoulders. Using the concept that the greater the friction, the greater the stability, the clinician flexes the patient's hips and knees so that only the feet rest flat on the bed. Depending on the level of dependence of the patient, the thighs may need to be supported with one or more pillows to maintain the position. The clinician and the assistant stand approximately opposite the patient's midchest level, facing toward the patient's head, and with the foot that is farthest from the bed in front of the other foot [VIDEO 10-2]. Using both

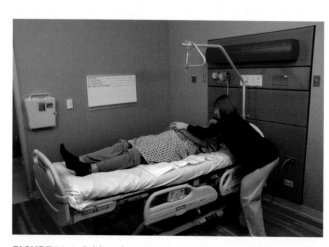

FIGURE 10-1 Folding the patient's arm in preparation for movement

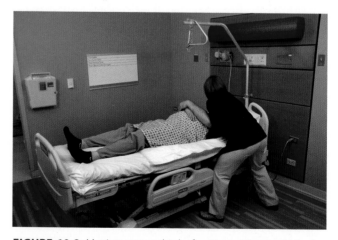

FIGURE 10-3 Moving upper third of patient sideways in bed—initial move

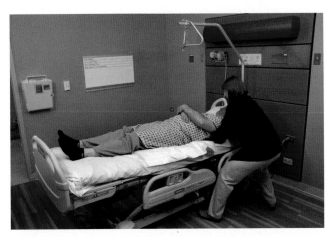

FIGURE 10-4 Moving upper third of patient sideways in bed—end of move

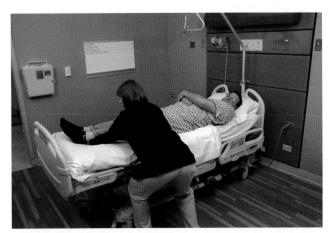

FIGURE 10-7 Moving the lower third of the patient—start position

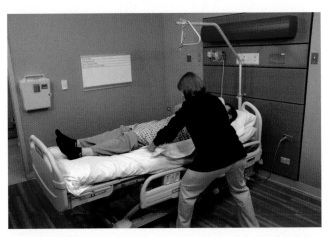

FIGURE 10-5 Moving the middle third of the patient using the bed mat

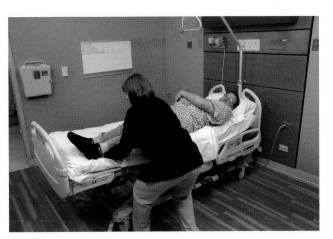

FIGURE 10-8 Moving the lower third of the patient—end position

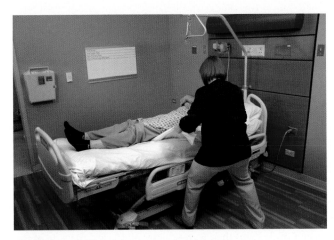

FIGURE 10-6 End of the move using the bed mat

arms, the lifting team grasps the bed mat and, keeping close to the patient's chest, the patient is slid upward approximately 6 inches. The technique is repeated until the required position is obtained.

Downward Movement. If the bed is adjustable, the portion that raises the head and trunk should be raised. The clinician and the assistant stand approximately opposite to the patient's waist or hips. Using both arms, the lifting team grasps the bed

mat and, keeping close to the patient's waist, the patient is slid downward. The technique is repeated until the required position is obtained.

Turning from Supine to Sidelying. To turn the patient to the right, the clinician stands on the side of the bed to which the patient is turning, and the patient is positioned close to the edge of the left side of the bed. The right arm is abducted to approximately 45°, and the left lower extremity is crossed over the right lower extremity at the ankle. Using the right hand, the clinician grasps the patient's left hip while holding the patient's left hand against the same hip. The clinician's left hand is used to grasp the patient's left shoulder, and then the patient is rolled into the sidelying position.

Turning from Supine to Prone. The need to move a patient from supine to prone in a hospital bed does not occur frequently because of the design of the modern mattress. Indeed, given the design of the mattress, placing a patient prone is likely to be hazardous because of the potential for breathing problems. Therefore, the following description is more likely to be used when the patient is on a mat table. The patient is positioned toward one edge of the mat table so that a full rolling movement to the prone position can occur without the patient coming too near the opposite edge. To roll to the right side, the patient is first moved to the left side of the bed using the technique described in Side-to-Side Movement. To roll a patient toward the right side:

▶ The patient's left lower extremity is crossed over the right lower extremity, with the left ankle resting on top of the right ankle.

▶ The patient's right upper extremity is abducted, placing the hand under the right hip, palm facing upward against the hip, while the hand and forearm of the left upper extremity are placed across the abdomen.

▶ The clinician stands on the side of the mat table to which the patient will be turned—in this case, on the patient's right-hand side.

▶ To initiate the rolling, the clinician's hands are positioned under the patient's left shoulder and lower back. At the point when the patient reaches the halfway position of the roll, the clinician rotates the hands, positioning them on the anterior surface of the patient in order to control the second half of the roll.

▶ At the completion of the roll, the head is repositioned first, placing it in a comfortable position facing to one side (normally toward the side of the roll direction) and ensuring that there is no pressure on the eyes, nose, or mouth. Where indicated, a pillow is placed under the trunk and adjusted as necessary (see Prone Position). The upper extremities are placed in a position of slight abduction—approximately 20° to 30°—and the feet are positioned approximately 6 to 8 inches apart. Generally speaking, rolling a patient from prone to supine is essentially the reverse of rolling the patient from supine to prone.

Independent Mobility

When performing these activities, it is important to instruct the patient to determine the body's position on the bed before any mobility activities are attempted. For example, depending on the width of the bed, it may be necessary for patient to adjust his or her position by moving forward or backward before attempting to roll. The following techniques may need to be modified based on the size of the patient and the patient's functional abilities.

Scooting Upward. If the bed is adjustable, the upper portion should be flat and the wheels should be locked. The patient is positioned in the hooklying position, with the heels close to the buttocks and the upper extremities beside the trunk. The patient is asked to elevate the pelvis using the lower extremities and to elevate the upper trunk by simultaneously pressing into the bed with the elbows and the back of the head, and then move upward by pressing down with the lower extremities and depressing the shoulders. The lower and upper extremities are then repositioned before successive movements are attempted. A number of other methods can be used to increase patient independence with moving up the bed. These methods are shown in [VIDEO 10-3 through 10-5].

Before discharge from the hospital, it is important that the clinician review any of the bed mobility skills that have been taught to the patient [VIDEO 10-6]. In addition to those previously described, the following should also be reviewed as appropriate.

Video Description

In Video 10-6, a number of bed mobility skills are reviewed with the patient. These include:

▶ *Hooklying.* Hooklying, which is the supine position with the hips and knees flexed so that the feet are flat on the bed, is a basic bed mobility position from which other skills are derived.

▶ *Bridging.* From the hooklying position, the patient lifts the hips and lower back off the bed. This skill can be used to provide pressure relief while also allowing items such as bedpans and bed linens to be placed underneath the patient.

▶ *Scooting in supine.* This skill, which is a precursor for such skills as rolling and getting out of bed, allows the patient to move up, down, and sideways in the bed. Scooting is made easier by lowering the part of the bed to which the patient is moving. For example, if the patient is moving up the bed, it is easier when the head of the bed is lowered.

▶ *Rolling.* This skill can be used to relieve pressure on body tissues, but also to help with air exchange in the lungs. From a functional point of view, the skill allows objects such as linens, slings, and bedpans to be placed under the supine patient. To assist with rolling, the patient can use head rotation, trunk rotation, and motions of the upper and lower extremities.

▶ *Supine to sitting.* The sitting position in bed can either occur with the legs extended (long sitting), or with the hips and knees flexed (short sitting). Long sitting is useful for positional adjustments, or when a patient has undergone a total hip arthroplasty and is not permitted to flex the hip beyond 60°. Short sitting is typically used to sit on the side of the bed, before standing. To move from supine to sitting requires upper extremity strength in patients with mobility limitations.

▶ *Sitting to supine.* This skill is essentially the reverse of supine to sitting, and the patient uses an upper extremity to control the descent of the trunk into the sidelying position before lifting both lower extremities onto the bed.

Side-to-side Movement. Side-to-side movements are best performed with the patient supine. The patient is asked to assume the hooklying position and to have one upper extremity next to the trunk, and the other upper extremity abducted approximately 6 inches from the trunk. The patient is asked to perform a bridge and then move the trunk toward the side of the abducted upper extremity before lowering the trunk (see Video 10-6). The lower and upper extremities are then repositioned to either move again or for comfort. The activity is practiced so that the patient can move to both the right and the left side.

Scooting Downward. If the bed is adjustable, the upper portion should be raised slightly and the wheels should be locked. The patient is positioned in the hooklying position with the heels approximately 12 inches distal to the buttocks and the upper extremities positioned next to the trunk. The patient is asked to elevate the pelvis using the lower extremities and to elevate the upper trunk by simultaneously pushing into the bed with the elbows and the back of the head, before moving down with by pulling with the lower extremities (concentric knee flexion), simultaneously pushing up with the shoulders and pulling down with the elbows (concentric shoulder extension) or forearms (see Video 10-6). The lower and upper extremities are then repositioned for successive movements.

Supine to Sidelying. The patient is asked to move to one side of the bed. To roll toward the left, the patient simultaneously reaches across the chest with the right upper extremity and lifts the right lower extremity diagonally over the left lower extremity, then uses a combination of neck flexors and the abdominal muscles to roll onto the side, or alternatively uses the right hand to grasp the edge of the bed/bed rail to pull themselves into the sidelying position (see Video 10-6). Once in the sidelying position, the BOS is increased by flexing the lower extremities and by reaching back with the right upper extremity. The activity is practiced so that the patient can move into both right and left sidelying.

Assuming Sitting. Moving directly from supine to sitting places extreme amounts of torque through the patient's spine. The better techniques do not overstress the patient's spine.

▶ *Supine to long sitting:* providing that the patient has enough strength, the long sitting position can be accomplished using a situp from a position propped up on the elbows (see Video 10-6). When minimal assistance is necessary, a trapeze bar can be used while the clinician provides assistance by placing an arm behind patient's back. In those situations where a trapeze bar is not available, the clinician's forearm can be used.

▶ *Supine to sitting:* if the patient is independent, the patient flexes the hips and knees to 60° to 90° and then moves the lower legs over the edge of the bed while using the upper extremities to push down on the table and raise the trunk (see Video 10-6). When minimal assistance is necessary, the clinician grasps the patient's lower extremities and lowers them over the edge of the bed, and helps lift the upper trunk as necessary.

Video Description

VIDEO 10-7, 10-8, 10-9, and **10-10** show a series of methods to teach a patient how to perform supine-to-sit and sit-to-supine skills based on patient ability. Notice how the clinician always tries to get the patient to do as much of the work as possible, thereby enhancing independence. The clinician also frequently asks the patient whether or not the instructions have been understood. This is particularly important in Video 10-10, when the patient's ability to transfer is limited by the postsurgical precautions. Again, the clinician reviews these precautions with the patient, a process that must occur as frequently as necessary.

Scooting in Sitting. Perhaps the most important scoot in sitting is the sideways scoot, which can be used for a patient who is about to return to lying supine in bed. To perform a sideways scoot on the edge of the bed, the patient abducts the arm on the side to which he or she is moving, thus creating a space for the patient's hips to move to. The patient is then asked to push down with both hands into the bed using a fisted hand (less stressful to the wrist than using an open palm with the wrist extended), to depress the shoulders, and to raise the hips off the bed and over to the new position (see Video 10-6). This technique is repeated until the desired position is achieved. To scoot backward or forward in a sitting position, one of two techniques can be used based on the patient's upper extremity strength:

▶ *Good upper extremity strength:* the patient is asked to lean the trunk slightly forward with the hands by the hips, and to press down into the bed. If the bed is at such a height that the patient's feet can touch the floor, this technique can be assisted by bringing the feet back toward the bed and pushing down on the feet while simultaneously pushing down with the upper extremities before the patient lifts the torso up and then either forward or backward.

▶ *Poor upper extremity strength:* the patient is asked to scoot forward or backward by weight shifting to one side and then moving the opposite hip forward or backward and then repeating this maneuver on the other side until the desired position is achieved.

PATIENT POSITIONING

Body weight produces pressure to the skin, subcutaneous tissue, bone, and the circulatory, neural, and lymphatic systems. Patient positioning is considered when a patient with limited bed mobility is to be at rest for an extended period.

CLINICAL PEARL

Deep venous thrombosis (DVT) and its sequela, pulmonary embolism, are the leading causes of preventable in-hospital mortality in the United States.[6] The Virchow triad, as first formulated (i.e., venous stasis, vessel wall injury, hypercoagulable state), is still the primary mechanism for the development of venous thrombosis.[6] Hypercoagulable states include:

▶ *Genetic:* includes antithrombin C deficiency, protein C deficiency, and protein S deficiency.

▶ *Acquired:* includes postoperative, postpartum, prolonged bed rest or immobilization, severe trauma, cancer, congestive heart failure, obesity, advanced age, and prior thromboembolism.

No single physical finding or combination of symptoms and signs is sufficiently accurate to establish the diagnosis of DVT.[6] The following is a list outlining the most sensitive and specific physical findings in DVT[6-9]:

▶ Edema, principally unilateral

▶ Tenderness, if present, is usually confined to the calf muscles or over the course of the deep veins in the thigh. Pain and/or tenderness away from these areas is not consistent with venous thrombosis and usually indicates another diagnosis.

▶ Venous distention and prominence of the subcutaneous veins.

▶ *Fever:* Patients may have a fever, usually low grade.

It is important to note that the Homan sign—discomfort in the calf muscles on forced dorsiflexion of the foot with the knee straight—which has been a time-honored sign of DVT, is found in more than 50% of patients without DVT and is present in less than one third of patients with confirmed DVT, making it very nonspecific.

Prophylactic treatment of DVT includes staying active and mobile whenever possible, medication (heparin, warfarin, aspirin, and dextran), and the use of mechanical modalities such as external pneumatic compression devices and compression stockings.

When appropriate, the clinician should introduce themselves to the patient and explain the purpose of the planned treatment, including how the patient is to be positioned. Whenever possible, the patient should be encouraged to be an active participant. To prevent injury to the patient, the patient's body and extremities should always be totally supported on the mat or table with no partial portion of the body or extremities projecting beyond the surface. The most effective way to position a patient is to position the proximal components (the center of the patient's mass) first. For example, if the pelvis is positioned correctly, the position of the head and extremities often occurs naturally.

Regular patient repositioning (at least every two hours when lying and every 10 minutes when sitting) is required for conditions including loss of or decreased sensory awareness, paralysis or inability to move independently, bowel and/or bladder incontinence, decreased skin integrity (friable), poor nutrition, severe weight loss (cachexia), impaired circulation, an inability to express or communicate discomfort, and a predisposition to contracture development (Table 10-3). In addition to the positioning of the patient, it is also necessary to inspect the patient's skin, especially over bony prominences (Table 10-4), before and immediately after the treatment session. It is also important to remove or reduce folds or wrinkles in the linen beneath the patient to avoid increased skin pressure.

CLINICAL PEARL

Factors to avoid when positioning a patient include:

- Compromising the patient's airway.
- Excessive, prolonged pressure to soft tissue, circulatory, and neurologic structures.
- Poor spinal alignment.

TABLE 10-3 — Soft Tissue Contracture Sites Associated with Prolonged Positioning

Position	Contracture Sites
Supine	Shoulder internal rotators, extensors, and adductors Forearm, elbow, wrist, and fingers (depending on the upper extremity position used) Hip and knee flexors Hip external rotators Ankle plantarflexors
Prone	Neck rotators, left or right Shoulder internal/external rotators, extensors, and adductors Forearm, elbow, wrist, and fingers (depending on the upper extremity position used) Ankle plantarflexors
Sidelying	Shoulder adductors and internal rotators Forearm, elbow, wrist, and fingers (depending on the upper extremity position used) Hip adductors and internal rotators Hip and knee flexors
Sitting	Shoulder adductors, internal rotators, and extensors Forearm, elbow, wrist, and fingers (depending on the upper extremity position used) Hip adductors and internal rotators Hip and knee flexors

- Positioning the patient's extremities beyond or below the support surface. Extremities that project beyond the support surface are at increased risk for injury, whereas extremities positioned below the support surface are prone to edema formation.
- Clothing or linen folds beneath the patient, which can produce skin breakdown.
- Excessive and prolonged pressure over bony prominences.
- Friction or shear forces. These can occur if the patient is dragged. A shear force is an applied force that tends to cause an opposite, but parallel, sliding motion of the planes of an object.
- Positioning a patient in a way that minimizes interaction with the environment.

The first time a patient is placed in a new position, it is recommended that the skin be checked after 5 to 10 minutes, and frequently thereafter, to determine tolerance for the new position.

TABLE 10-4 — Bony Prominences Associated with Pressure Ulcers

Supine	Prone	Sidelying	Seated
Occiput	Forehead	Ears	Spine of scapula
Spine of scapula	Anterior portion of the acromion process	Lateral portion of acromion process	Vertebral spinous processes
Inferior angle of scapula	Anterior head of humerus	Lateral head of humerus	Ischial tuberosities
Vertebral spinous processes	Sternum	Lateral epicondyle of humerus	
Medial epicondyle of humerus	Anterior superior iliac spine	Greater trochanter	
Posterior iliac crest	Patella	Head of fibula	
Sacrum	Dorsum of foot	Lateral malleolus	
Coccyx		Medial malleolus	

▶ When inspecting a patient's skin, red areas indicate areas of pressure, whereas pale (or blanched) areas may indicate severe, precarious pressure. A red or blanched area that does not return to a normal appearance within an hour must be monitored, and the use of the position that caused the problem should be avoided in the future.

▶ Subjective complaints of numbness or tingling are indicators of excessive pressure, as is localized edema or swelling.

▶ The use of supportive devices may cause perspiration, which may lead to skin maceration.

The goals of proper positioning are to:

▶ Support, stabilize, and provide proper alignment of the axial and appendicular skeletal segments in a position that promotes efficient function of the body systems.

▶ Provide correct positioning for the administration of effective, efficient, and safe treatment procedures.

▶ Make the patient as comfortable as possible. However, it is worth remembering that the position of patient comfort may be the position that could lead to the development of a soft tissue contracture. A contracture is a limitation in joint motion caused by adaptive shortening in the soft tissue structures, including ligaments, tendons, joint capsule, and muscles. Generally speaking, positions of flexion are positions of comfort—for example, hip flexion, knee flexion, and elbow flexion, all common sites for contractures.

▶ Position the patient based on current medical status. For example, it is worth remembering that patients with impaired cardiopulmonary systems do not tolerate prolonged positions and therefore require frequent monitoring.

▶ Prevent the development of secondary impairments such as deformities, edema, venous thrombosis, and/or pressure sores. Extra care must be taken with patients who are older, mentally incompetent, paralyzed, or agitated.

CLINICAL PEARL

A patient who is immobile does not have the ability to use the muscles to pump fluid throughout the body toward the heart. Therefore, any extremity that is positioned below the level of the heart (dependent position) is at increased risk for edema formation. In a similar fashion, a lack of muscle contraction can produce venous stasis, which increases the risk of the formation of a blood clot or thrombus.

▶ Provide the patient access to stimulation from the environment.

CLINICAL PEARL

A patient who is being turned or positioned must be lifted rather than dragged across the sheets to prevent skin breakdown.

Before positioning a patient, the clinician should assemble the necessary devices that are going be used to support or stabilize the patient. Such devices include pillows, rolled towels, or commercially available devices (e.g., bolsters, foam wedges). The pillows or rolled towels can be used to support body parts. If a sensitive area must be relieved of pressure, the limb segment can be supported just proximal and just distal to the sensitive area. If this type of "bridging" position is used, pressure is typically increased and circulation is decreased on the adjacent areas, meaning that the time spent in this position must be reduced.

CLINICAL PEARL

When attempting to position a patient, the clinician should have a number of alternatives that can be used based on the patient's condition and ability. For example, a patient who has congestive heart failure will not tolerate a supine flat position. The clinician should always consider the following factors when positioning a patient:

▶ Patient safety

▶ Patient comfort

▶ Whether the position provides sufficient access to the treatment area

Restraints, or safety straps, are often necessary to protect the patient from rolling or falling and to prevent injury. These devices are recommended for short-term use only and should not be used to hinder or restrain the patient for several hours. An exception to this rule would be the use of protective positioning for the patient who:

▶ Is comatose

▶ Is mentally or physically incapable of maintaining a safe position

▶ Is experiencing spasticity

▶ Has extensive paralysis

CLINICAL PEARL

Physical or pharmacologic restraints, or seclusion, cannot be used without the voluntary consent of the patient and the physician's ongoing order. Any patient who is restrained must be monitored at least every two hours. Rules, regulations, and guidelines related to the use of restraint and seclusion have been developed and are enforced by various state, local, and federal agencies, and by accreditation organizations including the Department of Public Health (DPH), the Centers for Medicare and Medicaid Services (CMS), and the Joint Commission (JC).

The clinician must be able to make a critical assessment of what is to be required and what the challenges will be before attempting the task. This includes clinician positioning for optimal body mechanics, appropriate adjustment of the bed height, control of the patient throughout the task, the application of appropriate contact with the patient, and communication with the rest of the rehabilitation team (e.g., establishing

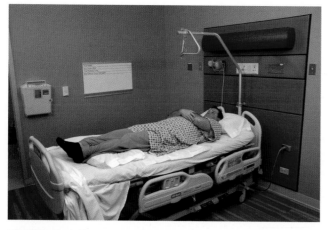

FIGURE 10-9 The supine position

The areas of greatest pressure in the supine position are:

► The occipital tuberosity of the skull
► The spine and inferior angle of the scapula
► The spinous processes of the vertebrae
► The posterior iliac crests
► The sacrum
► The posterior calcaneus

If the patient's hip is positioned in external rotation, the head of the fibula, the greater trochanter of the hip, and the lateral malleolus of the ankle should be regularly monitored.

that any lifting will follow a "1, 2, 3" count). Depending on the patient setting, the clinician may also have to take into account the presence of any lines, leads, and tubes attached to the patient. Where possible, it is advisable to include the nursing team in such scenarios.

Supine Position. The patient is positioned with the shoulders parallel to the hips and the spine straight (Figure 10-9). The upper extremities may be elevated on pillows by the patient's side or folded on the chest (Figure 10-10) to help prevent edema. The hands should be positioned in the open position to prevent contractures. The hip should be positioned in neutral flexion and/or extension, or slightly flexed. A rolled towel can be used to maintain the hips in a neutral position. A small pillow or a cervical roll can be placed under the patient's head while avoiding excessive neck and upper back flexion or scapula abduction (rounded shoulders). A small pillow may also be placed behind the knees to relieve strain on the lower back and to prevent knee hyperextension. However, because this position encourages hip and knee flexion that may contribute to lower extremity contractures of the iliopsoas and hamstring muscles, this position should not be maintained for a prolonged period. To relieve pressure to the heel (calcaneus), one of two methods can be used:

► A pillow can be placed under both legs (see Figure 10-9).
► A small, rolled towel can be placed under the patient's ankles while avoiding knee hyperextension.

Prone Position. The patient is positioned with the shoulders parallel to the hips and the spine straight. A small pillow or towel roll is placed under the patient's head, or the head is positioned to the left or right. The patient's upper extremities can be positioned in one of three ways:

► In a T-position with the arms overhead alongside the head (Figure 10-11). Placing the arms overhead increases the lumbar lordosis (see later).
► Along the sides of the patient (Figure 10-12). A folded towel should be placed under each anterior shoulder area to adduct the scapula, reduce the stress of the interscapular muscles, and protect the head of the humerus.
► With the hands under the head. It is worth remembering that if the upper extremities are positioned above shoulder height, there is an increased propensity for neurovascular compromise. Therefore this position should only be used when the patient has sensation in the arms, and when frequent testing for numbness or tingling can be performed.

The areas of greatest pressure in the prone position are:

► The forehead
► The lateral ear
► The tip of the acromion process

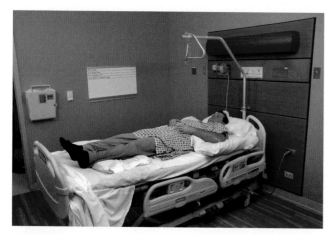

FIGURE 10-10 Using supports for the upper extremities

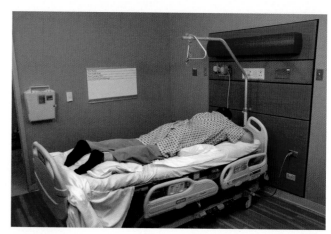

FIGURE 10-11 Prone position with the upper extremities in a T-position

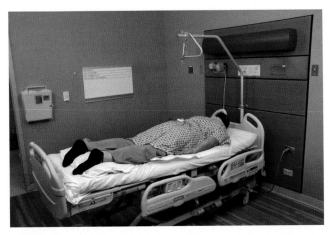

FIGURE 10-12 Prone position with the upper extremities along the sides of the patient

- ▶ The anterior head of the humerus
- ▶ The sternum
- ▶ The anterior superior iliac spine (ASIS)
- ▶ The patella
- ▶ The tibial crest
- ▶ The dorsum of the foot

The amount of lordosis and kyphosis of the spine can be controlled using padding. For example, a pillow placed under the patient's lower abdomen will reduce lumbar lordosis (see Figure 10-11), whereas a pillow placed under the middle or upper chest or positioned lengthwise from the pelvis to the thorax can be used to maintain the lordosis. To avoid positioning the patient's ankles in plantarflexion, the patient's feet can be positioned over the end of the bed, or a pillow can be used under the anterior portion of the patient's ankles to relieve stress on the hamstring muscles (see Figure 10-11). The latter position should not be maintained for a prolonged period as it promotes knee flexion, which can contribute to the development of a contracture of the knee flexors (hamstrings).

Sidelying Position. The patient is initially positioned in the center of the bed, with the head, trunk, and pelvis aligned and both of the lower extremities flexed at the hip and knee. The head is supported by a pillow (Figure 10-13). The uppermost

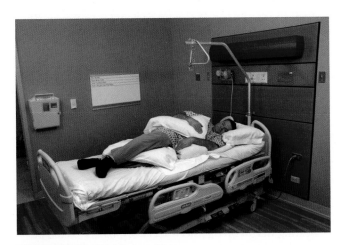

FIGURE 10-13 Sidelying position

lower extremity is supported on one or two pillows and positioned slightly forward compared to the lowermost extremity to avoid excessive pull on the lower trunk. It is the lowermost lower extremity that provides stability to the patient's pelvis and lower trunk. The upper trunk can be rotated forward or backward:

- ▶ If the patient is rotated backward, a pillow is placed behind the patient, and the uppermost upper extremity is extended and supported by that pillow (see Figure 10-13).
- ▶ If the patient is rotated forward, a pillow is placed in front of the patient and the uppermost upper extremity is flexed and supported by that pillow.

CLINICAL PEARL

The areas of greatest pressure in the sidelying position are:

- ▶ The lateral ear
- ▶ Lateral ribs
- ▶ The lateral acromion process
- ▶ The lateral and/or medial epicondyles of the humerus, depending on which upper extremity
- ▶ The epicondyles of the humerus
- ▶ The greater trochanter of the femur
- ▶ The lateral or medial condyle of the femur, depending on which lower extremity is uppermost or closest to the bed
- ▶ The lateral or medial malleolus, depending on which lower extremity is uppermost or closest to the bed

Sitting Position. It is important that the seated patient be positioned in a chair with adequate support and stability for the trunk and lower extremities. The patient's upper extremities can be supported on pillows, the chair armrests, a lap board, or a pillow in the patient's lap. It is important to remember that the patient should not be left unguarded in the sitting position when he or she cannot maintain the position safely.

CLINICAL PEARL

The areas of greatest pressure in the sitting position are:

- ▶ The ischial tuberosities
- ▶ The posterior areas of the thigh
- ▶ The sacrum
- ▶ The spinous processes of the vertebrae (if the patient is leaning against the chair back)
- ▶ The medial epicondyle of the humerus (if the elbow rests on a hard surface)

In general, a patient who is unable to alter his or her body positions should not be positioned for more than 30 minutes in the sitting position.

Preventative Positioning Based on Diagnosis. Certain diagnoses require specific positioning guidelines to avoid secondary complications related to short-term or prolonged positioning (Table 10-5).

TABLE 10-5	Preventative Positioning Based on Diagnosis	
Diagnosis	**Key Positions to Avoid**	**Recommendations**
Hemiplegia	*Upper Extremity* Shoulder adduction and internal rotation Elbow flexion Forearm supination or pronation Wrist, finger, or thumb flexion Finger and thumb adduction	The upper extremity should be positioned in varying amounts of shoulder abduction and external rotation, elbow extension, slight wrist extension, thumb abduction and extension, and finger extension and slight abduction.
	Lower Extremity Hip and knee flexion	The lower extremity should be positioned in varying amounts of hip and knee extension, hip abduction and internal rotation, and ankle dorsiflexion and eversion.
	Hip external rotation Ankle plantarflexion	The involved extremity must be exercised several times per day. The normal alignment of the patient's head and trunk should be maintained.
	Ankle inversion	The use of a sling to support the involved upper extremity should be avoided. Care should be taken when positioning the patient in sidelying on the affected side. For example the involved shoulder should be positioned slightly forward so that the scapula is protracted.
Recovering and grafted burn areas	Positions of comfort Flexion or adduction of most peripheral joints (if burn is located on the flexor or adductor surface of the joint)	Prevention is the key—once a contracture has developed, time, perseverance, and uncomfortable exercise will be necessary to return the joint to a normal position of functional use.
Transfemoral amputation	Hip flexion of the residual limb Hip abduction of the residual limb	Sitting should be limited to no more than 40 minutes of each hour. In the standing or lying position, the residual limb should be maintained in extension (prone lying when the patient is recumbent).
Transtibial amputation	Hip and knee flexion Leg crossing	Sitting should be limited to no more than 40 minutes of each hour. In the standing or lying position the residual limb should be maintained in extension (prone lying is recommended when the patient is recumbent).
Total hip arthroplasty	If a posterior lateral surgical approach was used, the following position should be avoided: ▶ Hip flexion beyond 60° to 90° ▶ Hip adduction beyond 0° ▶ Hip internal rotation beyond 0° Full sidelying is contraindicated.	Supine positioning with an abduction wedge or pillow between the legs to prevent hip adduction. Specific attention must be given to the sacral area, which is vulnerable to skin breakdown.

CLINICAL PEARL

A cerebrovascular accident (CVA), or stroke (see Chapter 6), can result in either increased or decreased muscle tone on one side of the body. An increase in muscle tone can result in contractures of the upper and/or lower extremity, whereas a decrease in muscle tone can make the affected joints more susceptible to distractive forces and to edema.

PATIENT DRAPING

When working with patients, including transport and treatment, attention must be paid to appropriate draping or dress. Draping involves covering the patient with a sheet(s), gown, or towel(s). Draping a patient appropriately during a therapy session is a seemingly simple yet very important component of a patient's care. When moving a patient, advance planning is required to maintain appropriate draping during movement. The purposes of draping are to:

▶ Expose or free a specific body segment for treatment. The patient should be draped with clean linen to expose only the areas or body parts to be treated, with the remainder of the patient's body covered to maintain modesty and warmth.

▶ Provide the clinician with the necessary access to specific areas of the body for examination and intervention.

▶ Absorb perspiration, water, and other various lubricants or to prevent the fluids from contacting the patient's clothing.

▶ Provide warmth and protection and to maintain a comfortable body temperature. For example, when patients are not ambulating, standing, or otherwise bearing weight on their feet, socks or slippers should be worn to provide adequate warmth and protection.

- Protect the skin and clothing from becoming soiled or damaged.
- Protect vulnerable skin areas such as wounds, scars, or stumps.

CLINICAL PEARL

Each patient has an individual sense of modesty and dignity, which is based on his or her cultural, religious, or personal beliefs. Thus it is important that the clinician initially assume that the patient is extremely modest, unless the patient says otherwise. In addition, any individual who has undergone some form of trauma (e.g., posttraumatic stress disorder) or abuse (physical, sexual, psychological, or any combination of these), may display an intense emotional reaction to bodily exposure, touch, or certain positions.[10–13]

Before draping, all restrictive clothing, splints, or other devices that will interfere with the treatment should be removed.

CLINICAL PEARL

Although hospital gowns are designed for ease in dressing and access during nursing care, they may not provide effective draping during the required movements and treatment positions.

A patient's cultural, religious, or personal preferences may affect the clinician's ability to appropriately drape the patient to expose the necessary areas of skin or body parts. It is therefore important that, before positioning or draping the patient, the clinician determine whether the patient has specific cultural, religious-based, or personal requests or preferences that would affect the draping process. Table 10-6 outlines some of the more common religious, cultural and ethnic preferences, although it is important to guard against stereotyping.

CLINICAL PEARL

The American Physical Therapy Association (APTA) has issued guidelines stating that physical therapists and physical therapist assistants are to "provide culturally sensitive care distinguished by trust, respect, and an appreciation for individual differences."

If draping becomes necessary, the clinician should inform the patient that clothing may need to be removed and the purpose of such removal, and obtain permission to proceed. The area to be treated must be exposed and have freedom of motion so that observation or palpation of the area can occur and so that the intervention can be performed effectively. It is important to stress that the body areas will be covered except for the area to be treated and that the amount of body area exposed and the length of time it is exposed will be kept to a minimum. Where possible, the patient should be educated on how to prepare themselves or be provided with an assistant of the same sex. The clinician should ask permission before entering the cubicle to ensure that the patient is appropriately draped. If, for whatever reason, the clinician needs to leave the treatment area, the patient should be dressed or draped

TABLE 10-6	Common Religious, Cultural, and Ethnic Preferences
Religious, Cultural, or Ethnic Group	**Preference**
African and Caribbean South Asian (Indian subcontinent) Chinese Hindu women Muslim women Some Latino groups	Strong preference for health-care provider of the same sex
Asian Chinese Romany traveler Orthodox Jewish women	Bodily exposure embarrassment
Some Mormons Rastafarian women	Taboos against wearing garments previously worn by others or against taking off garments that should not be removed
Traditional Egyptians Hindus Orthodox Jews Many North Americans Navajo women Children in many cultural or geographical groups Older individuals in some cultural or geographical groups	Restrictions on touching

Data from Mootoo JS: A guide to spiritual and cultural awareness. Nurs Stand 19:2-18, 2005.

so that the body is not unduly exposed. If the patient cannot remove items of clothing independently, the clinician must communicate clearly as to how he or she is going to provide assistance, and the clinician must proceed with a matter-of-fact and confident approach to help put the patient at ease, while observing the patient for any signs of discomfort or embarrassment.

CLINICAL PEARL

The American Medical Association (AMA) recommends that a chaperone be available to all patients on request and that this policy be communicated to the patient in a noticeable form. The APTA recommends providing a same-gender chaperone during patient examination and intervention if requested by the patient or deemed necessary by the clinician.

Only clean and previously unused linen and garments should be used for draping. At the conclusion of each treatment session, any soiled linen and garments must be properly disposed of. The clinician must wear gloves if body fluids have soiled the articles. A gown, sheet, or towel can be used to drape the patient's anterior chest and lower extremities while making sure not to restrict joint motion or access to the area to be treated.

CLINICAL PEARL

Hospital gowns, which open at the back, offer little to enhance patient modesty. However, if appropriate, two gowns can be used. By wearing an additional gown backward so that it opens in the front, better overall coverage of the body can be achieved.

When sheets or blankets are used for draping, they should not be tucked in tightly at the foot of the bed, as this can place the ankles into a position of plantarflexion. The correct draping for a supine patient is depicted in Figure 10-14 for treatment of the upper extremity. Figure 10-15 demonstrates the correct draping of the lower extremities for a supine patient. If a lower extremity is to be moved for treatment and there is potential for the patient's perineum (groin) to be exposed, the area must be covered with a sheet or towel applied high in the groin and under the thigh to ensure that the area is covered fully (Figure 10-16). Different techniques can be used to drape the trunk. For example, if ultrasound is to be applied to the lower back with the patient in prone, the entire trunk is first covered with a sheet (Figure 10-17), then a towel is placed over the sheet

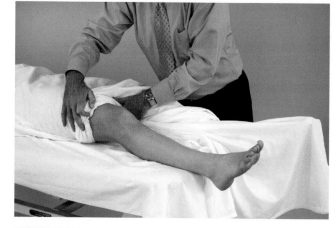

FIGURE 10-16 Correct draping for a supine patient for treatment of the lower extremity

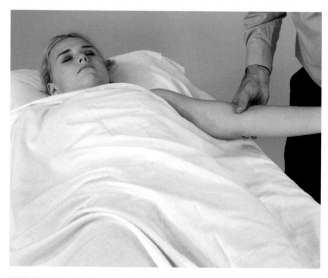

FIGURE 10-14 Correct draping for a supine patient for treatment of the upper extremity

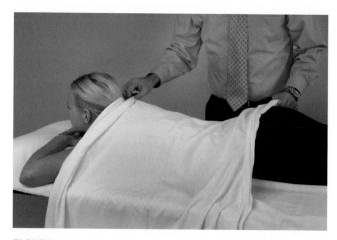

FIGURE 10-17 Draping the entire trunk with a sheet

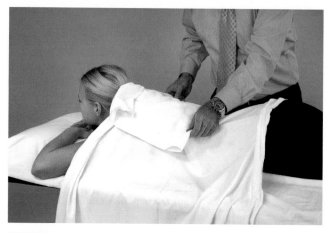

FIGURE 10-18 Towel placed over the sheet

(Figure 10-18), after which the sheet is withdrawn a sufficient amount (Figure 10-19) while simultaneously moving the towel over the treatment area (Figure 10-20).

At the termination of the treatment session, the materials used for draping must be placed in the appropriate laundry basket and must not be used with another patient, however clean they may appear. If the treatment procedure has involved the use of lotions or gels, the clinician should provide the patient with a towel to remove any residue.

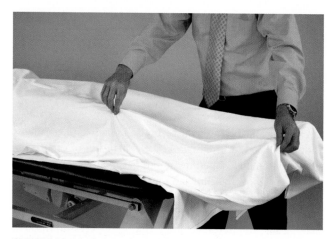

FIGURE 10-15 Correct draping for a supine patient

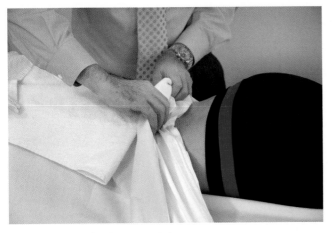

FIGURE 10-19 The sheet is withdrawn

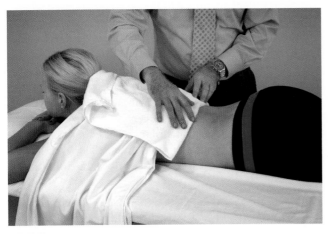

FIGURE 10-20 The towel replaces the sheet

REFERENCES

1. Bureau of Labor Statistics: Incidence rates for nonfatal occupational injuries and illnesses involving days away from work per 10,000 full-time workers by industry and selected events or exposures leading to injury or illness in 2006. Washington, DC, U.S. Department of Labor, 2007.
2. White AH: Principles for physical management of work injuries, in Isenhagen S (ed): Work Injury. Gaithersburg, Md Aspen, 1988.
3. Grandjean CK, McMullen PC, Miller KP, et al: Severe occupational injuries among older workers: demographic factors, time of injury, place and mechanism of injury, length of stay, and cost data. Nurs Health Sci 8:103-107, 2006.
4. Leigh JP, Waehrer G, Miller TR, et al: Costs of occupational injury and illness across industries. Scand J Work Environ Health 30:199-205, 2004.
5. Ogden CL, Carroll MD, Curtin LR, et al: Prevalence of overweight and obesity in the United States, 1999-2004. JAMA 295:1549-1555, 2006.
6. Motsch J, Walther A, Bock M, et al: Update in the prevention and treatment of deep vein thrombosis and pulmonary embolism. Curr Opin Anaesthesiol 19:52-58, 2006.
7. Bounameaux H, Reber-Wasem MA: Superficial thrombophlebitis and deep vein thrombosis: a controversial association. Arch Intern Med 157:1822-1824, 1997.
8. Gorman WP, Davis KR, Donnelly R: ABC of arterial and venous disease. Swollen lower limb—1: general assessment and deep vein thrombosis. BMJ 320:1453-1456, 2000.
9. Aschwanden M, Labs KH, Engel H, et al: Acute deep vein thrombosis: early mobilization does not increase the frequency of pulmonary embolism. Thromb Haemost 85:42-46, 2001.
10. Arias I, Dankwort J, Douglas U, et al: Violence against women: the state of batterer prevention programs. J Law Med Ethics 30:157-165, 2002.
11. Bemporad JR, Beresin E, Ratey JJ, et al: A psychoanalytic study of eating disorders: I. A developmental profile of 67 index cases. J Am Acad Psychoanal 20:509-531, 1992.
12. Elton D, Stanley G: Cultural expectations and psychological factors in prolonged disability. Adv Behav Med 2:33-42, 1982.
13. Sasano EM, Shepard KF: Sociocultural considerations in physical therapy education. Phys Ther 53:1269-1275, 1973.

Range of Motion

CHAPTER 11

CHAPTER OBJECTIVES

*At the completion of this chapter,
the reader will be able to:*

1. List the different types of physiologic motions

2. Describe the differences among active motions, active-assisted motions, and passive motions

3. Describe the purpose of range of motion exercises

4. List the different types of diagonal patterns of motion that can be incorporated therapeutically

5. Interpret the findings of active and passive range of motion testing

6. Perform a range of motion examination using a goniometer

7. Apply passive range of motion techniques to the upper extremity

8. Apply passive range of motion techniques to the lower extremity

OVERVIEW

Physiologic motions are joint and soft tissue movements that can be produced actively or passively. Active motions are those that can be produced by the patient alone, whereas passive motions are those motions that require assistance to complete. Active-assisted motions are those that are combination of active and passive motions (see Chapter 4).

RANGE OF MOTION EXERCISES

Range of motion exercises are designed to move the joint and soft tissues through the available physiologic ranges of motion.

CLINICAL PEARL

The purpose of range of motion exercises is to prevent the development of adaptive muscle shortening, contractures, and shortening of the capsule, ligaments, and tendons. In addition, range of motion exercises provide sensory stimulation.

- ► *Active range of motion (AROM):* performed by the patient independently. AROM exercises are used when the patient is able to voluntarily contract, control, and coordinate a movement when such a movement is not contraindicated. Contraindications to AROM include a healing fracture site, a healing surgical site, severe and acute soft tissue trauma, and cardiopulmonary dysfunction. The presence of a number of conditions requires caution with AROM exercises. These include acute rheumatoid arthritis, significant pain or joint swelling, or if the symptoms are intensified with the exercise. The benefits of AROM exercises are outlined in Table 11-1.

- ► *Active assisted range of motion (AAROM):* performed when the patient needs assistance with movement from an external force because of weakness, pain, or changes in muscle tone. The assistance may be applied mechanically, manually, or by gravity while the patient performs a voluntary muscle contraction to the extent he or she is able. AAROM exercises are used in the presence of muscular weakness, fatigue, or pain.

- ► *Passive range of motion (PROM):* usually performed when the patient is unable or not permitted to move the body segment, and the clinician, or family member, moves the body segment. PROM exercises are typically used where there is paralysis, when the patient is comatose, in the presence of a healing fracture, or if pain is elicited during an active muscle contraction. One of the primary goals of PROM is to counteract the detrimental effects of immobilization. However, it is important to remember that PROM exercises cannot prevent muscle atrophy.

Diagonal Patterns of Motion

Diagonal patterns of motion, which can be performed using PROM, AAROM, or AROM, or with more advanced techniques using resistance, were first incorporated with the techniques of proprioceptive neuromuscular facilitation (PNF), which were based on the theory that the muscles of the body function around three planes of movement in a three-dimensional fashion, with each movement associated with an antagonistic motion. These motions and their antagonists are as follows:

TABLE 11-1	The Benefits of Active Range of Motion (AROM) Exercises

Maintaining the elasticity, strength, and contractile endurance of the muscle

Enhancing local blood circulation

Providing increased sensory awareness

Possible improvements in cardiopulmonary functions if performed at the correct intensity

Possible prevention of thrombus formation

Enhancing bone strength if performed in weight-bearing

- ▶ Flexion or extension
- ▶ Adduction or abduction in the extremities and lateral movement in the trunk
- ▶ Internal or external rotation

Combinations of these movements work together in spiral and diagonal patterns. The patterns, which integrate the motions of sports and daily living, are based on the infant developmental sequences such as rolling, crawling, and walking. The advantages of diagonal patterns include:

- ▶ All of the movements involve a combination of motions.
- ▶ Rotation is incorporated with all movements.
- ▶ Many of the movements involve crossing of the midline of the body.
- ▶ The movements are more functional than movements performed in a planar direction.

There are two fundamental diagonal patterns for the lower extremity (Table 11-2) and for the upper extremity and scapula (Table 11-3), which are referred to as the diagonal 1 (D1) and diagonal 2 (D2) patterns.

These patterns are subdivided into D1 and D2 patterns that move into flexion (diagonal 1 flexion and diagonal 2 flexion) and D1 and D2 patterns that move into extension (diagonal 1 extension and diagonal 2 extension). Based on whether the upper extremity or lower extremity is being used, the terminology can be expanded to diagonal 1 flexion lower extremity, diagonal one flexion upper extremity, and so on. The patterns are named according to the position of the proximal joint of the pattern (i.e., the shoulder or the hip) at the end position of the pattern. This means the pattern is initiated with the proximal joint positioned opposite to its end position. For example, to initiate a D1 flexion diagonal of the upper extremity, which involves flexion, abduction, and external rotation, the shoulder is positioned in the D1 extension position of the upper extremity (extension, abduction, and internal rotation).

CLINICAL PEARL

Although it would appear that the use of diagonal patterns for range of motion exercises is more efficient than ranging a joint through its anatomic planes because these patterns employ a number of planes simultaneously, they do not produce the same amount of range of motion to the muscles and joints as when the anatomic planes are used.

TABLE 11-2	Lower Extremity Proprioceptive Neuromuscular Facilitation Patterns

Start Position for D1 Pattern	
D1 Extension	**D1 Flexion**
Hip flexed, adducted, and externally rotated	Hip extended, abducted, and internally rotated
Knee flexed	Knee extended
Tibia internally rotated	Tibia externally rotated
Ankle and foot dorsiflexed and inverted	Ankle and foot plantarflexed and everted
Toes extended	Toes flexed
Movement into hip extension, abduction, and internal rotation; ankle plantarflexion; foot eversion; toe flexion	Movement into hip flexion, adduction, and external rotation; ankle dorsiflexion; foot inversion; toe extension

Start Position for D2 Pattern	
D2 Flexion	**D2 Extension**
Hip extended, adducted, and externally rotated	Hip flexed, abducted, and internally rotated
Knee extended	Knee flexed
Tibia externally rotated	Tibia internally rotated
Ankle and foot plantarflexed and inverted	Ankle and foot dorsiflexed and everted
Toes flexed	Toes extended
Movement into hip flexion, abduction, and internal rotation; ankle dorsiflexion; foot eversion; toe extension	Movement into hip extension, adduction, and external rotation; ankle plantarflexion; foot inversion; toe flexion

D1, diagonal 1; D2, diagonal 2.

TABLE 11-3   Upper Extremity and Scapular Proprioceptive Neuromuscular Facilitation Patterns

Start Position for D1 Pattern	
D1 Flexion	**D1 Extension**
Scapula depressed and adducted	Scapula elevated and abducted
Shoulder extended, abducted, and internally rotated	Shoulder flexed, adducted, and externally rotated
Elbow extended	Elbow extended
Forearm pronated	Forearm supinated
Wrist extended and ulnarly deviated	Wrist flexed and radially deviated
Fingers abducted and extended	Fingers adducted and flexed
Thumb extended and abducted	Thumb flexed and adducted
Movement into shoulder flexion, adduction, and internal rotation; scapular elevation and abduction; forearm supination; wrist flexion and radial deviation; finger flexion	Movement into shoulder extension, abduction, and internal rotation; scapular depression and adduction; forearm pronation; wrist extension and ulnar deviation; finger extension

Start Position for D2 Pattern	
D2 Extension	**D2 Flexion**
Scapula elevated and adducted	Scapula depressed and abducted
Shoulder flexed, abducted, and externally rotated	Shoulder extended, adducted, and internally rotated
Elbow extended	Elbow extended
Forearm supinated	Forearm pronated
Wrist extended and radially deviated	Wrist flexed and ulnarly deviated
Fingers extended and abducted	Fingers adducted and flexed
Thumb extended and adducted	Thumb flexed and abducted
Movement into shoulder extension, adduction, and internal rotation; scapular depression and abduction; forearm pronation; wrist flexion and ulnar deviation; finger flexion	Movement into shoulder flexion, abduction, and external rotation; scapular elevation and adduction; forearm supination; wrist extension and radial deviation; finger extension

D1, diagonal 1; D2, diagonal 2.

When performing PNF patterns involving patient contribution (active or resisted motions), the clinician's hand placement is designed to provide a tactile contact and stimulus to the major muscles involved in producing the desired movement, so the hands of the clinician are placed over the muscle or muscles that are to contract while avoiding contact with the muscle or muscles that are to relax during the exercise. When performing the diagonal patterns without patient contribution (passive motion), hand placement is not as critical.

Before prescribing any of the range of motion exercises, it is important that the clinician determine the purpose of the exercise, the amount support necessary for the patient, whether stabilization is necessary, the ability of the patient to perform the exercise, and the effect of gravity.

Purpose. The most common purpose for range of motion exercises is to enhance the functional capacity of the patient by maintaining or improving joint motion and range. Active range of motion can affect strength, endurance, and coordination, whereas the benefits of passive range of motion are limited to maintaining or improving joint motion range and assisting in the maintenance of local circulation.

Support Necessary. Support is used to relieve stress on a joint or body segment by controlling the weight of the extremity or body part, or to compensate for the loss of muscle strength.

Stabilization. Stabilization, which is used to avoid, limit, or prevent movement, is typically used to protect the site of a healing fracture or extensive tissue trauma, and during the acute stage of healing.

Ability of the Patient. Whenever possible, the patient must be allowed to perform at a level that is challenging without being detrimental. To make such a determination, the clinician must have knowledge of the musculoskeletal, neuromuscular, and cardiopulmonary systems of the patient. In addition, the clinician must have a working knowledge of the various stages of healing, and biomechanical concepts such as stress, force, torque, levers, and axes of motion.

Effect of Gravity. Gravity can affect an exercise based on the angle at which the exercise is performed:

▶ An active exercise performed perpendicular to the ground is working against gravity if the exercise is performed in a direction away from the ground.

▶ An active exercise performed perpendicular to the ground is working with gravity if the exercise is performed in a direction toward the ground.

▶ An active exercise performed parallel to the ground negates the effect of gravity if the limb is supported.

INTERPRETATION OF ACTIVE AND PASSIVE RANGE OF MOTION

Both active and passive motions can provide the clinician with valuable information.

Active Physiologic Range of Motion of the Extremities. Active movements of the involved area are performed before passive movements if possible. During the history, the clinician should have deduced the general motions that aggravate or provoke the pain. Any movements that are known to be painful are performed last. The range of motion examination should be used to confirm the exact directions of motion that elicit the symptoms. The diagnosis of restricted movement in the extremities can usually be simplified by comparing both sides, provided that at least one side is uninvolved. Under normal circumstances, the normal (uninvolved) side is tested first as this allows the clinician to establish a baseline, while also showing the patient what to expect. Active range of motion testing may be deferred if small and unguarded motions provoke intense pain, because this may indicate a high degree of joint irritability, or other serious condition. The normal active range of motion for each of the joints is depicted in Table 11-4.

Active range of motion testing gives the clinician information about the following:

▶ Quantity of available physiologic motion
▶ Presence of muscle substitutions
▶ Willingness of the patient to move
▶ Integrity of the contractile and inert tissues
▶ Quality of motion
▶ Symptom reproduction
▶ Pattern of motion restriction (e.g., capsular or noncapsular)

TABLE 11-4	Active Ranges of Joint Motions			
Joint	**Action**	**Available Degrees of Motion**	**Expected Range**	**Possible Substitutions**
Shoulder	Flexion	0–180	120° of pure GH flexion 150° with GH, AC, SC, and ST contribution 180° if lumbar hyperextension permitted	Lumbar hyperextension Scapular tipping NB: Maintain slight elbow flexion so that long head of triceps does not restrict motion
	Extension	0–40	40°	Lumbar flexion
	Abduction	0–180	90° of pure GH abduction 150° with GH, AC, SC, and ST contribution 180° if lumbar side bending is allowed	Lumbar side bending Excessive scapular upward rotation can contribute to movement
	Internal/external rotation	Internal: 0–70 External: 0–90	70° internal rotation; 90° external rotation	The amount of motion available is influenced by the position of abduction in the frontal plane and whether the measurement is performed in the scapular or frontal planes.
	Horizontal adduction	Varies	45°	Trunk rotation
Elbow	Flexion	0–150	150°	Position of forearm (supination/pronation) can affect results
	Extension	Varies according to gender	Males: 0° Females: 10–15°	Towel roll may need to be placed posterior to elbow to allow hyperextension to occur
Forearm	Pronation	80–90	80–90°	Wrist flexion and/or ulnar deviation, abduction and IR of the shoulder, and/or contralateral trunk side bending
	Supination	80–90	80–90°	Wrist extension and/or radial deviation, adduction and ER of the shoulder, and ipsilateral trunk side bending

(continued)

		Available Degrees of		
TABLE 11-4	**Active Ranges of Joint Motions** (continued)			
Joint	**Action**	**Motion**	**Expected Range**	**Possible Substitutions**
Wrist	Flexion	0–75	Varies according to generalized hypermobility	Excessive radial or ulnar deviation
	Extension	0–75	75°	Excessive radial or ulnar deviation
	Radial deviation	0–20	20°	MCP abduction or adduction
	Ulnar deviation	0–30	30°	MCP abduction or adduction
Hip	Flexion	0–120	Typically decreases with age	Lumbar spine flexion
	Extension	0–30	Typically decreases with age	Lumbar spine extension
	Abduction	0–45	45°	Hip external rotation, knee flexion/internal rotation, or lateral pelvic tilt
	Adduction	0–30	30°	Hip internal rotation or lateral pelvic tilt
	Internal rotation	0–45	45° (can be decreased in elderly population secondary to osteoarthritis)	Thigh adduction
	External rotation	0–45	45°	Thigh abduction
Knee	Flexion	0–150	135° (depends on degree of musculature)	May be decreased with adaptive shortening of the rectus femoris
Ankle	Plantarflexion	0–50	30–50°	None
	Dorsiflexion	0–20	10° with knee extended 20° with knee flexed	Affected by degree of gastrocnemius adaptive shortening
Subtalar	Inversion	0–20	20°	None
	Eversion	0–10	10°	None

GH: glenohumeral; AC: acromioclavicular; SC: sternoclavicular; ST: scapulothoracic.

Capsular and Noncapsular Patterns of Restriction. Cyriax[1] introduced us the terms *capsular* and *noncapsular* patterns of restriction, which link impairment to pathology (Table 11-5). A capsular pattern of restriction is a limitation of pain and movement in a joint-specific ratio, which is usually present with arthritis or following prolonged immobilization.[1] It is worth remembering that a consistent capsular pattern for a particular joint might not exist and that these patterns are based on empirical findings and tradition, rather than on research.[2,3] Significant degeneration of the articular cartilage presents with crepitus (joint noise) on movement when compression of the joint surfaces is maintained.

A noncapsular pattern of restriction is a limitation in a joint in any pattern other than a capsular one and may indicate the presence of a joint derangement, a restriction of one part of the joint capsule, or an extra-articular lesion that obstructs joint motion.[1]

A positive finding for joint hypomobility would be a reduced range in a capsular or noncapsular pattern. The hypomobility can be painful, suggesting an acute sprain of a structure, or painless, suggesting a contracture or adhesion of the tested structure.

Although abnormal motion is typically described as being reduced, abnormal motion may also be excessive. Excessive motion is often missed and is erroneously classified as normal motion. To help determine whether the motion is normal or excessive, passive range of motion, in the form of passive overpressure, and the end-feel are assessed (see next section).

CLINICAL PEARL

Apprehension from the patient during active range of motion that limits a movement at near or full range suggests instability, whereas apprehension in the early part of the range suggests anxiety caused by pain.

Full and pain-free active range of motion suggests normalcy for that movement, although it is important to remember

TABLE 11-5	Capsular Patterns of Restriction
Joint	**Limitation of Motion (Passive Angular Motion)**
Glenohumeral	External rotation > abduction > internal rotation (3:2:1)
Acromioclavicular	No true capsular pattern; possible loss of horizontal adduction and pain (and sometimes slight loss of end range) with each motion
Sternoclavicular	See acromioclavicular joint
Humeroulnar	Flexion > extension (±4:1)
Humeroradial	No true capsular pattern; possible equal limitation of pronation and supination
Superior radioulnar	No true capsular pattern; possible equal limitation of pronation and supination with pain at end ranges
Inferior radioulnar	No true capsular pattern; possible equal limitation of pronation and supination with pain at end ranges
Wrist (carpus)	Flexion = extension
Radiocarpal	See wrist (carpus)
Carpometacarpal	
Midcarpal	
Carpometacarpal 1	Retroposition
Carpometacarpals 2–5	Fan > fold
Metacarpophalangeal 2–5	Flexion > extension (±2:1)

Interphalangeal
  Proximal (PIP)
  Distal (DIP)
	Flexion > extension (±2:1)

Hip	Internal rotation > flexion > abduction = extension > other motions
Tibiofemoral	Flexion > extension (±5:1)
Superior tibiofibular	No capsular pattern; pain at end range of translatory movements
Talocrural	Plantar flexion > dorsiflexion
Talocalcaneal (subtalar)	Varus > valgus
Midtarsal	Inversion (plantar flexion, adduction, supination)
Talonavicular calcaneocuboid	> Dorsiflexion
Metatarsophalangeal 1	Extension > flexion (±2:1)
Metatarsophalangeals 2–5	Flexion ≥ extension

Interphalangeals 2–5
  Proximal
  Distal
	Flexion ≥ extension
	Flexion ≥ extension

Data from Cyriax J: Textbook of Orthopaedic Medicine, Diagnosis of Soft Tissue Lesions (ed 8). London, Bailliere Tindall, 1982.

that normal *range* of motion is not synonymous with normal motion.[4] Normal motion implies that the control of motion must also be present. This control is a factor of muscle flexibility, joint stability, and central neurophysiologic mechanisms. These factors are highly specific in the body.[5] A loss of motion at one joint may not prevent the performance of a functional task, although it may result in the task being performed in an abnormal manner. For example, the act of walking can still be accomplished in the presence of a knee joint that has been fused into extension. Because the essential mechanisms

of knee flexion in the stance period and foot clearance in the swing period are absent, the patient compensates for these losses by hiking the hip on the involved side, by side bending the lumbar spine to the uninvolved side, and through excessive motion of the foot.

Single motions in the cardinal planes are usually tested first. These tests are followed by dynamic and static testing. Dynamic testing involves repeated movements. Static testing involves sustaining a position. Sustained static positions may be used to help detect postural syndromes.[6] McKenzie advocates the use of repeated movements in specific directions in the spine and the extremities. Repeated movements can give the clinician some valuable insight into the patient's condition[6]:

- ▶ Symptoms of a postural dysfunction remain unchanged with repeated motions.
- ▶ Pain from a dysfunction syndrome is increased with tissue loading but ceases at rest.
- ▶ Repeated motions can indicate the irritability of the condition.
- ▶ Repeated motions can indicate to the clinician the direction of motion to be used as part of the intervention. If pain increases during repeated motion in a particular direction, exercising in that direction is not indicated. If pain only worsens in part of the range, repeated motion exercises can be used for that part of the range that is pain free or that does not worsen the symptoms.
- ▶ Pain that is increased after the repeated motions may indicate a retriggering of the inflammatory response, and repeated motions in the opposite direction should be explored.

Combined motion testing may be used when the symptoms are not reproduced with the cardinal plane motions (flexion, extension, abduction, etc.), repeated motions, or sustained positions. Compression and distraction also may be added to all of the active motion tests in an attempt to reproduce the symptoms.

CLINICAL PEARL

It must be remembered that in order for full joint motion to occur, multijoint muscles (the muscles that cross two or more joints such as the hamstrings, gastrocnemius, and long flexor and extensors of the hands and feet) must not be lengthened simultaneously over the joints they cross so that they do not prevent full joint motion from occurring. For example, if the clinician is performing passive range of motion of ankle dorsiflexion, if the knee is maintained in full extension, the gastrocnemius will prevent full dorsiflexion from occurring. Instead, the clinician should ensure that the knee is flexed.

Active Physiologic Range of Motion of the Spine. Active physiologic intervertebral mobility, or active mobility, tests of the spine were originally designed by osteopaths to assess the ability of each spinal joint to move actively through its normal range of motion, by palpating over the transverse processes of a joint during the motion. Theoretically, by palpating over the transverse processes, the clinician can indirectly assess the motions occurring at the zygapophysial joints at either side of the intervertebral disk. However, the clinician must remember that, although it is convenient to describe the various motions of the spine occurring in a certain direction, these involve the integration of movements of a multijoint complex.

The human zygapophysial joints are capable of only two major motions: gliding upward and gliding downward. If these movements occur in the same direction, flexion or extension of the spine occurs, whereas if the movements occur in opposite directions, side flexion occurs.

Osteopaths use the terms *opening* and *closing* to describe flexion and extension motions, respectively, at the zygapoph-

ysial joint. Under normal circumstances, an equal amount of gliding occurs at each zygapophysial joint with these motions.

- ▶ During flexion, both zygapophysial joints glide superiorly (open).
- ▶ During extension, both zygapophysial joints glide inferiorly (close).
- ▶ During side flexion, one joint is gliding inferiorly (closing), while the other joint is gliding superiorly (opening). For example, during right side flexion, the right joint is gliding inferiorly (closing), while the left joint is gliding superiorly (opening).

By combining flexion or extension movements with side flexion, the joint can be "opened" or "closed" to its limits. Thus, flexion and right side flexion of a segment assesses the ability of the left joint to maximally open (flex), whereas extension and left side flexion of a segment assesses the ability of the left joint to maximally close (extend).

There is a point that may be considered as the center of segmental rotation, about which all segmental motion must occur. In the case of a zygapophysial joint impairment (hypermobility or hypomobility), it is presumed that this center of rotation will be altered.

If one zygapophysial joint is rendered hypomobile (i.e., the superior facet cannot move to the extreme of superior or inferior motion), then the pure motions of flexion and extension cannot occur. This results in a relative asymmetric motion of the two superior facets, as the end of range of flexion or extension is approached (i.e., a side-flexion motion will occur). However, this side-flexion motion will not be about the normal center of segmental rotation. The structure responsible for the loss of zygapophysial joint motion, whether it is a muscle, disk protrusion, or the zygapophysial joint itself, will become the new axis of vertebral motion, and a new component of rotation about a vertical axis, normally unattainable, will be introduced into the segmental motion. The degree of this rotational deviation is dependent on the distance of the impairment from the original center of rotation.

Because the zygapophysial joints in the spine are posterior to the axis of rotation, an obvious rotational change occurring between full flexion and full extension (in the position of a vertebral segment) is indicative of zygapophysial joint motion impairment.

By observing any marked and obvious rotation of a vertebral segment occurring between the positions of full flexion and full extension, one may deduce the probable pathologic impairment.

CLINICAL PEARL

Active motion induced by the contraction of the muscles determines the so-called physiologic range of motion,[7] whereas passively performed movement causes stretching of noncontractile elements, such as ligaments, and determines the anatomic range of motion.

Passive Physiologic Range of Motion of the Extremities. Passive motions are movements performed by the clinician without the assistance of the patient. Passive movements

TABLE 11-6   Normal End-Feels

Type	Cause	Characteristics and Examples

Bony	Produced by bone-to-bone approximation	Abrupt and unyielding; gives impression that further forcing will break something
		
		Examples:
		  Normal: elbow extension
		  Abnormal: cervical rotation (may indicate osteophyte)

Elastic	Produced by muscle–tendon unit; may occur with adaptive shortening	Stretches with elastic recoil and exhibits constant-length phenomenon; further forcing feels as if it will snap something
		
		Examples:
		  Normal: wrist flexion with finger flexion, the straight-leg raise, and ankle dorsiflexion with the knee extended
		  Abnormal: decreased dorsiflexion of the ankle with the knee flexed

Soft-tissue approximation	Produced by contact of two muscle bulks on either side of a flexing joint where joint range exceeds other restraints	Very forgiving end feel that gives impression that further normal motion is possible if enough force could be applied
		
		Examples:
		  Normal: knee flexion and elbow flexion in extremely muscular subjects
		  Abnormal: elbow flexion with obese subject

Capsular	Produced by capsule or ligaments	Various degrees of stretch without elasticity; stretch ability is dependent on thickness of tissue
		Strong capsular or extracapsular ligaments produce hard capsular end-feel, whereas thin capsule produces softer one
		Impression given to clinician is that if further force is applied, something will tear
		
		Examples:
		  Normal: wrist flexion (soft), elbow flexion in supination (medium), and knee extension (hard)
		  Abnormal: inappropriate stretch ability for specific joint; if too hard, may indicate hypomobility due to arthrosis; if too soft, hypermobility

Data from Meadows JTS: Manual Therapy: Biomechanical Assessment and Treatment, Advanced Technique. Calgary, Swodeam Consulting, 1995.

are performed in the anatomic range of motion for the joint and normally demonstrate slightly greater range of motion than active motion—the barrier to active motion should occur earlier in the range than the barrier to passive motion.

If the patient can complete the active physiologic range of motion easily, without presenting pain or other symptoms, then passive testing of that motion is usually unnecessary. However, if the active motions do not reproduce the patient's symptoms, because the patient avoids going into the painful part of the range, or the active range of motion appears incomplete, it is important to perform gentle passive overpressure. Pain during passive overpressure is often due to moving, stretching, or pinching of noncontractile structures. Pain that occurs at the mid-end range of active and passive movement is suggestive of a capsular contraction or scar tissue that has not been adequately remodeled.[6] Pain occurring at the end of PROM may be due to stretching contractile structures, as well as noncontractile structures.[8] Thus, PROM testing gives the clinician information about the integrity of the contractile and inert tissues, and with gentle overpressure, the *end-feel*. Cyriax[1] introduced the concept of the end-feel, which is the quality of resistance at end range. To execute the end-feel, the point at which resistance is encountered is evaluated for quality and tenderness. Additional forces are needed as the end range of

a joint is reached and the elastic limits are challenged. This space, termed the *end-play zone*, requires a force of overpressure to be reached so that, when that force is released, the joint springs back from its elastic limits. The end-feel can indicate to the clinician the cause of the motion restriction (Tables 11-6 and 11-7).

CLINICAL PEARL

One study that looked at the intra- and inter-rater reliability of assessing end-feel, and pain and resistance sequence in subjects with painful shoulders and knees, found the end-feel to have good intrarater reliability, but unacceptable inter-rater reliability.[2]

Although some clinicians feel that overpressure should not be applied in the presence of pain, this is erroneous. Most, if not all, of the end-feels that suggest acute or serious pathology are to be found in the painful range, including spasm and the empty end-feel.

The end-feel is very important in joints that have only very small amounts of normal range, such as those of the spine. The type of end-feel can help the clinician determine the presence of dysfunction. For example, a hard, capsular end-feel indicates a pericapsular hypomobility, whereas a jammed or

TABLE 11-7	Abnormal End-Feels	
Type	**Causes**	**Characteristics and Examples**
Springy	Produced by articular surface rebounding from intra-articular meniscus or disk; impression is that if forced further, something will collapse	Rebound sensation as if pushing off from a rubber pad *Examples:* Normal: axial compression of cervical spine Abnormal: knee flexion or extension with displaced meniscus
Boggy	Produced by viscous fluid (blood) within joint	"Squishy" sensation as joint is moved toward its end range; further forcing feels as if it will burst joint *Examples:* Normal: none Abnormal: hemarthrosis at knee
Spasm	Produced by reflex and reactive muscle contraction in response to irritation of nociceptor, predominantly in articular structures and muscle; forcing it further feels as if nothing will give	Abrupt and "twangy" end to movement that is unyielding while the structure is being threatened but disappears when threat is removed (kicks back) With joint inflammation, it occurs early in range, especially toward close-packed position, to prevent further stress With irritable joint hypermobility, it occurs at end of what should be normal range, as it prevents excessive motion from further stimulating the nociceptor Spasm in grade II muscle tears becomes apparent as muscle is passively lengthened and is accompanied by a painful weakness of that muscle *Note:* Muscle guarding is not a true end-feel, as it involves co-contraction *Examples:* Normal: none Abnormal: significant traumatic arthritis, recent traumatic hypermobility, and grade II muscle tears
Empty	Produced solely by pain; frequently caused by serious and severe pathologic changes that do not affect joint or muscle and so do not produce spasm; demonstration of this end-feel is, with exception of acute subdeltoid bursitis, de facto evidence of serious pathology; further forcing simply increases pain to unacceptable levels	Limitation of motion has no tissue resistance component, and resistance is from patient being unable to tolerate further motion due to severe pain; it is not same feeling as voluntary guarding, but rather it feels as if patient is both resisting and trying to allow movement simultaneously *Examples:* Normal: none Abnormal: acute subdeltoid bursitis and sign of the buttock
Facilitation	Not truly an end-feel, as facilitated hypertonicity does not restrict motion; it can, however, be perceived near end range	Light resistance as from constant light muscle contraction throughout latter half of range that does not prevent end of range being reached; resistance is unaffected by rate of movement *Examples:* Normal: none Abnormal: spinal facilitation at any level

Data from Meadows JTS: Manual Therapy: Biomechanical Assessment and Treatment, Advanced Technique. Calgary, Swodeam Consulting, 1995.

pathomechanical end-feel indicates a pathomechanical hypomobility. A normal end-feel would indicate normal range, whereas an abnormal end-feel would suggest abnormal range, either hypomobile or hypermobile. An association between an increase in pain and abnormal pathologic end-feels compared with normal end-feels has been demonstrated.[9]

The planned intervention, and its intensity, is based on the type of tissue resistance to movement, demonstrated by the end-feel, and on the acuteness of the condition (Table 11-8).[1] This information may indicate whether the resistance is caused by pain, muscle, capsule ligament, disturbed mechanics of the joint, or a combination.

CLINICAL PEARL

According to Cyriax, if active and passive motions are limited or painful in the same direction, the lesion is in the inert tissue, whereas if the active and passive motions are limited or painful in the opposite direction, the lesion is in the contractile tissue.[1]

The quantity and quality of movement refer to the ability to achieve end range without deviation from the intended movement plane.

Both the passive and active physiologic ranges of motion can be measured using a goniometer, which has been shown

Barrier	End-Feel	Technique
TABLE 11-8	**Abnormal Barriers to Motion and Recommended Manual Techniques**	
Pain	Empty	None
Pain	Spasm	None
Pain	Capsular	Oscillations (I, IV)
Joint adhesions	Early capsular	Passive articular motion stretch (I–V)
Muscle adhesions	Early elastic	Passive physiologic motion stretch
Hypertonicity	Facilitation	Muscle energy (hold/relax, etc.)
Bone	Bony	None

to have a satisfactory level of intraobserver reliability.[10–12] Visual observation in experienced clinicians has been found to be equal to measurements by goniometry.[13]

The recording of range of motion varies. The American Medical Association recommends recording the range of motion on the basis of the neutral position of the joint being zero, with the degrees of motion increasing in the direction the joint moves from the zero starting point.[14] A plus sign (+) is used to indicate joint hyperextension and a minus sign (–) to indicate an extension lag. The method of recording chosen is not important, provided the clinician chooses a recognized method and documents it consistently with the same patient.

Passive Physiologic Range of Motion of the Spine. The passive physiologic intervertebral mobility, or passive mobility, tests use the same principles as the active physiologic intervertebral mobility tests to assess the ability of each joint in the spine to move passively through its normal range of motion, while the clinician palpates over the interspinous spaces. During extension, the spinous processes should approximate, whereas during flexion, they should separate.

If pain is reproduced, it is useful to associate the pain with the onset of tissue resistance to gain an appreciation of the acuteness of the problem.

RANGE OF MOTION TECHNIQUES

As previously discussed, range of motion can be assessed to provide the clinician with information, but it can also be used therapeutically when a patient is unable to independently maintain his or her mobility whether globally or at a specific joint. The measurement of range of motion is described in the Goniometry section later in the chapter.

Range of Motion—Upper Extremity

For all of the following techniques, it is assumed that the patient is in the supine position, unless otherwise stated.

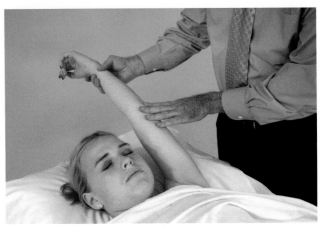

FIGURE 11-1 Shoulder flexion

Glenohumeral Joint

Flexion and Extension. Glenohumeral flexion/extension occurs in the sagittal plane around the frontal axis (see Chapter 4).

Pure glenohumeral motion can be assessed by stabilizing the scapula which will significantly limit motion at the glenohumeral joint to approximately 90°. In the following example, the scapular is not stabilized.

Hand Placement. The clinician uses one hand to grasp the patient's wrist, while using the other hand to grasp the patient's elbow (Figure 11-1).

Technique. The clinician lifts the patient upper extremity through the available range of motion (Figure 11-1) and then returns to the start position. Shoulder extension beyond the midline of the body can be accomplished by lowering the arm below the table or bed.

Normal End-feel. The normal end-feel for glenohumeral flexion is firm, resulting from tension in the posterior joint capsule, the posterior band of the coracohumeral ligament, teres major, teres minor, and infraspinatus muscles. If the scapular is stabilized, the end-feel for shoulder complex flexion is also firm, but results from tension in the latissimus dorsi muscle and the costosternal fibers of the pectoralis major muscle. The normal end-feel for glenohumeral extension is firm because of the tension in the anterior band of the coracohumeral ligament and the anterior joint capsule. For shoulder complex extension, the end-feel is also firm as a result of the tension in the clavicular fibers of the pectoralis major muscle and the serratus anterior muscle.

CLINICAL PEARL

When performing range of motion exercises to the shoulder in flexion and extension, it is important to remember the two joint muscles:

▶ *Biceps brachii.* The arm, which is positioned with the elbow extended and the forearm pronated, should be lowered below the level of the bed or table until maximal tension is felt.

▶ *Triceps brachii (long head).* Stretching of this muscle can be achieved by first flexing the shoulder to its point of available motion and then flexing the elbow maximally until the point of maximal tension.

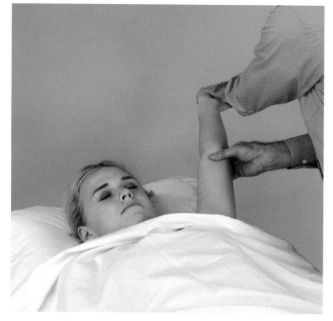

FIGURE 11-2 Shoulder abduction

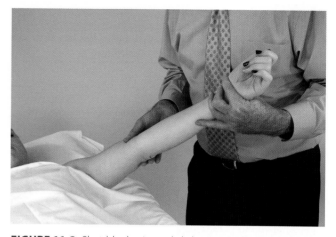

FIGURE 11-3 Shoulder horizontal abduction and adduction

Abduction and Adduction. Motion occurs in the frontal plane around an anterior-posterior (A-P) axis (see Chapter 4).

Hand Placement. The clinician uses one hand to grasp the patient's wrist and the other hand to grasp the patient's elbow (Figure 11-2). The patient's elbow may be extended or flexed.

Technique. The clinician moves the extremity away from the patient's trunk and returns to the start position while avoiding shoulder flexion by maintaining the arm horizontal to the floor (Figure 11-2). If the elbow is extended, the clinician must move his or her feet and step toward the patient's head (Figure 11-2). To avoid impingement of the humeral head on the acromion process, it is important to externally rotate the humerus during this technique. The technique may be modified to prevent excessive elevation of the scapula by using one hand to stabilize the scapula over its superior border.

Normal End-feel. The end-feel for pure glenohumeral abduction is usually firm because of the tension in the middle and inferior bands of the glenohumeral ligament, the inferior joint capsule, and latissimus dorsi and pectoralis major muscles. For shoulder abduction, the end-feel is also firm because of tension in the middle and inferior portion of the trapezius muscle, and the rhomboid major and minor muscles.

Horizontal Abduction and Adduction

Hand Placement. Using one hand, the clinician grasps the wrist of the patient while using the other hand to grasp the patient's elbow (Figure 11-3). The patient's elbow can be flexed or extended.

Technique. The technique begins with the patient's shoulder abducted to 90° and parallel to the floor. The clinician lifts the arm up and across the upper chest of the patient (Figure 11-3) and then returns to the start position. If possible, the patient's arm is lowered below the height of the bed or table to achieve full horizontal abduction.

External Rotation. With the patient in the reference position, external rotation of the shoulder occurs in the transverse plane around a longitudinal axis.

Hand Placement. Using one hand, the clinician grasps the patient's elbow, while grasping the patient's wrist with the other hand (Figure 11-4). The patient's arm is typically positioned in 90° of abduction and 90° of elbow flexion. However, if this is not possible, the patient's arm can be positioned by the side with the elbow extended or flexed.

Technique. The clinician moves the patient's forearm backward toward the floor so that the humerus externally rotates to a point when the forearm is horizontal to the floor (Figure 11-4) or at the point when the shoulder girdle is felt to move into retraction, and is then returned to the start position. If the technique requires the arm to be by the patient's side and the elbow extended, the clinician uses one hand to grasp the humerus just above the epicondyles and the other hand to grasp the forearm of the wrist and then rotates or rolls the entire upper extremity in an outward direction. If the technique requires the arm to be by the patient's side and the elbow flexed, the clinician uses one hand to grasp the patient's elbow and the other hand to grasp the distal end of the forearm, and the forearm is moved away from the chest without abducting or abducting the shoulder.

Normal End-feel. Using the described motion, the end-feel is firm because of tension in the three bands of the glenohumeral ligament, the coracohumeral ligament, the anterior joint capsule, and the latissimus dorsi, pectoralis major, subscapularis, and teres major muscles. The end-feel for pure

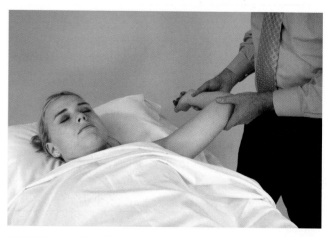

FIGURE 11-4 Shoulder external rotation

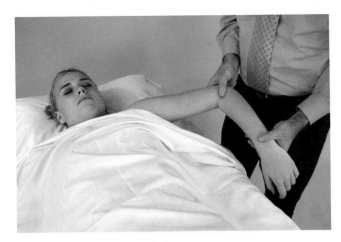

FIGURE 11-5 Shoulder internal rotation

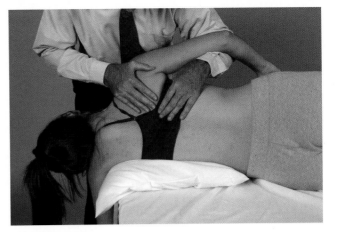

FIGURE 11-6 Scapular elevation and depression

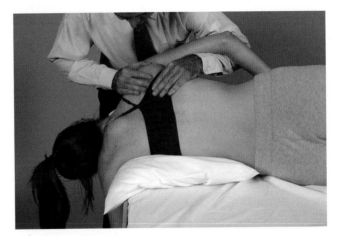

FIGURE 11-7 Scapular protraction and retraction

glenohumeral external rotation is also firm because of tension in the pectoralis minor and serratus anterior muscles.

Internal Rotation. With the patient in the reference position, external rotation of the shoulder occurs in the transverse plane around a longitudinal axis.

Hand Placement. Using one hand, the clinician grasps the patient's elbow, while grasping the patient's wrist with the other hand (Figure 11-5). The patient's arm is typically positioned in 90° of abduction and 90° of elbow flexion. However, if this is not possible, the patient's arm can be positioned differently (see below).

Technique. The clinician moves the patient's forearm forward toward the floor so that the humerus internally rotates to a point when the acromion process rises toward the ceiling, signifying that the humeral head is being blocked by the acromion (Figure 11-5) and the shoulder is beginning to move into protraction, and is then returned to the start position. If the technique requires the arm to be by the patient's side and the elbow extended, the clinician uses one hand to grasp the humerus just above the epicondyles and the other hand to grasp the forearm of the wrist and then rotates or rolls the entire upper extremity in an inward direction. It is not advised to use the technique where the patient's arm is by the side and the elbow is flexed, as the motion of internal rotation is blocked by the patient's body, thereby preventing the attainment of complete range of motion.

Normal End-feel. Using the described motion, the end-feel is firm because of tension in the middle and inferior portions of the trapezius muscle, and the rhomboid major and minor muscles. The end-feel for pure glenohumeral internal rotation is also firm because of tension in the posterior joint capsule and the teres minor and infraspinatus muscles.

Scapulothoracic Joint

Mobilization of the scapulothoracic joint is not commonly performed with the inpatient population. However, in cases of shoulder impingement syndrome, these techniques can prove useful in helping improve the scapular humeral rhythm. For these techniques, the patient is positioned in sidelying. The hand placement for the first two of these techniques is essentially the same; the only difference is the direction of force applied to the scapula.

Scapular Elevation and Depression

Hand Placement. Using one hand, the clinician cups the inferior angle of the scapula while placing the other hand on the superior border of the scapula.

Technique. The scapular is moved in an upward and downward direction (Figure 11-6).

Scapular Protraction (Abduction) and Retraction (Adduction)

Hand Placement. Using one hand, the clinician cups the inferior angle of the scapula while placing the other hand on the superior border of the scapula.

Technique. The scapula is moved toward and away from the spinous processes (Figure 11-7).

Scapular Winging. The patient is positioned in sidelying.

Hand Placement. Using one hand, the clinician slides the fingertips under the vertebral (medial) border of the scapula (Figure 11-8).

Technique. The clinician gently lifts the scapula from the ribs. This technique is made easier if the patient's arm is placed behind the trunk.

Elbow Joint

Flexion and Extension. Motion occurs in the sagittal plane around the frontal axis.

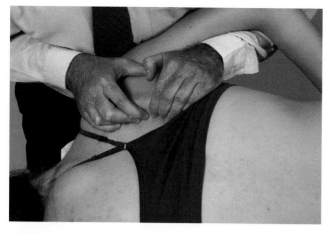

FIGURE 11-8 Scapular winging

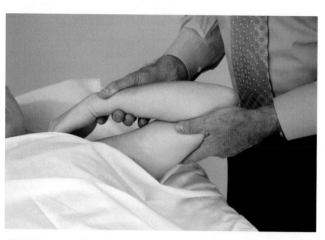

FIGURE 11-9 Elbow flexion

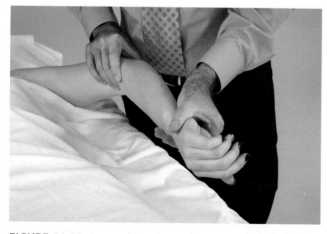

FIGURE 11-10 Approaching the end range of elbow extension and pronation

Hand Placement. Using one hand, the clinician grasps the distal forearm and hand of the patient while using the other hand to support and stabilize the distal end of the patient's humerus.

Technique. While preventing any shoulder motion, the clinician flexes and extends the patient's elbow with the patient's forearm positioned in neutral (Figure 11-9), then with the patient's forearm positioned in pronation (Figure 11-10), and finally with the patient's forearm positioned in supination (Figure 11-11).

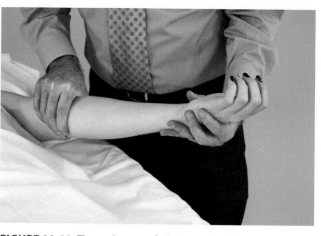

FIGURE 11-11 The end range of elbow extension and supination

Normal End-feel. The end-feel for elbow flexion is normally one of soft tissue approximation due to compression of the muscle bulk of the anterior forearm with that of the anterior upper arm. However, in a very slight individual with a small muscle bulk, the end-feel may be either:

▶ Hard because of the contact between the coronoid process of the ulna and the coronoid fossa of the humerus, and contact between the head of the radius and the radial fossa of the humerus

▶ Firm because of the tension in the posterior joint capsule and the triceps brachii muscle

The end-feel for elbow extension is typically hard because of contact between the olecranon process of the ulna and the olecranon fossa of the humerus. On occasion, the end-feel can be firm because of tension in the anterior joint capsule, the collateral ligaments, and the biceps brachii and brachialis muscles.

Forearm Pronation and Supination. With the patient in the anatomic reference position, motion occurs in the transverse plane around a longitudinal axis.

Hand Placement. The clinician uses one hand to grasp the patient's distal forearm and the patient's hand while using the other hand to support and stabilize the patient's humerus.

Technique. The technique can be performed with the patient's elbow flexed or extended. While ensuring that no motion is occurring at the shoulder, the clinician supinates (Figure 11-11) and pronates (Figure 11-10) the patient's forearm.

Normal End-feel. The normal end-feel for forearm pronation is either hard because of contact between the ulna and the radius, or firm because of tension in the posterior (dorsal) radioulnar ligament of the distal (inferior) radioulnar joint, the supinator and biceps brachii muscles, and the interosseous membrane. The normal end-feel for forearm supination is firm as a result of tension in the anterior radioulnar ligament of the distal radioulnar joint, interosseous membrane, and the pronator teres and pronator quadratus muscles.

Wrist Joint

Flexion and Extension. Motion occurs in the sagittal plane around a frontal axis.

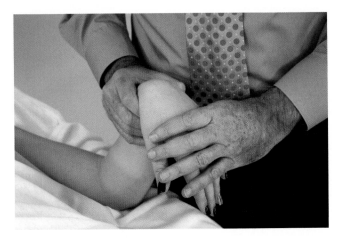

FIGURE 11-12 Wrist flexion

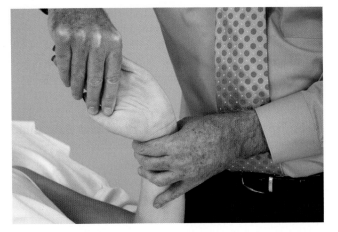

FIGURE 11-14 Radial deviation

Hand Placement. Using one hand, the clinician grasps the patient's hand over the posterior and anterior surfaces, while using the other hand to support and stabilize the forearm.

Technique. The technique can be performed with the patient's elbow flexed or extended. While allowing the patient's fingers to relax, the clinician moves the patient's palm toward the forearm (flexion) (Figure 11-12) and then the posterior aspect of the hand toward the forearm (extension) (Figure 11-13). The technique can then be repeated with the patient's fingers fully flexed in a closed fist position.

Normal End-feel. The end-feel for wrist flexion is firm because of tension in the posterior (dorsal) radio carpal ligament and the posterior (dorsal) joint capsule. The end-feel for wrist extension is usually firm because of the tension in the anterior (palmar) radiocarpal ligament and the anterior (palmar) joint capsule, but it can be hard as a result of contact between the radius and the carpal bones.

CLINICAL PEARL

While performing range of motion exercises at the wrist, it is important to remember those muscles/tendons that cross multiple joints:

▶ *Extensor digitorum.* This technique can be performed with the patient's elbow flexed or extended. While plac-

ing one hand over the posterior aspect of all of the fingers and the patient's hand, the clinician uses the other hand to support and stabilize the forearm. The clinician then sequentially flexes the DIP, PIP, and MCP joints (see later), and then gently flexes the wrist.

▶ *Flexor digitorum superficialis and profundus.* This technique can be performed with the patient's elbow flexed or extended. The clinician places one hand over the anterior surface of all of the fingers of the patient's hand, while using the other hand support and stabilize the forearm. The clinician then sequentially extends the DIP, PIP, and MCP joints, and then gently extends the wrist to the point of maximal tension.

Radial and Ulnar Deviation

Hand Placement. While maintaining the patient's wrist in neutral flexion-extension, the clinician uses one hand to grasp the patient's hand over the posterior and anterior surfaces, while using the other hand to support and stabilize the forearm.

Technique. While avoiding any wrist flexion-extension, the clinician moves the patient's hand in a radial (Figure 11-14) and ulnar (Figure 11-15) direction.

Normal End-feel. The end-feel for radial deviation is typically hard because of contact between the radial styloid process and

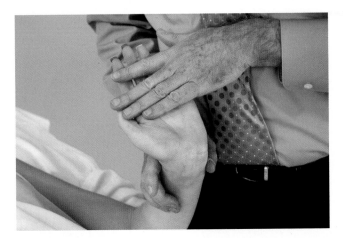

FIGURE 11-13 Wrist extension

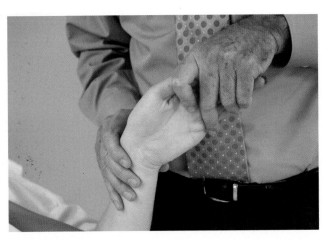

FIGURE 11-15 Ulnar deviation

the scaphoid. However, if there is tension in the ulnar collateral ligament, the ulnar carpal ligament, and the ulnar portion of the joint capsule, the end-feel may be firm. The end-feel for ulnar deviation is firm because of tension in the radial collateral ligament and the radial portion of the joint capsule.

Hand and Thumb Joints

Metacarpophalangeal (MCP) Flexion and Extension.
Motion occurs in the sagittal plane around a frontal axis.

Hand Placement. Using the thumb and index finger of one hand, the clinician grasps the posterior and anterior surfaces of a metacarpal just proximal to the metacarpal head, while using the thumb and index finger of the other hand to grasp the posterior and anterior surfaces of a proximal phalanx (Figure 11-16).

Technique. While stabilizing the metacarpal with one hand, the other hand moves the phalanx in an upward and downward direction (Figure 11-16). The technique is repeated for each MCP of the fingers on each hand.

Normal End-feel. The end-feel for MCP flexion can vary from hard because of contact between the palmar aspect of the proximal phalanx and metacarpal, to firm because of tension in the posterior joint capsule and the collateral ligaments. The end-feel for MCP extension is firm as a result of tension in the anterior (palmar) joint capsule and anterior (palmar) fibrocartilaginous plate.

Metacarpophalangeal (MCP) Joint of the Thumb Flexion and Extension.
Motion occurs in the frontal plane around an A-P axis, when the patient is in the anatomic reference position.

Hand Placement. Using one hand, the clinician stabilizes the first metacarpal to prevent wrist motion, and flexion and opposition of the CMC joint of the thumb, while using the other hand to move the thumb at the MCP joint.

Technique. Once correct stabilization is attained, the clinician moves the thumb around the MCP joint into flexion, toward the palm (Figure 11-17), and then into extension (Figure 11-18), away from the hand.

Normal End-feel. The end-feel for MCP flexion is either hard because of contact between the anterior aspect of the proximal phalanx and the first metacarpal, or firm because of tension in

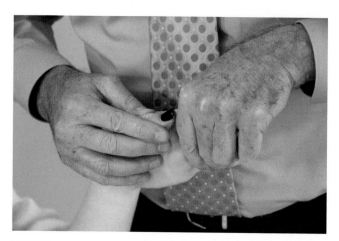

FIGURE 11-17 MCP flexion of the thumb

the posterior joint capsule, the extensor policies brevis muscle, and the collateral ligaments. The end-feel for MCP extension is firm, resulting from tension in the anterior joint capsule, anterior (palmar) fibrocartilaginous plate, and the flexor pollicis brevis muscle.

Metacarpophalangeal (MCP) Abduction.
Motion occurs in the frontal plane around an A-P axis.

Hand Placement. The clinician uses one hand to grasp and stabilize the PIP joints of the first, second, and third fingers, while using the other hand to grasp the forefinger.

Technique. While maintaining the MCP and IP joint in extension, the clinician gently moves the fourth finger away from the third finger. Then, the clinician stabilizes the first and second fingers and moves the third finger away from the second finger. Next, the second finger can be moved to the left and to the right without stabilization of any of the other fingers.

Normal End-feel. The normal end-feel for MCP abduction is firm because of tension in the collateral ligaments of the MCP joints, the anterior (palmar) interossei muscles, and the fascia of the web space between the fingers.

Thumb (Carpometacarpal) Abduction and Adduction.
Motion occurs in the sagittal plane around a frontal axis, when the patient is in the anatomic reference position.

FIGURE 11-16 MCP flexion of the index finger

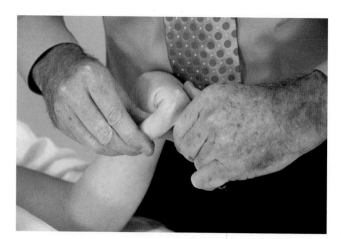

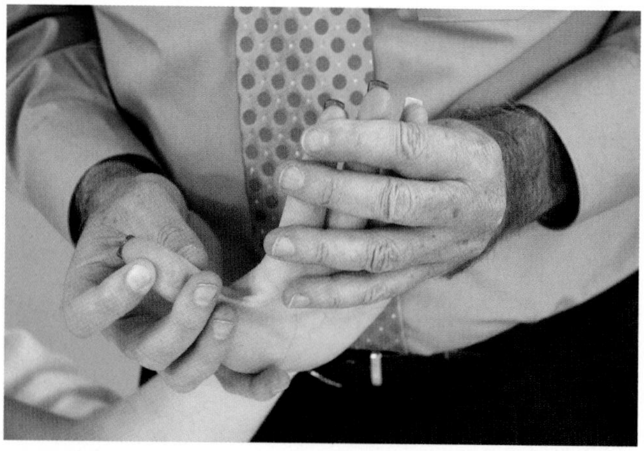

FIGURE 11-18 MCP extension of the thumb

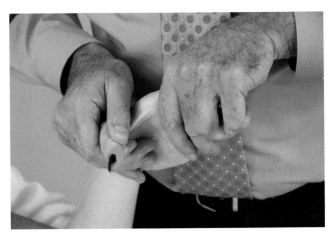

FIGURE 11-19 Thumb abduction

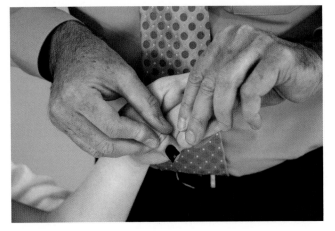

FIGURE 11-20 Thumb opposition

Hand Placement. Using the fingers and thumb of one hand, the clinician grasps the patient's thumb, while using the other hand to stabilize the second metacarpal.

Technique. The clinician lifts the thumb away from the palm so that it is perpendicular to the palm while maintaining the MCP and IP joint in extension (Figure 11-19). The thumb is then returned to the palm parallel to the second metatarsal.

Normal End-feel. The end-feel for carpometacarpal (CMC) joint abduction is firm because of tension in the fascia and skin of the web space between the thumb and index finger, and tension in the adductor pollicis and first posterior interossei muscles.

Thumb (CMC) Extension and Flexion. Motion occurs in the frontal plane around an A-P axis, when the patient is in the anatomic reference position.

Hand Placement. Using the fingers and thumb of one hand, the clinician grasps the patient's thumb, while using the other hand to stabilize the second metacarpal.

Technique. The clinician moves the thumb away from the index finger and horizontal to the palm, thereby widening the web space to its maximum. The thumb is then returned so that it rests next to the side of the second metacarpal.

Normal End-feel. The end-feel for CMC joint flexion can be either soft because of contact between the muscle bulk of the thenar eminence in the palm of the hand, or firm because of tension in the posterior joint capsule and the extensor pollicis brevis and abductor pollicis brevis muscles. The end-feel for CMC joint extension is firm as a result of tension in the anterior joint capsule and the adductor pollicis, flexor pollicis brevis, opponens pollicis, and the first posterior interossei muscles.

Thumb Opposition. This motion is a combination of flexion, abduction, and medial-axial rotation.

Hand Placement. The clinician uses the thumb and index finger of one hand to grasp the patient's thumb, while using the other hand to grasp the fifth metacarpal and finger.

Technique. The clinician rolls the patient's thumb toward the fifth finger while maintaining the MCP and IP joint in extension

(Figure 11-20), and then returns the thumb to a position of full extension.

Normal End-feel. The end-feel can be soft because of contact between the muscle bulk of the thenar eminence and the palm, or firm because of tension in the joint capsule, extensor pollicis brevis muscle, and transverse metacarpal ligament (when moving the fifth finger).

Interphalangeal (IP) Joint of the Thumb Flexion and Extension. Motion occurs in the frontal plane around an A-P axis, when the patient is in the anatomic reference position.

Hand Placement. The clinician uses one hand to stabilize the proximal phalanx to prevent flexion or extension of the MCP joint and the other hand to flex the thumb about the IP joint.

Technique. Using the tip of the index finger and the thumb of one hand, the clinician flexes the tip of thumb around the IP joint into flexion (Figure 11-21), and extension.

Normal End-feel. The normal end-feel for IP flexion is firm because of tension in the collateral ligaments and the posterior joint capsule. The normal end-feel for IP extension is firm because of tension in the anterior joint capsule and the anterior (palmar) fibrocartilaginous plate.

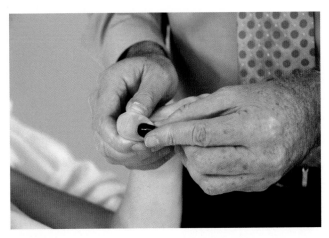

FIGURE 11-21 Flexion of the thumb interphalangeal joint

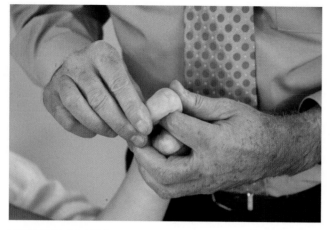

FIGURE 11-22 PIP flexion

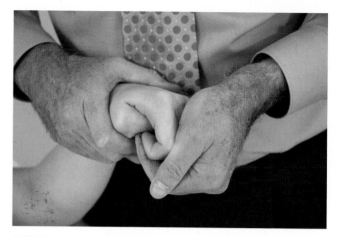

FIGURE 11-24 Combined flexion of the PIP and DIP joints

Finger Joints

Flexion and Extension of the Proximal Interphalangeal (PIP) and Distal Interphalangeal (DIP) Joints.
Motion occurs in the sagittal plane around a frontal axis.

Hand Placement. Using the thumb and index finger of one hand, the clinician grasps the more proximal phalanx, while using the thumb and index finger of the other hand to grasp the more distal phalanx. The same technique is used for the PIP (Figure 11-22) and the DIP (Figure 11-23) joints.

Technique. While stabilizing the more proximal phalanx, the clinician moves the more distal phalanx in an upward (extension) and downward (flexion) direction. The technique is repeated for each articulation on each hand, including the thumb. Depending on the intent, the PIP and DIP joints can be flexed (Figure 11-24) and extended as a unit.

Normal End-feel. The end-feel for PIP flexion can be either hard because of contact between the anterior aspect of the middle phalanx and the proximal phalanx, or soft because of compression of soft tissue between the anterior aspect of the middle and proximal phalanges. The end-feel for PIP extension is firm as a result of tension in the anterior (palmar) joint capsule and anterior (palmar) fibrocartilaginous plate. The end-feel for DIP flexion is firm because of tension in the posterior (dorsal) joint capsule, the contralateral ligaments, and the oblique retinacular ligament. The end-feel for DIP

extension is firm as a result of tension in the anterior (palmar) joint capsule and the anterior (palmar) fibrocartilaginous plate.

Diagonal Patterns of the Upper Extremity

Diagonal patterns of motion, incorporating the PNF patterns, can be performed using AROM, AAROM, or PROM as part of a range of motion regime, although it must always be remembered that because these patterns employ a number of planes simultaneously, they do not produce the same amount of range of motion to the muscles and joints as when the anatomic planes are used. However, there are times when these more functional movements are appropriate, particularly in the case where a patient is able to participate. As described in the Diagonal Patterns of Motion section earlier, there are four major patterns of motions that are commonly used, two for the upper extremities (D1 and D2 flexion and extension), and two for the lower extremities (D1 and D2 flexion and extension). Perhaps the major benefit of using PNF patterns as opposed to the standard anatomic range of motion exercises is that they induce some degree of spinal rotation, which can be particularly beneficial for the immobile patient. When used as a method of applying range of motion to a patient, hand placement is not as critical. The two patterns for the upper extremities are depicted in Figs. 11-25 through 11-28 and VIDEO 11-1 and 11-2.

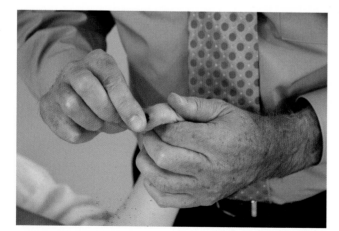

FIGURE 11-23 DIP flexion

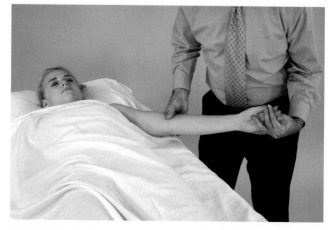

FIGURE 11-25 Upper extremity D1 extension

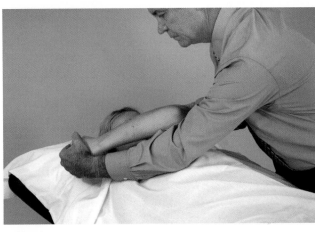

FIGURE 11-26 Upper extremity D1 flexion

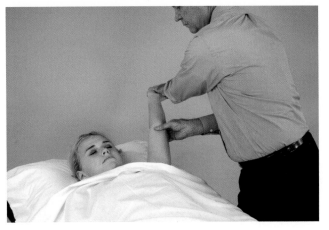

FIGURE 11-28 Upper extremity D2 extension

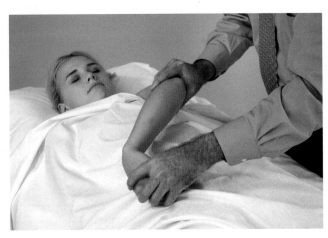

FIGURE 11-27 Upper extremity D2 flexion

Video Description

While the proprioceptive neuromuscular facilitation (PNF) techniques are typically performed using a rigid set of hand positions by the clinician and precise movements of the patient's upper or lower extremities, there are occasions when these techniques can be modified based on any range of motion restriction found with the patient. If you look closely at Video 11-1, you will notice that the clinician introduces the correct direction of forearm rotation toward the end of the technique to illustrate that there are occasions when the components of the technique may have to be modified.

Range of Motion—Lower Extremity

For all of the following techniques, it is assumed that the patient is in the supine position, unless otherwise stated.

Hip Joint

Hip Flexion. Motion occurs in the sagittal plane around a frontal axis.

The range of motion exercises for the hip can incorporate motion at the knee and at the pelvis. Although the knee motion is more obvious, it is important to remember that hip flexion can induce posterior pelvic rotation and hip extension can induce anterior pelvic rotation. Based on the desired

outcome of the range of motion exercise, the clinician may determine that the end ranges of hip motion that induce pelvic motion may be necessary.

Hand Placement. The clinician uses one hand to grasp the patient's ankle, and the other hand to support the patient's knee.

Technique. The clinician moves the patient's lower extremity into a combination of hip and knee flexion (Figure 11-29) to the appropriate end-feel. Ankle dorsiflexion can also be included. In addition, the clinician may decide to omit the knee flexion and perform hip flexion with knee extension, also known as a straight leg raise (Figure 11-30). This particular maneuver serves the function of lengthening the multijoint muscles of the posterior thigh (the hamstrings) across both the knee and the hip. The straight leg maneuver can be performed in neutral hip rotation, adduction, and abduction, or can be performed with varying degrees of these motions. For example, the clinician may decide to perform the straight leg raise with the hip in internal rotation and adduction in order to stretch a specific structure, or group of structures.

Normal End-feel. The normal end-feel for hip flexion is usually soft tissue approximation because of contact between the muscle bulk of the anterior thigh and the lower abdomen.

Hip Extension. Motion occurs in the sagittal plane around a frontal axis.

The patient is positioned in prone.

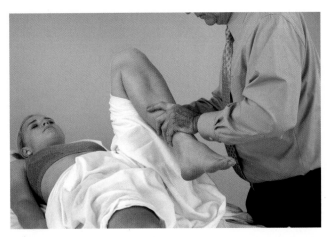

FIGURE 11-29 Hip and knee flexion

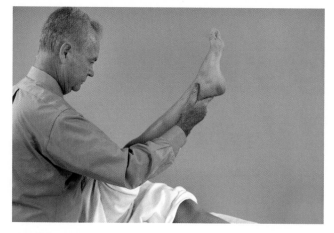

FIGURE 11-30 Hip flexion and knee extension

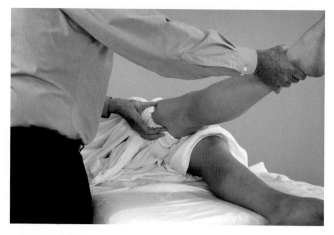

FIGURE 11-32 Hip adduction

Hand Placement. The clinician uses one hand to grasp the patient's knee while using the other hand to stabilize the patient's pelvis.

Technique. The clinician raises the patient's thigh from the bed to the point when the pelvis is felt to begin to rotate anteriorly.

This technique can also be performed with the patient in sidelying, with the lower extremity to be treated uppermost. As before, the clinician uses one hand to monitor the pelvis while using the other hand and arm to support the patient's lower extremity. A modification to the sidelying technique can be used to apply tension to the tensor fasciae latae by using a combination of hip extension and hip adduction while stabilizing the pelvis.

Normal End-feel. The end-feel is firm as a result of tension in the anterior joint capsule, iliofemoral ligament, and, to a lesser degree, the ischiofemoral and pubofemoral ligaments.

Hip Abduction and Adduction. Motion occurs in a frontal plane around an A-P axis.

Hand Placement. The clinician uses one hand to grasp the patient's foot and ankle, and the other hand to support the patient's knee, or to stabilize the pelvis to prevent rotation and lateral tilting.

Technique. The clinician moves the patient's lower extremity so that the hip is abducted (Figure 11-31) and then adducted (Figure 11-32). In order to ensure that hip abduction occurs

beyond the midline, the patient's contralateral lower extremity may need to be elevated or positioned in hip abduction.

Normal End-feel. The end-feel for abduction is firm because of tension in the inferior-medial joint capsule, pubofemoral ligament, ischiofemoral ligament, and the inferior band of the iliofemoral ligament. In addition, depending on the degree of adaptive shortening, the adductor magnus, adductor longus, adductor brevis, pectineus, and gracilis muscles may contribute to the firmness of the end-feel. The end-feel for adduction is firm because of tension in the superior-lateral joint capsule and the superior band of the iliofemoral ligament. In addition, depending on the degree of adaptive shortening, the gluteus medius and minimus and the tensor fascia latae muscles may also contribute to the firmness of the end-feel.

Hip External and Internal Rotation. Motion occurs in a transverse plane around a longitudinal axis, when the subject is in the anatomic reference position.

Hand Placement. The clinician uses one hand to grasp the patient's foot and ankle, and the other hand to support the patient's knee. The patient's hip and knee are positioned in approximately 90°.

Technique. The clinician moves the foot of the patient toward the midline for external rotation of the hip (Figure 11-33), and away from the midline for internal rotation of the hip (Figure 11-34).

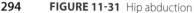

FIGURE 11-31 Hip abduction

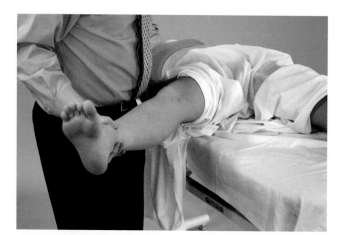

FIGURE 11-33 Hip external rotation

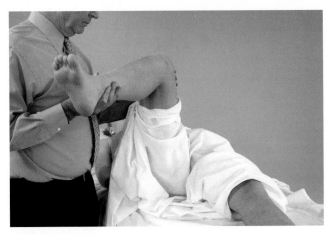

FIGURE 11-34 Hip internal rotation

Normal End-feel. The end-feel for internal rotation is firm because of tension in the posterior joint capsule and the ischiofemoral ligament, and muscle tension from the external rotators of the hip (piriformis, obturator internis and externus, gemelli superior and inferior, quadratus femoris, and the posterior fibers of the gluteus medius and gluteus maximus). The end-feel for external rotation is also firm as a result of tension in the anterior joint capsule, iliofemoral ligament, and pubofemoral ligament. In addition, tension from the internal rotators of the hip (the anterior portion of the gluteus medius, the gluteus minimus, the adductor magnus and longus, and the pectineus muscles) may also enhance the firmness of the end-feel.

Knee Joint

Knee Flexion and Extension. Motion occurs in the sagittal plane around a frontal axis.

Hand Placement. The clinician uses one hand to grasp the patient's foot and ankle, and the other hand to support the patient's knee.

Technique. The patient's knee is flexed (Figure 11-35) to the appropriate end-feel. This technique can be modified by positioning the patient prone (with a pillow under the hips to maintain pelvic neutral) in order to stretch the two joint muscles of the hip and knee, especially the rectus femoris. The clinician uses one hand to grasp the patient's ankle and the other hand to monitor the patient's pelvis. The clinician flexes

the patient's knee to the point where anterior pelvic rotation motion is felt to occur.

Normal End-feel. The end-feel for knee flexion is normally one of soft tissue approximation because of contact between the muscle bulk of the posterior calf and thigh, or between the heel and the buttocks. However, if there is significant adaptive shortening of the rectus femoris muscle, the end-feel is firm because of tension in this muscle. The end-feel for knee extension is firm because of tension in the posterior joint capsule, the oblique and arcuate popliteal ligaments, collateral ligaments, and the anterior posterior cruciate ligaments.

Ankle Joint

Dorsiflexion and plantarflexion motions occur in the sagittal plane around a frontal axis. The motions of inversion and eversion consist of a combination of motions:

▶ *Inversion:* a combination of supination, adduction, and plantarflexion occurring in varying degrees throughout the various joints of the ankle and foot.

▶ *Eversion:* a combination of pronation, abduction, and dorsiflexion occurring in varying degrees throughout the various joints of the ankle and foot.

Dorsiflexion

Hand Placement. Using one hand, the clinician stabilizes the patient's lower leg, while using the other hand on the sole of the patient's foot.

Technique. The clinician uses the hand on the sole of the patient's foot to apply motion into dorsiflexion (Figure 11-36).

Normal End-feel. The end-feel is firm because of tension in the joint capsules, the calcaneofibular ligament, the anterior and posterior talofibular ligament, the posterior calcaneal ligaments, the anterior, posterior, lateral, and interosseous talocalcaneal ligaments, the posterior talonavicular ligament, the posterior calcaneocuboid ligament, the lateral band of the bifurcate ligament, the transverse metatarsal ligament, and various anterior and posterior and interosseous ligaments of the smaller joints of the foot. In addition, tension from the fibularis longus and brevis muscles can also enhance the firmness of the end-feel.

Plantarflexion

Hand Placement. Using one hand, the clinician stabilizes the patient's lower leg, while placing the other hand on the posterior aspect of the patient's foot.

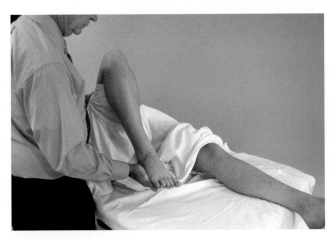

FIGURE 11-35 Knee flexion

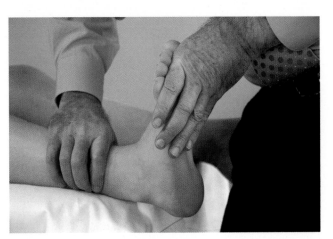

FIGURE 11-36 Ankle dorsiflexion

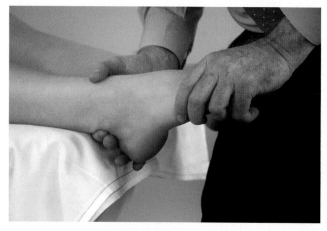

FIGURE 11-37 Ankle plantarflexion

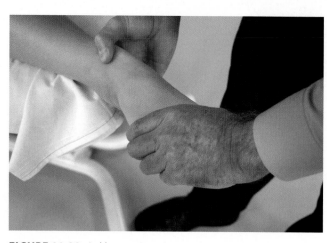

FIGURE 11-39 Ankle eversion

Technique. The clinician uses the hand on the posterior aspect of the patient's foot to apply motion into plantarflexion (Figure 11-37).

Normal End-feel. The end-feel can be either hard because of contact between the calcaneus and the floor of the sinus tarsi, or firm because of tension in the joint capsules, the deltoid ligament, the plantar calcaneonavicular and calcaneocuboid ligaments, the medial talocalcaneal ligament, the medial band of the bifurcate ligament, the transverse metatarsal ligament, the posterior talonavicular ligament and, various posterior, anterior and interosseous ligaments of the smaller joints of the foot. In addition, tension from the tibialis posterior muscle can also enhance the firmness of the end-feel.

Inversion

Hand Placement. Using one hand, the clinician stabilizes the patient's lower leg, while placing the other hand around the patient's foot.

Technique. The clinician uses the hand around the patient's foot to apply motion into inversion (Figure 11-38).

Normal End-feel. The end-feel is firm because of tension in the lateral joint capsule, the calcaneofibular ligament, the anterior and posterior talofibular ligaments, and the lateral, posterior, anterior, and interosseous talocalcaneal ligaments.

Eversion

Hand Placement. Using one hand, the clinician stabilizes the patient's lower leg, while placing the other hand around the patient's foot.

Technique. The clinician uses the hand around the patient's foot to apply motion into eversion (Figure 11-39).

Normal End-feel. The end-feel is either hard because of contact between the calcaneus and the floor of the sinus tarsi, or firm because of tension in the deltoid ligament, the medial talocalcaneal ligament, and the tibialis posterior muscle.

Toe Joints

Flexion and extension of the toe joints occurs in the sagittal plane around a frontal axis.

Metatarsophalangeal (MTP) Flexion

Hand Placement. Using one hand, the clinician stabilizes the patient's foot, while using the other hand to grasp the patient's toes.

Technique. The clinician moves the toes into flexion around the MTP joint (Figure 11-40). This technique can be performed at each of the MTP joints for more specificity.

Normal End-feel. The end-feel is firm because of tension in the posterior joint capsule and the collateral ligaments, in addition to tension in the extensor digitorum brevis muscle.

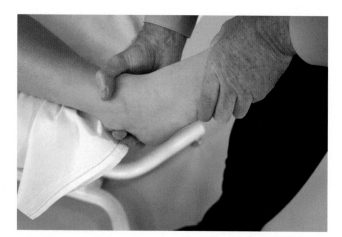

FIGURE 11-38 Ankle inversion

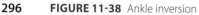

FIGURE 11-40 MTP flexion

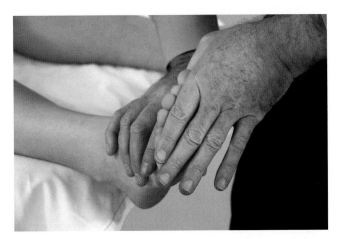

FIGURE 11-41 MTP extension

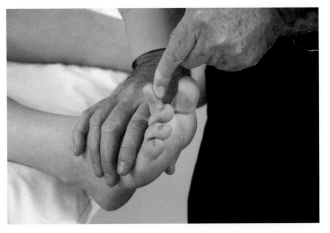

FIGURE 11-43 Interphalangeal joint extension

Metatarsophalangeal (MTP) Extension

Hand Placement. Using one hand, the clinician stabilizes the patient's foot, while using the other hand to grasp the patient's toes.

Technique. The clinician moves the toes into extension around the MTP joint (Figure 11-41). The technique can be performed at each of the MTP joints for more specificity.

Normal End-feel. The end-feel is firm because of tension in the plantar joint capsule, the plantar fibrocartilaginous plate, and the flexor hallucis brevis, flexor digitorum brevis, and flexor digiti minimi muscles.

Interphalangeal (IP) Flexion and Extension

Hand Placement. Using one hand, the clinician stabilizes the patient's foot, while using the other hand to grasp the patient's toes.

Technique. The clinician moves each toe into flexion (Figure 11-42) and extension (Figure 11-43). The technique is repeated with the great toe into flexion (Figure 11-44) and extension (Figure 11-45).

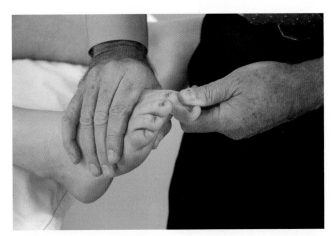

FIGURE 11-44 Great toe flexion

Diagonal Patterns of the Lower Extremity

As with the upper extremity, diagonal patterns of motion, incorporating the PNF patterns, can be performed using AROM, AAROM, or PROM as part of a range of motion of a regime [VIDEO 11-3 and 11-4]. The diagonal patterns of the lower extremity have a greater potential for inducing motion

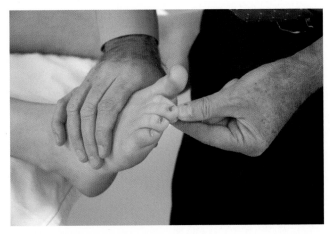

FIGURE 11-42 Interphalangeal joint flexion

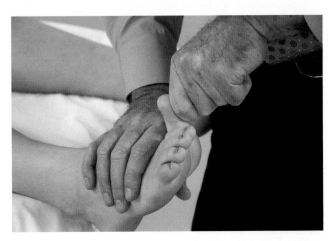

FIGURE 11-45 Great toe extension

at the lumbar and thoracic spine, particularly at the extremes of range. The clinician must determine whether range of motion into these regions is desired or not and place limits on the range of motion accordingly. As stated earlier, although it would appear that the use of diagonal patterns is a more efficient method of applying range of motion to a series of joints rather than ranging a series of individual joints, these PNF patterns do not produce the same amount of range of motion to the muscles and joints as when the individual joints are moved through their various ranges of motion. When used as a method of applying range of motion to a patient, hand

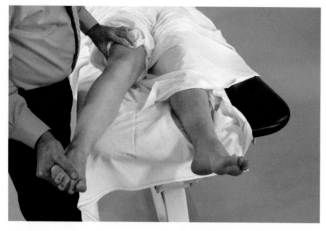

FIGURE 11-46 Lower extremity D1 extension

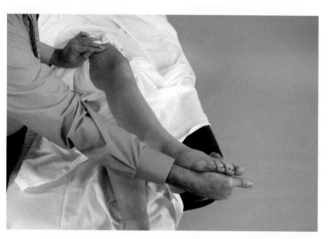

FIGURE 11-47 Lower extremity D1 flexion

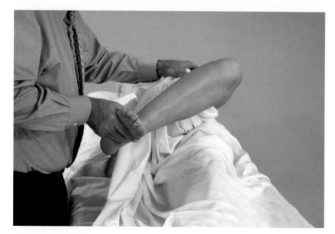

FIGURE 11-48 Lower extremity D2 flexion

placement is not as critical. The two patterns for the lower extremities are depicted in Figures 11-46 through 11-49.

Combined Ranges of Motion

When performing passive range of motion exercises, the clinician may decide to apply combined motions simultaneously (VIDEO 11-5). For example, when performing range of motion to the lower extremities, the clinician may use a

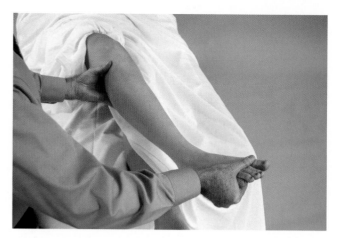

FIGURE 11-49 Lower extremity D2 extension

technique that incorporates ankle dorsiflexion, knee flexion, and hip flexion. In addition, the clinician may decide to superimpose hip internal rotation and hip external rotation to the technique.

Video Description

In Video 11-5, the clinician demonstrates a combined technique of hip flexion, knee flexion, and dorsiflexion for the lower extremity. Notice how the clinician adds internal rotation and external rotation of the hip to the technique. Also note how the clinician uses the larger trunk muscles to perform the range of motion rather than just the muscles of the upper extremities.

Range of Motion—The Spine

Cervical Spine

Hand Placement. Standing at the foot of the bed, the clinician uses both hands to support patient's head.

Technique. While supporting the patient's head, the clinician moves the patient's head and cervical spine into flexion (Figure 11-50), rotation to the right (Figure 11-51) and left, and side flexion to the right (Figure 11-52) and left.

Wherever possible, cervical spine motion should be tested actively in either the sitting or standing position (VIDEO 11-6),

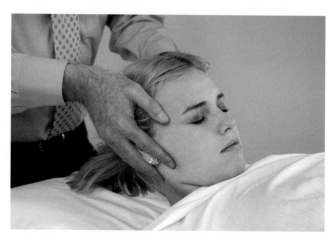

FIGURE 11-50 Cervical flexion

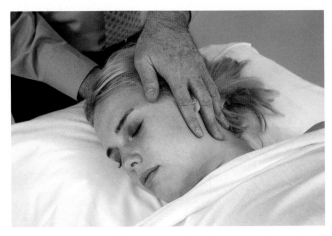

FIGURE 11-51 Cervical rotation to the right

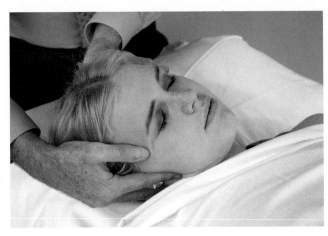

FIGURE 11-52 Cervical side bending to the right

so that the effect of the compression of the head on the range of motion can be noted.

Video Description

In Video 11-6, the patient demonstrates active range of motion of the cervical spine. To the trained eye, this patient demonstrates a loss of range of motion in one direction. Can you spot it?

Lumbar Spine

Although passive range of motion can be applied to the lumbar spine, to achieve end ranges of motion is very difficult. Whenever possible, active range of motion of the lumbar spine in the sitting or standing position (VIDEO 11-7) should be assessed so that the effect of the compression of the trunk and head on the range of motion can be noted.

Video Description

In Video 11-7, the patient performs active range of motion of the lumbar spine. What do you consider the cause of the apparent decrease in lumbar flexion?

GONIOMETRY

The term goniometry is derived from two Greek words, *gonia*, meaning angle, and *metron*, meaning measure. Thus, a goniometer is an instrument used to measure angles. Within the field of physical therapy, goniometry is used to measure the total amount of available motion at a specific joint. Goniometry can be used to measure both active and passive range of motion.

Goniometers are produced in a variety of sizes and shapes and are usually constructed of either plastic or metal (Figure 11-53). The two most common types of instruments used to measure joint angles are the bubble inclinometer and the traditional goniometer.

▶ *Bubble goniometer* (Figure 11-54). The bubble goniometer, which has a 360° rotating dial and scale with fluid indicator, can be used for flexion and extension; abduction and adduction; and rotation in the neck, shoulder, elbow, wrist, hip, knee, ankle, and spine.

▶ *Traditional goniometer.* The traditional goniometer, which can be used for flexion and extension; abduction and adduction; and rotation in the shoulder, elbow, wrist, hip, knee, and ankle, consists of three parts:

■ *A body.* The body of the goniometer is designed like a protractor and may form a full or half circle. A measuring scale is located around the body. The scale can extend either from 0° to 180° and 180° to 0° for the half-circle models, or from 0° to 360° and from 360° to 0° on the full-circle models. The intervals on the scales can vary from 1° to 10°.

■ *A stationary arm.* The stationary arm is structurally a part of the body and therefore cannot move independently of the body.

■ *A moving arm.* The moving arm is attached to the fulcrum in the center of the body by a rivet or screwlike device that allows the moving arm to move freely on the body of the device. In some instruments, the screwlike device can be tightened to fix the moving arm in a certain position or loosened to permit free movement.

The correct selection of which goniometer device to use depends on the joint angle to be measured. The length of arms varies among instruments and can range from 3 to 18 inches. Extendable goniometers (Figure 11-55) allow varying ranges from 9½ inches to 26 inches. The longer armed goniometers or the bubble inclinometer are recommended when the landmarks are farther apart, such as when measuring hip, knee, elbow, and shoulder movements. In the smaller joints such as the wrist, hand, foot, and ankle, a traditional goniometer with a shorter arm is used.

The general procedure for measuring range of motion involves the following:

1. The patient is positioned in the recommended testing position close to the edge of the treatment table or bed and should be correctly draped. While stabilizing the proximal joint component, the clinician gently moves the distal joint component through the available range of motion until the end-feel is determined (see

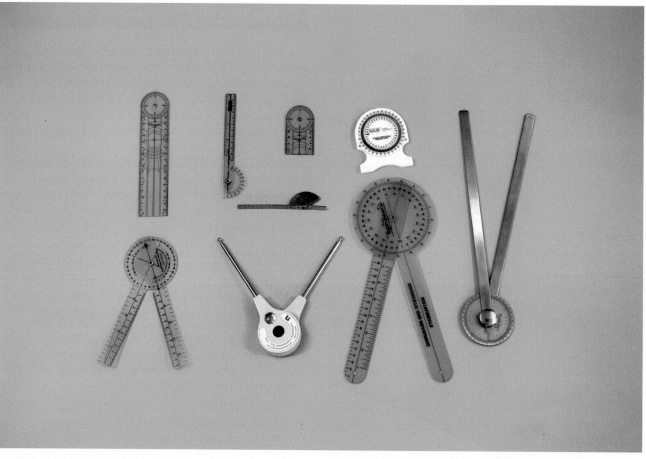

FIGURE 11-53 The various types of goniometers

Range of Motion Examination). An estimate is made of the available range of motion, and the distal joint component is returned to the starting position. For the sake of brevity, the following descriptions of goniometric measurements do not include assessment of passive range of motion, but the reader should consider it as read.

2. The clinician palpates the relevant bony landmarks and aligns the goniometer.

3. A record is made of the starting measurement. The goniometer is then removed and the patient moves the joint through the available range of motion. Once the joint has been moved through the available range of motion, the goniometer is replaced and realigned, and a measurement is read and recorded.

The standard testing procedures for each of the upper and lower extremity joints are outlined in Tables 11-9 and 11-10.

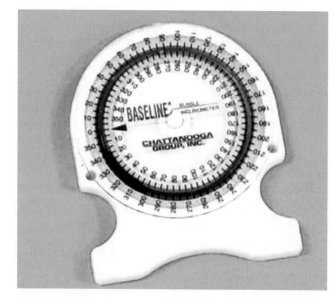

FIGURE 11-54 Bubble goniometer

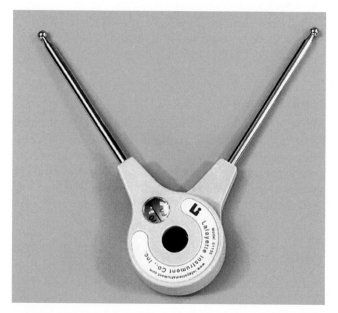

FIGURE 11-55 Extendable goniometer

TABLE 11-9	Goniometric Techniques for the Upper Extremity			
Joint	**Motion**	**Fulcrum**	**Proximal Arm**	**Distal Arm**
Shoulder	Flexion	Acromion process	Mid-axillary line of the thorax	Lateral midline of the humerus using the lateral epicondyle of the humerus for reference
	Extension	Acromion process	Mid-axillary line of the thorax	Lateral midline of the humerus using the lateral epicondyle of the humerus for reference
	Abduction	Anterior aspect of the acromion process	Parallel to the midline of the anterior aspect of the sternum	Medial midline of the humerus
	Adduction	Anterior aspect of the acromion process	Parallel to the midline of the anterior aspect of the sternum	Medial midline of the humerus
	Internal rotation	Olecranon process	Parallel or perpendicular to the floor	Ulna using the olecranon process and ulnar styloid for reference
	External rotation	Olecranon process	Parallel or perpendicular to the floor	Ulna using the olecranon process and ulnar styloid for reference
Elbow	Flexion	Lateral epicondyle of the humerus	Lateral midline of the humerus using the center of the acromion process for reference	Lateral midline of the radius using the radial head and radial styloid process for reference
	Extension	Lateral epicondyle of the humerus	Lateral midline of the humerus using the center of the acromion process for reference	Lateral midline of the radius using the radial head and radial styloid process for reference
Forearm	Pronation	Lateral to the ulnar styloid process	Parallel to the anterior midline of the humerus	Dorsal aspect of the forearm, just proximal to the styloid process of the radius and ulna
	Supination	Medial to the ulnar styloid process	Parallel to the anterior midline of the humerus	Ventral aspect of the forearm, just proximal to the styloid process of the radius and ulna
Wrist	Flexion	Lateral aspect of the wrists over the triquetrum	Lateral midline of the ulna using the olecranon and ulnar styloid process for reference	Lateral midline of the fifth metacarpal
	Extension	Lateral aspect of the wrists over the triquetrum	Lateral midline of the ulna using the olecranon and ulnar styloid process for reference	Lateral midline of the fifth metacarpal
	Radial deviation	Over the middle of the posterior aspect of the wrist over the capitate	Posterior midline of the forearm using the lateral epicondyle of the humerus for reference	Posterior midline of the third metacarpal
	Ulnar deviation	Over the middle of the posterior aspect of the wrist over the capitate	Dorsal midline of the forearm using the lateral epicondyle of the humerus for reference	Posterior midline of the third metacarpal
Thumb	Carpometacarpal flexion	Over the anterior aspect of the first carpometacarpal joint	Anterior midline of the radius using the anterior surface of the radial head and radial styloid process for reference	Anterior midline of the first metacarpal
	Carpometacarpal extension	Over the anterior aspect of the first carpometacarpal joint	Anterior midline of the radius using the anterior surface of the radial head and radial styloid process for reference	Anterior midline of the first metacarpal

(continued)

TABLE 11-9	Goniometric Techniques for the Upper Extremity (continued)			
Joint	Motion	Fulcrum	Proximal Arm	Distal Arm
	Carpometacarpal abduction	Over the lateral aspect of the radial styloid process	Lateral midline of the second metacarpal using the center of the second metacarpal or phalangeal joint for reference	Lateral midline of the first metacarpal using the center of the first metacarpal or phalangeal joint for reference
	Carpometacarpal adduction	Over the lateral aspect of the radial styloid process	Lateral midline of the second metacarpal using the center of the second metacarpal or phalangeal joint for reference	Lateral midline of the first metacarpal using the center of the first metacarpal or phalangeal joint for reference
Fingers	Metacarpophalangeal flexion	Over the posterior aspect of the metacarpophalangeal joint	Over the posterior midline of the metacarpal	Over the posterior midline of the proximal phalanx
	Metacarpophalangeal extension	Over the posterior aspect of the metacarpophalangeal joint	Over the posterior midline of the metacarpal	Over the posterior midline of the proximal phalanx
	Metacarpophalangeal abduction	Over the posterior aspect of the metacarpophalangeal joint	Over the posterior midline of the metacarpal	Over the posterior midline of the proximal phalanx
	Metacarpophalangeal adduction	Over the posterior aspect of the metacarpophalangeal joint	Over the posterior midline of the metacarpal	Over the posterior midline of the proximal phalanx
	Proximal interphalangeal flexion	Over the posterior aspect of the proximal interphalangeal joint	Over the posterior midline of the proximal phalanx	Over the posterior midline of the middle phalanx
	Proximal interphalangeal extension	Over the posterior aspect of the proximal interphalangeal joint	Over the posterior midline of the proximal phalanx	Over the posterior midline of the middle phalanx
	Distal interphalangeal flexion	Over the posterior aspect of the proximal interphalangeal joint	Over the posterior midline of the middle phalanx	Over the posterior midline of the distal phalanx
	Distal interphalangeal extension	Over the posterior aspect of the proximal interphalangeal joint	Over the posterior midline of the middle phalanx	Over the posterior midline of the distal phalanx

Upper Extremity

The following sections describe in detail how to measure joint range of motion for the major joints of the upper extremity.

Shoulder Complex

Shoulder motion occurs at the glenohumeral, scapulothoracic, acromioclavicular, and sternoclavicular joints. In addition, for full shoulder motion to occur, there must also be available motion in the cervical and upper thoracic spine. For the following measurements, the patient is positioned in supine with both hips and knees flexed and the feet placed on the bed to flatten the lumbar spine, unless otherwise stated.

Shoulder Flexion. When measuring glenohumeral flexion, allowing motion to occur at the other joints provides a more functional reading. However, if the clinician requires a measurement of pure glenohumeral motion, the other joints must be manually blocked. This is best achieved by stabilizing the scapula to prevent it from elevating, upwardly rotating, and posteriorly tilting. In the following description, the scapula is not stabilized; instead the thorax is stabilized to prevent extension of the spine.

Upper Extremity Position. The glenohumeral joint is initially positioned in 0° of abduction, adduction, and rotation, and the forearm is positioned in 0° of supination and pronation so that the palm of the hand faces the body.

Goniometer Placement. The fulcrum is centered close to the acromion process, the proximal arm is aligned with the mid-axillary line of the thorax, and the distal arm is aligned with the lateral midline of the humerus, using the lateral epicondyle of the humerus as a landmark.

Technique. The shoulder is moved passively or actively to the end range of available shoulder flexion (Figure 11-56), and a measurement is made (Figure 11-57).

Shoulder Extension. The patient is positioned in prone.

Upper Extremity Position. The glenohumeral joint is positioned in 0° of abduction and rotation, the elbow is positioned in slight flexion, and the forearm is positioned in 0° of supination and pronation. If a measurement of pure glenohumeral extension is required, the scapula must be stabilized prevent elevation and anterior tilting.

Goniometer Placement. The fulcrum is centered close to the acromion process, the proximal arm is aligned with the midaxillary line of the thorax, and the distal arm is aligned

TABLE 11-10 Goniometric Techniques for the Lower Extremity

Joint	Motion	Fulcrum	Proximal Arm	Distal Arm
Hip	Flexion	Over the lateral aspect of the hip joint using the greater trochanter of the femur for reference	Lateral midline of the pelvis	Lateral midline of the femur using the lateral epicondyle for reference
	Extension	Over the lateral aspect of the hip joint using the greater trochanter of the femur for reference	Lateral midline of the pelvis	Lateral midline of the femur using the lateral epicondyle for reference
	Abduction	Over the anterior superior iliac spine (ASIS) of the extremity being measured	Aligned with imaginary horizontal line extending from one ASIS to the other ASIS	Anterior midline of the femur using the midline of the patella for reference
	Adduction	Over the anterior superior iliac spine (ASIS) of the extremity being measured	Aligned with imaginary horizontal line extending from one ASIS to the other ASIS	Anterior midline of the femur using the midline of the patella for reference
	Internal rotation	Anterior aspect of the patella	Perpendicular to the floor or parallel to the supporting surface	Anterior midline of the lower leg using the crest of the tibia and a point midway between the two malleoli for reference
	External rotation	Anterior aspect of the patella	Perpendicular to the floor or parallel to the supporting surface	Anterior midline of the lower leg using the crest of the tibia and a point midway between the two malleoli for reference
Knee	Flexion	Lateral epicondyle of the femur	Lateral midline of the femur using the greater trochanter for reference	Lateral midline of the fibula using the lateral malleolus and fibular head for reference
	Extension	Lateral epicondyle of the femur	Lateral midline of the femur using the greater trochanter for reference	Lateral midline of the fibula using the lateral malleolus and fibular head for reference
Ankle	Dorsiflexion	Lateral aspect of the lateral malleolus	Lateral midline of the fibula using the head of the fibula for reference	Parallel to the lateral aspect of the fifth metatarsal
	Plantarflexion	Lateral aspect of the lateral malleolus	Lateral midline of the fibula using the head of the fibula for reference	Parallel to the lateral aspect of the fifth metatarsal
	Inversion	Anterior aspect of the ankle midway between the malleoli	Anterior midline of the lower leg using the tibial tuberosity for reference	Anterior midline of the second metatarsal
	Eversion	Anterior aspect of the ankle midway between the malleoli	Anterior midline of the lower leg using the tibial tuberosity for reference	Anterior midline of the second metatarsal
Subtalar	Inversion	Posterior aspect of the ankle midway between the malleoli	Posterior midline of the lower leg	Posterior midline of the calcaneus
	Eversion	Posterior aspect of the ankle midway between the malleoli	Posterior midline of the lower leg	Posterior midline of the calcaneus

with the lateral midline of the humerus, using the lateral epicondyle of the humerus as a landmark.

Technique. The shoulder is moved passively or actively to the end range of available shoulder extension (Figure 11-58). The clinician can take a measurement of active range of motion (Figure 11-59) or passive range of motion, or both if a comparison is to be made.

Shoulder Abduction. Although measured here with the patient positioned in supine, shoulder abduction can be measured with the patient in sitting or prone, which has the advantage of allowing free motion of the scapula.

Upper Extremity Position. The glenohumeral joint is positioned in 0° of flexion and extension, and full external rotation so that the palm of the hand faces anteriorly to prevent the greater tubercle of the humerus from impacting on the upper portion of the glenoid fossa or acromion process. Pure glenohumeral abduction can be measured by stabilizing the scapula to prevent its upward rotation and elevation.

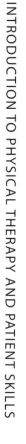

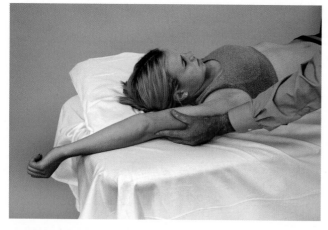

FIGURE 11-56 Passive shoulder flexion

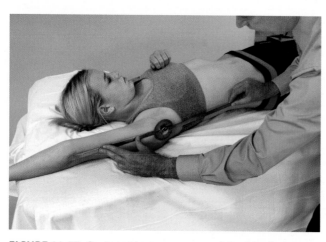

FIGURE 11-57 Goniometric measurement of shoulder flexion

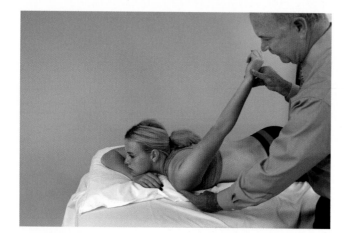

FIGURE 11-58 Passive shoulder extension

Goniometer Placement. The fulcrum is centered close to the anterior aspect of the acromion process, the proximal arm is aligned so that it is parallel to the midline of the anterior aspect of the sternum, and the distal arm is aligned with the medial midline of the humerus using the medial epicondyle as a landmark. If shoulder abduction is measured with the patient in the seated position, the fulcrum is centered close to the posterior aspect of the acromion process, the proximal arm is aligned parallel to the spinous processes of the vertebral column, and the distal arm is aligned with the lateral midline of the humerus, using the lateral epicondyle as a landmark.

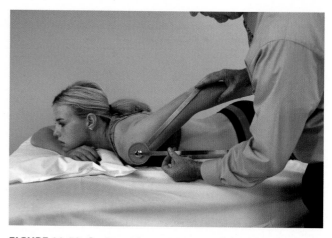

FIGURE 11-59 Goniometric measurement of shoulder extension

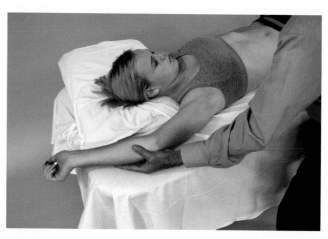

FIGURE 11-60 Passive shoulder abduction

Technique. The shoulder is moved passively or actively to the end range of available shoulder abduction (Figure 11-60), and a goniometric measurement is made (Figure 11-61).

CLINICAL PEARL

Shoulder adduction is not typically measured, as it represents the patient's arm by the side. Further motion toward the patient's midline is considered horizontal adduction.

Shoulder Internal Rotation

Upper Extremity Position. The patient is positioned in prone. The glenohumeral joint is positioned in 90° of shoulder abduction with the forearm perpendicular to the supporting surface and in 0° of supination/pronation so that the palm of the hand faces the feet. If necessary, a rolled-up towel can be placed under the humerus so that the humerus is positioned level with the acromion process.

Goniometer Placement. The fulcrum is centered over the olecranon process, the proximal arm is aligned so that it is either parallel to or perpendicular to the floor, and the distal arm is aligned with the ulna, using the olecranon process and ulnar styloid as landmarks.

Technique. The shoulder is moved passively or actively to the end range of shoulder internal rotation (Figure 11-62), and a measurement is taken (Figure 11-63).

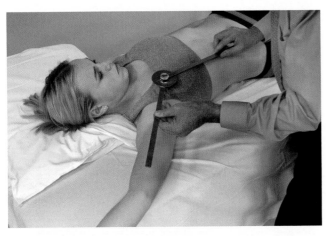

FIGURE 11-61 Goniometric measurement of shoulder abduction

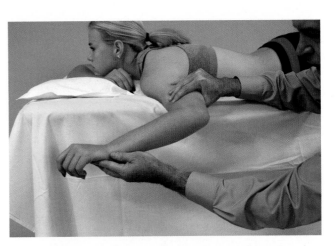

FIGURE 11-64 Passive shoulder external rotation

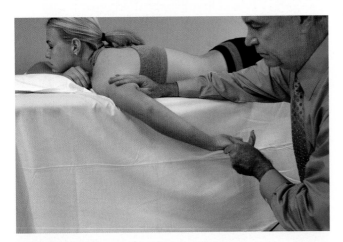

FIGURE 11-62 Passive shoulder internal rotation

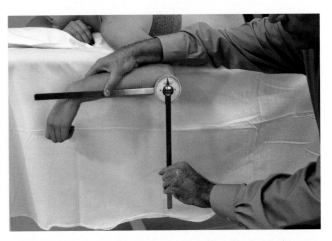

FIGURE 11-65 Goniometric measurement of shoulder external rotation

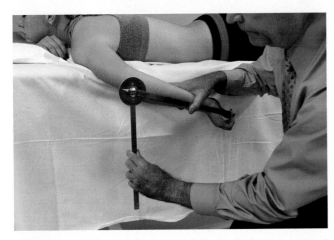

FIGURE 11-63 Goniometric measurement of shoulder internal rotation

Shoulder External Rotation. The patient position is the same as for internal rotation of the shoulder.

Goniometer Placement. The goniometer alignment is the same as for shoulder internal rotation.

Technique. The shoulder is moved passively or actively to the end range of shoulder external rotation (Figure 11-64), and a measurement is taken (Figure 11-65).

Alternatively, shoulder internal rotation can be measured with the patient in supine (Figure 11-66), as can shoulder

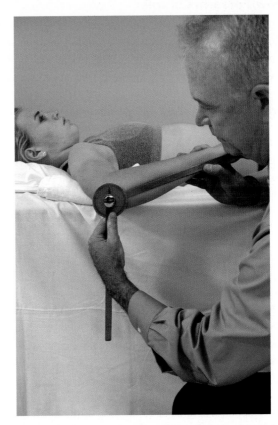

FIGURE 11-66 Goniometric measurement of shoulder internal rotation with the patient in supine

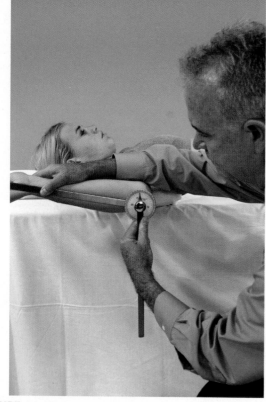

FIGURE 11-67 Goniometric measurement of shoulder external rotation with the patient in supine

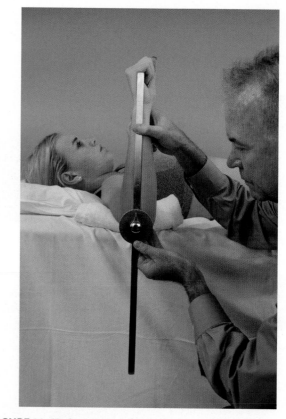

FIGURE 11-68 Start position for the goniometer to measure internal and external rotation with the patient in supine

external rotation (Figure 11-67), using the start position for the goniometer as depicted in Figure 11-68.

Elbow/Forearm Complex

For the following measurements, the patient is positioned in supine with both hips and knees flexed and the feet placed on the bed to flatten the lumbar spine, unless otherwise stated.

Flexion/Extension. A pad can be placed under the distal end of the humerus to allow for elbow extension.

Upper Extremity Position. The glenohumeral joint is positioned in 0° of flexion, extension, and abduction, so that the arm is close to the side of the body.

Goniometer Placement. The goniometer placement is the same for flexion and extension. The fulcrum is centered over the lateral epicondyle of the humerus, the proximal arm is aligned with the lateral midline of the humerus (using the acromion process as a landmark), and the distal arm is aligned with the lateral midline of the radius, using the styloid process as a landmark.

Technique. The elbow is passively or actively flexed to the end of the available range, and a measurement is taken (Figure 11-69). To measure elbow extension, the upper extremity is positioned correctly and a measurement is taken (Figure 11-70).

Forearm Pronation. This measurement can also be performed with the patient in sitting.

Upper Extremity Position. The glenohumeral joint is positioned in 0° of flexion, extension, abduction, and rotation so that the upper arm is close to the side of the body, and the elbow is flexed to 90° with the forearm midway between supination and pronation.

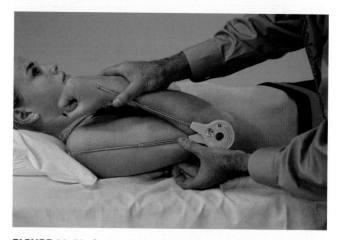

FIGURE 11-69 Goniometric measurement of elbow flexion

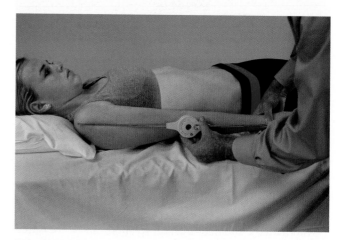

FIGURE 11-70 Goniometric measurement of elbow extension

Goniometer Placement. The fulcrum is centered lateral to the ulnar styloid process, the proximal arm is aligned parallel to the anterior midline of the humerus, and the distal arm is aligned across the posterior aspect of the forearm, just proximal to the styloid processes of the radius and ulna (Figure 11-71).

Technique. The forearm is moved passively or actively to the end of the available range of motion (Figure 11-72), and a measurement is taken (Figure 11-73).

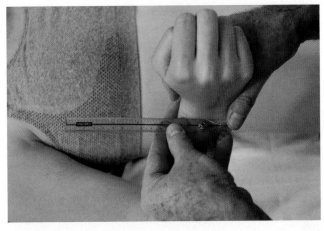

FIGURE 11-71 Start position for goniometric measurement of forearm supination/pronation

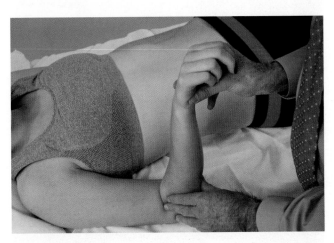

FIGURE 11-72 Passive forearm pronation

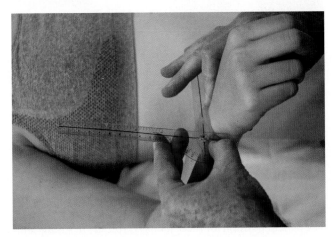

FIGURE 11-73 Goniometric measurement of forearm pronation

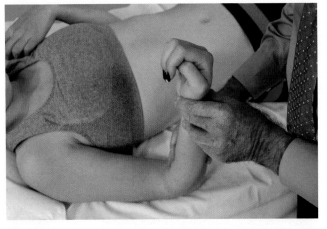

FIGURE 11-74 Passive forearm supination

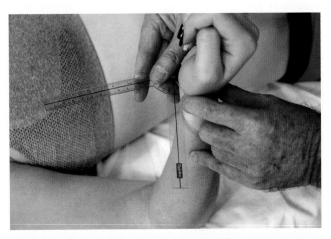

FIGURE 11-75 Goniometric measurement of forearm supination

Forearm Supination. The patient position is the same as for forearm pronation.

Goniometer Placement. The fulcrum is aligned medial to the ulnar styloid process, the proximal arm is aligned parallel to the anterior midline of the humerus, and the distal arm is aligned across the anterior aspect of the forearm, just proximal to the styloid process (Figure 11-71).

Technique. The forearm is moved passively or actively to the end of the available range of motion (Figure 11-74), and a measurement is taken (Figure 11-75).

An alternative technique to measure forearm supination and pronation involves having the patient holding a pen or pencil in a close-fisted hand. The goniometer can then be aligned using the end of the pen as a landmark (Figure 11-76).

Wrist Joints

For the following measurements, the patient is positioned in sitting next to a supporting surface so that the forearm is supported but the hand is free to move.

Wrist Flexion and Extension. The clinician should stabilize the forearm to prevent supination or pronation.

Goniometer Placement. The goniometer placement is the same for wrist flexion and wrist extension. The fulcrum is centered over the lateral aspect of the wrist close to the triquetrum, the proximal arm is aligned with the lateral midline

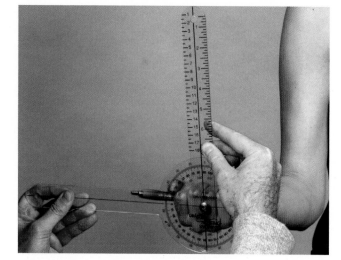

FIGURE 11-76 Alternative method for measuring forearm supination/pronation

of the ulna, using the olecranon process as a landmark, and the distal arm is aligned with the lateral midline of the fifth metacarpal. The palm of the patient is moved downward for wrist flexion, and upward for wrist extension while avoiding extension of the fingers.

Technique. To measure wrist flexion, the wrist is actively or passively flexed to the end of the available range of motion (Figure 11-77), and a measurement is taken (Figure 11-78). To measure wrist extension, the wrist is actively or passively extended to the end of the available range of motion (Figure 11-79), and a measurement is taken (Figure 11-80).

Radial Deviation and Ulnar Deviation. The patient position is the same as for wrist flexion/extension.

Goniometer Placement. The goniometer placement is the same for radial deviation and ulnar deviation. The fulcrum is centered over the middle of the posterior aspect of the wrist close to the capitate, the proximal arm is aligned with the posterior midline of the forearm, using the lateral epicondyles as a landmark, and the distal arm is aligned with the posterior midline of the third metacarpal. For radial deviation, the patient's hand moves toward the patient's body, whereas for ulnar deviation, the patient's hand moves away from the patient's body.

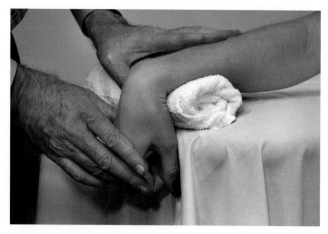

FIGURE 11-77 Passive wrist flexion—more motion occurs if the fingers are extended

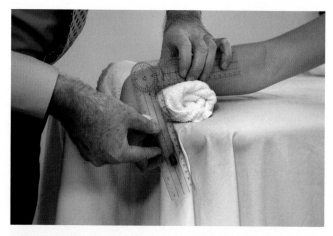

FIGURE 11-78 Goniometric measurement of wrist flexion

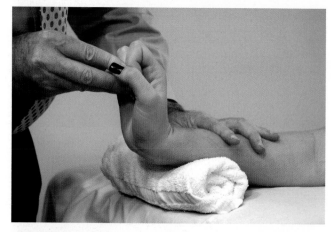

FIGURE 11-79 Passive wrist extension—less motion occurs if the fingers are extended

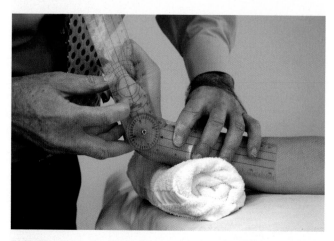

FIGURE 11-80 Goniometric measurement of wrist extension

Technique. To measure radial deviation, the wrist is passively or actively moved to the end of the available range of motion for radial deviation (Figure 11-81), and a measurement is taken (Figure 11-82). To measure ulnar deviation, the wrist is passively or actively moved to the end of the available range of motion for ulnar deviation (Figure 11-83), and a measurement is taken (Figure 11-84).

Finger Joints

The patient position for these joints is typically in sitting, with the forearm supported and midway between pronation and

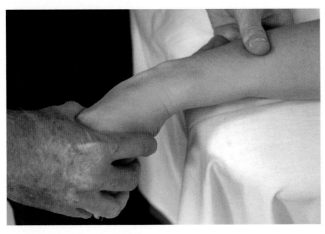

FIGURE 11-81 Passive radial deviation

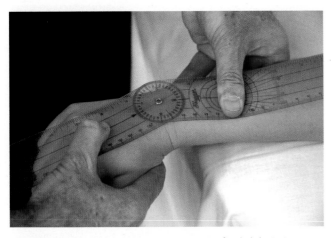

FIGURE 11-82 Goniometric measurement of radial deviation

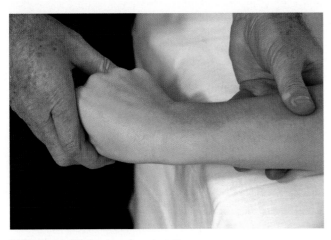

FIGURE 11-83 Passive ulnar deviation

supination, the wrist positioned in 0° of flexion and extension, and in neutral radial and ulnar deviation.

Metacarpophalangeal (MCP) Joint Flexion/Extension. While performing these measurements, the clinician must ensure that the MCP joint is maintained in a neutral position relative to abduction and adduction and to avoid too much motion occurring at the proximal interphalangeal and distal interphalangeal joints. The same technique is used for all of the MCP joints of the fingers.

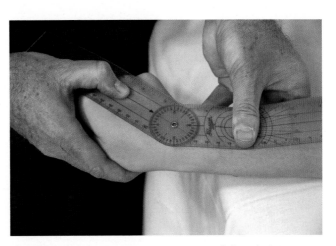

FIGURE 11-84 Goniometric measurement of ulnar deviation

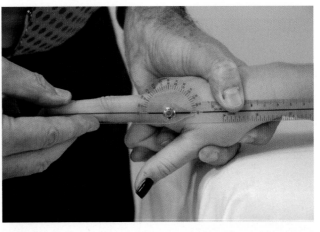

FIGURE 11-85 Goniometer placement for MCP flexion/extension

Goniometer Placement. The goniometer placement is the same for MCP flexion and MCP extension. The fulcrum is centered over the posterior aspect of the MCP joint, the proximal arm is aligned over the posterior midline of the metacarpal, and the distal arm is aligned over the posterior midline of the proximal phalanx. For the index finger, the fulcrum is centered over the thumb side of the MCP joint, the proximal arm is aligned with the radial styloid, and the distal arm is aligned over the thumb side of the phalanx (Figure 11-85).

Technique. A measurement is taken for MCP flexion (Figure 11-86), and MCP extension (Figure 11-87).

Metacarpophalangeal (MCP) Joint Abduction/Adduction. The same technique is used for all of the MCP joints of the fingers.

Goniometer Placement. The goniometer placement is the same for MCP joint abduction and MCP joint adduction. The fulcrum is centered over the posterior aspect of the MCP joint, the proximal arm is aligned over the posterior midline of the metacarpal, and the distal arm is aligned over the posterior midline of the proximal phalanx (Figure 11-88).

Technique. A measurement is taken for MCP abduction (Figure 11-89), and for MCP abduction (Figure 11-90).

Proximal Interphalangeal (PIP) Joint Flexion/Extension. The clinician attempts to stabilize the proximal phalanx to prevent motion at the wrist and MCP joint.

309

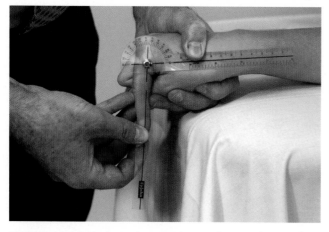

FIGURE 11-86 Goniometric measurement for MCP flexion of the index finger

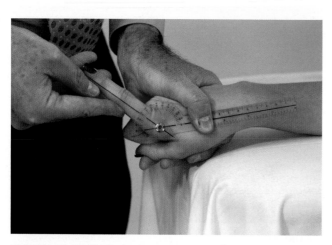

FIGURE 11-87 Goniometric measurement for MCP extension of the index finger

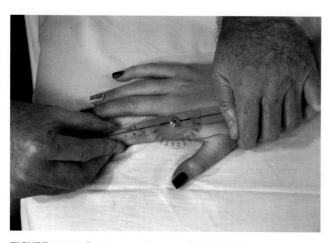

FIGURE 11-88 Goniometer placement for MCP abduction/adduction

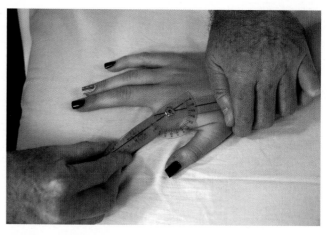

FIGURE 11-89 Goniometric measurement for MCP abduction

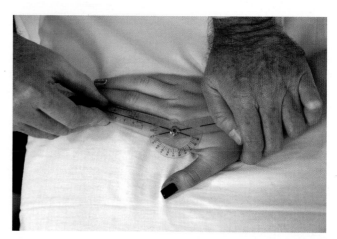

FIGURE 11-90 Goniometric measurement for MCP adduction

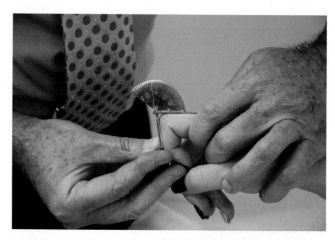

FIGURE 11-91 Goniometric measurement for PIP joint flexion

Goniometer Placement. The goniometer placement is the same for PIP joint flexion and PIP joint extension. The fulcrum is centered over the posterior aspect of the PIP joint, the proximal arm is aligned over the posterior midline of the proximal phalanx, and the distal arm is aligned over the posterior midline of the middle phalanx. The same technique is used for each of the PIP joints of the fingers. It is questionable whether a measurement of PIP joint extension is possible, as

any loss of PIP extension is technically a measurement of PIP flexion.

Technique. A measurement is taken for PIP joint flexion (Figure 11-91).

Distal Interphalangeal (DIP) Joint Flexion/Extension. The MCP joint is positioned in 0° of flexion, extension, abduction, and adduction, with the PIP joint positioned in approximately 70° to 90° of flexion. The clinician attempts to stabilize the middle phalanx to prevent further flexion or extension of the wrist, MCP joints, and PIP joints.

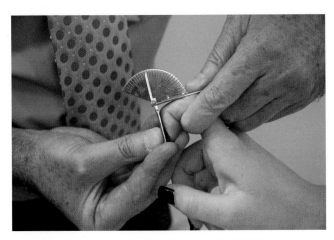

FIGURE 11-92 Goniometric measurement for DIP joint flexion

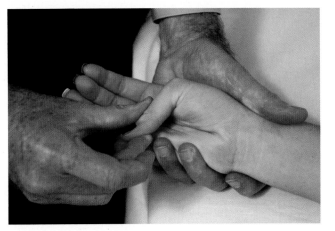

FIGURE 11-93 Passive thumb CMC joint flexion

Goniometer Placement. The goniometer placement is the same for DIP joint flexion and DIP joint extension. The fulcrum is centered over the posterior aspect of the PIP joint, the proximal arm is aligned over the posterior midline of the middle phalanx, and the distal arm is aligned over the posterior midline of the distal phalanx. The same technique is used for each of the DIP joints of the fingers. As with PIP joint extension, it is questionable whether a measurement of DIP joint extension is possible, as any loss of DIP extension is technically a measurement of DIP flexion.

Technique. A measurement is taken for DIP joint flexion (Figure 11-92).

Thumb Joints

The patient position for these joints is typically in sitting, with the forearm supported in supination, the wrist positioned in 0° of flexion and extension, and in neutral radial and ulnar deviation. The MCP and IP joints of the thumb are positioned in 0° of flexion and extension.

Carpometacarpal (CMC) Flexion and Extension

Goniometer Placement. The goniometer placement is the same for CMC flexion and CMC extension. The fulcrum is centered over the anterior aspect of the first CMC joint, the proximal arm is aligned parallel to the anterior midline of the radius, and the distal arm is aligned with the anterior midline of the first metacarpal. CMC flexion occurs when the thumb moves toward the palm of the hand, and CMC extension occurs when the thumb moves away from the palm of the hand.

Technique. The CMC joint is passively or actively moved into the available range of motion for flexion (Figure 11-93), and a measurement is taken (Figure 11-94). The CMC joint is passively or actively moved into the available range of motion for extension (Figure 11-95), and a measurement is taken (Figure 11-96).

Carpometacarpal (CMC) Abduction and Adduction.
The patient positioning is the same as for CMC flexion and extension.

Goniometer Placement. The goniometer placement is the same for CMC abduction and CMC adduction. The fulcrum is centered midway between the posterior aspect of the first

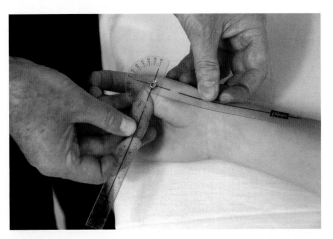

FIGURE 11-94 Goniometric measurement of thumb CMC joint flexion

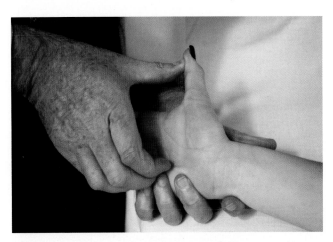

FIGURE 11-95 Passive thumb CMC joint extension

and second carpometacarpal joints, the proximal arm is aligned with the lateral midline of the second metacarpal, and the distal arm is aligned with the lateral midline of the first metacarpal. CMC abduction occurs when the thumb moves away from the hand, whereas CMC adduction occurs when the thumb moves toward the hand.

Technique. The CMC joint is passively or actively moved into the available range of motion for abduction (Figure 11-97), and a measurement is taken (Figure 11-98).

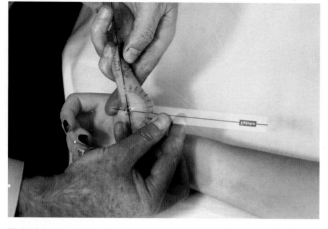

FIGURE 11-96 Goniometric measurement of thumb CMC joint extension

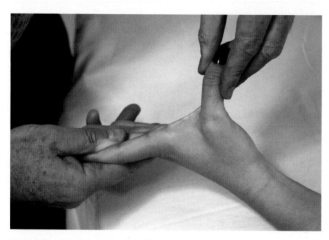

FIGURE 11-97 Passive thumb CMC joint abduction

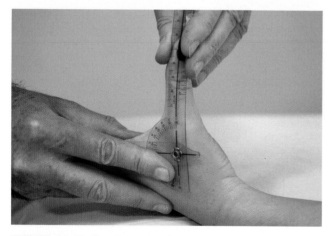

FIGURE 11-98 Goniometric measurement of thumb CMC joint abduction

Thumb Opposition. The patient positioning is the same as for CMC flexion and extension.

Goniometer Placement. The ruler component of a goniometer is typically used to measure the amount of thumb opposition by calculating the distance between the tip of the thumb and the tip of the fifth digit.

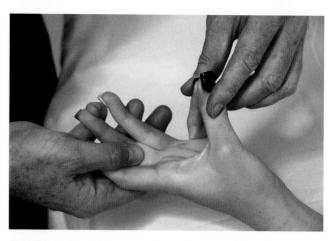

FIGURE 11-99 Passive opposition of thumb and little finger

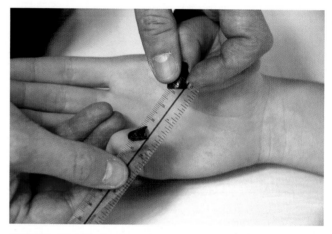

FIGURE 11-100 Goniometric measurement of active thumb opposition

Technique. The thumb and little finger are actively or passively moved together in the direction of opposition (Figure 11-99), and a measurement is taken (Figure 11-100).

Metacarpophalangeal (MCP) Joint of the Thumb Flexion and Extension. The patient positioning is the same as for CMC flexion and extension.

Goniometer Placement. The goniometer placement is the same for MCP joint flexion and MCP joint extension. The fulcrum is centered over the posterior aspect of the MCP joint, the proximal arm is aligned over the posterior midline of the metacarpal, and the distal arm is aligned with the posterior midline of the proximal phalanx.

Technique. The MCP joint of the thumb is actively or passively flexed to the end of the available range of motion, and a measurement is taken (Figure 11-101).

Interphalangeal (IP) Joint of the Thumb Flexion and Extension. The patient positioning is the same as for CMC flexion and extension.

Goniometer Placement. The goniometer placement is the same for IP flexion and IP extension. The fulcrum is centered over the posterior surface of the IP joint, the proximal arm is aligned over the posterior aspect of the proximal phalanx, and the distal arm is aligned with the posterior midline of the distal phalanx.

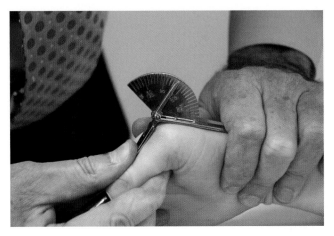

FIGURE 11-101 Goniometric measurement of thumb MCP flexion

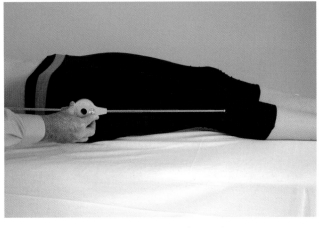

FIGURE 11-102 Goniometer position for hip flexion

Technique. The IP joint of the thumb is actively or passively flexed to the end of the available range of motion, and a measurement is taken.

Lower Extremity

The following sections describe in detail how to measure joint range of motion for the major joints of the lower extremity.

Hip Joint

The patient is positioned in supine to measure hip flexion, hip abduction, and hip adduction, seated to measure hip internal rotation and external rotation, and prone to measure hip extension.

Hip Flexion. Hip flexion can be measured in one of two ways, with the knee allowed to flex, or with the knee extended. Measuring hip flexion with the knee extended is merely an indication of the length of the patient's hamstrings rather than a true measurement of hip joint motion. Hip flexion with the knee flexed is described here.

Lower Extremity Position. The hip is positioned in 0° of abduction, abduction, and rotation, with the knee motion unrestricted.

Goniometer Placement. The fulcrum is centered over the lateral aspect of the hip joint using the greater trochanter of the femur as a landmark, the proximal arm is aligned with the lateral midline of the pelvis, and the distal arm is aligned with the lateral midline of the femur, using the lateral epicondyle of the femur as a landmark (Figure 11-102).

Technique. The hip is actively or passively flexed to the end of the available range of motion, and a measurement is taken (Figure 11-103).

Hip Extension. The patient is positioned in prone. As with hip flexion, hip extension can be measured in one of two ways, with the knee allowed to flex, or with the knee extended. Measuring hip extension with the knee flexed can be misleading due to tension from the rectus femoris muscle which can restrict motion.

Lower Extremity Position. The hip is positioned in 0° of abduction, abduction, and rotation, with the knee motion unrestricted.

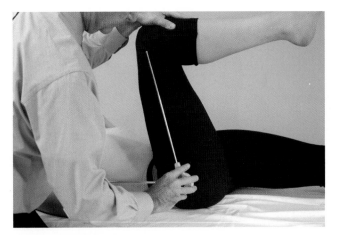

FIGURE 11-103 Goniometric measurement of hip flexion

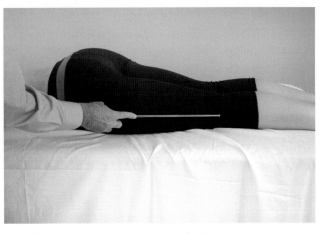

FIGURE 11-104 Goniometer position for hip extension

Goniometer Placement. The goniometer placement and alignment is the same as for hip flexion, except that the patient is positioned in prone (Figure 11-104).

Technique. The hip is actively or passively extended to the end of the available range of motion, and a measurement is taken (Figure 11-105).

Hip Abduction/Adduction

Lower Extremity Position. The lower extremity is kept as straight as possible. It is worth remembering that, in order for

313

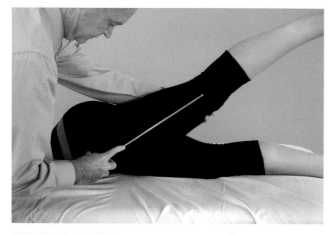

FIGURE 11-105 Goniometric measurement of hip extension

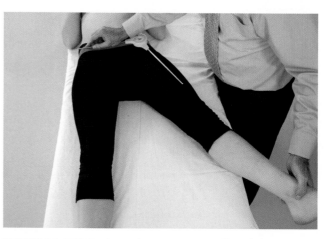

FIGURE 11-107 Goniometric measurement of hip abduction

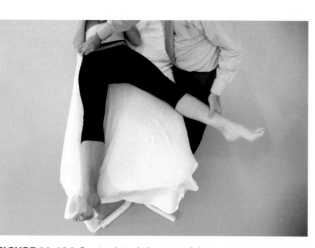

FIGURE 11-106 Passive hip abduction while monitoring contralateral ASIS

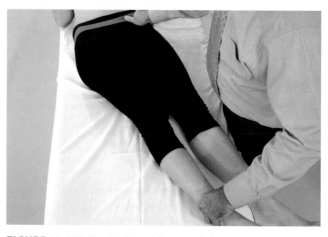

FIGURE 11-108 Passive hip adduction while monitoring contralateral ASIS

full hip adduction to take place, the contralateral hip must be abducted to allow the hip being measured to complete its full range of motion.

Goniometer Placement. The goniometer placement for hip abduction and hip adduction is the same. The fulcrum is centered over the anterior superior iliac spine (ASIS) of the extremity being measured, the proximal arm is aligned with an imaginary horizontal line extending from one ASIS to the other ASIS, and the distal arm is aligned with the anterior midline of the femur using the midline of the patella as a landmark.

Technique. The hip is actively or passively abducted to the end of the available range of motion (Figure 11-106), and a measurement is taken (Figure 11-107). To measure hip adduction, the hip is actively or passively adducted to the end of the available range of motion (Figure 11-108), and a measurement is taken (Figure 11-109).

Hip Internal Rotation/External Rotation. The patient is positioned in sitting on the supporting surface, with the knee flexed over the edge of the table surface.

Lower Extremity Position. The hip is in 0° of abduction and adduction and 90° of flexion. If necessary, a towel roll is placed under the distal end of the femur to maintain the femur in a horizontal plane.

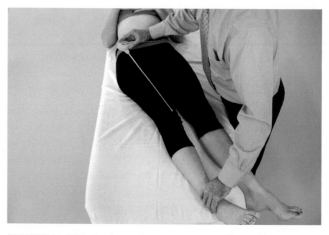

FIGURE 11-109 Goniometric measurement of hip adduction

Goniometer Placement. The goniometer placement for hip internal rotation and hip external rotation is the same. The fulcrum is centered over the anterior aspect of the patella, the proximal arm is aligned so that it is perpendicular to the floor all parallel to the supporting surface, and the distal arm is aligned with the anterior midline of the lower leg, using the tibial crest and a point midway between the two malleoli as reference points.

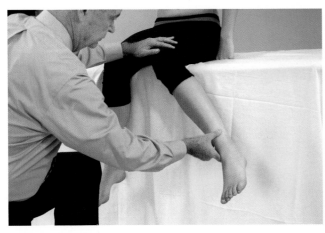

FIGURE 11-110 Passive hip internal rotation

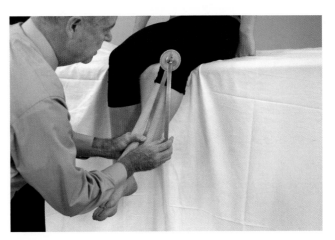

FIGURE 11-113 Goniometric measurement of hip external rotation

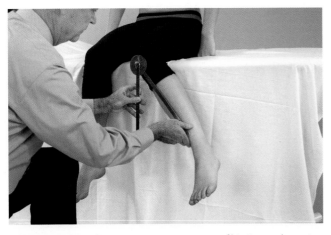

FIGURE 11-111 Goniometric measurement of hip internal rotation

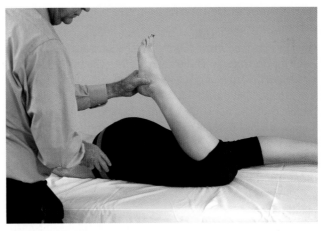

FIGURE 11-114 Passive knee flexion

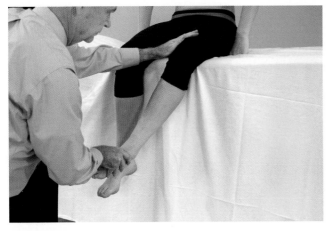

FIGURE 11-112 Passive hip external rotation

Technique. The hip is actively or passively internally rotated to the end of the available range of motion (Figure 11-110), and a measurement is taken (Figure 11-111). To measure external rotation of the hip, the hip is actively or passively externally rotated to the end of the available range of motion (Figure 11-112), and a measurement is taken (Figure 11-113).

Tibiofemoral Joint

To assess tibiofemoral joint flexion and extension, the patient is typically positioned in prone. However, in the presence of significant adaptive shortening of the rectus femoris muscle, knee flexion can be measured with the patient in supine.

Tibiofemoral Joint Flexion/Extension. During these measurements, it is important to stabilize the femur to prevent rotation, flexion, or extension of the hip.

Lower Extremity Position. The hip is positioned in 0° of abduction, adduction, flexion, extension, and rotation.

Goniometer Placement. The goniometer placement for tibiofemoral flexion and tibiofemoral extension is the same. The fulcrum is centered over the lateral epicondyle of the femur, the proximal arm is aligned with the lateral midline of the femur, using the greater trochanter at a landmark, and the distal arm is aligned with the lateral midline of the fibula, using the lateral malleolus as a landmark.

Technique. The knee is actively or passively flexed to the end of the available range of motion (Figure 11-114), and a measurement is taken (Figure 11-115).

Ankle Joint

The ankle joint can be assessed with the patient in sitting, prone or supine. For a more accurate measurement of ankle motion, the patient's knee should be flexed to at least 30° to remove any influence from the gastrocnemius complex.

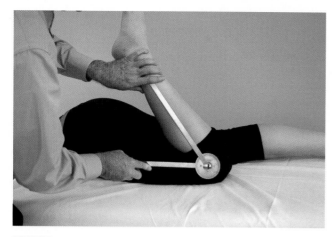

FIGURE 11-115 Goniometric measurement of knee flexion with the patient prone

Dorsiflexion and Plantarflexion. The patient is positioned in sitting or supine.

Goniometer Placement. The goniometer placement is the same for dorsiflexion and plantarflexion. The fulcrum is centered over the lateral aspect of the lateral malleolus, the proximal arm is aligned with the lateral midline of the fibula, using the head of the fibula as a landmark, and the distal arm is aligned parallel to the lateral aspect of the fifth metatarsal, or parallel to the inferior aspect of the calcaneus.

Technique. The ankle is actively or passively dorsiflexed to the end of the available range of motion (Figure 11-116), and a measurement is taken (Figure 11-117). To measure ankle plantarflexion, the ankle is actively or passively plantarflexed to the end of the available range of motion (Figure 11-118), and a measurement is taken (Figure 11-119).

Subtalar Joint Inversion and Eversion. The patient is positioned in sitting or prone.

Goniometer Placement. The goniometer placement is the same for inversion and eversion. The fulcrum is centered over the posterior aspect of the ankle, midway between the malleoli, the proximal arm is aligned with the posterior midline of the lower leg, and the distal arm is aligned with the posterior midline of the calcaneus.

Technique. The ankle is actively or passively inverted to the end of the available range of motion (Figure 11-120), and a

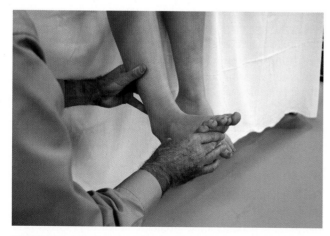

FIGURE 11-116 Passive ankle dorsiflexion

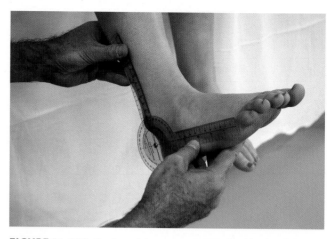

FIGURE 11-117 Goniometric measurement of ankle dorsiflexion

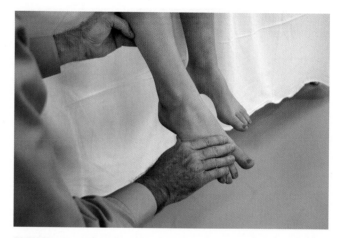

FIGURE 11-118 Passive ankle plantarflexion

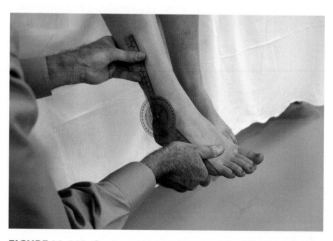

FIGURE 11-119 Goniometric measurement of ankle plantarflexion

measurement is taken (Figure 11-121). For ankle eversion, the ankle is actively or passively everted to the end of the available range of motion (Figure 11-122), and a measurement is taken (Figure 11-123).

Tarsal Joint Inversion and Eversion. The patient is positioned in sitting.

Goniometer Placement. The goniometer placement is the same for inversion and eversion. The fulcrum is centered over the anterior aspect of the ankle midway between the malleoli,

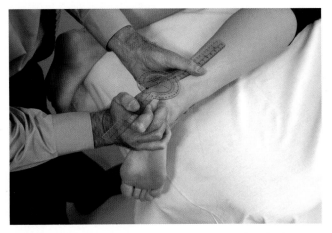

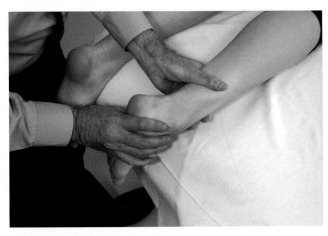

FIGURE 11-120 Passive subtalar joint inversion

FIGURE 11-123 Goniometric measurement of subtalar joint eversion

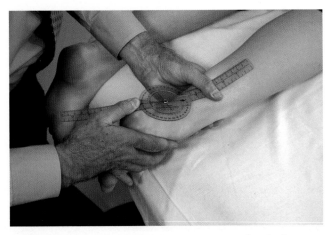

FIGURE 11-121 Goniometric measurement of subtalar joint inversion

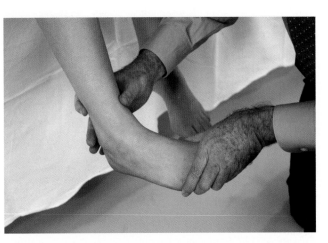

FIGURE 11-124 Passive tarsal joint inversion

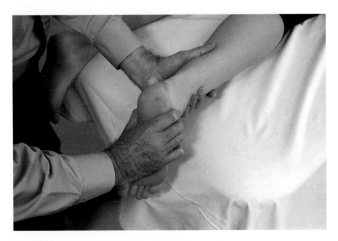

FIGURE 11-122 Passive subtalar joint eversion

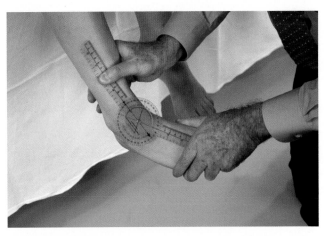

FIGURE 11-125 Goniometric measurement of tarsal joint inversion

the proximal arm is aligned with the anterior midline of the lower leg, using the tibial crest for reference, and the distal arm is aligned with the anterior midline of the second metatarsal.

Technique. The tarsal joints are actively or passively inverted to the end of the available range of motion (Figure 11-124), and a measurement is taken (Figure 11-125). For tarsal joint eversion, the tarsal joints are actively or passively everted to the end of the available range of motion (Figure 11-126), and a measurement is taken (Figure 11-127).

Toe Joints

Metatarsophalangeal (MTP) Joint Flexion and Extension. The patient is positioned in sitting or supine with the MTP and IP joints positioned in 0° of flexion and extension.

Goniometer Placement. The goniometer placement is the same for MTP joint flexion and MTP joint extension. The fulcrum is aligned over the posterior aspect of the MTP joint, the proximal arm is aligned over the posterior midline of the

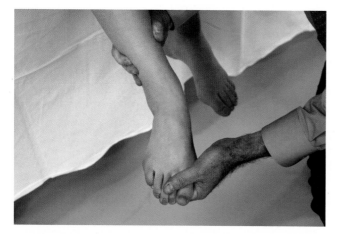

FIGURE 11-126 Passive tarsal joint eversion

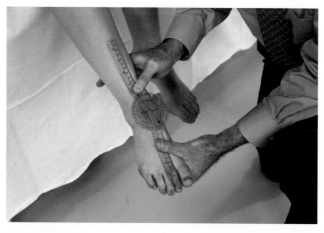

FIGURE 11-127 Goniometric measurement of tarsal joint eversion

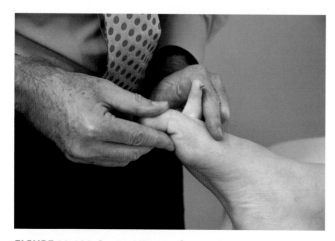

FIGURE 11-128 Passive MTP joint flexion of the great toe

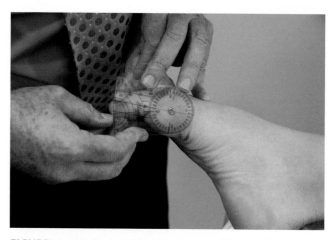

FIGURE 11-129 Goniometric measurement of flexion of the great toe

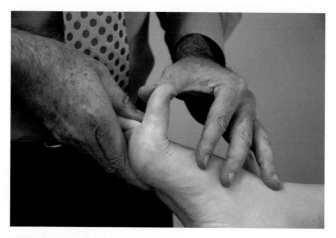

FIGURE 11-130 Passive MTP joint extension of the great toe

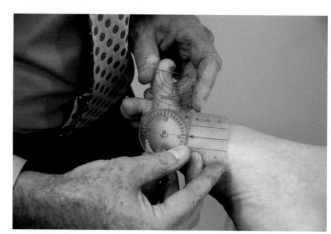

FIGURE 11-131 Goniometric measurement of extension of the great toe

metatarsal, and the distal arm is aligned over the posterior midline of the proximal phalanx.

Technique. The MTP joint is actively or passively flexed to the end of the available range of motion (Figure 11-128), and a measurement is taken (Figure 11-129). To measure MTP joint extension, the MTP joint is actively or passively extended to the end of the available range of motion (Figure 11-130), and a measurement is taken (Figure 11-131).

CLINICAL PEARL

Although motions such as abduction of the great toe (Figure 11-132), flexion/extension of the individual proximal interphalangeal (PIP) joints, and flexion/extension of the individual distal interphalangeal (DIP) joint can theoretically be measured, one has to question the usefulness of these measurements. A more practical approach is to perform a visual assessment of

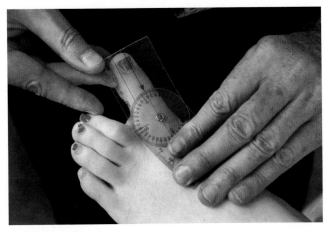

FIGURE 11-132 Goniometric measurement of great toe abduction

combined PIP and DIP joint flexion/extension, and great toe abduction (if the patient is able to perform such an action).

The Spine

Goniometric measurement of spinal motion brings its own set of challenges. Over the years, various methods have been put forward that have incorporated the use of a tape measure, the use of standard goniometers, and the use of specialized goniometers, such as the bubble goniometer. Most of the problems have stemmed from determining the best appropriate landmarks, the wide variations in body types, and whether such measurements have sufficient inter-rater and intrarater reliability.

Whichever method is chosen, it is important remember that, as with other joints in the body, the range of motion in the spine may vary according to a number of factors including structural alterations, the individual's age, neck girth and length, body habitus, diurnal changes,[15] neurologic disease, or other factors unrelated to the disability for which the exam is being performed. Without taking body size into account, measurements may underestimate or overestimate range of motion.[16]

Cervical Spine

Cervical Rotation

Traditional Goniometer Method. The fulcrum is centered over the center of the superior aspect of the head, the proximal arm is aligned parallel to an imaginary line between the two acromion processes, and the distal arm is aligned with the tip of the nose.

Tape Measure Method. A tape measure can be used to measure the distance between the tip of the chin and the acromion process.

Bubble Goniometer Method. The dual inclinometer method, using two bubble goniometers is the approach recommended in the American Medical Association's *Guides to the Evaluation of Permanent Impairment*[14] and is often considered the clinical standard for assessing cervical ROM in the clinic.[17,18] This method requires accurate identification of anatomic landmarks (Table 11-11). Both inter- and intrarater reliability studies have shown the inclinometry method to be reliable.[19–22] Others dispute this conclusion and contend that the inclinometer method is flawed and should not be used in clinical settings.[23,24] The normal range of motion using this method is 80° or greater from the neutral position for active motion. To measure cervical rotation using a bubble goniometer, the patient is positioned in prone, and the goniometer is aligned over the crown of the head in the transverse plane (Figure 11-133). The goniometer is zeroed out and the patient is asked to rotate the head to the right (Figure 11-134), and then to the left (Figure 11-135).

> ## CLINICAL PEARL
>
> Using the bubble goniometer method, the full arc of passive cervical rotation range depends on the age of the patient[7]:
>
> ▶ 20–29: 183° ± 11
> ▶ 30–49: 172° ± 13
> ▶ >50: 155° ± 15

TABLE 11-11	The American Medical Association Inclinometer Technique for Measuring Cervical ROM
Range	**Method**
Flexion	Two inclinometers are used, which are aligned in the sagittal plane. The center of the first inclinometer is placed over the T1 spinous process. The center of the second one is placed on top of the head, parallel to a line drawn from the corner of the eye to the ear, where the temple of eyeglasses would sit. The patient is asked to flex the neck, and both inclinometer angles are recorded. The cervical flexion angle is calculated by subtracting the T1 from the calvarium inclinometer angle.
Extension	Two inclinometers can be used, which are aligned as for measuring cervical flexion. The patient is asked to extend the neck, and both inclinometer angles are recorded. The cervical extension angle is calculated by subtracting the T1 from the calvarium inclinometer angle.
Rotation	The patient is positioned supine. One inclinometer is used, and it is aligned in the transverse plane. The base of the inclinometer is placed over the forehead. The patient is asked to rotate the neck, and the inclinometer angle is recorded. The test is repeated on the other side.
Side bending	Two inclinometers are used, which are aligned in the frontal plane. The center of the first inclinometer is placed over the T1 spinous process. The center of the second one is placed on top of the head, over the calvarium. The patient is asked to side bend the neck, and both inclinometer angles are recorded. The cervical side-bending angle is calculated by subtracting the T1 from the calvarium inclinometer angle.

ROM: range of motion

Data from American Medical Association: Guides to the Evaluation of Permanent Impairment (ed 5). Chicago, American Medical Association, 2001.

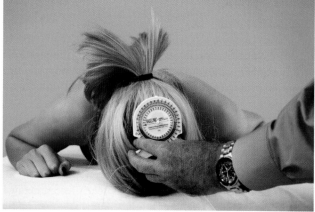

FIGURE 11-133 Bubble goniometer placement for cervical rotation

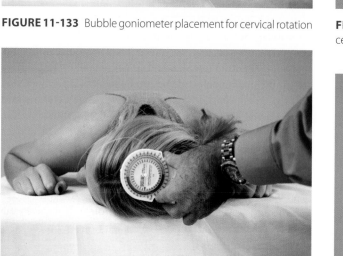

FIGURE 11-134 Goniometric measurement for right cervical rotation

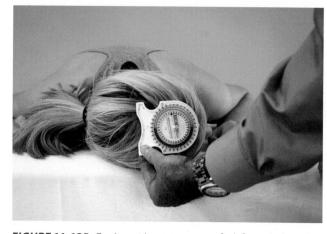

FIGURE 11-135 Goniometric measurement for left cervical rotation

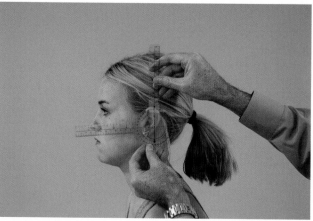

FIGURE 11-136 Goniometer placement for the start position for cervical flexion

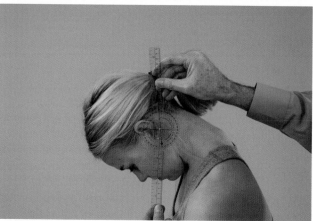

FIGURE 11-137 Goniometric measurement of cervical flexion

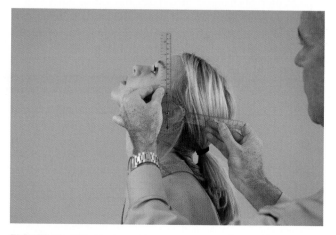

FIGURE 11-138 Goniometric measurement of cervical extension

Cervical Flexion and Extension

Traditional Goniometer Method. The fulcrum is centered over the external auditory meatus, the proximal arm is aligned so that it is either perpendicular or parallel to the ground, and the distal arm is aligned with the base of the skull or with the end of the eye brow (the tip of the nose can also be used). (Figure 11-136). The patient is then asked to flex the cervical spine (Figure 11-137) and to extend the cervical spine (Figure 11-138).

Tape Measure Method. A tape measure can be used to measure the distance between the tip of the chin and the sternal notch, while making sure that the patient's mouth remains closed.

Bubble Goniometer Method. See Table 4-11. The normal range of motion for cervical flexion using this technique is 60° or greater from the neutral position, and 75° or greater from the neutral position for active motion.[7] From the start position (Figure 11-139), the patient is asked to flex the cervical spine (Figure 11-140), and then to extend the cervical spine (Figure 11-141).

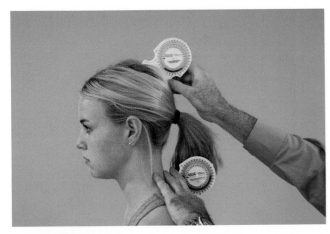

FIGURE 11-139 Bubble goniometer placement for the start position for cervical flexion

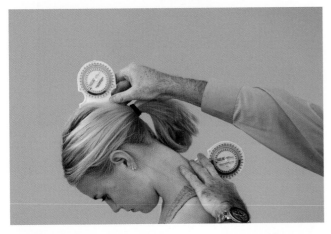

FIGURE 11-140 Goniometric measurement of cervical flexion

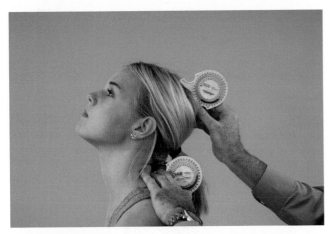

FIGURE 11-141 Goniometric measurement of cervical extension

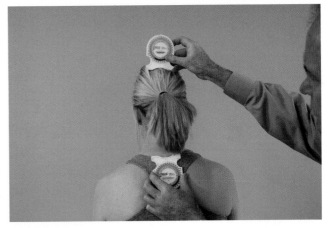

FIGURE 11-142 Bubble goniometer placement for the start position for cervical side bending

Cervical Side Bending. When measuring cervical side bending, the clinician should stabilize the shoulder girdle to prevent lateral flexion of the thoracic and lumbar spine.

Traditional Goniometer Method. The fulcrum is centered over the spinous process of the C7 vertebra, the proximal arm is aligned with the spinous processes of the thoracic vertebra so that the arm is perpendicular to the ground, and the distal arm is aligned with the posterior midline of the head, using the occipital protuberance as a landmark.

Tape Measure Method. A tape measure can be used to measure the distance between the mastoid process and the acromion process.

Bubble Goniometer Method. See Table 11-11. The normal range of cervical side bending using this method is 45° or greater from the neutral position for active motion. From the start position (Figure 11-142), the patient is asked to side bend the cervical spine to the left (Figure 11-143), and then to the right (Figure 11-144).

Thoracic Spine

Oftentimes, thoracic spine motion is measured simultaneously with lumbar spine motion using a variety of methods, none of which are really satisfactory. To objectively measure thoracic motion and differentiate thoracic spine motion from lumbar spine motion, the bubble goniometer techniques recommended by the American Medical Association are recommended.[14]

Flexion. To measure thoracic flexion, two inclinometers are used and are aligned in the sagittal plane. The center of the first inclinometer is placed over the T1 spinous process.

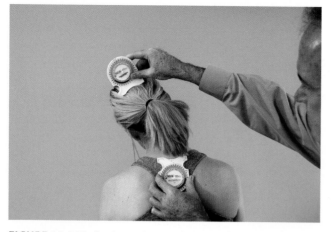

FIGURE 11-143 Goniometric measurement of cervical side bending to the left

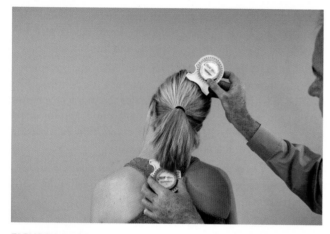

FIGURE 11-144 Goniometric measurement of cervical side bending to the right

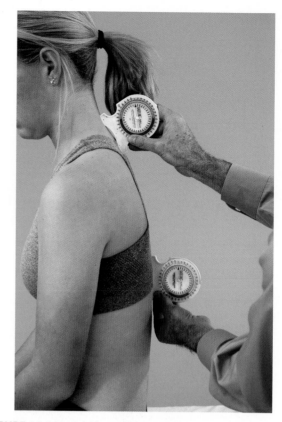

FIGURE 11-145 Bubble goniometer placement for the start position of thoracic flexion and extension

The center of the second one is placed over the T12 or L1 spinous process (Figure 11-145). The patient is asked to slump forward as though trying to place the forehead on the knees (Figure 11-146), and both inclinometer angles are recorded. The thoracic flexion angle is calculated by subtracting the T12 from the T1 inclinometer angle. The patient should be able to flex approximately 50° from the neutral position.[25,26] The clinician observes for any paravertebral fullness during flexion, which might alter the measurement. The thoracic spine during flexion should curve forward in a smooth and even manner, and there should be no evidence of segmental rotation or side bending. To decrease pelvic and hip movements, McKenzie advocates examining thoracic flexion with the patient seated.[27]

Extension. Clinical guidelines for measurements of thoracic extension recommend that range of motion be defined with reference to the magnitude of the kyphosis measured in standing. However, to date, the relationship between the magnitude of the thoracic kyphosis and the amount of thoracic extension movement has not been reported.[28] Thoracic extension may be measured using the same technique and inclinometer positions as described for flexion (Figure 11-147). The thoracic extension angle is calculated by subtracting the T12 or L1 from the T1 inclinometer angle. The patient should be able to extend approximately 15° to 20° from the neutral

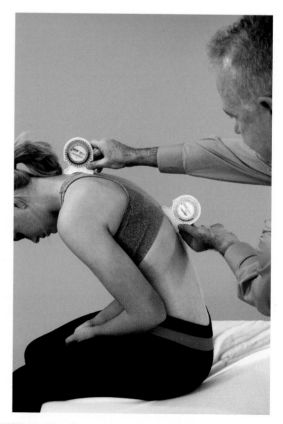

FIGURE 11-146 Goniometric measurement of thoracic flexion

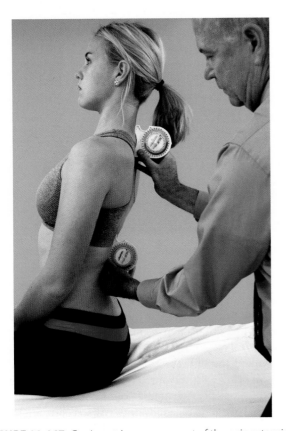

FIGURE 11-147 Goniometric measurement of thoracic extension

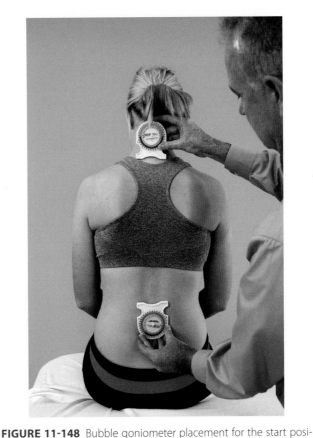

FIGURE 11-148 Bubble goniometer placement for the start position of thoracic side bending

position.[26] Alternatively, thoracic extension can be measured using a tape measure. The distance between two points (the C7 and T12 spinous processes) is measured. A 2.5-cm difference between neutral and extension measurements is considered normal.[29,30] During thoracic extension, the thoracic curve should curve backward or straighten. As with flexion, there should be no evidence of segmental rotation or side bending.

Rotation. Rotation is a primary movement of the thoracic spine and a key component of functional activities. Thoracic rotation can be measured objectively using a tape measure, or two bubble goniometers.

Tape Measure Method. Pavelka[31] devised a simple objective clinical method to measure thoracolumbar rotation using a tape measure that can be used to detect asymmetries in rotation. The tape is placed over the L5 spinous process and over the jugular notch on the superior aspect of the manubrium. A measurement is taken before and after full trunk rotation. The measurements from each side are then compared.

Bubble Goniometer Method. The patient is positioned in sitting, and is then asked to flex forward as close to horizontal as possible. One bubble goniometer is positioned at the T1 level and the other at the T12 level, both in the frontal plane. Both goniometers are zeroed out, and then the patient is instructed to rotate the trunk to one side. The clinician records both the T1 and the T12 inclinations and subtracts the T12 from the T1 inclination to arrive at the thoracic rotation angle. The technique is then repeated to the opposite side. The patient should be able to rotate 30° or greater from the neutral position.[32,33] Active thoracic rotation of less than 20° can result in an

impairment of function during activities of daily living involving the thoracic spine.[29]

Side Bending. Side bending can be measured objectively using a tape measure,[34] or using two bubble goniometers.

Tape Measure Method. Two ink marks are placed on the skin of the lateral trunk. The upper mark is made at a point where a horizontal line through the xiphisternum crosses the frontal line. The lower mark is made at the highest point on the iliac crest. The distance between the two marks is measured in centimeters, with the patient standing erect, and again after full ipsilateral side bending. The second measurement is subtracted from the first, and the remainder is taken as an index of lateral spinal mobility.

Bubble Goniometer Method. The patient is positioned in standing, and one goniometer is placed flat against the T1 spinous process and the other flat against the T12/L1 spinous process (Figure 11-148). Both goniometers are zeroed out, and then the patient is asked to side bend the thoracic spine to the left side (Figure 11-149) and then to the right side (Figure 11-150). The T1 inclination angle is subtracted from the T12/L1 inclination angle to arrive at the thoracic side bending angle. The patient should be able to side bend 20° to 40° from the neutral position.

Lumbar Spine

Lumbar spine motion can be measured using a variety of methods.

Flexion and Extension. Flexion and extension can be measured using two bubble goniometers or a tape measure.

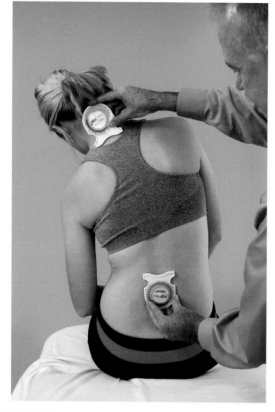

FIGURE 11-149 Goniometric measurement of thoracic side bending to the left

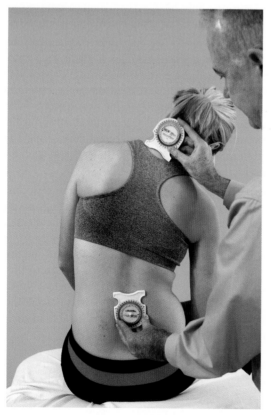

FIGURE 11-150 Goniometric measurement of thoracic side bending to the right

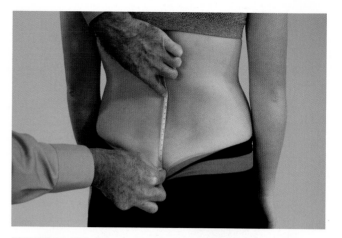

FIGURE 11-151 Start position for the modified Schober technique

Tape Measure Method. Using the modified Schober technique, the patient is positioned in relaxed standing. A point is drawn with the skin marker at the spinal intersection of a line joining S1. Additional marks are made 10 cm above and 5 cm below S1 (Figure 11-151). The patient is then asked to bend forward and the distance between the marks 10 cm above and 5 cm below S1 is measured (Figure 11-152). Despite this method's simplicity, Reynolds[35] found this measurement of motion to have good reliability, with Pearson correlation coefficients of 0.59 for lumbar flexion and 0.75 for extension. In another study by Fitzgerald and colleagues,[36] the Pearson correlation coefficient was found to be 1.0 for lumbar flexion and 0.88 for lumbar extension in a study of young healthy subjects.

Bubble Goniometer Method. The patient is positioned in standing with the lumbar spine in a neutral position. The clinician places one bubble goniometer over the T12/L1 spinous process in the sagittal plane, and the other goniometer at the level of the sacrum, also in the sagittal plane (Figure 11-153). Both goniometers are zeroed out, and the patient is then asked to flex the trunk forward (Figure 11-154). The clinician notes the inclinations of both goniometers and subtracts the sacral inclination from the T12/L1 inclination to obtain the lumbar flexion angle. The patient is then asked to extend the trunk (Figure 11-155). The clinician subtracts the sacral inclination from the T12/L1 inclination to obtain the lumbar extension angle. The normal ranges of motion for flexion and extension vary according to patient age and gender[37] (Table 11-12).

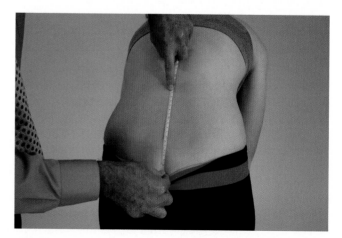

FIGURE 11-152 End position for the modified Schober technique

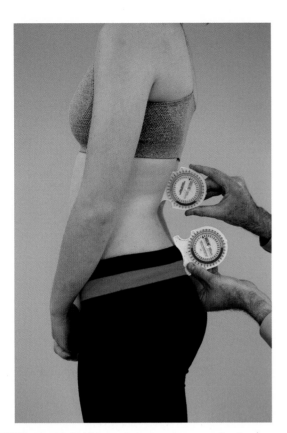

FIGURE 11-153 Bubble goniometer placement for the start position of lumbar spine flexion and extension

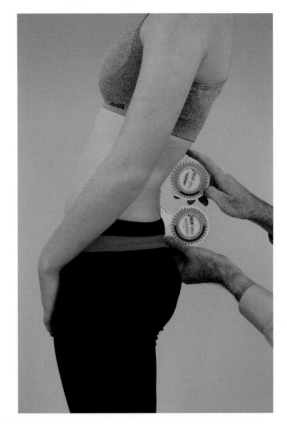

FIGURE 11-155 Goniometric measurement for lumbar spine extension

Side Bending. Side bending can be measured with the patient standing with the feet together using a standard goniometer, a tape measure, or two bubble goniometers.

Standard Goniometer Method. The fulcrum is centered over the posterior aspect of the spinous process of S1, the proximal arm is aligned so that it is perpendicular to the ground, and the distal arm is aligned with the posterior aspect of the spinous process of C7.

Tape Measure Method. A tape measure is used to measure the distance between the tip of the middle finger and the floor.

TABLE 11-12	Normal Ranges of Motion for Lumbar Spine Flexion and Extension Based on Patient Age and Gender		
Gender	**Age Range**	**Normal Range of Flexion in Degrees**	**Normal Range of Extension in Degrees**
Male	15–30 years old	66	38
	31–60 years old	58	35
	>61 years old	49	33
Female	15–30 years old	67	42
	31–60 years old	60	40
	>61 years old	44	36

Data from Loebl WY: Measurement of spinal posture and range of spinal movement. Ann Phys Med 9:103-110, 1967.

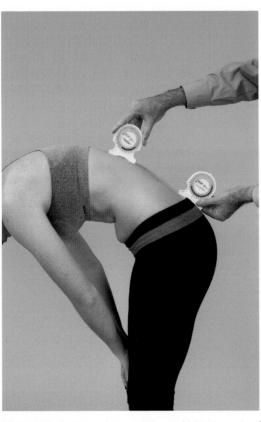

FIGURE 11-154 Goniometric measurement for lumbar spine flexion

RANGE OF MOTION

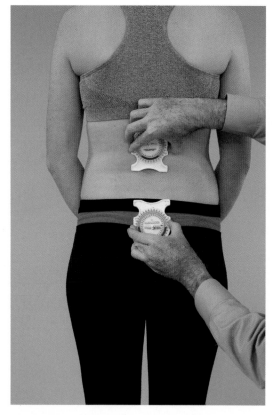

FIGURE 11-156 Bubble goniometer placement for the start position of lumbar spine side bending

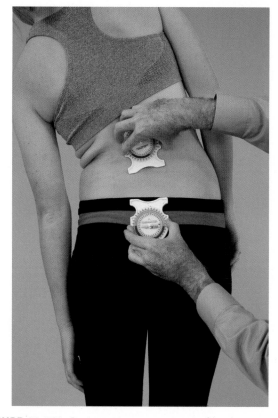

FIGURE 11-158 Goniometric measurement of lumbar spine side bending to the left

Bubble Goniometer Method. The clinician places one a goniometer flat at the T12/L1 spinous process in the frontal plane and the other goniometer at the superior aspect of the sacrum, also in the frontal plane (Figure 11-156). Both goniometers are zeroed out, and then the patient is asked to side bend the trunk to the right side (Figure 11-157) and the inclination is recorded from both goniometers. The clinician subtracts the sacral inclination from the T12/L1 inclination to obtain the lumbar side bending angle. The technique is then repeated to the left side (Figure 11-158). The normal ranges of motion for flexion and extension vary according to patient age and gender (Table 11-13).[36,38]

TABLE 11-13	Normal Ranges of Motion for Lumbar Side Bending Based on Gender and Age	
Gender	**Age Range**	**Normal Range of Flexion in Degrees**
Male	20–29 years old	38 ± 5.8
	31–60 years old	29 ± 6.5
	>61 years old	19 ± 4.8
Female	15–30 years old	35 ± 6.4
	31–60 years old	30 ± 5.8
	>61 years old	23 ± 5.4

Data from Fitzgerald GK, Wynveen KJ, Rheault W, et al: Objective assessment with establishment of normal values for lumbar spinal range of motion. Phys Ther 63:1776-1781, 1983; Einkauf DK, Gohdes ML, Jensen GM, et al: Changes in spinal mobility with increasing age in women. Phys Ther 67:370-375, 1987.

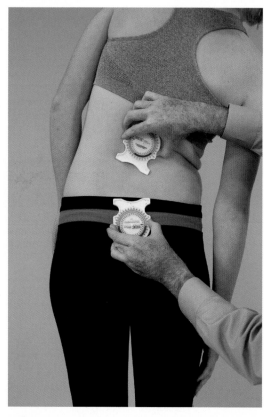

FIGURE 11-157 Goniometric measurement of lumbar spine side bending to the right

REFERENCES

1. Cyriax J: Textbook of Orthopaedic Medicine, Diagnosis of Soft Tissue Lesions (ed 8). London, Bailliere Tindall, 1982.

2. Hayes KW: An examination of Cyriax's passive motion tests with patients having osteoarthritis of the knee. Phys Ther 74:697, 1994.

3. Rothstein JM: Cyriax reexamined. Phys Ther 74:1073, 1994.

4. Farfan HF: The scientific basis of manipulative procedures. Clin Rheum Dis 6:159-177, 1980.

5. Harris ML: Flexibility. Phys Ther 49:591-601, 1969.

6. McKenzie R, May S: Physical examination, in McKenzie R, May S (eds): The Human Extremities: Mechanical Diagnosis and Therapy. Waikanae, New Zealand, Spinal Publications New Zealand, 2000, pp 105-121.

7. Dvorak J, Antinnes JA, Panjabi M, et al: Age and gender related normal motion of the cervical spine. Spine 17:S393-S398, 1992.

8. White DJ: Musculoskeletal examination, in O'Sullivan SB, Schmitz TJ (eds): Physical Rehabilitation (ed 5). Philadelphia, FA Davis, 2007, pp 159-192.

9. Petersen CM, Hayes KW: Construct validity of Cyriax's selective tension examination: association of end-feels with pain at the knee and shoulder. J Orthop Sports Phys Ther 30:512-527, 2000.

10. Boone DC, Azen SP, Lin C-M, et al: Reliability of goniometric measurements. Phys Ther 58:1355-1360, 1978.

11. Mayerson NH, Milano RA: Goniometric measurement reliability in physical medicine. Arch Phys Med Rehabil 65:92-94, 1984.

12. Riddle DL, Rothstein JM, Lamb RL: Goniometric reliability in a clinical setting: shoulder measurements. Phys Ther 67:668-673, 1987.

13. Williams JG, Callaghan M: Comparison of visual estimation and goniometry in determination of a shoulder joint angle. Physiotherapy 76:655-657, 1990.

14. American Medical Association: Guides to the Evaluation of Permanent Impairment (ed 5). Chicago, American Medical Association, 2001.

15. Wing P, Tsang I, Gagnon F: Diurnal changes in the profile shape and range of motion of the back. Spine 17:761-766, 1992.

16. Chibnall JT, Duckro PN, Baumer K: The influence of body size on linear measurements used to reflect cervical range of motion. Phys Ther 74:1134-1137, 1994.

17. Mayer TG, Kondraske G, Beals SB, et al: Spinal range of motion. Accuracy and sources of error with inclinometric measurement. Spine 22:1976-1984, 1997.

18. Mayer T, Brady S, Bovasso E, et al: Noninvasive measurement of cervical tri-planar motion in normal subjects. Spine 18:2191-2195, 1993.

19. Capuano-Pucci D, Rheault W, Aukai J, et al: Intratester and intertester reliability of the cervical range of motion device. Arch Phys Med Rehabil 72:338-340, 1991.

20. Ordway NR, Seymour R, Donelson RG, et al: Cervical sagittal range-of-motion analysis using three methods. Cervical range-of-motion device, 3space, and radiography. Spine 22:501-508, 1997.

21. Nilsson N, Christensen HW, Hartvigsen J: The interexaminer reliability of measuring passive cervical range of motion, revisited. J Manipulative Physiol Ther 19:302-305, 1996.

22. Nilsson N: Measuring passive cervical motion: a study of reliability. J Manipulative Physiol Ther 18:293-297, 1995.

23. Youdas JW, Carey JR, Garrett TR: Reliability of measurements of cervical spine range of motion: comparison of three methods. Phys Ther 71:98-104, 1991.

24. Chen SP, Samo DG, Chen EH, et al: Reliability of three lumbar sagittal motion measurement methods: surface inclinometers. J Occup Environ Med 39:217-223, 1997.

25. Raou RJP: Recherches sur la mobilité vertebrale en fonction des types rachidiens. Paris, Thèse, 1952.

26. Lawrence DJ, Bakkum B: Chiropractic management of thoracic spine pain of mechanical origin, in Giles LGF, Singer KP (eds): Clinical Anatomy and Management of Thoracic Pain. Oxford, Butterworth-Heinemann, 2000, pp 244-256.

27. McKenzie RA: The Cervical and Thoracic Spine: Mechanical Diagnosis and Therapy. Waikanae, New Zealand, Spinal Publications, 1990.

28. Edmondston SJ, Waller R, Vallin P, et al: Thoracic spine extension mobility in young adults: influence of subject position and spinal curvature. J Orthop Sports Phys Ther 41:266-273, 2011.

29. Evans RC: Illustrated Essentials in Orthopedic Physical Assessment. St. Louis, Mosby-Year book, 1994.

30. Magee DJ: Orthopedic Physical Assessment. Philadelphia, WB Saunders, 1997.

31. Pavelka K, Von: Rotationsmessung der Wirbelsaule. A Rheumaforschg 29:366, 1970.

32. Gonon JP, Dimnet J, Carret JP, et al: Utilité de l'analyse cinématique de radiographies dynamiques dans le diagnostic de certaines affections de la colonne lombaire, in Simon L, Rabourdin JP (eds): Lombalgies et médecine de rééducation. Paris, Masson, 1983, pp 27-38.

33. White AA: An analysis of the mechanics of the thoracic spine in man. Acta Orthop Scand 127 (Suppl):8-92, 1969.

34. Moll JMH, Wright V: Measurement of spinal movement, in Jayson MIV (ed): The Lumbar Spine and Back Pain. New York, Grune and Stratton, 1981, pp 93-112.

35. Reynolds PM: Measurement of spinal mobility: a comparison of three methods. Rheumatol Rehabil 14:180-185, 1975.

36. Fitzgerald GK, Wynveen KJ, Rheault W, et al: Objective assessment with establishment of normal values for lumbar spinal range of motion. Phys Ther 63:1776-1781, 1983.

37. Loebl WY: Measurement of spinal posture and range of spinal movement. Ann Phys Med 9:103-110, 1967.

38. Einkauf DK, Gohdes ML, Jensen GM, et al: Changes in spinal mobility with increasing age in women. Phys Ther 67:370-375, 1987.

Manual Muscle Testing

CHAPTER 12

OVERVIEW

Movement occurs through the interaction between the nervous and musculoskeletal systems. The nervous system provides cognition, perception, and sensory integration and is primarily involved in the control of movement, while the musculoskeletal system provides the power for movement. A basic overview of the neurologic structures is provided in Chapter 4. This chapter provides an overview of the anatomy and physiology of the musculoskeletal system and then describes how the muscular system can be assessed.

GROSS MUSCLE SCREENING

Muscle testing requires that the patient be able to voluntarily control the tension developed in the muscles. A patient with a disorder of the central nervous system who demonstrates spasticity is not an appropriate candidate for muscle testing.

A gross muscle screening is performed on a patient when a quick assessment of the patient's general level of muscle strength is required. If any weakness is found during the gross muscle screening test, a specific muscle test is then performed. It is important to remember that the gross muscle screening does not detail the determination of strength; it only provides the clinician with information as to whether a region of the body is either normal or weak. An example when a gross muscle screening would be used is when the clinician is preparing the patient to get out of a wheelchair and to ambulate using a standard walker—the clinician needs to determine whether the patient has sufficient strength to weight bear through the lower extremities and to weight bear through the upper extremities. Regardless of the type of muscle testing used, the procedure is innately subjective and depends on the subject's ability to exert a maximal contraction. This ability can be negatively affected by such factors as pain, poor comprehension, motivation, cooperation, fatigue, and fear.

The gross muscle testing procedures for each of the main regions of the body are described in Table 12-1. As mentioned, one of the more common gross muscle testing procedures is the one performed by the clinician before gait training with an assisted device when the clinician is not sure of the patient's capabilities. In this scenario, the clinician must efficiently assess the strength of the major muscle groups that are used when using an assistive device. The muscle groups tested include the shoulder abductors (Figure 12-1), the shoulder flexors (Figure 12-2), the shoulder extensors (Figure 12-3), the elbow flexors (Figure 12-4), the elbow extensors (Figure 12-5), the wrist extensors (Figure 12-6), the wrist flexors (Figure 12-7), the hip flexors (Figure 12-8), the knee extensors (Figure 12-9), the knee flexors and hip extensors (the hamstrings) (Figure 12-10), the hip abductors (Figure 12-11), the ankle dorsiflexors (Figure 12-12), and the ankle plantarflexors (Figure 12-13).

TABLE 12-1	Gross Muscle Screening	
Patient Position	**Tested Muscle Group**	**Procedure**
Supine	Hip flexors	The patient is instructed to raise both legs off the supporting surface simultaneously while keeping both legs straight. The position is held for 10 seconds. The hip flexors can also be tested in the sitting position.
	Hip abductors	The patient is instructed to abduct the legs to each side, then to hold the position while the clinician attempts to bring the legs together.
	Hip adductors	The patient is instructed to keep the legs together while the clinician attempts to separate the legs.
	Hip extensors	The patient is instructed to flex the hips and the knees, keeping the soles of the feet on the supporting surface, and to raise the pelvis from the supporting surface. This position is held for 10 seconds.
	Shoulder flexors and scapular upward rotators	The patient is instructed to flex the shoulder to 90° with the elbow straight and to hold the position while the clinician attempts to push the arms into extension.
	Shoulder extensors and scapula downward rotators	The patient is instructed to flex the shoulder to 90° with the elbow straight and to hold the position while the clinician attempts to push the arms into flexion.
	Shoulder horizontal abductors	The patient is instructed to flex the shoulder to 90° with the elbow straight and to hold the position while the clinician attempts to push the arms together into horizontal adduction
	Shoulder adductors	The patient is instructed to bring the hands together in front of the chest, keeping the elbow straight, and to hold this position. The clinician attempts to separate the arms into horizontal abduction.
	Neck and trunk flexors	The patient is instructed to hold both arms straight in front of the body and then to raise the head and shoulders off the supporting surface, and to hold this position.
Supine or sitting	Shoulder abductors	The patient is instructed to abduct the shoulder to the side up to shoulder level with the elbows straight. The clinician attempts to push the arms down to the patient's sides into shoulder adduction.
	Shoulder adductors	The patient is instructed to abduct the shoulder to the side up to shoulder level with the elbows straight. The clinician attempts to push the arms over the patient's head into shoulder abduction.
	Shoulder internal rotators	The patient is instructed to hold the arms at the sides, flex the elbows to approximately 90°, and place the forearms in neutral. The clinician attempts to push the arms outward into external rotation of the shoulder.
	Shoulder external rotators	The patient is instructed to hold the arms at the sides, flex the elbows to approximately 90°, and place the forearms in neutral. The clinician attempts to push the arms inward into internal rotation of the shoulder.
	Elbow flexors	The patient is instructed to hold the arms at the sides, flex the elbows to approximately 90°, and place the forearms in neutral. The clinician attempts to push the forearms toward the supporting surface into elbow extension.
	Elbow extensors	The patient is instructed to hold the arms at the sides, flex the elbows to approximately 90°, and place the forearms in neutral. The clinician attempts to push the forearms toward the shoulders into elbow flexion.
	Forearm supinators	The patient is instructed to hold the arms at the sides, flex the elbows to approximately 90°, and place the forearms in neutral. The clinician attempts to turn the palms toward the body into pronation.
	Forearm pronators	The patient is instructed to hold the arms at the sides, flex the elbows to approximately 90°, and place the forearms in neutral. The clinician attempts to turn the palms away from the body into supination.
	Wrist flexors	The patient is instructed to hold the arms at the sides, flex the elbows to approximately 90°, and place the forearms in neutral. The clinician attempts to push the palms upward into wrist extension.

(continued)

TABLE 12-1	Gross Muscle Screening (continued)	
Patient Position	**Tested Muscle Group**	**Procedure**
	Wrist extensors	The patient is instructed to hold the arms at the sides, flex the elbows to approximately 90°, and place the forearms in neutral. The clinician attempts to push the hand downward into wrist flexion.
	Finger flexors	The patient is instructed to hold the arms at the sides, flex the elbows to approximately 90°, and place the forearms in neutral. The clinician places his or her index and middle fingers into the patient's hand and the patient is asked to squeeze the fingers. The clinician then attempts to pull the fingers out.
	Finger extensors	The patient is instructed to hold the arms at the sides, flex the elbows to approximately 90°, and place the forearms in neutral. The patient is asked to straighten the fingers, and then the clinician attempts to push the fingers into flexion.
	Anterior interossei	The patient is instructed to hold the arms at the sides, flex the elbows to approximately 90°, and place the forearms in neutral. The patient is asked to adduct the fingers, and then the clinician attempts to pull the fingers into abduction.
	Posterior interossei	The patient is instructed to hold the arms at the sides, flex the elbows to approximately 90°, and place the forearms in neutral. The patient is asked to abduct the fingers, and then the clinician attempts to push the fingers into adduction.
	Opponens pollicis	The patient is instructed to hold the arms at the sides, flex the elbows to approximately 90°, and place the forearms in neutral. The clinician places his or her index finger between the patient's thumb and each finger one at a time while asking the patient to pinch the finger.
Sitting	Latissimus dorsi and triceps	The patient is instructed to place both hands on the supporting surface next to the hips, keeping the elbows straight and the shoulder shrugged. The patient is then asked to depress the scapular by lifting the buttocks off the supporting surface.
	Upper trapezius and levator scapulae	The patient is instructed to shrug the shoulders toward the ears and to hold the position. The clinician attempts to push the shoulders down into depression.
	Internal rotators of the hip and evertors of the feet	The patient is instructed to evert the foot and to hold the position while the clinician pushes on the lateral border of each foot, into inversion and external rotation of the hip.
	External rotators of the hip and invertors of the feet	The patient is instructed to invert the foot and to hold the position while the clinician pushes on the medial border of each foot, into eversion and internal rotation of the hip.
Prone	Rhomboids, middle trapezius, and posterior deltoid	The patient is instructed to flex the elbows level with the shoulders, pinch or adduct the scapulae together, and raise the arms from the supporting surface. The clinician attempts to push the arms downward.
	Elbow and shoulder extensors	The patient is instructed to raise the arm off the supporting surface while keeping the arms at the sides and the elbows straight. The clinician attempts to push the arms downward.
	Extensors of the hips, back, neck, and shoulders	The patient is instructed to keep the arms at the sides and to raise the head and shoulders and arms and legs off the supporting surface simultaneously by arching the back. The position is held for 10 seconds.
Prone or sitting	Hamstrings	The patient is instructed to flex the knees to about 90°. The clinician attempts to pull the knees into extension.
	Quadriceps	The patient is instructed to flex the knees to about 90°. The clinician attempts to push the knees into flexion.
Standing	Gastrocnemius/soleus	The patient is instructed to stand on one leg with one finger on the supporting surface for balance. The patient is then asked to rise up on tiptoes and to repeat 10 times. The other leg is then tested.
	Dorsiflexors	The patient is instructed to walk on the heel for 10 steps.
	Hip and knee extensors	The patient is instructed to do five partial deep-knee bends.

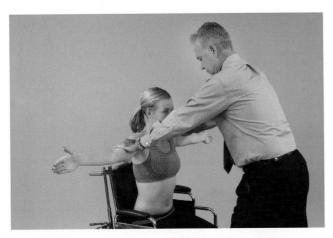

FIGURE 12-1 Gross muscle testing of the shoulder abductors

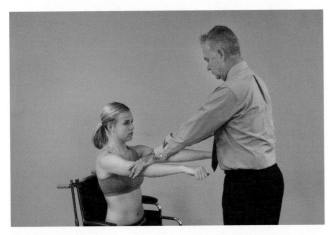

FIGURE 12-2 Gross muscle testing of the shoulder flexors

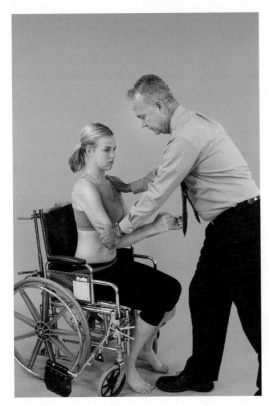

FIGURE 12-3 Gross muscle testing of the shoulder extensors

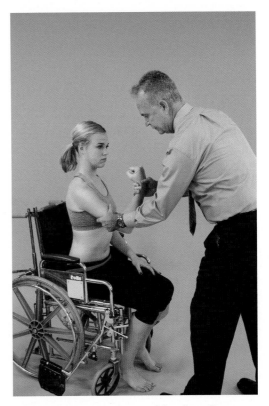

FIGURE 12-4 Gross muscle testing of the elbow flexors

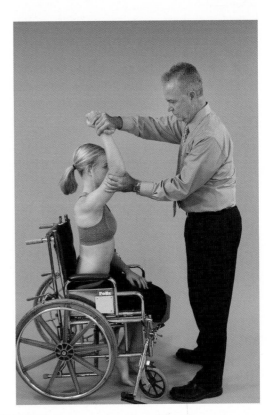

FIGURE 12-5 Gross muscle testing of the elbow extensors

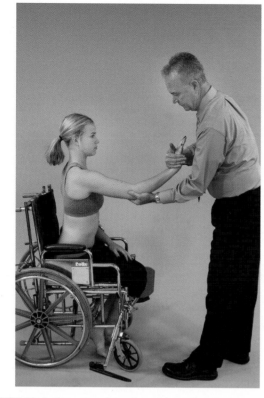

FIGURE 12-6 Gross muscle testing of the wrist extensors

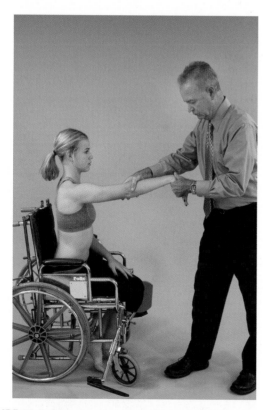

FIGURE 12-7 Gross muscle testing of the wrist flexors

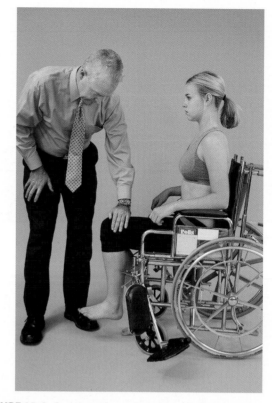

FIGURE 12-8 Gross muscle testing of the hip flexors

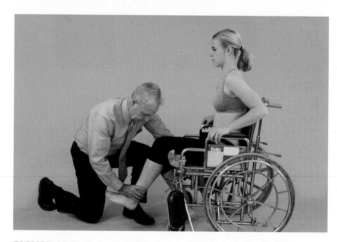

FIGURE 12-9 Gross muscle testing of the knee extensors

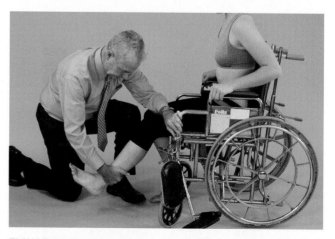

FIGURE 12-10 Gross muscle testing of the knee flexors and hip extensors

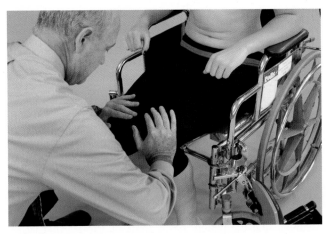

FIGURE 12-11 Gross muscle testing of the hip abductors

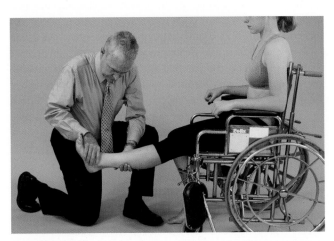

FIGURE 12-12 Gross muscle testing of the ankle dorsiflexors

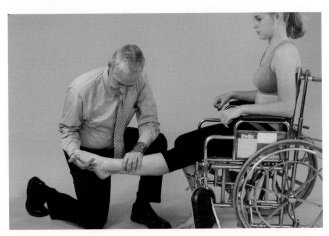

FIGURE 12-13 Gross muscle testing of the ankle plantarflexors

SPECIFIC MUSCLE TESTING

Specific muscle testing, also called manual muscle testing (MMT) is a procedure for the evaluation of the voluntary function and strength of individual muscles and muscle groups based on effective performance of limb movement in relation to the forces of gravity and manual resistance.

MMT is typically used when the gross muscle screening shows specific muscle weakness. From a physiologic viewpoint, MMT measures the ability of the musculotendinous units to act across a bone-joint lever-arm system to actively generate motion, or passively resist movement against gravity and variable resistance.[1]

The results from MMT can be influenced by a number of factors:

▶ The length of the muscle at the time of the contraction. The amount of tension a muscle produces depends on its length as it contracts. Each muscle has its own optimal length to produce optimal tension—for some muscles the lengthened position is more favorable than the shortened position. Generally speaking, as a muscle continues to lengthen, it eventually reaches a point of passive insufficiency, where it is not capable of generating its maximum force output (see active and passive insufficiency in Chapter 4).

▶ Whether the muscle acts on one joint or multiple joints. As a one-joint muscle shortens, or as the distal and proximal attachments of a two-joint muscle approach each other during a concentric contraction, the tension diminishes.

▶ The type of muscle contraction. Physiologically, a muscle is capable of generating its greatest tension during an eccentric contraction, less tension when contracting isometrically, and even less tension when contracting concentrically.[2]

▶ The speed of contraction. The faster a muscle produces a concentric contraction, the less ability the muscle has to generate tension—as velocity increases, tension decreases.

▶ The length of the moment arm. As a muscle moves through its range of motion, the torque generated varies with the length of the moment arm (distance from the axis of rotation—see Chapter 4). For example, as the elbow moves from full extension into flexion, the moment arm increases, reaching its maximum at approximately 90° of flexion, and then decreases throughout the remainder of the range of motion.

▶ Whether the muscle is working against gravity or with gravity. The force of gravity has the greatest leverage and therefore is able to produce the greatest toll on the body segment when the segment is horizontal.

To assess strength, strength values using MMT have traditionally been used between similar muscle groups on opposite extremities, or antagonistic ratios. This information is then used to determine whether a patient is fully rehabilitated. An agonist muscle contracts to produce the desired movement.

From a rehabilitation viewpoint, knowledge of a specific muscle's synergists and antagonists is very important:

▶ *Synergist.* Synergist muscles are muscle groups that work together with the agonist to produce a desired movement.[3] In essence, a synergist muscle can be viewed as a muscle's helper muscle, as the force generated by the synergists works in the same direction. Synergist muscles may need to be strengthened so that they can assist the agonist muscle.

▶ *Antagonists.* The antagonist muscle can oppose the desired movement. Antagonists allow movement by relaxing and lengthening in a gradual manner to ensure that the desired motion occurs, and that it does so in a coordinated and controlled fashion. Care must be taken to ensure that the antagonist muscles are not adaptively shortened and to monitor whether the antagonist muscles are not overpowering the agonist muscle.

To assist the clinician, for each of the specific muscle tests, the synergists and antagonist are provided.

To accurately perform a specific muscle test, the clinician must have knowledge of the following:

▶ The origin and insertion of the muscle being tested.

▶ The function of the muscle being tested. Muscles rarely perform one single action; instead they form groups of actions that overlap with the functions of other muscles. For that reason, if a component of a muscle's function is lost, other muscles that have duplicate functions can compensate for that loss.

▶ How to eliminate substitute or trick motions. This is best accomplished by using standardized testing positions. Where appropriate, these motions are included in each of the test procedures so that the clinician is aware of what to avoid.

▶ How to skillfully apply resistance. Pressure should be applied slowly, very gently, and gradually before progressing to the maximum resistance tolerable.

▶ The standard positions for each muscle test based on the effects of gravity. Typically the patient is positioned in either an antigravity or a gravity-eliminated position (see later).

▶ The standard methods of grading muscle strength. A number of grading methods have been described (see later).

It should be noted that there is considerable variability in the amount of resistance that normal muscles can hold against. The application of resistance throughout the arc of motion (referred to as a make test or active resistance test) in addition to resistance applied at only one point in the arc of motion (referred to as a break test) can help in judging the strength of a muscle.[4]

The main purposes of specific muscle testing are as follows:

▶ To help determine a diagnosis. For example, specific muscle testing can aid in precisely localizing a lesion in the peripheral nervous system.

▶ To establish a baseline for muscle reeducation and exercise.

▶ To determine a patient's need for supportive apparatus (orthosis, assistive device of ambulation, or splints).

▶ To help determine a patient's progress.

CLINICAL PEARL

Manual muscle testing has been shown to be less sensitive in detecting strength deficits in stronger muscles compared to weaker muscles.[4]

Several scales have been devised to assess muscle strength, including numerical, descriptive, and fractional (Table 12-2). The patient is positioned in an antigravity position for grades 3 to 5 and in a gravity-eliminated position for grades 0 to 2. If the muscle strength is less than grade 3, then the methods advocated in muscle testing manuals must be used.[4] For the testing methods and positions described in this chapter, it is assumed that the patient has a grade of 3 to 5. Alternative, gravity-eliminated/minimized positions will also be provided.

A number of problems exist with the grading systems. The grading systems for MMT produce ordinal data with unequal rankings between grades. For example, a muscle grade of 4 is not equivalent to 75% of the strength represented by a grade 5; it is a natural grade determined by the effect of gravity, manual resistance, the patient's age, and so forth. In general, the grades 5 (normal) and 4 (good) typically encompass a large range of a muscle's strength—although a score of 5 does not mean that the muscle is normal in every circumstance (e.g., when at the onset of fatigue or in a state of exhaustion)— whereas the grades of 3 (fair), 2 (poor), and 1 (trace) include a much narrower range.[4] As a result, scores of 4 or 5 require some subjectivity, which can increase the variability between testers, whereas the precise definitions for 0 to 3 scores produce little tester-to-tester variability. Some of the confusion arises from the descriptions of maximal, moderate, and minimal, or considerable, which removes much of the objectivity from the tests. It has been advocated by some to add + or – to the scales. The – is used to describe that the test range is not complete but the motion is over one-half the standard test range of motion (e.g., a grade of 2– with a patient who achieves more than one half of the standard range, with gravity eliminated). The + is used to describe the test range that is less than one half of the test range (e.g., a grade of 2+ with a patient who achieves less than one half of the standard range, in the anti-gravity position).

CLINICAL PEARL

If the clinician is having difficulty differentiating between a grade 4 and a grade 5, the eccentric "break" method of muscle testing may be used. This procedure starts as an isometric contraction, but then the clinician applies sufficient force to cause an eccentric contraction or a "break" in the patient's isometric contraction.

CLINICAL PEARL

Studies have demonstrated that reliability in MMT is dependent on the specific muscle being examined. For example, Florence and colleagues[5] found high reliability in the proximal muscles as opposed to the distal muscles, and Barr and colleagues[6] found the upper body muscles to be more reliably tested than the lower body ones.[7]

TABLE 12-2   Manual Muscle Grading

Numerical	Descriptive	Fractional	Description
10	Normal	5/5	Ability to complete test movement and/or hold test position against gravity and maximum (strong) pressure
9	Good +	4+/5	Ability to complete test movement and/or hold test position against gravity and slightly less than maximum (moderate to strong) pressure
8	Good	4/5	Ability to complete test movement and/or hold test position against gravity and moderate pressure
7	Good –	4–/5	Ability to complete test movement and/or hold test position against gravity and slightly less than moderate (slight to moderate) pressure
6	Fair +	3+/5	Ability to complete test movement and/or hold test position against gravity and minimal (slight) pressure
5	Fair	3/5	Ability to complete test movement and/or hold test position against gravity but cannot hold if even slight pressure is applied
4	Fair –	3–/5	Ability to complete at least 1/2 of test movement against gravity. Cannot complete full test movement against gravity. NOTE: Kendall and colleagues[a] refer to this as a very gradual release from antigravity test position
3	Poor +	2+/5	Ability to initiate test movement against gravity, but completes less than 1/2 of test movement range OR Ability to complete test movement in a gravity lessened position against resistance throughout the range OR Ability to complete test movement and hold test position in a gravity-lessened position against pressure
2	Poor	2/5	Ability to complete test movement in gravity lessened position with friction reduced. No movement against gravity
1	Poor –	2–/5	Ability to initiate or complete partial test movement in a gravity-lessened position with friction reduced; unable to complete full range of test movement.
T	Trace	1/5	Feeble but palpable muscle contraction or prominent tendon during muscle contraction with no visible motion of the part
0	Zero	0/5	No palpable muscle contraction

[a]Data from Kendall FP, McCreary EK, Provance PG: Muscles: Testing and Function. Baltimore, Williams & Wilkins, 1993.

To be a valid test, strength testing must elicit a maximum contraction of the muscle being tested. The following strategies ensure that this occurs:

1. *Comparing the passive range of motion to the active range of motion.* To achieve a grade of 3 to 5, the muscle must move through the entire available range. One of the most common mistakes is to overgrade or undergrade a muscle by assessing a muscle in a patient who is unable to achieve the full available range of motion.

2. *Placing the joint which the muscle to be tested crosses in, or close to, its open packed position.* This strategy helps protect the joint from excessive compressive forces, and the surrounding inert structures from excessive tension. The body area or segment to be evaluated is exposed, and the subject is properly draped. It is important to remember that the position used is dependent on the overall condition and comfort of the patient.

3. *Placing the muscle to be tested in a shortened position.* This puts the muscle in an ineffective physiologic position and has the effect of increasing motor neuron activity. Three basic factors must be considered with

specific muscle testing: (1) the weight of the limb or distal segment with a minimal effect of gravity on the moving segment; (2) the weight of the limb plus the effects of gravity on the limb or segment; and (3) the weight of the limb or segment plus the effects of gravity plus manual resistance.

4. *Using standardized positions.* If the muscle to be tested is not isolated, the clinician is merely testing a muscle group rather than an individual muscle. Initially, the standardized gravity-minimized positions may be necessary to avoid the effect of the weight of the moving body segment on the force measurement. For example, to test the strength of the hip abductors, the patient is positioned in supine so that the muscle action pulls in a horizontal plane relative to the ground.[4]

5. *Stabilizing the appropriate parts of the body.* When performing a specific muscle test, emphasis is placed on correct stabilization of the body part on which the muscle originates in addition to careful avoidance of substitution by other muscle groups to enhance accuracy. Substitutions by other muscle groups during

testing indicate the presence of weakness. It does not, however, tell the clinician the cause of the weakness.

6. *Apply force at the appropriate location.* The force is typically applied distally on the segment to where the muscle insertion occurs, except when a longer lever is needed. The application of force is usually made at the end of range with one-joint muscles and at midrange with two-joint muscles. Resistance is always applied at right angles to the long axis of the segment. The force is applied by the clinician in a direction opposite to the torque (the rotary force around an axis, which is a combination of the force along the longitudinal axis of the segment on which the muscle attaches and another force that is at right angles to the axis of motion) exerted by the muscle being tested.

7. *Give consideration to the patient's age, size, strength, occupation, and neuromuscular condition.* It is important to remember that the standardized positions are applicable to the adult population and may need to be adjusted for the aged or younger subjects. In addition, the clinician should know his or her own limitations.

8. *For grades 3 to 5, ask the patient to perform an eccentric muscle contraction.* This can be accomplished by using the command "Don't let me move you." Because the tension at each cross-bridge and the number of active cross-bridges are greater during an eccentric contraction, the maximum eccentric muscle tension developed is greater with an eccentric contraction than with a concentric one.

9. *Breaking the contraction.* It is important to break the patient's muscle contraction, in order to ensure that the patient is making a maximal effort and that the full power of the muscle is being tested. Although force values determined with *make* and *break* tests are highly correlated, break tests usually result in greater force values than make tests,[8,9] so they should not be used interchangeably.

10. *Holding the contraction for at least 5 seconds.* Weakness resulting from nerve palsy has a distinct fatigability. The muscle demonstrates poor endurance, because usually it is only able to sustain a maximum muscle contraction for about 2 to 3 seconds before complete failure occurs. This strategy is based on the theories behind muscle recruitment, wherein a normal muscle, while performing a maximum contraction, uses only a portion of its motor units, keeping the remainder in reserve to help maintain the contraction. A palsied muscle, with its fewer functioning motor units, has very few, if any, motor units in reserve. If a muscle appears to be weaker than normal, further investigation is required, as follows:

    a. The test is repeated three times. Muscle weakness resulting from disuse will be consistently weak and should not become weaker with several repeated contractions.

    b. Another muscle that shares the same innervation is tested. Knowledge of both spinal and peripheral nerve innervation will aid the clinician in determining which muscle to select.

11. *Comparing findings with uninvolved side.* One study found no statistically significant difference in force between the dominant and nondominant lower extremities, but did find the difference between the dominant and nondominant upper extremities.[10] Sapega[11] states that a difference in muscle force between sides of greater than 20% probably indicates abnormality, whereas a difference of 10% to 20% possibly indicates abnormality.

As always, these tests cannot be evaluated in isolation but have to be integrated into a total clinical profile before drawing any conclusion about the patient's condition. Many factors can influence the results from MMT, including:

- Age
- Type of contraction (isometric, concentric, or eccentric)
- Muscle size
- Speed of contraction
- Training effect
- Joint position
- Fatigue
- Nutrition status
- Level of motivation
- Pain
- Body type
- Limb dominance

CLINICAL PEARL

MMT is an ordinal level of measurement[11] and has been found to have both inter- and intrarater reliability, especially when the scale is expanded to include plus or minus a half or a full grade.[12–14] Training in standardized testing positions, stabilization, and grading criteria resulted in higher agreement and correlation coefficients between testers.

Although the grading of muscle strength has its role in the clinic, and the ability to isolate the various muscles is very important in determining the source of nerve palsy, specific grading of individual muscles does not give the clinician much information on the ability of the structure to perform functional tasks. In addition, measurements of isometric muscle force are specific to a point or small range in the joint range excursion and thus cannot be used to predict dynamic force capabilities.[15–17]

More recently, the use of quantitative muscle testing (QMT) has been recommended to assess strength, as it produces interval data that describe force production. QMT methods include:

- *The use of handheld dynamometers.* Although more costly and time-consuming than manual muscle testing, handheld dynamometry can be used to improve objectivity and sensitivity. Patients are typically asked to push against the dynamometer in a maximal isometric contraction (make test), or hold a position until the clinician overpowers the muscle producing an eccentric contraction (break tests).[4] Normative force values for particular muscle groups by patient age and gender have been reported, with some authors including regression equations that take into account body weight and height.[18]

CLINICAL PEARL

Depending on the study, handheld dynamometers have demonstrated good to excellent intratester reliability and poor to excellent intertester reliability.[19–23]

▶ *The use of an isokinetic dynamometer.* This is a stationary, electromechanical device that controls the velocity of the moving body segment by resisting and measuring the patient's effort so that the body segment cannot accelerate beyond a preset angular velocity.[4] Isokinetic dynamometers measure torque and range of motion as a function of time and can provide an analysis of the ratio between the eccentric contraction and concentric contraction of a muscle at various positions and speeds.[24] This ratio is aptly named the *eccentric/concentric ratio.*[25] The ratio is calculated by dividing the eccentric strength value by the concentric strength value. Various authors[26,27] have demonstrated that the upper limit of this ratio is 2.0 and that lower ratios indicate pathology.[25,28] Alternatively, the same recommendations for manual muscle testing advocated by Sapega[11] can be used: a difference in muscle force between sides of greater than 20% probably indicates abnormality, whereas a difference of 10% to 20% possibly indicates abnormality. To ensure the validity of isokinetic dynamometry measurements, calibration of equipment is necessary and should be performed each day of testing, at the same speed and damp setting to be used during the testing.[29]

One of the major criticisms of muscle testing is the overestimation of strength when a muscle is weak as identified by QMT, compared to the same muscle being graded as normal by MMT, such that a theoretical percentage score based on MMT is likely to grossly overestimate the strength of a patient.[7]

Studies that compare the reliability of MMT and QMT often come to the conclusion that MMT may be consistent and reliable, but it is unable to detect subtle differences in strength.[30,31] Thus, although MMT results are more consistent, the variation produced by QMT can appreciate differences in strength undetectable in MMT.[7] For example, Beasley[2] showed that 50% of the knee extensor strength needed to be lost before MMT was able to identify weakness.

CLINICAL PEARL

Voluntary muscle strength testing will remain somewhat subjective until a precise way of measuring muscle contraction is generally available.[1] This is particularly true when determining normal and good values.

MUSCLE TESTING OF THE SHOULDER COMPLEX

A number of significant muscles control motion at the shoulder and provide dynamic stabilization. Rarely does a single muscle act in isolation at the shoulder. For simplicity, the

TABLE 12-3	Muscles of the Shoulder Complex
Scapular pivoters	
Trapezius	
Serratus anterior	
Levator scapulae	
Rhomboid major	
Rhomboid minor	
Humeral propellers	
Latissimus dorsi	
Teres major	
Pectoralis major	
Pectoralis minor	
Humeral positioners	
Deltoid	
Shoulder protectors	
Rotator cuff (supraspinatus, infraspinatus, teres minor, and subscapularis)	
Long head of the biceps brachii	

muscles acting at the shoulder may be described in terms of their functional roles: scapular pivoters, humeral propellers, humeral positioners, and shoulder protectors (Table 12-3).[32]

Scapular Pivoters

The scapular pivoters comprise the trapezius, serratus anterior, levator scapulae, rhomboid major, and rhomboid minor.[32] As a group, these muscles are involved with motions at the scapulothoracic articulation, and their proper function is vital to the normal biomechanics of the whole shoulder complex. The scapular muscles can contract isometrically, concentrically, or eccentrically, depending on the desired movement and whether the movement involves acceleration or deceleration. To varying degrees, the serratus anterior and all parts of the trapezius cooperate during the upward rotation of the scapula.

Trapezius. The trapezius muscle (Figure 12-14) originates from the medial third of the superior nuchal line, the external occipital protuberance, the ligamentum nuchae, the apices of the seventh cervical vertebra, all the thoracic spinous processes, and the supraspinous ligaments of the cervical and thoracic vertebrae. This muscle traditionally is divided into middle, upper, and lower parts (see Figure 12-14), according to anatomy and function.

▶ The upper fibers descend to attach to the lateral third of the posterior border of the clavicle.

▶ The middle fibers of the trapezius run horizontally to the medial acromial margin and superior lip of the spine of the scapula.

▶ The inferior fibers ascend to attach to an aponeurosis gliding over a smooth triangular surface at the medial end of the spine of the scapula to a tubercle at the scapular lateral apex.

The nerve supply to the trapezius is from the spinal accessory (cranial nerve [CN] XI) and from the anterior ramus of C2-4.

Upper Trapezius. The upper portion of the trapezius originates from the external occipital protuberance, medial

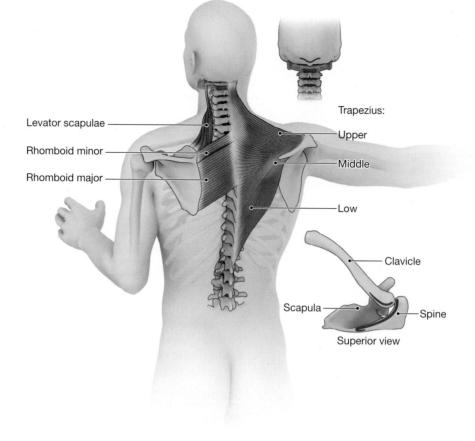

FIGURE 12-14 Trapezius muscle and its relationship to some of the other scapular pivoters

one-third of the superior nuchal line, the ligamentum nuchae, and the spinous process of the seventh cervical vertebra (see Figure 12-14). It inserts on the lateral one third of the clavicle and acromion processes of the scapula. It has been suggested that the upper fibers of this muscle have a different motor supply than the middle and lower portions.[33,34] Recent clinical and anatomic evidence seems to suggest that the spinal accessory nerve (CN XI) provides the most important and consistent motor supply to all portions of the trapezius muscle, and that although the C2-4 branches of the cervical plexus are present, no particular elements of innervation within the trapezius have been determined.[35]

One of the functions of the upper trapezius is to produce shoulder girdle elevation on a fixed cervical spine. For the trapezius to perform its actions, the cervical spine must be stabilized by the anterior neck flexors to prevent simultaneous occipital extension from occurring. Failure to prevent this occipital extension would allow the head to translate anteriorly, resulting in a decrease in the length, and therefore the efficiency, of the trapezius,[36] and an increase in the cervical lordosis. The synergists for the upper trapezius include the rhomboid major and minor, the middle trapezius, the levator scapulae, and the serratus anterior. The antagonists for the upper trapezius include the lower trapezius, pectoralis minor, subclavius, pectoralis major (sternal portion), serratus anterior, and latissimus dorsi. Weakness of the upper trapezius results in a decrease in the ability to approximate the acromial end of the scapula and the occiput, difficulty raising the head from a prone position, and difficulty with abduction

and flexion of the humerus above shoulder level.[37] Adaptive shortening of the muscle results in elevation of the shoulder girdle. Unilateral contracture of this muscle is frequently seen in torticollis cases. This muscle is a common location for trigger points.

CLINICAL PEARL

Complete paralysis of the trapezius usually causes moderate to marked difficulty in elevating the arm over the head. The task, however, can usually be completed through full range as long as the serratus anterior remains totally innervated.[38]

To specifically test this muscle, the patient is seated with the arm relaxed at the sides. The patient is asked to raise the shoulder as high as possible, and to extend and rotate the occiput toward the elevated shoulder (Figure 12-15). The clinician stabilizes the top of the shoulders with one hand, and applies resistance against the head in the direction of cervical flexion anterolaterally (see Figure 12-15). The command given to the patient is "Don't let me separate your head and shoulder." Substitution or trick motions can include abduction and upward rotation of the scapula (serratus anterior), elevation and downward rotation of the scapula (rhomboid major and minor), anterior tilting of the scapula (pectoralis minor), and elevation of the first and second ribs (scalenus muscle group). The gravity minimized/eliminated position for this muscle is with the patient positioned in supine or prone with the upper limb and shoulder supported.

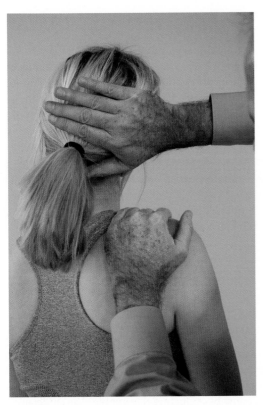

FIGURE 12-15 Test position for the upper portion of the trapezius

Middle Trapezius. The middle portion of the trapezius originates from the spinous processes of the first through fifth thoracic vertebrae and inserts on the medial margin of the acromion and the superior lip of the spine of the scapula (see Figure 12-14) forming the cervicothoracic part of the muscle. Working alone, this muscle produces scapular adduction (retraction). The synergists for the middle trapezius include the rhomboid major and minor, the upper and lower trapezius, the levator scapulae, and the serratus anterior (depending on its action). The antagonists for the middle trapezius include the lower trapezius (depending on its action), serratus anterior, pectoralis minor, and pectoralis major (sternal portion).

To specifically test this muscle, the patient is positioned in prone with the shoulder abducted to 90°, the elbow extended, and the upper extremity externally rotated so that the thumb points toward the ceiling (Figure 12-16). The clinician applies

pressure against the forearm in a downward direction toward the table. The command given to the patient is "Don't let me push your arm down while keeping your elbow straight and your thumb pointing upward." Substitution or trick motions can include trunk rotation, horizontal abduction of the shoulder (posterior deltoid) elevation and downward rotation of the scapula (rhomboid major and minor), depression and downward rotation of the scapula (lower trapezius), synergistic contraction of the upper and lower fibers of the trapezius muscle, and synergistic contraction of the lower trapezius and the rhomboids. The gravity-minimized/eliminated position for this muscle is with the patient positioned in sitting with the upper limb supported on a friction-free surface in a position of 90° of abduction and 90° of elbow flexion.

Lower Trapezius. The lower fibers of this muscle originate from the spinous processes of the 6th through 12th thoracic vertebrae (see Figure 12-14) and insert at the tubercle of the apex of the spine of the scapula. Working alone, the lower trapezius muscle stabilizes the scapula against lateral displacement (abduction) produced by the serratus anterior and to stabilize the scapula against scapular elevation produced by the levator scapulae. The synergists for the lower trapezius include the rhomboid major and minor, the middle and upper trapezius, the pectoralis minor, and the latissimus dorsi. The antagonists for the lower trapezius include the upper trapezius, levator scapulae, rhomboid major and minor, and serratus anterior.

To specifically test this muscle, the patient is positioned in prone with the arm placed diagonally overhead, and the shoulder is externally rotated (Figure 12-17). The clinician applies pressure against the forearm downward toward the table. The command given to the patient is "Don't let me push your arm down while keeping your arm diagonally upward and your thumb facing upward." Substitution or trick motions can include assistance from the posterior deltoid, latissimus dorsi, or pectoralis major. The gravity-minimized/eliminated position for this muscle is with the patient positioned in prone with the arms by the sides and the upper extremity supported by the clinician. The patient is asked to depress and adduct the scapula through full range of motion.

Serratus Anterior. The muscular digitations of the serratus anterior (Figure 12-18) originate from the upper 8 to 10 ribs

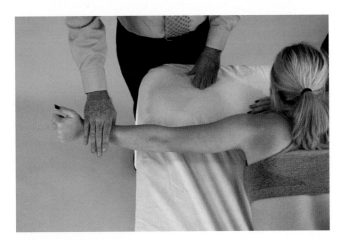

FIGURE 12-16 Test position for the middle trapezius

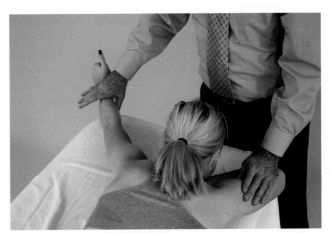

FIGURE 12-17 Test position for the lower trapezius

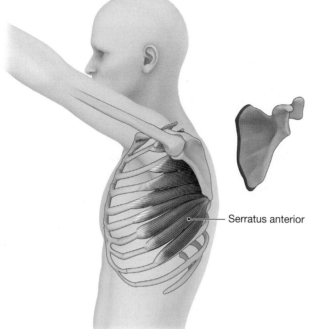

FIGURE 12-18 Serratus anterior muscle

and fascia over the intercostals. The muscle is composed of three functional components[39,40]:

▶ The upper component originates from the first and second ribs and inserts on the superior angle of the scapula.

▶ The middle component arises from the second, third, and fourth ribs and inserts along the anterior aspect of the medial scapular border.

▶ The lower component is the largest and most powerful, originating from the fifth through ninth ribs. It runs anterior to the scapula and inserts on the medial border of the scapula.

The serratus anterior is activated with all shoulder movements, but especially during shoulder flexion and abduction.[40] Working in synergy with the upper and lower trapezius, as part of a force couple, the main function of the serratus anterior is to protract and upwardly rotate the scapula,[41,42] while providing a strong, mobile base of support to position the glenoid optimally for maximum efficiency of the upper extremity.[43] Its lower fibers draw the lower angle of the scapula forward to rotate the scapula upward while maintaining the scapula on the thorax during arm elevation.[44] This moves the coracoacromial arch out of the path of the advancing greater tuberosity and opposes the excessive elevation of the scapula by the levator scapulae and trapezius muscles.[45] Without upward rotation and protraction of the scapula by the serratus anterior, full glenohumeral (G-H) elevation is not possible. In fact, in patients with complete paralysis of the serratus anterior, Gregg and colleagues[43] reported that abduction is limited to 110°.

Dysfunction of serratus anterior muscle causes winging of the scapula as the patient attempts to elevate the arm.[46,47] Scapulothoracic dysfunction can also contribute to G-H

instability, as the normal stable base of the scapula is destabilized during abduction or flexion.[47-49]

The serratus anterior muscle is innervated by the long thoracic nerve (C5–7). The synergists for the serratus anterior include the upper and lower trapezius, pectoralis minor, latissimus dorsi, and subclavius. The antagonists for the serratus anterior include the middle trapezius, levator scapulae, and rhomboids.

CLINICAL PEARL

Paralysis or weakness of the serratus anterior muscle results in disruption of normal shoulder kinesiology. The disability may be slight with partial paralysis, or profound with complete paralysis. As a rule, persons with complete or marked paralysis of the serratus anterior cannot elevate the arms above 110° of abduction.[38]

To specifically test this muscle, the patient is positioned in supine, standing, or sitting.

▶ *Supine:* the patient is asked to flex the shoulder to 90° with slight abduction and with the elbow in extension. From this position, the patient moves the arm upward toward the ceiling by abducting the scapula. The clinician applies resistance by grasping around the forearm and elbow and applying a downward and inward pressure toward the table (Figure 12-19). The command given to the patient is "Try to lift your arm higher by moving your shoulder forward while I push down on it."

▶ *Standing:* the patient places a hand against the wall with the shoulder in forward flexion to 80° to 90° and the

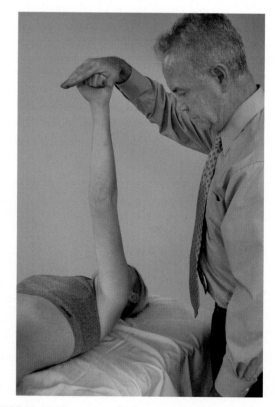

FIGURE 12-19 Test position for the serratus anterior—patient supine

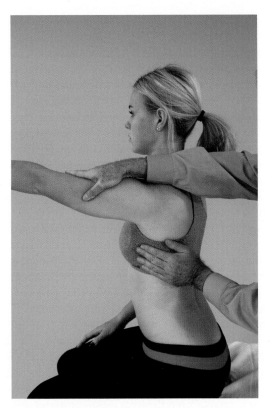

FIGURE 12-20 Test position for the serratus anterior—patient sitting

provides eccentric control of scapular upward rotation in the higher ranges of motion.[51]

Both the trapezius and levator scapulae muscles are activated with increased upper extremity loads.[36,40,52]

The levator scapulae muscle is innervated by the posterior (dorsal) scapular nerve (C3–5). The synergists for the levator scapulae include all portions of the trapezius and the rhomboid major and minor. The antagonists for the levator scapulae include the lower trapezius, pectoralis minor, pectoralis major (lower portion), subclavius, serratus anterior, and latissimus dorsi.

To specifically test this muscle, the patient is positioned in sitting with the arms relaxed at the sides. The patient is asked to raise the shoulder as high as possible while the clinician generates resistance downward on top of the shoulder (see Figure 12-15). The command given to the patient is "Don't let me push your shoulder down." It is worth remembering that it is difficult to differentiate the strength of the levator scapulae from that of the upper trapezius. For this reason, the levator scapulae strength is often assessed together with the rhomboids, or with the upper trapezius.

Rhomboid Major and Minor. The rhomboid muscles help control scapular positioning, particularly with horizontal flexion and extension of the shoulder complex.[51] Based on anatomy and function, the rhomboids are divided into a major and a minor muscle.

▶ The rhomboid major muscle (see Figure 12-14) originates from the second to fifth thoracic spinous processes and the overlying supraspinous ligaments. The fibers descend to insert on the medial scapular border between the root of the scapular spine and the inferior angle of the scapula.

▶ The rhomboid minor muscle (see Figure 12-14) originates from the lower ligamentum nuchae and the seventh cervical and first thoracic spinous processes and attaches to the medial border of the scapula at the root of the spine of the scapula.

The rhomboid muscles are innervated by the posterior (dorsal) scapular nerve (C4–5). Working together, the rhomboid muscles adduct and elevate the scapula and downwardly rotate the scapula. The rhomboid major muscle helps stabilize the scapula against the rib cage. The synergists for the rhomboids include all portions of the trapezius muscle and the levator scapulae. The antagonists for the rhomboids include the lower trapezius, pectoralis major and minor, serratus anterior, and latissimus dorsi.

To specifically test this muscle, the patient is positioned in prone with the head turned toward the tested side, the elbow flexed, and the ipsilateral humerus abducted, slightly extended, and externally rotated (Figure 12-21a). The clinician applies pressure with one hand against the patient's arm in the direction of abducting the scapula and externally rotating the inferior angle, while the other hand is placed against the patient's shoulder in the direction of depression (see Figure 12-21a). The command given to the patient is "Don't let me push your arm down." Substitution or trick motions can include assistance from the wrist extensors, middle trapezius, posterior deltoid, latissimus dorsi, teres major, and levator scapulae. An alternative test can be performed with the patient positioned in prone

elbows locked in extension. While monitoring the inferior angle of the scapula for any winging, the command given to the patient is "Push against the wall."

▶ *Sitting:* this test focuses on the upward rotation action of the serratus in the abducted position. The patient is asked to move the humerus into approximately 120° to 130° of flexion. Using one hand, the clinician wraps the thumb and index finger around the inferior aspect of the scapula and the other hand is placed on the anterior aspect of the arm (Figure 12-20). The command given to the patient is "Keep your arm still while I try and push it down," as the clinician pushes downwardly on the arm while applying a resistive force with the other hand into internal rotation of the inferior angle of the scapula.

Substitution or trick motions typically occur in sitting and can include flexion of the vertebrae or rotation of the vertebrae.

The gravity-minimized/eliminated position for this muscle is with the patient positioned in sitting with the upper limb resting on a table, with the shoulder positioned in 90° of flexion, and the elbow extended.

Levator Scapulae. The levator scapulae muscle (see Figure 12-14) originates by tendinous strips from the transverse processes of the atlas, axis, and C3 and C4 vertebrae and descends diagonally to insert on the medial superior angle of the scapula.

The levator scapulae can act on either the cervical spine or the scapula. If it acts on the cervical spine, it can produce extension, side bending, and rotation of the cervical spine to the same side.[50] When acting on the scapula during upper extremity flexion or abduction, the levator scapula muscle acts as an antagonist to the lower trapezius muscle and

341

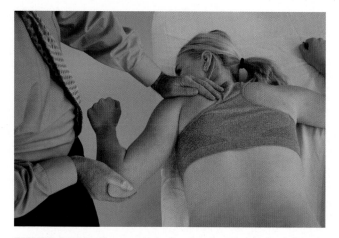

FIGURE 12-21a Test position for the rhomboids (and levator scapulae)

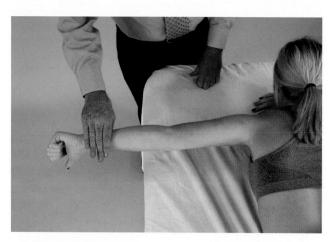

FIGURE 12-21b Alternate test position for the rhomboids

with the upper extremity positioned in 90° of abduction and internally rotated so that the thumb is pointing down (Figure 12-21b). The patient is asked to raise the arm toward the ceiling and to hold the position while the clinician applies a downward force to the patient's forearm. The gravity-minimized/eliminated position for this muscle is with the patient positioned in sitting with the hand resting on the lumbar spine.

Humeral Propellers

The total muscle mass of the shoulder's internal rotators (subscapularis, anterior deltoid, pectoralis major, latissimus dorsi, and teres major) is much greater than that of the external rotators (infraspinatus, teres minor, and posterior deltoid).[38] This fact explains why the shoulder internal rotators produce about 1.75 times greater isometric torque than the external rotators.[53] Peak torques of the internal rotators also exceed the external rotators when measured isokinetically, under both concentric and eccentric conditions.[38,54]

Latissimus Dorsi. The latissimus dorsi muscle (Figure 12-22) originates from the spinous processes of the last six thoracic vertebrae, the lower three or four ribs, the lumbar and sacral spinous processes through the thoracolumbar fascia, the posterior third of the external lip of the iliac crest, and a slip from the inferior scapular angle. The scapular slip allows the

latissimus dorsi to act at the scapulothoracic articulation. The latissimus dorsi inserts on the intertubercular sulcus of the humerus. The latissimus dorsi functions as an extensor, adductor, and powerful internal rotator of the shoulder, and also assists in scapular depression, retraction, and downward rotation.[55] It is innervated by the thoracodorsal nerve (C6-8). The synergists for the latissimus dorsi include the teres major, anterior and posterior deltoid, triceps brachii, erector spinae, subscapularis, and pectoralis major. The antagonists for the latissimus dorsi include the middle trapezius, supraspinatus, infraspinatus, teres minor, anterior and posterior deltoid, coracobrachialis, biceps brachii, and pectoralis major (clavicular portion).

To specifically test this muscle, the patient is positioned in prone with the shoulder internally rotated and adducted and the palm facing upward (Figure 12-23). The patient is asked to extend the shoulder while keeping the elbow straight. The command given to the patient is "While keeping your palm facing the ceiling, don't let me push your arm down." The clinician stabilizes the thorax, and resistance is given proximal to the elbow joint using a force that is a combination of shoulder abduction and minimal flexion (see Figure 12-23). Substitution or trick motions can include scapular adduction with no shoulder motion, anterior tipping and abduction of the scapula, assistance from the teres major, posterior deltoid, or pectoralis major (sternal head). The gravity-minimized/eliminated position for this muscle is with the patient positioned in sidelying, with the upper limb supported in 90° of shoulder flexion and internal rotation, and with the elbow flexed.

Teres Major. The teres major (see Figure 12-22) originates from the inferior third of the lateral border of the scapula and just superior to the inferior angle. The teres major tendon inserts on the medial lip of the intertubercular groove of the humerus. The teres major functions to complement the actions of the latissimus dorsi in that it extends, adducts, and internally rotates the G-H joint. It is innervated by the lower subscapular nerve (C5, C6). The synergists for the teres major include the latissimus dorsi, anterior and posterior deltoid, triceps brachii (long head), pectoralis major, and subscapularis. The antagonists for the teres major are numerous and include the middle deltoid, supraspinatus, infraspinatus, teres minor, coracobrachialis, biceps brachii, anterior and posterior deltoid, and pectoralis major (clavicular portion).

To specifically test this muscle, the patient is positioned in prone with the upper extremity extended, abducted, and medially rotated and with the back of the hand resting on the small of the back. The clinician places a hand against the arm proximal to the elbow (Figure 12-24), and the command given to the patient is "Keeping your hand against your back, don't let me move your arm toward the table," while the clinician generates a force into flexion and abduction of the upper extremity. Substitution or trick motions can include scapular adduction without shoulder motion, external rotation of the glenohumeral joint, and assistance from the latissimus dorsi, pectoralis major, and teres minor. In general, the teres major muscle is not tested in a gravity-eliminated position, because it will only contract against resistance.

Pectoralis Major. The pectoralis major (Figure 12-25) originates from the sternal half of the clavicle, half of the

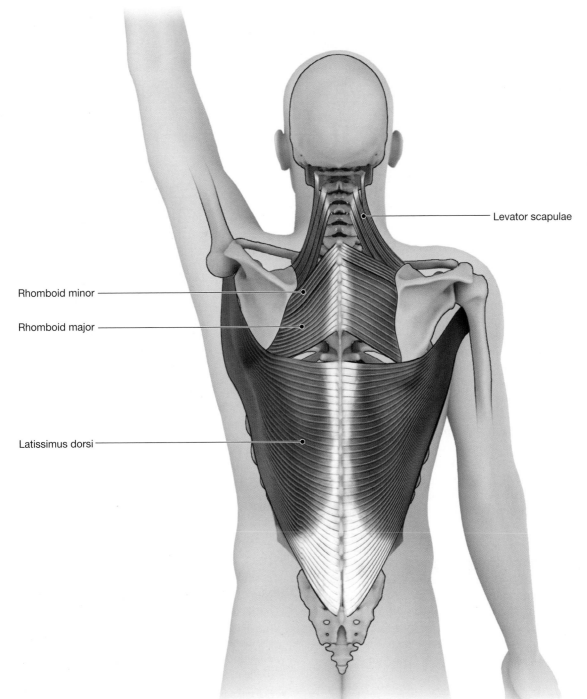

Levator scapulae

Rhomboid minor

Rhomboid major

Latissimus dorsi

FIGURE 12-22 Latissimus dorsi and teres major muscles—their relation to each other and to the rhomboids and levator scapulae

anterior surface of the sternum to the level of the sixth or seventh costal cartilage, the sternal end of the sixth rib, and the aponeurosis of the obliquus externus abdominis. The fibers of the pectoralis major converge to form a tendon that inserts on the lateral lip of the intertubercular sulcus of the humerus. Although this muscle does not insert on the scapula, it does act on the scapulothoracic articulation through its insertion on the humerus. The function of the pectoralis muscle depends on which fibers are activated:

▶ *Upper fibers (clavicular head)*—internal rotation, horizontal adduction, flexion, abduction (once the humerus is abducted 90°, the upper fibers assist in further abduction), and adduction (with the humerus below 90° of abduction) of the G-H joint

▶ *Lower fibers (sternal head)*—internal rotation, horizontal adduction, extension, and adduction of the G-H joint

From a functional perspective, this muscle is important with crutch walking or ambulation within the parallel bars.

343

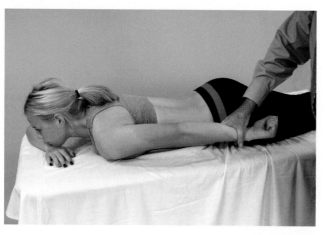

FIGURE 12-23 Test position for the latissimus dorsi–stabilization of the thorax not shown

The pectoralis major is innervated by the medial (lower fibers) and lateral (upper fibers) pectoral nerves (C8-T1 and C5-7, respectively). The synergists for the clavicular portion include the sternal portion of the pectoralis major, subscapularis, latissimus dorsi, teres major, anterior and middle deltoid, coracobrachialis, pectoralis minor, serratus anterior, and biceps brachii. The antagonists for the clavicular portion include the latissimus dorsi, teres major, middle and posterior deltoid, infraspinatus, triceps brachii (long head), teres minor, and supraspinatus. The synergists for the sternal portion include the clavicular portion of the pectoralis major, posterior deltoid, latissimus dorsi, teres major, triceps brachii (long head), and pectoralis minor. The antagonists for the sternal portion include the supraspinatus, deltoid, trapezius, serratus anterior, levator scapulae, and rhomboids.

CLINICAL PEARL

The pectoralis major and latissimus dorsi muscles are referred to as *humeral propeller* muscles as they have been shown to be the only muscles in the upper extremity to have a positive correlation between peak torque and pitching velocity, and during the propulsive phase of the swim stroke.

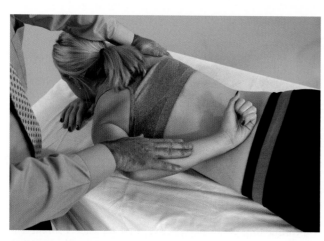

FIGURE 12-24 Test position for the teres major

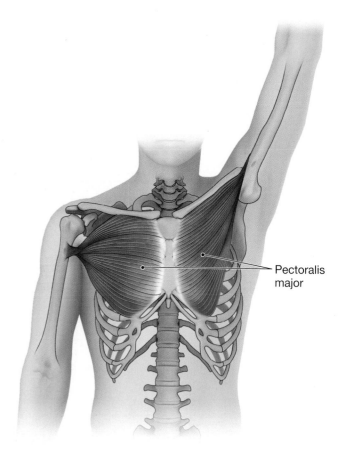

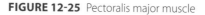
Pectoralis major

FIGURE 12-25 Pectoralis major muscle

To specifically test this muscle, the patient is positioned in supine. The patient's arm position depends on which portion of the muscle is being tested:

▶ *Clavicular portion (upper fibers):* the patient arm is positioned in 60° to 90° of shoulder abduction and the elbow is slightly flexed. The patient is then asked to horizontally adduct the shoulder as the clinician applies resistance at the forearm (or proximal to the elbow if the elbow flexors are weak) in a downward and outward direction (Figure 12-26). The coracobrachialis, a synergist of the upper fibers, can also be assessed (Figure 12-26a).

▶ *Sternal portion (lower fibers):* the patient arm is positioned in 120° of shoulder abduction with the elbow slightly flexed. The patient is asked to move the arm down and in across the body as the clinician applies resistance at the elbow in an up and outward direction (Figure 12-27).

Substitution or trick motions can include trunk rotation and assistance from the anterior deltoid, coracobrachialis, and biceps brachii. The gravity-minimized/eliminated position for this muscle is with the patient positioned in sitting with the shoulder positioned in neutral rotation and in 90° of abduction, the elbow flexed to 90°, and the upper limb supported.

Pectoralis Minor. The pectoralis minor (Figure 12-28) originates from the outer surface of the upper margins of the third to fifth ribs near their cartilage. The fibers of the pectoralis minor ascend laterally, converging to a tendon that inserts on the coracoid process of the scapula.

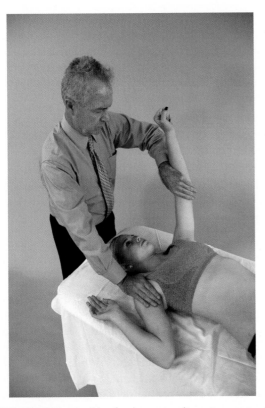

FIGURE 12-26 Test position for the pectoralis major—upper fibers

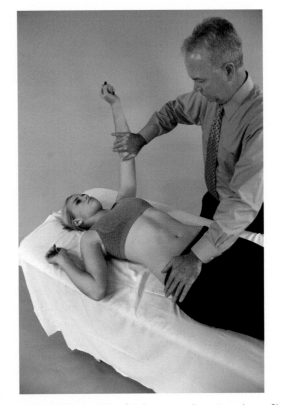

FIGURE 12-27 Test position for the pectoralis major—lower fibers

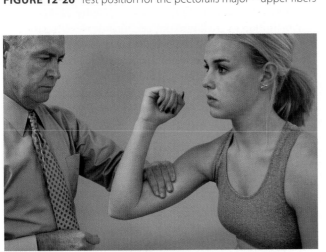

FIGURE 12-26a Test position for the coracobrachialis

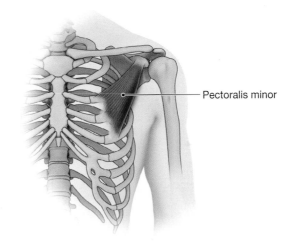

FIGURE 12-28 Pectoralis minor muscle

Working alone, this muscle depresses the shoulder, downwardly rotates the scapula, and protracts the scapula. This muscle can also assist with elevation of the ribs during forced inspiration. The pectoralis minor muscle is innervated by the medial pectoral nerve (C6–8). The pectoralis minor is prone to adaptive shortening, particularly if the patient commonly adopts a rounded shoulder posture, which in turn can result in impingement on the cords of the brachial plexus or the axillary vessels. The synergists to this muscle include the pectoralis major, lower trapezius, serratus anterior, latissimus dorsi, levator scapulae, rhomboid major and minor, and middle trapezius. The antagonists of this muscle are the trapezius, levator scapulae, latissimus dorsi, serratus anterior, and the rhomboid major and minor.

To specifically test this muscle, the patient is positioned in supine with the arms at the sides and the patient is asked to lift the shoulder girdle from the table (without using force from the elbow or hand) and to hold the position while the clinician applies resistance against the anterior aspect of the shoulder (Figure 12-29) in a downward direction toward the table. Substitution or trick motions can include flexion of the wrist or fingers, which can give the appearance of anterior tipping of the scapula. The gravity-minimized/eliminated position for this muscle is with the patient positioned in sitting with the hand resting on the small of the back.

Humeral Positioners

Deltoid. The deltoid muscle originates from the lateral third of the clavicle, the superior surface of the acromion, and the spine of the scapula (Figure 12-30). It inserts into the deltoid

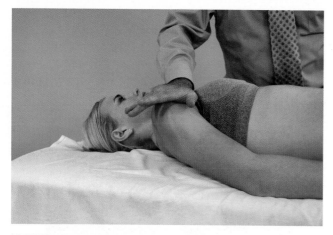

FIGURE 12-29 Test position for pectoralis minor

tuberosity of the humerus. The deltoid can be described as three separate muscles—anterior, middle, and posterior—all of which function as humeral positioners, positioning the humerus in space.[32]

Working alone, the three separate muscles of the deltoid can produce shoulder horizontal adduction, shoulder flexion, internal rotation of the shoulder, and shoulder scaption (arm elevated in the plane of the scapula). Working in a combined fashion, the deltoid can produce shoulder abduction. The deltoid muscle is innervated by the axillary nerve (C5-6). The synergists and antagonists of this muscle depend on which of the three portions is being used:

▶ *Anterior deltoid (see Figure 12-30).* The synergists include the middle and posterior deltoid, subscapularis, biceps brachii, pectoralis major, coracobrachialis, and supraspinatus. The antagonists include the triceps brachii (long head), posterior deltoid, latissimus dorsi, teres major, infraspinatus, and teres minor.

▶ *Middle deltoid (see Figure 12-30).* The synergists are the supraspinatus, posterior deltoid, and anterior deltoid. The antagonists are latissimus dorsi, teres major, coracobrachialis, and triceps brachii (long head).

▶ *Posterior deltoid (see Figure 12-30).* The synergists are the teres minor, latissimus dorsi, teres major, triceps brachii (long head), and infraspinatus.

To specifically test this muscle, the patient's arm position used depends on which portion of the muscle is being tested:

▶ *Anterior deltoid.* The patient is positioned in sitting or supine with the shoulder abducted in minimal flexion and external rotation. The command given to the patient is "Place your arm diagonally outward from your body and hold it against my resistance." While stabilizing the patient's shoulder with one hand, the clinician uses the other hand to apply resistance to the anterior and medial aspect of the arm proximal to the elbow in the direction of abduction and minimal extension (Figure 12-31). Substitution or trick motions can include elevating the shoulder and leaning backward; assistance from the biceps brachii, coracobrachialis, or pectoralis major (clavicular head); or moving the scapula. The gravity-minimized/eliminated position for this muscle is with the patient positioned in sidelying with the upper extremity

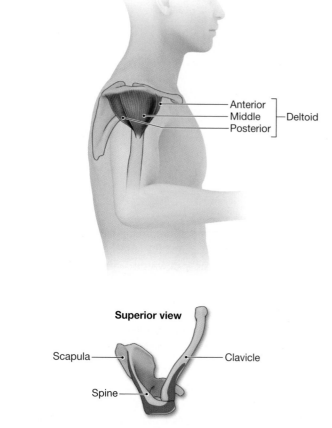

FIGURE 12-30 Deltoid muscle

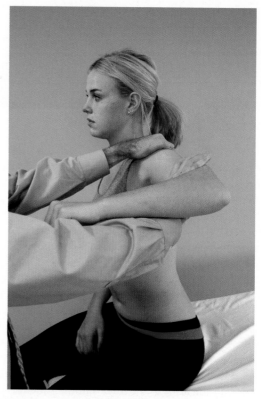

FIGURE 12-31 Test position for the anterior deltoid

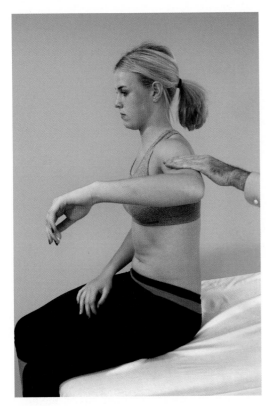

FIGURE 12-32 Test position for the middle deltoid

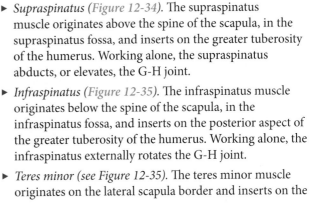

FIGURE 12-33 Test position for the posterior deltoid

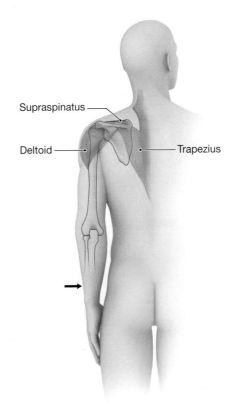

supported and the shoulder positioned in neutral, and the elbow flexed.

▶ *Middle deltoid.* The patient is positioned in sitting with the arm abducted to 90° and the elbow flexed to approximately 90°. The patient is asked to hold this position while the clinician applies resistance just proximal to the elbow in a downward direction (Figure 12-32). Substitution or trick motions can include trunk flexion to the opposite side, or assistance from the biceps brachii, supraspinatus, or serratus anterior. The gravity-minimized/eliminated position for this muscle is with the patient positioned in supine with the upper extremity supported and the elbow flexed to 90°.

▶ *Posterior deltoid.* The patient positioned in sitting with the shoulder abducted to approximately 90° and positioned in minimal shoulder extension and internal rotation. The patient is asked to push the arms back toward the clinician as the clinician uses one hand to stabilize the shoulder and the other hand to apply resistance to the posterolateral aspect of the arm, proximal to the elbow, in the direction of shoulder abduction and slight flexion (Figure 12-33). Substitution or trick motions can include assistance from the long head of the triceps or adduction of the scapula without horizontally abducting the shoulder. The gravity-minimized/eliminated position for this muscle is with the patient positioned in sitting with the upper extremity supported on a table, and the shoulder and elbow flexed to 90°.

Shoulder Protectors

Rotator Cuff. The rotator cuff (RC) muscles consist of the supraspinatus, infraspinatus, teres minor, and the subscapularis:

▶ *Supraspinatus (Figure 12-34).* The supraspinatus muscle originates above the spine of the scapula, in the supraspinatus fossa, and inserts on the greater tuberosity of the humerus. Working alone, the supraspinatus abducts, or elevates, the G-H joint.

▶ *Infraspinatus (Figure 12-35).* The infraspinatus muscle originates below the spine of the scapula, in the infraspinatus fossa, and inserts on the posterior aspect of the greater tuberosity of the humerus. Working alone, the infraspinatus externally rotates the G-H joint.

▶ *Teres minor (see Figure 12-35).* The teres minor muscle originates on the lateral scapula border and inserts on the

Supraspinatus

Deltoid

Trapezius

FIGURE 12-34 Supraspinatus muscle

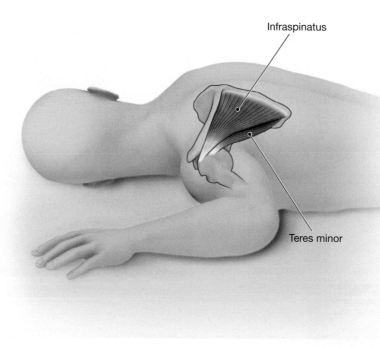

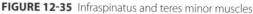

FIGURE 12-35 Infraspinatus and teres minor muscles

inferior aspect of the greater tuberosity of the humerus. Working alone, the teres minor muscle externally rotates the G-H joint.

▶ *Subscapularis (Figure 12-36).* The subscapularis muscle originates on the anterior surface of the scapula, sitting directly over the ribs, and inserts on the lesser tuberosity of the humerus. Working alone, the subscapularis is an internal rotator of the shoulder. It also depresses the head of the humerus, allowing it to move freely in the G-H joint during elevation of the arm. Internal rotation of the shoulder dominates over external rotation secondary to the greater muscle mass of the subscapularis.

The RC muscles are referred to as the protectors of the shoulder because, in addition to working individually to move the humerus, they have an important role in the function of the shoulder and serve the following roles[32]:

▶ *Assist in the rotation of the shoulder and arm.* At the G-H joint, elevation through abduction of the arm requires that the greater tuberosity of the humerus pass under the coracoacromial arch. For this to occur, the humerus must externally rotate, and the acromion must elevate.[56] External rotation of the humerus is produced actively by a contraction of the infraspinatus and teres minor, and by a twisting of the joint capsule. A force couple exists in the transverse plane between the subscapularis anteriorly and the infraspinatus and teres minor posteriorly in which co-contraction of the infraspinatus, teres minor, and subscapularis muscles both depresses and compresses the humeral head during overhead movements.

CLINICAL PEARL

The importance of the external rotation during humeral elevation can be demonstrated clinically. If the humerus is held in full internal rotation, only about 60° of G-H abduction is passively possible before the greater tuberosity impinges against the coracoacromial arch and blocks further abduction. This helps explain why individuals with marked internal rotation contractures cannot abduct fully, but can elevate the arm in the sagittal plane.

In the frontal plane, there is another force couple between the deltoid and the inferior rotator cuff muscles (infraspinatus, subscapularis, and teres minor). With the arm fully adducted, contraction of the deltoid produces a vertical force in a superior direction, resulting in an upward translation of the humeral head relative to the glenoid. Co-contraction of the inferior rotator cuff muscles produces both a compressive force and a downward translation of the humerus that counterbalances the force of the deltoid, thereby stabilizing the humeral head.

FIGURE 12-36 Subscapularis muscle

Electromyography (EMG) studies have shown that during casual elevation of the arm in normal shoulders, the deltoid and the rotator cuff act continuously throughout the motion of abduction, each reaching a peak of activity between 120° and 140° of abduction.[57,58] However, during more rapid and precise movements such as those involved with throwing, a more selective pattern emerges with specific periods of great intensity.[59] Weakening of the rotator cuff appears to allow the deltoid to elevate the proximal part of the humerus in the absence of an adequate depressor effect from the rotator cuff. A decrease in the subacromial space is created, and impingement of the rotator cuff on the anterior aspect of the acromion occurs.[60,61]

▶ *Reinforce the G-H capsule.* The rotator cuff muscles, together with the glenohumeral ligament (and the long head of the biceps—often referred to as the fifth rotator cuff muscle), enhance stability. For example, firing of the rotator cuff muscles increases the tension of the middle G-H ligament when the arm is abducted to 45° and externally rotated.[62]

▶ *Control much of the active arthrokinematics of the G-H joint.* Contraction of the horizontally oriented supraspinatus produces a compression force directly into the glenoid fossa.[60] This compression force holds the humeral head securely in the glenoid cavity during its superior roll, which provides stability to the joint, and also maintains a mechanically efficient fulcrum for elevation of the arm.[60] In the shoulder's midrange position, when all of the passive restraints are lax, joint stability is achieved almost entirely by the rotator cuff. In addition, as previously mentioned, without adequate supraspinatus force, the near-vertical line of force of a contracting deltoid tends to jam or impinge the humeral head superiorly against the coracoacromial arch.[38]

The synergists and antagonists of the rotator cuff muscles depend on the individual muscles of the group:

▶ *Teres minor.* The synergists are the infraspinatus and the posterior deltoid. The antagonists are the anterior deltoid, subscapularis, pectoralis major, latissimus dorsi, and teres major.

▶ *Subscapularis.* The synergists are the pectoralis major, anterior deltoid, teres major, and latissimus dorsi. The antagonists are the infraspinatus, posterior deltoid, and teres minor.

▶ *Supraspinatus.* The synergist is the middle deltoid. The antagonists are the teres major, latissimus dorsi, and pectoralis major.

▶ *Infraspinatus.* The synergists are the teres minor and posterior deltoid. The antagonists are the subscapularis, pectoralis major, latissimus dorsi, anterior deltoid, and teres major.

Each of the muscles of the rotator cuff can be specifically tested, with the patient setup dependent on which muscle is being tested:

▶ *Teres minor.* The patient is positioned in prone with the shoulder abducted to 90° and the arm supported by the table so that the forearm is permitted to move freely

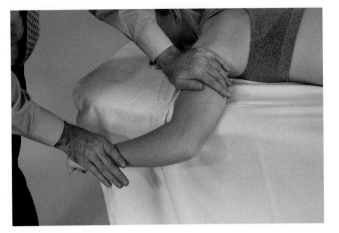

FIGURE 12-37 Test position for the shoulder external rotators—teres minor and infraspinatus—patient prone

(Figure 12-37). The patient is asked to externally rotate the shoulder so that the forearm moves toward the ceiling. The patient is asked to hold this position while the clinician applies resistance at the patient's wrist in a downward direction with one hand, while using the other hand to support the patient's elbow (see Figure 12-37). The teres minor can also be tested with the patient in supine with the humerus in external rotation and the elbow held at a right angle. Using one hand, the clinician stabilizes the upper arm, while using the other arm to apply pressure in the direction of internal rotation of the humerus (Figure 12-38).

▶ *Subscapularis.* The patient is positioned in prone with the shoulder abducted to 90° and the upper arm resting on the table so that the forearm is permitted to move freely (Figure 12-39). The patient is asked to internally rotate the shoulder so that the forearm moves toward the ceiling. The patient is asked to hold the position while the clinician applies resistance at the wrist in a downward direction with one hand, while using the other hand to support the patient's arm (see Figure 12-39). The subscapularis can also be tested with the patient in supine with the upper arm at the side and the elbow held at a right angle (Figure 12-40). Using one hand to stabilize

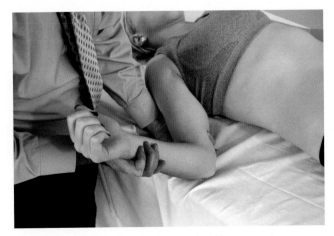

FIGURE 12-38 Test position for the shoulder external rotators—teres minor and infraspinatus—patient supine

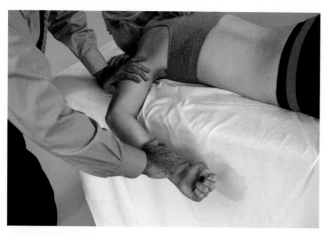

FIGURE 12-39 Test position for the shoulder internal rotators—subscapularis

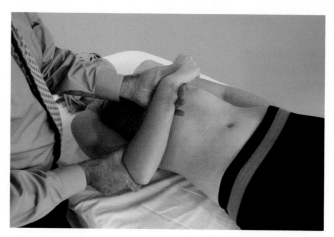

FIGURE 12-40

the patient's upper arm, the clinician uses the other hand to apply force against the inner aspect of the patient's wrist and forearm in a direction of external rotation. Substitution or trick motions can include scapular abduction, pronation of the forearm, and assistance from the pectoralis major, teres major, and latissimus dorsi. The gravity-minimized/eliminated position for this muscle is with the patient positioned in prone with the shoulder flexed over the edge of the table.

▶ *Supraspinatus.* The patient is positioned in sitting with the arm by the side and the head rotated ipsilaterally and extended. Using one hand, the clinician palpates the supraspinatus; the other hand applies resistance at the elbow into shoulder adduction while the patient is asked to raise the arm up into shoulder abduction. This is a difficult muscle to isolate as it works in conjunction with the middle deltoid.

▶ *Infraspinatus.* The patient is positioned in prone with the shoulder abducted to 90° and the arm supported by the table so that the forearm is permitted to move freely (see Figure 12-37). The patient is asked to externally rotate the shoulder so that the forearm moves toward the ceiling and to hold that position. Using one hand, the clinician stabilizes the patient's elbow while using the other hand to apply resistance in a downward direction at the patient's wrist (see Figure 12-37). The infraspinatus can also be tested with the patient in supine with the humerus in external rotation and the elbow held at a right angle. Using one hand, the clinician stabilizes the upper arm, while using the other arm to apply pressure in the direction of internal rotation of the humerus (see Figure 12-38).

Long Head of the Biceps Brachii. The biceps brachii muscle is a large fusiform muscle in the anterior compartment of the upper extremity, which has two tendinous origins from the scapula (Figure 12-40a). The medial head and long head of the biceps (LHB) normally originate from the coracoid process and supraglenoid tubercle of the scapula, respectively. However, researchers have noted that the origin

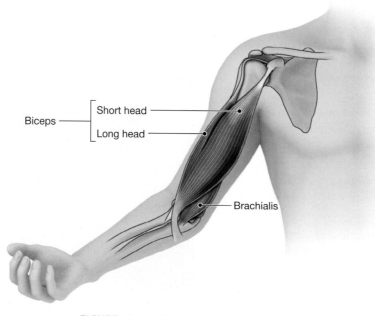

Biceps — Short head
Long head

Brachialis

FIGURE 12-40a Biceps brachii and brachialis muscles

of the biceps tendon varies, not only in the type of insertion (single, bifurcated, or trifurcated), but also in the specific anatomic location where it inserts.[63,64] The proximal LHB tendon receives some arterial supply from labral branches of the suprascapular artery.[65] As it leaves its origin, the LHB tendon is surrounded by a synovial sheath, which ends at the distal end of the bicipital groove, making the tendon an intra-articular but extrasynovial structure.[63] As the LHB tendon moves between the greater and lesser tuberosities, it is stabilized in position by the tendoligamentous sling made up of the coracohumeral ligament, superior G-H ligament, and fibers from the supraspinatus and subscapularis.[63,66] Once in the bicipital groove, the LHB tendon passes under the transverse humeral ligament, which bridges the groove.[67] After coursing through the groove, the two heads join to form the biceps muscle belly at the level of the deltoid insertion.[68] The medial tendon is interarticular, lying inside the G-H capsule.[69-71] This tendon is not as common a source of shoulder pain as the long tendon, and it rarely ruptures.[69-71]

The function of the biceps as a forearm supinator and secondarily as an elbow flexor is well known (see Muscle Testing of the Elbow).[72] At the shoulder joint, however, the function of the LHB tendon is less clear, with most references regarding it as a weak flexor of the shoulder.[73] Cadaveric studies have suggested that the LHB tendon functions as a humeral head depressor (in full external rotation), an anterior stabilizer, a posterior stabilizer, a limiter of external rotation, a lifter of the glenoid labrum, and a humeral head compressor of the shoulder.[74-77] The muscle has also been described as having important role in decelerating the rapidly moving arm during activities such as forceful overhand throwing.[63] In the anatomic position, the biceps has no ability to elevate the humerus. If the arm is rotated 90° externally, the tendon of the long head aligns with the muscle belly to form a straight line across the humeral head. As the biceps contracts in this position, the humeral head rotates beneath the tendon, resisting external rotation of the humeral head and increasing the anterior stability of the G-H joint.[78-80] Contraction of the long head of the biceps when the arm is abducted and externally rotated fixes the humeral head snugly against the glenoid cavity, as the resultant force passes obliquely through the center of rotation of the humeral head and at right angles to the glenoid.[78] The humeral head is prevented from moving upward by the hoodlike action of the biceps tendon, which exerts a downward force and assists the depressor function of the cuff.[81-83] Interestingly, the biceps tendon was found to be wider in cuff-deficient shoulders in one study.[84]

The biceps brachii muscle is innervated by the musculocutaneous nerve.

CLINICAL PEARL

A number of pathologic conditions have been associated with the LHB tendon including LHB tendon degeneration, superior labral tear from anterior to posterior (SLAP) lesions, LHB tendon anchor abnormalities, and LHB tendon instability.[67]

The strength of the LHB is assessed in combination with the short head of the biceps (see Elbow Flexors later).

MUSCLE TESTING OF THE ELBOW

A summary of the muscles of the elbow is outlined in Table 12-4.

Elbow Flexors

Anatomic, biomechanic, and electromyographic analyses have demonstrated that the prime movers of elbow flexion are the biceps, brachialis, and brachioradialis (see Table 12-4).[85] The pronator teres, flexor carpi radialis (FCR), flexor carpi ulnaris (FCU), and extensor carpi radialis longus (ECRL) muscles are considered to be weak flexors of the elbow.[86] Most elbow flexors, and essentially all the major supinator and pronator muscles, have their distal attachments on the radius.[87] Contraction of these muscles, therefore, pulls the radius proximally against the humeroradial joint.[88,89] The combined efforts of all the elbow flexors can create large amounts of elbow flexion torque. The interosseous membrane transfers a component of this muscle force to the radius and to the ulna, thereby dissipating some of the force.[87] The reverse action of the elbow flexors can be used in a closed chain perspective (see Chapter 4) by bringing the upper arm closer to the forearm, such as when performing a pull-up.[90]

Biceps Brachii. The biceps is a two-headed muscle that spans two joints. The short head of the biceps arises from the tip of the coracoid process of the scapula, whereas the long head arises from the supraglenoid tuberosity of the scapula (see Figure 12-40a). The biceps has two insertions: the radial tuberosity and by the lacertus fibrosus (see Figure 12-40a).

At the elbow, the biceps is the dominant flexor, but its secondary function is supination of the forearm.[91] The supination action of the biceps increases the more the elbow is flexed and is maximal at 90°. It diminishes again when the elbow is fully flexed. No,[92] or limited,[93] biceps muscle activity has been demonstrated during elbow flexion, with the forearm pronated.[86] The biceps, via its long head, also functions as a shoulder flexor (see Muscles of the Shoulder earlier).

The biceps brachii muscle is innervated by the musculocutaneous nerve.

The synergists of this muscle include the brachialis and brachioradialis, supinator, anterior deltoid, coracobrachialis, pectoralis major (clavicular portion), FCR, FCU, pronator teres, and extensor carpi radialis longus and brevis. The antagonists include the triceps brachii and anconeus, pronator teres, pronator quadratus, posterior deltoid, and latissimus dorsi.

To specifically test this muscle the patient is positioned in sitting with the elbow flexed to approximately 90° and the forearm in supination. Using one hand to stabilize the patient's shoulder, the clinician uses the other hand to apply resistance over the anterior aspect of the patient's forearm while asking the patient to hold the position of elbow flexion against the resistance (Figure 12-41). As with all of the elbow flexors, the gravity-minimized/eliminated position is with the patient positioned in sitting with the arm supported on a table at 90° of abduction, the shoulder in neutral rotation, and the elbow extended. Substitution or trick motions when testing any of the elbow flexors can include shoulder extension and assistance from the pronator teres or the wrist and finger extensors and flexors.

TABLE 12-4	Muscles of the Elbow, Forearm, Wrist, and Hand: Their Actions, Nerve Supply, and Nerve Root Derivation		
Muscles	**Nerve Supply**	**Nerve Root Derivation**	**Action**
Triceps	Radial	C7-C8	Elbow extension
Anconeus	Radial	C7-C8, (T1)	
Brachialis	Musculocutaneous	C5-C6, (C7)	Elbow flexion
Biceps brachii	Musculocutaneous	C5-C6	
Brachioradialis	Radial	C5-C6, (C7)	
Biceps brachii	Musculocutaneous	C5-C6	Supination of the forearm
Supinator	Posterior interosseous (radial)	C5-C6	
Pronator quadratus	Anterior interosseous (median)	C8, T1	Pronation of the forearm
Pronator teres	Median	C6-C7	
Flexor carpi radialis	Median	C6-C7	
Extensor carpi radialis longus	Radial	C6-C7	Extension of the wrist
Extensor carpi radialis brevis	Posterior interosseous (radial)	C7-C8	
Extensor carpi ulnaris	Posterior interosseous (radial)	C7-C8	
Flexor carpi radialis	Median	C6-C7	Flexion of the wrist
Flexor carpi ulnaris	Ulnar	C7-C8	
Flexor carpi ulnaris	Ulnar	C7-C8	Ulnar deviation of the wrist
Extensor carpi ulnaris	Posterior interosseous (radial)	C7-C8	
Flexor carpi radialis	Median	C6-C7	Radial deviation of the wrist
Extensor carpi radialis longus	Radial	C6-C7	
Abductor pollicis longus	Posterior interosseous (radial)	C7-C8	
Extensor pollicis brevis	Posterior interosseous (radial)	C7-C8	
Extensor digitorum communis	Posterior interosseous (radial)	C7-C8	Extension of the fingers
Extensor indicis	Posterior interosseous (radial)	C7-C8	
Extensor digiti minimi	Posterior interosseous (radial)	C7-C8	
Flexor digitorum profundus	Lateral: Anterior interosseous (median)	C8, T1	Flexion of the fingers (lateral aspect flexes the 2nd and 3rd digits; medial aspect flexes the 4th and 5th digits
	Medial: Ulnar	C8, T1	
Flexor digitorum superficialis	Median	C7-C8, T1	Flexion of the fingers

Brachialis. The brachialis (see Figure 12-41) originates from the lower two-thirds of the anterior surface of the humerus and inserts on the ulnar tuberosity and the coronoid process. The brachialis is the workhorse of the elbow and functions to bend the elbow regardless of the degree of pronation and supination of the forearm,[93] It is the most powerful flexor of the elbow when the forearm is pronated.[94]

The brachialis muscle is innervated by the musculocutaneous and radial nerves.

The synergists of the brachialis include the biceps brachii, brachioradialis, extensor carpi radialis longus and brevis,

pronator teres, FCR, and FCU. The antagonists of this muscle include the triceps brachii and anconeus.

To specifically test this muscle the patient is positioned in sitting or supine with the elbow flexed and the forearm pronated (Figure 12-42). Using one hand to stabilize the patient's elbow, the clinician places the other hand over the posterior surface of the patient's forearm proximal to the wrist and applies a force in the direction of elbow extension while asking the patient to try and prevent the motion (see Figure 12-42).

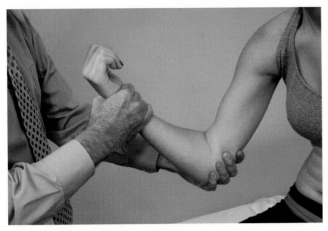

FIGURE 12-41 Test position for the biceps brachii

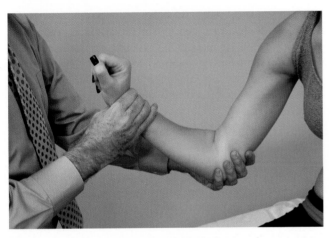

FIGURE 12-42 Test position for the brachialis

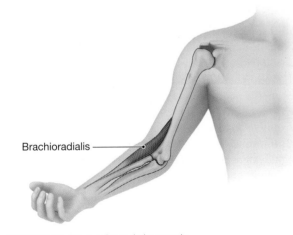

Brachioradialis

FIGURE 12-43 Brachioradialis muscle

Brachioradialis. The brachioradialis (Figure 12-43) arises from the proximal two-thirds of the lateral supracondylar ridge of the humerus and the lateral intermuscular septum. It travels down the forearm and inserts on the lateral border of the styloid process on the distal aspect of the radius.

The brachioradialis appears to have a number of functions, two of which occur with rapid movements of elbow flexion. Initially it functions as a shunt muscle, overcoming centrifugal forces acting on the elbow, and then by adding power to increase the speed of flexion.[91]

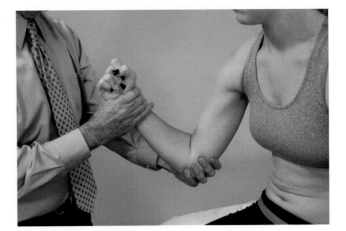

FIGURE 12-44 Test position for the brachioradialis

The brachioradialis also functions to bring a pronated or supinated forearm back into the neutral position of pronation and supination. In the neutral or pronated position, the muscle acts as a flexor of the elbow, an action that diminishes when the forearm is held in supination.[93,95]

The brachioradialis muscle is innervated by the radial nerve.

The synergists of the brachioradialis include the biceps brachii, brachialis, supinator, pronator teres, pronator quadratus, FCR, FCU, palmaris longus, and flexor digitorum superficialis. The antagonists include the triceps brachii and anconeus, extensor carpi radialis longus and brevis, extensor carpi ulnaris, and extensor digitorum communis.

To specifically test this muscle, the patient is positioned in sitting or supine with the elbow flexed and the forearm placed in a neutral position half way between supination and pronation (Figure 12-44). Using one hand to stabilize the patient's elbow, the clinician places the other hand proximal to the patient's wrist and applies a force into elbow extension while asking the patient to resist the movement.

Pronator Teres. The pronator teres (Figure 12-45) has two heads of origin: a humeral head and an ulnar head. The humeral head arises from the medial epicondylar ridge of the humerus and common flexor tendon, whereas the ulnar head arises from the medial aspect of the coronoid process of the ulna. The pronator teres inserts on the anterolateral surface of the

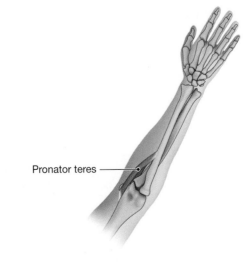

Pronator teres

FIGURE 12-45 Pronator teres muscle

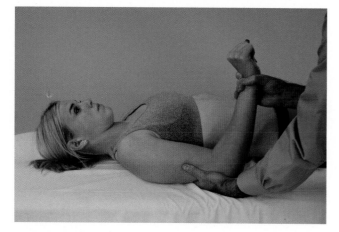

FIGURE 12-46 Test position for the pronator teres

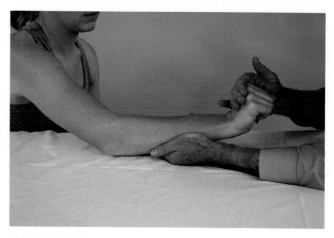

FIGURE 12-48 Test position for the extensor carpi radialis longus and brevis

midpoint of the radius. The muscle functions predominantly to pronate the forearm, but can also assist with elbow flexion.[94-96]

The pronator teres is innervated by the median nerve.

The synergists of this muscle include the biceps brachii, brachioradialis, brachialis, FCR, FCU, palmaris longus, flexor digitorum superficialis, and the pronator quadratus. The antagonists of this muscle include the triceps brachii and anconeus, biceps brachii, brachioradialis, and supinator.

To specifically test this muscle, the patient is positioned in sitting or supine with the elbow flexed to approximately 60° and the forearm fully pronated (Figure 12-46). Using one hand, the clinician stabilizes the patient's elbow against the patient's thorax while placing the other hand proximal to the patient's wrist (see Figure 12-46). The patient is asked to maintain the position while the clinician generates a force into forearm supination. Substitution or trick motions can include trunk flexion to the contralateral side, and abduction and internal rotation of the shoulder. The gravity-minimized/eliminated position for this muscle is with the patient positioned in sitting with the shoulder supported on a table at 90° of flexion, the elbow flexed to 90°, and the forearm perpendicular to the table.

Extensor Carpi Radialis Longus. The ECRL arises from a point superior to the lateral epicondyle of the humerus on the lower third of the supracondylar ridge, just distal to the brachioradialis. It travels down the forearm to insert on the posterior surface of the base of the second metacarpal (Figure 12-47). The muscle functions as a weak flexor of the elbow, as well as providing wrist extension and radial deviation.

The ECRL is innervated by the radial nerve. The synergists of this muscle include the extensor carpi ulnaris, FCR, extensor digitorum communis, extensor indicis, extensor pollicis longus, extensor pollicis brevis, and abductor pollicis longus. The antagonists of this muscle include the extensor carpi ulnaris, FCU, FCR, palmaris longus, flexor digitorum profundus, flexor digitorum superficialis, and flexor pollicis longus.

To specifically test this muscle the patient is positioned in sitting or supine with the elbow extended and the forearm just short of full pronation. Using one hand, the clinician supports the patient's forearm and the patient is asked to extend the wrist in a radial direction (Figure 12-48). Using the other hand, the clinician applies pressure on the posterior aspect of the patient's hand along the second through fourth metacarpal bones in an ulnar direction while asking the patient to prevent the movement (Figure 12-48).

Flexor Carpi Radialis. The FCR (Figure 12-49) arises from the common flexor tendon on the medial epicondyle of the humerus and inserts on the base of the second and third metacarpal bones. The FCR functions to flex the elbow and wrist but also assists in pronation and radial deviation of the wrist.

The FCR is innervated by the median nerve. The synergists of this muscle include the FCU, palmaris longus, flexor digitorum profundus, flexor digitorum superficialis, flexor pollicis longus, extensor carpi radialis longus and brevis, extensor pollicis brevis, and abductor pollicis longus. The antagonists of this muscle include the FCU, extensor carpi ulnaris, flexor

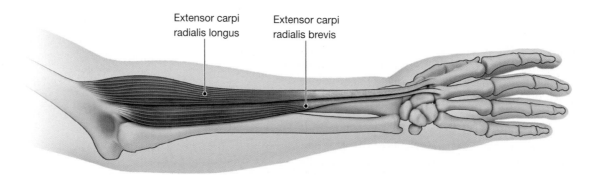

Extensor carpi radialis longus   Extensor carpi radialis brevis

FIGURE 12-47 Extensor carpi radialis longus and brevis

INTRODUCTION TO PHYSICAL THERAPY AND PATIENT SKILLS

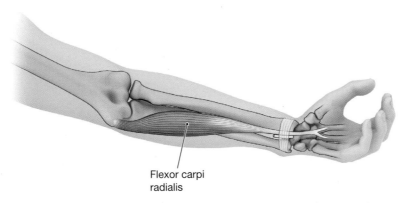

Flexor carpi
radialis

FIGURE 12-49 Flexor carpi radialis muscle and the palmaris longus (cut)

pollicis longus, extensor carpi radialis longus and brevis, extensor digitorum communis, extensor indicis, and extensor pollicis longus.

To specifically test this muscle the patient is positioned in sitting or supine, with the wrist flexed and ulnarly deviated and the forearm in supination. Using one hand, the clinician supports the patient forearm, while using the index and middle finger of the other hand to apply pressure on the thenar eminence in an ulnar and extension direction (Figure 12-50). The patient is asked to prevent this motion.

Flexor Carpi Ulnaris. The FCU (Figure 12-51) arises from two heads. The humeral head arises from the medial humeral epicondyle as part of the common flexor tendon, while the ulnar head arises from the proximal portion of the subcutaneous

border of the ulna. The FCU inserts directly onto the pisiform, the hamate via the pisohamate ligament, and onto the anterior surface of the base of the fifth metacarpal, via the pisometacarpal ligament. The FCU functions to assist with elbow flexion in addition to flexion and ulnar deviation of the wrist.

The FCU is innervated by the ulnar nerve. The synergists of this muscle include the FCR, palmaris longus, flexor digitorum profundus, flexor digitorum superficialis, flexor pollicis longus, extensor carpi ulnaris, biceps brachii, brachialis, pronator teres, brachioradialis, and extensor carpi radialis longus and brevis. The antagonists of this muscle include the triceps brachii and anconeus, extensor carpi radialis longus and brevis, extensor carpi ulnaris, extensor digitorum communis, extensor indicis, extensor digiti minimi, extensor pollicis longus, extensor pollicis brevis, FCR, and abductor pollicis longus.

To specifically test this muscle, the patient is positioned in supine or sitting with the forearms supported, the wrist flexed, and the fingers relaxed. The patient is asked to flex and ulnarly deviate the wrist. While stabilizing the wrist with one hand, the clinician generates a radial and extension force with the other on the medial aspect of the patient's hand (Figure 12-52).

Forearm Pronators

Pronator Teres. See earlier discussion.

Pronator Quadratus. The fibers of the pronator quadratus run perpendicular to the direction of the arm, running from

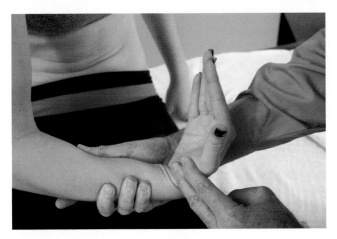

FIGURE 12-50 Test position for the flexor carpi radialis

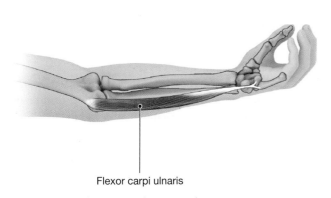

Flexor carpi ulnaris

FIGURE 12-51 Flexor carpi ulnaris muscle

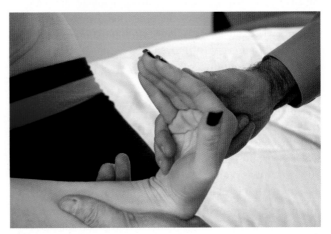

FIGURE 12-52 Test position for the flexor carpi ulnaris

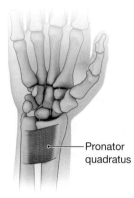

FIGURE 12-53 Pronator quadratus muscle

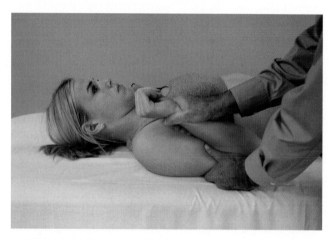

FIGURE 12-54 Test position for the pronator quadratus

the most distal quarter of the anterior ulna to the distal quarter of the anterior radius (Figure 12-53). It is the only muscle that attaches only to the ulna at one end and the radius at the other end.

The pronator quadratus, which is the main pronator of the hand, is innervated by the anterior interosseous branch of the median nerve. The synergists for this muscle include the pronator teres, brachioradialis, and FCR. The antagonists include the biceps brachii, brachioradialis, and supinator.

To specifically test this muscle the patient is positioned in sitting or supine with the elbow completely flexed and the forearm pronated. Using one hand to stabilize the patient's elbow, the clinician places the other hand proximal to the patient's wrist and applies a force into supination while asking the patient to prevent the movement (Figure 12-54).

Flexor Carpi Radialis. See earlier discussion.

Forearm Supinators

Biceps. See earlier discussion. It is important to remember that the effectiveness of the biceps as a supinator is greatest when the elbow is flexed to 90°, placing the biceps tendon at a 90° angle to the radius. In contrast, with the elbow flexed only 30°, much of the rotational efficiency of the biceps is lost.[90]

Supinator. The supinator (Figure 12-55) originates from the lateral epicondyle of the humerus, the lateral collateral ligament (LCL), the annular ligament, the supinator crest, and

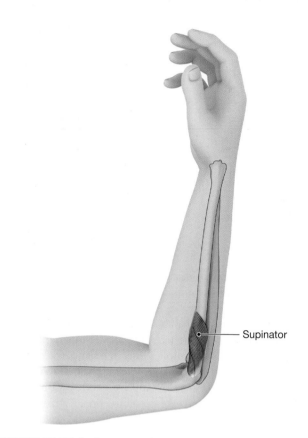

FIGURE 12-55 Supinator muscle

the ulnar fossa. It inserts on the superior third of the anterior and lateral surface of the radius. The supinator muscle is a relentless forearm supinator, similar to the brachialis during elbow flexion. The supinator functions to supinate the forearm in any elbow position, whereas the previously mentioned ECRL and brevis work as supinators during fast movements, and against resistance.

The nervous system usually recruits the supinator muscle for low-power tasks that require a supination motion only, while the biceps remains relatively inactive—a fine example of the law of parsimony.[87]

CLINICAL PEARL

The muscles about the elbow help provide stability by compressing the joint surfaces through muscular contraction.[97] The flexor and pronator muscles, which originate at the medial epicondyle, provide additional static and dynamic support to the medial elbow,[96] with the FCU and flexor digitorum superficialis being the most effective in this regard.[98]

The supinator is innervated by the radial nerve.

The synergists for the supinator include the biceps brachii, and the brachioradialis. The antagonists include the pronator teres, pronator quadratus, brachioradialis, and FCR.

To specifically test this muscle the patient is positioned in standing or sitting. The patient's arm can be positioned in one of two ways:

▶ The shoulder flexed to 90°, the elbow fully flexed, and the forearm fully supinated (Figure 12-56).

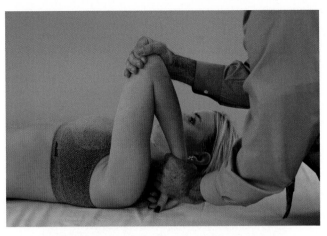

FIGURE 12-56 Test position for the supinator

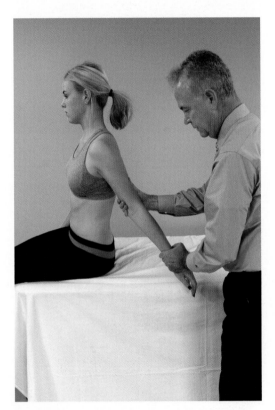

FIGURE 12-57 Alternate test position for the supinator

▶ The shoulder and elbow extended behind the patient and the forearm supinated (Figure 12-57).

Using one hand to stabilize the patient's upper arm at the elbow, the clinician places the other hand just proximal to the patient's wrist and applies a force into pronation while asking the patient to prevent the motion.

Elbow Extensors

There are two muscles that extend the elbow: the triceps and the anconeus (see Table 12-4).

Triceps Brachii. The triceps brachii (Figure 12-58) has three heads of origin. The long head arises from the infraglenoid tuberosity of the scapula, the lateral head from the posterior and lateral surface of the humerus, and the medial head

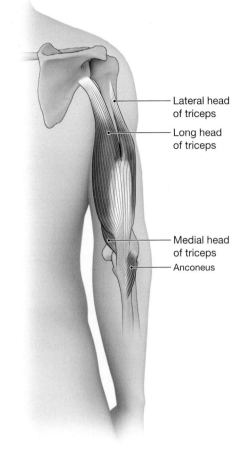

FIGURE 12-58 Triceps brachii and anconeus

from the lower posterior surface of the humerus. The muscle inserts on the superoposterior surface of the olecranon and deep fascia of the forearm. The triceps has its maximal force in movements that combine both elbow extension and shoulder extension. Like the biceps, it is a two-joint muscle. The medial head of the triceps is the workhorse of elbow extension, with the lateral and long heads recruited during heavier loads.[75] During strong contractions of the triceps—for example, a push-up, which involves a combination of elbow extension and shoulder flexion—as the triceps strongly contracts to extend the elbow, the shoulder simultaneously flexes by action of the anterior deltoid, which overpowers the shoulder extension torque of the long head of the triceps.[90]

Anconeus. The anconeus arises from the lateral epicondyle of the humerus and inserts on the lateral aspect of the olecranon and posterior surface of the ulna (see Figure 12-58). The exact function of the anconeus in humans has yet to be determined, although it appears as a fourth head of the elbow extension mechanism, similar to the quadriceps of the knee.[87] It has been suggested that in addition to assisting with elbow extension, the anconeus functions to stabilize the ulnar head in all positions (except radial deviation) and to pull the sub-anconeus bursa and the joint capsule out of the way during extension, thus avoiding impingement.[96,99] The anconeus has also been found to stabilize the elbow during forearm pronation and supination.[93]

The triceps brachii and anconeus are innervated by the radial nerve.

The synergists of the triceps brachii and anconeus include the latissimus dorsi, teres major, and posterior deltoid. The antagonists include the biceps brachii, brachioradialis, brachialis, FCR, FCU, pronator teres, and the extensor carpi radialis longus and brevis.

To specifically test the triceps brachii and anconeus, three different positions can be used:

► *Patient prone.* The patient abducts the shoulder to 90°, extends the elbow fully, and then unlocks it slightly (Figure 12-59).

► *Patient supine.* The patient abducts the shoulder to 90°, extends the elbow fully, and then unlocks it slightly (Figure 12-60).

► *Patient sitting.* The patient abducts the shoulder to 160–180°, extends the elbow fully, and then unlocks it slightly (Figure 12-61). This position is the one used most commonly.

With each of the foregoing positions, the clinician uses one hand to stabilize the upper arm and places the other hand proximal to the patient's wrist. The patient is asked to hold the arm position while the clinician applies a force into elbow flexion.

Substitution or trick motions can include flexion of the shoulder. The gravity-minimized/eliminated position for this

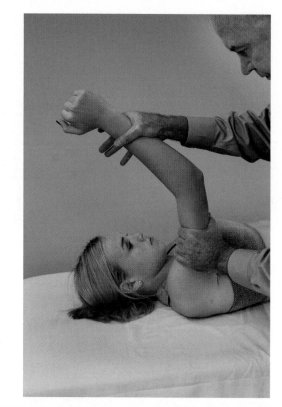

FIGURE 12-60 Test position for the triceps brachii—patient supine

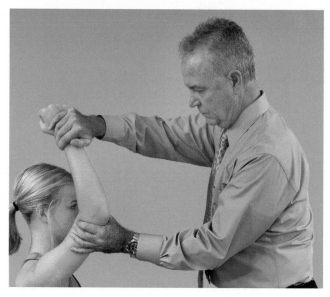

FIGURE 12-61 Test position for the triceps brachii—patient sitting

muscle is with the patient positioned in sitting with the shoulder supported in 90° of abduction and internal rotation and with the elbow flexed and the forearm in neutral.

MUSCLE TESTING OF THE WRIST AND FOREARM

The muscles of the forearm are contained within three major fascial compartments, the anterior forearm, the posterior forearm, and the compartment referred to as the mobile wad (Table 12-5), all of which can be described as the 18 extrinsic

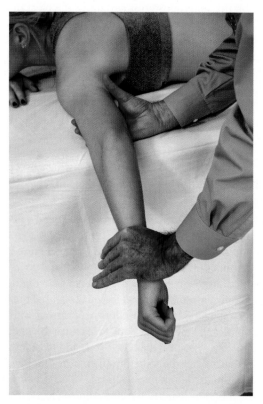

FIGURE 12-59 Test position for the triceps brachii—patient prone

TABLE 12-5	Muscle Compartments of the Forearm
Compartment	**Principal Muscles**
Anterior	Pronator teres
	Flexor carpi radialis
	Palmaris longus
	Flexor digitorum superficialis
	Flexor digitorum profundus
	Flexor pollicis longus
	Flexor carpi ulnaris
	Pronator quadratus
Posterior	Abductor pollicis longus
	Extensor pollicis brevis
	Extensor pollicis longus
	Extensor digitorum communis
	Extensor digitorum proprius
	Extensor digiti quinti
	Extensor carpi ulnaris
Mobile wad	Brachioradialis
	Extensor carpi radialis longus
	Extensor carpi radialis brevis

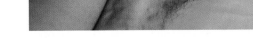

FIGURE 12-62 Test position for the palmaris longus

muscles that originate in the forearm and insert within the hand.[101] The flexors, which are located in the anterior compartment, flex the wrist and digits, whereas the extensors, located in the posterior compartment, extend the wrist and the digits.

The extrinsic group, whose muscle bellies lie proximal to the wrist, join with the intrinsic muscles located entirely within the hand. This design provides for a large number of muscles to act on the hand without excessive bulkiness. The extrinsic tendons enhance wrist stability by balancing flexor and extensor forces and compressing the carpals.

The amount of tendon excursion determines the available range of motion at a joint. To calculate the amount of tendon excursion needed to produce a certain number of degrees of joint motion involves an appreciation of geometry. A circle's radius equals approximately 1 radian (57.29°). The mathematical radius, which is equivalent to the moment arm, represents the amount of tendon excursion required to move the joint through 1 radian.[102] For example, if a joint's moment arm is 10 mm, the tendon must glide 10 mm to move the joint 60° (approximately 1 radian) or 5 mm to move the joint 30° (½ radian).[103]

Anterior Compartment of the Forearm

Superficial Muscles

Pronator Teres. See earlier discussion.

Flexor Carpi Radialis (FCR). See earlier discussion.

Palmaris Longus. The inconsistent palmaris longus (see Figure 12-49) arises from the medial humeral epicondyle as part of the common flexor tendon and inserts on the transverse carpal ligament and palmar aponeurosis. The function of the palmaris longus is to flex the wrist, and it may play a role in thumb abduction in some people.[104]

The palmaris longus is innervated by the median nerve. The synergists of this muscle include the FCR, FCU, flexor digitorum profundus, flexor digitorum superficialis, and

flexor pollicis longus. The antagonists of this muscle include the extensor carpi ulnaris, extensor carpi radialis longus and brevis, extensor digitorum communis, extensor pollicis longus, and extensor indicis.

To specifically test this muscle, the patient is positioned in sitting or supine with the forearm supinated and is asked to flex the wrist and cup the palm (Figure 12-62). While supporting the patient's forearm with one hand, the clinician uses the other hand to apply an uncupping and wrist extension force to the thenar and hypothenar eminences of the patient's hand (see Figure 12-62).

Flexor Carpi Ulnaris (FCU). See earlier discussion.

Intermediate Muscle

Flexor Digitorum Superficialis (FDS). The FDS has a three-headed origin (Figure 12-63). The humeral head arises from the medial humeral epicondyle as part of the common flexor tendon. The ulnar head arises from the coronoid process of the ulna. The radial head arises from the oblique line of the radius. The FDS inserts on the middle phalanx of the medial four digits via a split, "sling" tendon. The FDS serves to flex the proximal and middle interphalangeal joints of the medial four digits and assist with elbow flexion and wrist flexion. The FDS possesses tendons that are capable of relatively independent action at each finger.

The FDS is innervated by the median nerve. The synergists of this muscle include the flexor digitorum profundus, FCR, FCU, palmaris longus, lumbricals, interossei, abductor digiti minimi, flexor digiti minimi, and opponens digiti minimi. The antagonists to this muscle include the extensor carpi radialis longus and brevis, extensor carpi ulnaris, extensor digitorum communis, extensor indicis, lumbricals, and interossei.

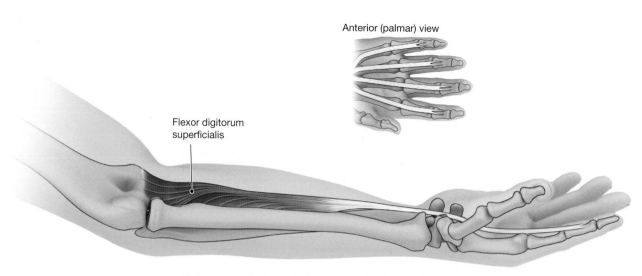

Anterior (palmar) view

FIGURE 12-63 Flexor digitorum superficialis muscle

To specifically test this muscle the patient is positioned in sitting or supine with the forearm supported in supination and the metacarpophalangeal (MCP) joint stabilized by the clinician. The patient is asked to bend the middle phalanx of the finger (Figure 12-64) while the patient maintains the three fingers not being tested into extension and prevents the wrist from excessive flexing (see Figure 12-64). The clinician tests each finger individually by applying an extension force to the anterior aspect of the middle phalanx while asking the patient to prevent the movement.

Deep Muscles

Flexor Pollicis Longus (FPL). The FPL has its origin on the anterior surface of the radius, medial border of the coronoid process of the ulna, and the adjacent interosseous membrane. It inserts on the distal phalanx of the thumb (Figure 12-65). The FPL functions to flex the thumb.

The FPL is innervated by the anterior interosseous branch of the median nerve. The synergists of this muscle include the FCR, FCU, palmaris longus, flexor digitorum profundus, FDS, flexor pollicis brevis, abductor pollicis brevis, and adductor pollicis. The antagonists to this muscle include the extensor carpi radialis longus and brevis, extensor carpi ulna-ris, extensor digitorum communis, extensor indicis, extensor pollicis longus, extensor pollicis brevis, abductor pollicis brevis, and abductor pollicis longus.

To specifically test this muscle, the patient is positioned in sitting or supine with the hand resting on a surface and the forearm in supination. Using one hand, the clinician stabilizes the MCP joint of the thumb into extension (Figure 12-66) and uses the other hand to generate an extension force to the anterior aspect of the distal phalanx of the thumb (see Figure 12-66).

Flexor Digitorum Profundus (FDP). The FDP arises from the medial and anterior surfaces of the proximal ulna, the adjacent interosseous membrane, and the deep fascia of the forearm (Figure 12-67). The FDP inserts on the base of the distal phalanges of the medial four digits. The FDP functions to flex the distal interphalangeal (DIP) joints, after the FDS flexes the second phalanges, and assists with flexion of the wrist. The tendons of the FDS and FDP are held against the phalanges by a fibrous sheath. At strategic locations along the sheath, five dense annular pulleys (designated A1, A2, A3, A4, and A5) and three thinner cruciform pulleys (designated C1, C2, and C3) prevent the tendons from bowstringing.[105]

CLINICAL PEARL

Tendinous connections between the FDP and the FPL are a common anatomic anomaly, which has been linked to a condition causing chronic forearm pain, called Linburg syndrome,[106] although the association is by no means conclusive.[107]

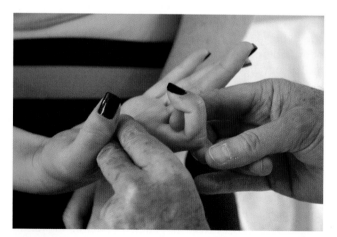

FIGURE 12-64 Test position for the flexor digitorum superficialis

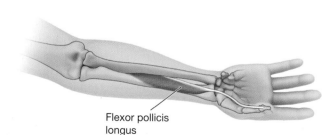

Flexor pollicis longus

FIGURE 12-65 Flexor pollicis longus muscle

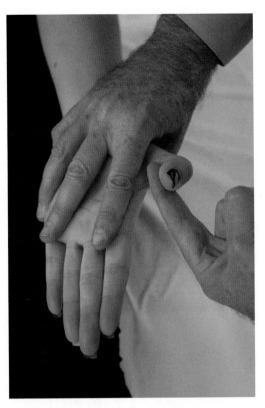

FIGURE 12-66 Test position for flexor pollicis longus

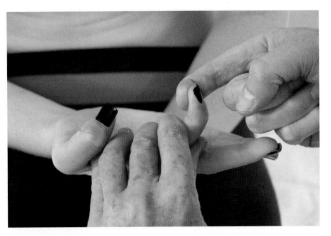

FIGURE 12-68 Test position for flexor digitorum profundus muscle

To specifically test this muscle, the patient is positioned in sitting or supine with the wrist in a neutral position or slightly extended. Using one hand, the clinician stabilizes the proximal and middle phalanges of the finger to be tested. The patient is asked to flex the DIP joint of the finger while the clinician applies an extension force to the anterior aspect of the DIP (Figure 12-68).

Pronator Quadratus. See earlier discussion.

Posterior Compartment of the Forearm

Superficial Muscles

Extensor Carpi Radialis Longus (ECRL). See earlier discussion.

Extensor Carpi Radialis Brevis (ECRB). The ECRB arises from the common extensor tendon on the lateral epicondyle of the humerus, and from the radial collateral ligament (see Figure 12-47). It inserts on the posterior surface of the base of the third metacarpal bone. The muscle stretches across the radial head during pronation, resulting in increased tensile stress when the forearm is pronated, the wrist is flexed, and

The FDP has a dual nerve supply: the medial two heads are supplied by the ulnar nerve, whereas the lateral two heads are supplied by the anterior interosseous branch of the median nerve. The synergists of this muscle include the FCR, FCU, palmaris longus, FDS, FPL, lumbricals, interossei, abductor digiti minimi, flexor digiti minimi, and opponens digiti minimi. The antagonists of this muscle include the extensor carpi radialis longus and brevis, extensor carpi ulnaris, extensor digitorum communis, extensor indicis, extensor pollicis longus, lumbricals, and interossei.

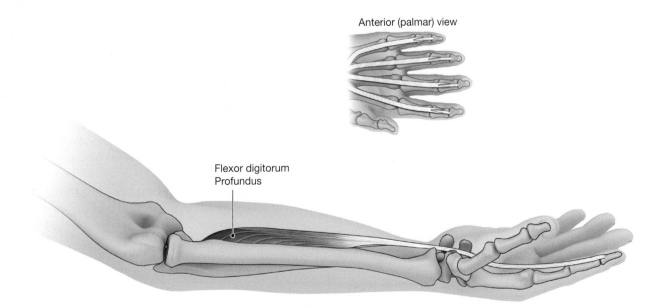

Anterior (palmar) view

Flexor digitorum
Profundus

FIGURE 12-67 Flexor digitorum profundus muscle

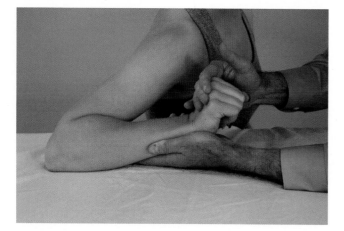

FIGURE 12-69 Test position for the extensor carpi radialis brevis

the elbow is extended. The more medial location of the ECRB compared to the ECRL makes it the primary wrist extensor, but it has also a slight action of radial deviation.

CLINICAL PEARL

The ECRB and ECRL are commonly considered to be similar muscles, but in fact they differ in many respects.[108] The ECRB, because of its origin on the epicondyle, is not affected by the position of the elbow, so that all of its action is on the wrist.[109] Taken together, both ECR tendons comprise about 10% of the muscle mass of the forearm and 76% of the muscle mass of the extensors of the wrist.[110] The ECRL has longer muscular fibers, mostly at the level of the elbow.

The ECRB receives its nerve supply from the posterior interosseous branch of the radial nerve. The synergists and antagonists of this muscle are similar to those of the ECRL except for those that cross the elbow.

To specifically test this muscle, the patient is positioned in sitting or supine with the elbow fully flexed (to place the ECRL in a position of mechanical insufficiency), and the forearm just short of full pronation supported by the examiner or the table (Figure 12-69). The patient is asked to extend the wrist in a radial direction and to hold that position while the clinician applies pressure on the posterior aspect of the hand along the second and third metacarpal bones.

Extensor Digitorum Communis (EDC). The EDC, which consists of the extensor indices, extensor digiti minimi, and extensor digitorum, arises from the lateral humeral epicondyle, part of the common extensor tendon and inserts on the lateral and posterior aspect of the medial four digits (Figure 12-70). The EDC functions to extend the medial four digits.

The EDC is innervated by the posterior interosseous branch of the radial nerve. The synergists of this muscle include the extensor carpi radialis longus and brevis, extensor carpi ulnaris, extensor indicis, extensor pollicis longus, lumbricals, and interossei. The antagonist of this muscle include the FCR, FCU, palmaris longus, FDP, FDS, flexor pollicis longus, lumbricals, interossei, abductor digiti minimi, flexor digiti minimi, and opponens digiti minimi.

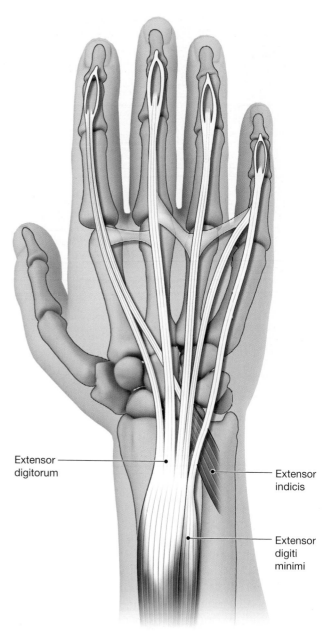

Extensor digitorum

Extensor indicis

Extensor digiti minimi

FIGURE 12-70 Extensor digitorum communis muscle

To specifically test this muscle the patient is positioned supine or sitting with the forearm pronated, the wrist positioned in neutral—halfway between flexion and extension—and the MCP and proximal interphalangeal (PIP) joints slightly flexed. The patient is asked to extend the MCP of the finger to be tested and to hold that position. The clinician uses one hand to stabilize the wrist and, using two fingers of the other hand, applies pressure against the posterior surfaces of the patient's proximal phalanges (Figure 12-71).

Extensor Digiti Minimi (EDM). The EDM arises from a muscular slip from the ulnar aspect of the extensor digitorum muscle and inserts on the proximal phalanx of the fifth digit. The EDM extends the MCP of the fifth digit and, in conjunction with the lumbricals and interossei, extends the interphalangeal joints of the fifth digit. The EDM also assists in abduction of the fifth digit.

The EDM is innervated by the posterior interosseous branch of the radial nerve.

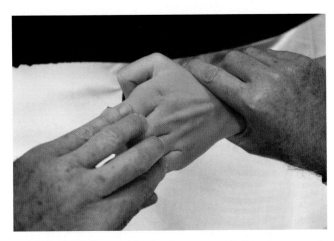

FIGURE 12-71 Test position for the extensor digitorum communis

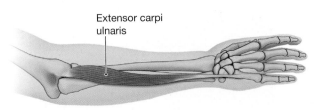

Extensor carpi
ulnaris

FIGURE 12-72 Extensor carpi ulnaris muscle

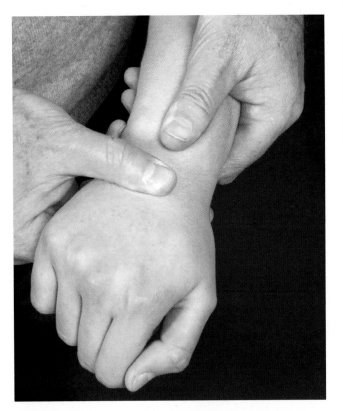

FIGURE 12-73 Test position for the extensor carpi ulnaris

To specifically test this muscle the patient is positioned supine or sitting with the forearm pronated, the wrist positioned in neutral—halfway between flexion and extension—and the MCP and PIP joints slightly flexed. The patient is asked to extend the MCP of the fifth digit and to hold that position. The clinician uses one hand to stabilize the wrist and, using two fingers of the other hand, applies pressure against the posterior surface of the patient's proximal phalange.

Extensor Carpi Ulnaris (ECU). The ECU arises from the common extensor tendon on the lateral epicondyle of the humerus and the posterior border of the ulna (Figure 12-72). It inserts on the medial side of the base of the fifth metacarpal bone. The ECU is an extensor of the wrist in supination, and primarily causes ulnar deviation of the wrist in pronation,

working in synergy with the FCU to prevent radial deviation during pronation.[109]

The ECU is innervated by the posterior interosseous branch of the radial nerve. The synergists for this muscle include the FCU, FPL, extensor carpi radialis longus and brevis, EDC, extensor indicis, and extensor pollicis longus. The antagonist of this muscle include the FCR, extensor carpi radialis longus and brevis, extensor pollicis brevis, abductor pollicis longus, FCU, palmaris longus, FDP, FDS, and FPL.

To specifically test this muscle, the patient is positioned sitting or supine with the forearm positioned in complete pronation. The patient is asked to extend the wrist in an ulnar direction and to hold this position. Using one hand to stabilize the patient's forearm, the clinician uses the other hand to apply pressure to the posterior aspect of the patient's hand along the fifth metacarpal bone in a radial direction (Figure 12-73).

Deep Muscles

Abductor Pollicis Longus (APL). The APL arises from the dorsal surface of the proximal portion of the radius, ulna, and interosseous membrane and inserts on the ventral surface of the base of the first metacarpal (Figure 12-74). The APL functions in abduction, extension, and external rotation of the first metacarpal.

The APL is innervated by the posterior interosseous branch of the radial nerve. The synergists of this muscle include the FCR, extensor carpi radialis longus and brevis, abductor pollicis brevis, and extensor pollicis brevis. The antagonists of this muscle include the FCU, extensor carpi ulnaris, FPL, flexor pollicis brevis, and adductor pollicis.

CLINICAL PEARL

Extension of the wrist is dependent on three muscles:

▶ Extensor carpi radialis longus (ECRL).

▶ Extensor carpi radialis brevis (ECRB).

▶ Extensor carpi ulnaris (ECU).

The ECRL only becomes a wrist extensor after radial deviation is balanced against the ulnar forces of the ECU.

The ECU, the antagonist of the extensor pollicis longus (EPL), has the weakest moment of extension, which becomes zero when the wrist is in complete pronation.

Thus, the three wrist extensors have very different moment arms of extension. The ECRB is the most effective extensor of the wrist, because it has the greatest tension and the most favorable moment arm.[109]

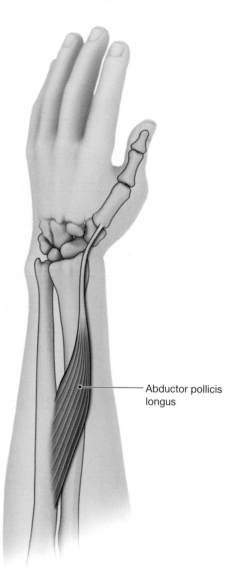

Abductor pollicis longus

FIGURE 12-74 Abductor pollicis longus muscle

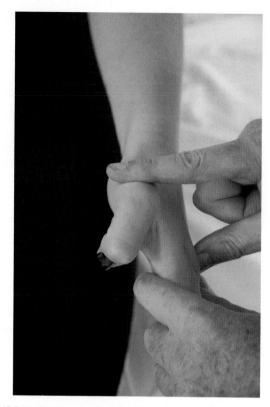

FIGURE 12-75 Test position for the abductor pollicis longus

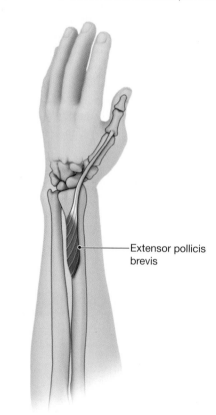

Extensor pollicis brevis

FIGURE 12-76 Extensor pollicis brevis muscle

To specifically test this muscle, the patient is positioned sitting or supine. The patient is asked to abduct and slightly extend the thumb and to hold that position. Using one hand, the clinician stabilizes the patient's hand and uses the other hand to apply an adduction and flexion force against the lateral aspect of the distal first metacarpal (Figure 12-75).

Extensor Pollicis Brevis (EPB). The EPB arises from the posterior surface of the radius and interosseous membrane, just distal to the origin of the APL. It inserts on the posterior surface of the proximal phalanx of the thumb via the extensor expansion (Figure 12-76). The EPB functions in extension of the proximal phalanx of the thumb.

The EPB is innervated by the posterior interosseous branch of the radial nerve. The synergists of this muscle include the FCR, extensor carpi radialis longus and brevis, abductor pollicis longus, and abductor pollicis brevis. The antagonists of this muscle include the FCU, extensor carpi ulnaris, flexor pollicis longus, flexor pollicis brevis, and adductor pollicis.

To specifically test this muscle, the patient is positioned sitting or supine with the MCP joint of the thumb extended. Using one hand, the clinician stabilizes the patient's hand,

while using a finger from the other hand to apply a flexion force against the proximal phalanx of the thumb (Figure 12-77).

Extensor Pollicis Longus (EPL). The EPL arises from the posterior surface of the midportion of the ulna and interosseous membrane. It inserts on the posterior surface of the

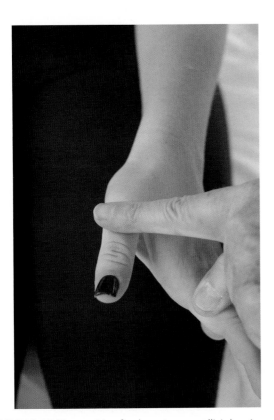

FIGURE 12-77 Test position for the extensor pollicis brevis

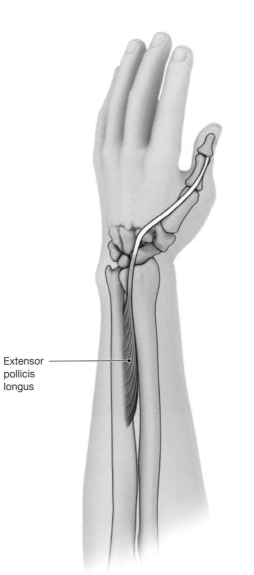

Extensor pollicis longus

FIGURE 12-78 Extensor pollicis longus muscle

distal phalanx of the thumb via the extensor expansion (Figure 12-78). The EPL functions in extension of the distal phalanx of the thumb and is thus involved in extension of the middle phalanx and the MCP joint of the thumb.

The EPL is innervated by the posterior interosseous branch of the radial nerve. The synergists of this muscle include the abductor pollicis brevis, flexor pollicis brevis, adductor pollicis, extensor carpi radialis longus and brevis, extensor carpi ulnaris, extensor digitorum communis, extensor indicis, and first anterior interosseous. The antagonists of this muscle include the flexor pollicis longus, flexor pollicis brevis, abductor pollicis brevis, FCR, FCU, palmaris longus, FDP, and FDS.

To specifically test this muscle, the patient is positioned in sitting or supine with the thumb extended. The clinician uses one hand to stabilize the patient's hand and uses the other to apply a flexion force to the distal phalanx of the posterior surface of the patient's thumb (Figure 12-79).

Extensor Indicis (EI). The EI arises from the posterior surface of the ulna, distal to the other deep muscles, and inserts on the extensor expansion of the index finger. The EI is involved in extension of the proximal phalanx of the index finger.

The EI is innervated by the posterior interosseous branch of the radial nerve. The synergists of this muscle include the extensor carpi radialis longus and brevis, extensor carpi ulnaris, EDC, EPL, lumbricals, and interossei. The antagonists of this muscle include the FCR, FCU, palmaris longus, FDP, FDS, FPL, lumbricals, and interossei.

To specifically test this muscle, the patient is positioned in sitting or supine and is asked to extend the index finger.

The clinician uses one hand to stabilize the patient's hand and uses the other hand to generate a flexion force to the posterior aspect of the proximal phalanx of the index finger (see Figure 12-71).

MUSCLE TESTING OF THE HAND

The muscles of the hand are those that originate and insert within the hand and are responsible for the fine finger movements.

Short Muscles of the Thumb

Abductor Pollicis Brevis (APB). The APB arises from the flexor retinaculum and the trapezium bone and inserts on the radial aspect of the proximal phalanx of the thumb (Figure 12-80). The APB functions to abduct the first metacarpal and proximal phalanx of the thumb.

The APB is innervated by the median nerve. The synergists of this muscle include the abductor pollicis longus, flexor pollicis longus, and flexor pollicis brevis. The antagonists of

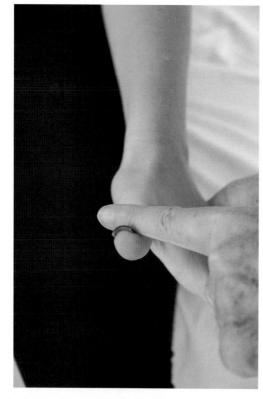

FIGURE 12-79 Test position for the extensor pollicis longus

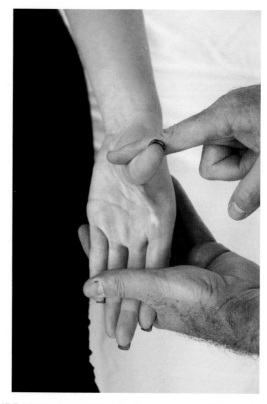

FIGURE 12-81 Test position for the abductor pollicis brevis

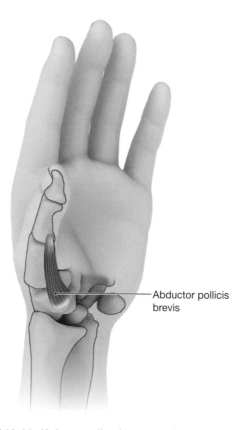

Abductor pollicis brevis

FIGURE 12-80 Abductor pollicis brevis muscle

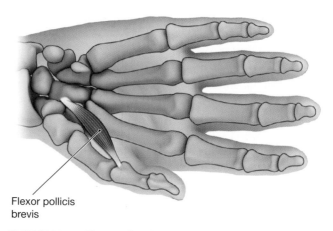

Flexor pollicis brevis

FIGURE 12-82 Flexor pollicis brevis muscle

uses the other hand to generate a downward force against the proximal phalanx of the patient's thumb (Figure 12-81).

Flexor Pollicis Brevis (FPB). The FPB arises from two heads. The superficial head arises from the flexor retinaculum and the trapezium bone, whereas the deep head arises from the floor of the carpal canal (Figure 12-82). The FPB inserts on the base of the proximal phalanx of the thumb. The FPB functions to flex the proximal phalanx of the thumb.

The FPB has dual innervation—the superficial head receives its innervation from the median nerve, whereas the deep head is innervated by the ulnar nerve. The synergists to this muscle include the flexor pollicis longus, abductor pollicis brevis, and adductor pollicis. The antagonists of this muscle include the extensor pollicis longus and extensor pollicis brevis.

this muscle include the abductor pollicis and extensor pollicis longus.

To specifically test this muscle, the patient is positioned in sitting or supine and is asked to abduct the thumb. Using one hand, the clinician stabilizes the patient's wrist and hand and

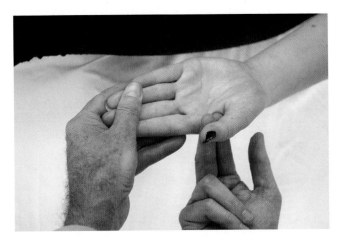

FIGURE 12-83 Test position for the flexor pollicis brevis

To specifically test this muscle, the patient is positioned in sitting or supine and is asked to flex the thumb. Using one hand, the clinician stabilizes the patient's wrist and hand and uses the other hand to apply an extension force to the anterior surface of the proximal phalanx of the patient's thumb (Figure 12-83).

Opponens Pollicis (OP). The OP arises from the flexor retinaculum and the trapezium bone and inserts along the radial surface of the first metacarpal (Figure 12-84). The OP functions to flex, rotate, and slightly abduct the first metacarpal across the palm to allow for opposition to each of the other digits.

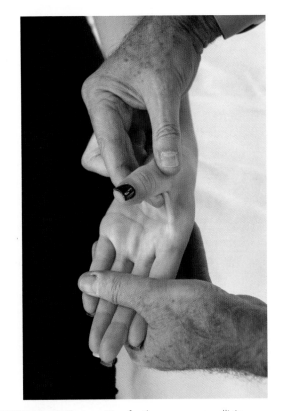

FIGURE 12-85 Test position for the opponens pollicis

The OP is innervated by the median nerve. The synergists of this muscle include the flexor pollicis brevis and adductor pollicis. The antagonists include the extensor pollicis longus and extensor pollicis brevis.

To specifically test this muscle, the patient is positioned in sitting or supine and is asked to touch his or her thumb to the little finger (a combination of flexion, abduction, and slight internal rotation). The clinician uses one hand to stabilize the patient's wrist and hand, and the other hand to generate pressure to the metacarpal bone of the thumb in an adduction and external rotation and extension direction (Figure 12-85).

Adductor Pollicis (AP). The AP arises from two heads. The transverse head originates from the ventral surface of the shaft of the third metacarpal, whereas the oblique head originates from the trapezium, trapezoid, and capitate bones (Figure 12-86) and the base of the second and third metacarpal bone. The AP inserts on the ulnar side of the base of the proximal phalanx of the thumb. The AP functions to adduct the carpometacarpal joint and adducts and assists in flexion of the MCP joints and opposition of the thumb. The AP may also assist in extending the interphalangeal joint.

The AP is innervated by the deep branch of the ulnar nerve. The synergists of this muscle include the extensor pollicis longus, flexor pollicis longus, flexor pollicis brevis, opponens pollicis, and first anterior interossei. The antagonists include the abductor pollicis brevis, abductor pollicis longus, flexor pollicis longus, and extensor pollicis brevis.

To specifically test this muscle, the patient is positioned in sitting or supine and is asked to move the thumb toward the palm. Using one hand, the clinician stabilizes the patient's wrist and hand, while using the other to apply an abduction force to the inner aspect of the thumb (Figure 12-87).

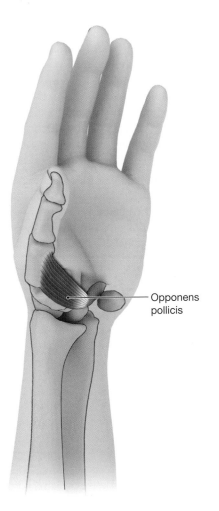

Opponens pollicis

FIGURE 12-84 Opponens pollicis muscle

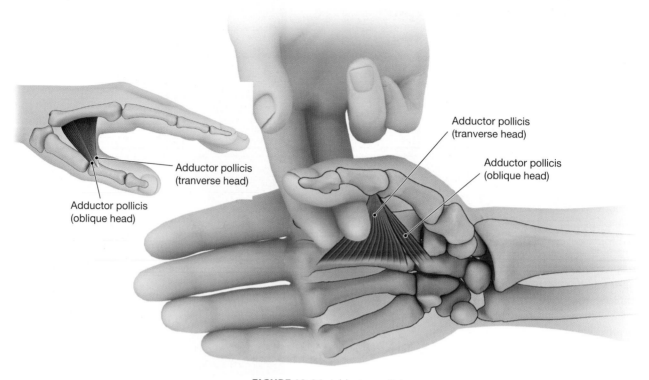

FIGURE 12-86 Adductor pollicis

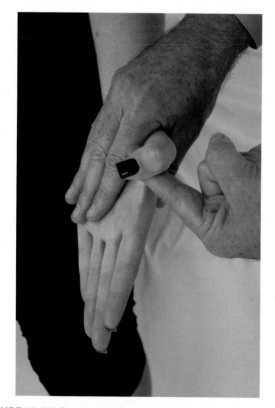

FIGURE 12-87 Test position for the adductor pollicis

Short Muscles of the Fifth Digit

Abductor Digiti Minimi (ADM). The ADM arises from the pisiform bone and the tendon of the flexor carpi ulnaris. It inserts on the ulnar aspect of the base of the proximal phalanx of the fifth digit, together with the flexor digiti minimi brevis (Figure 12-88). The ADM functions to abduct the fifth digit.

The ADM is innervated by the deep branch of the ulnar nerve. The synergists for this muscle include the interossei, FDP, FDS, and fourth lumbrical. The antagonists to this muscle include the anterior interossei, extensor digitorum communis, and extensor digiti minimi.

To specifically test this muscle, the patient is positioned sitting or supine and is asked to abduct the little finger. The clinician uses one hand to stabilize the patient's wrist and hand, and the other to apply an adduction force against the ulnar aspect of the middle phalanx of the patient's fifth digit (Figure 12-89).

Flexor Digiti Minimi (FDM). The FDM originates from the flexor retinaculum and the hook of the hamate bone (Figure 12-90). It inserts on the ulnar aspect of the base of the proximal phalanx of the fifth digit, together with the abductor digiti minimi. The FDM functions to flex the proximal phalanx of the fifth digit.

CLINICAL PEARL

Deep branches of the ulnar artery and nerve enter the thenar mass, and course into the deep region of the hand by passing between the ABD and the FDM.

The FDM is innervated by the deep branch of the ulnar nerve. The synergists for this muscle include the opponens digiti minimi, lumbricals 3 and 4, interossei, flexor digitorum profundus, and flexor digitorum superficialis. The antagonists include the extensor digitorum communis and extensor digiti minimi.

To specifically test this muscle, the patient is positioned sitting or supine and is asked to flex the little finger at the MCP joint while maintaining the interphalangeal joint in extension. Using

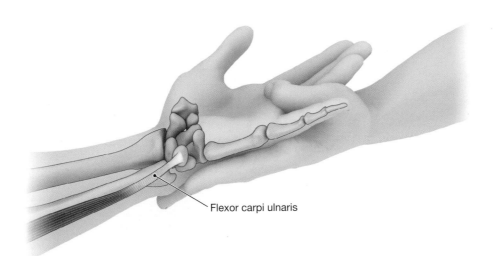

FIGURE 12-88 Abductor digiti minimi muscle

one hand, the clinician stabilizes the patient's hand, while using the other to apply an extension force against the flexed proximal phalanx of the patient's fifth digit (Figure 12-91).

Opponens Digiti Minimi (ODM). The ODM arises from the flexor retinaculum and the hook of the hamate bone and inserts on the ulnar border of the shaft of the fifth metacarpal bone (Figure 12-92). The ODM functions to provide a small amount of flexion and external rotation of the fifth digit.

The ODM is innervated by the deep branch of the ulnar nerve. The synergists of this muscle include the flexor digiti minimi, abductor digiti minimi, fourth lumbricals, third and fourth anterior interossei, flexor digitorum superficialis, and flexor digitorum profundus. The antagonists include the extensor digitorum communis, extensor digiti minimi, and abductor digiti minimi.

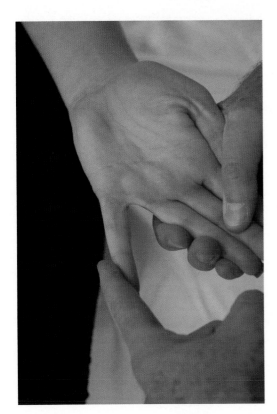

FIGURE 12-89 Test position for the abductor digiti minimi

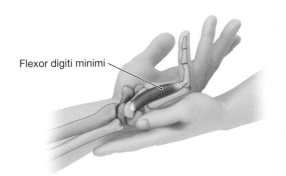

FIGURE 12-90 Flexor digiti minimi muscle

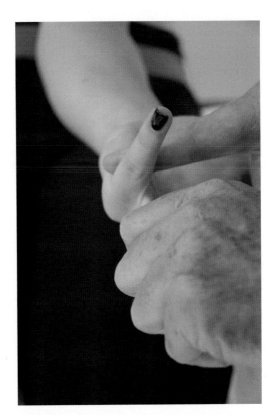

FIGURE 12-91 Test position for the flexor digiti minimi

369

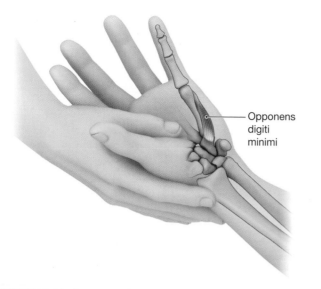

FIGURE 12-92 Opponens digiti minimi muscle

To specifically test this muscle, the patient is positioned in sitting or supine and is asked to try to cup the fifth metacarpal toward the thumb. Using one hand, the clinician stabilizes the patient's hand, while using the index finger of the other hand to push against the first metacarpal of the fifth digit and apply a downward force (Figure 12-93).

Interosseous Muscles of the Hand

The interossei muscles of the hand are divided by anatomy and function into anterior (palmar) and posterior (dorsal) interossei.

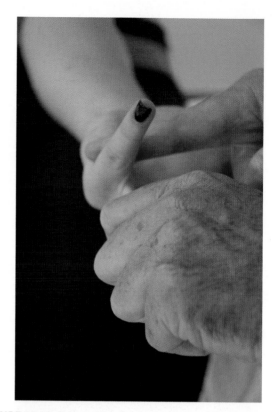

FIGURE 12-93 Test position for the opponens digit minimi

Anterior Interossei. The three anterior (palmar) interossei have a variety of origins and insertions (Figure 12-94). The first interosseus originates from the ulnar surface of the second metacarpal bone and inserts on the ulnar side of the proximal phalanx of the second digit. The second palmar

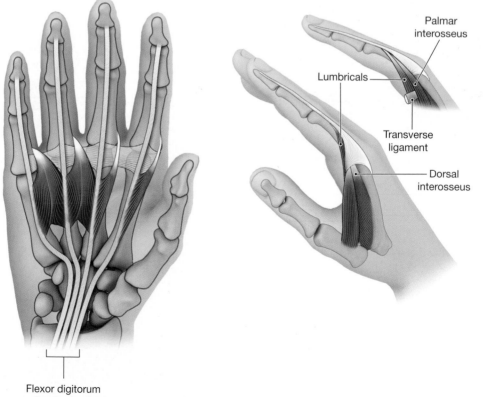

FIGURE 12-94 Lumbricals, anterior and posterior interossei

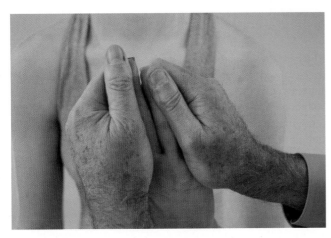

FIGURE 12-95 Test position for the anterior interossei

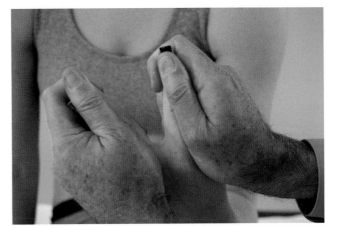

FIGURE 12-96 Test position for the posterior interossei

interosseus arises from the radial side of the fourth metacarpal bone and inserts into the radial side of the proximal phalanx of the fourth digit. The third palmar interosseus originates from the radial side of the fifth metacarpal bone and inserts into the radial side of the proximal phalanx of the fifth digit. Each of the anterior interossei functions to adduct the digit to which it is attached toward the middle digit. The anterior interossei also function to extend the distal and then the middle phalanges.

The anterior interossei are innervated by the deep branch of the ulnar nerve. The synergists to the anterior interossei include the posterior interossei, lumbricals, flexor digitorum profundus and superficialis, extensor indicis, extensor digitorum communis, extensor digiti minimi, abductor digiti minimi, flexor digiti minimi, opponens digiti minimi, and adductor pollicis. The antagonists to the anterior interossei include the posterior interossei, extensor digitorum communis, extensor indicis, extensor digiti minimi, abductor digiti minimi, flexor digitorum profundus and superficialis, and lumbricals.

To specifically test this muscle group, the patient is positioned sitting or supine with the digits not being tested stabilized, and the finger being tested brought toward midline. One by one, the clinician applies pressure in an abduction direction against the appropriate phalanx of the thumb, index, ring, and little finger (Figure 12-95).

Posterior Interossei. The four posterior (dorsal) interossei have a varied origin and insertion similar to those of their anterior counterparts (see Figure 12-94). The posterior interossei originate via two heads from adjacent sides of the metacarpal bones. The first posterior interosseus muscle inserts into the radial side of the proximal phalanx of the second digit. The second inserts into the radial side of the proximal phalanx of the third digit. The third inserts into the ulnar side of the proximal phalanx of the third digit, and the fourth inserts into the ulnar side of the proximal phalanx of the fourth digit. The posterior interossei abduct the index, middle, and ring fingers from the midline of the hand.

The posterior interossei receive their innervation from the deep branch of the ulnar nerve.

To specifically test this muscle group, the patient is positioned sitting or supine with the digits not being tested stabilized, and the finger being tested moved away from midline. One by one, the clinician applies pressure in the direction

of adduction against the appropriate phalanx of the thumb, index, ring, and little finger (Figure 12-96).

Lumbricals

The lumbrical muscles are usually four small intrinsic muscles of the hand that originate from the FDP tendons and insert into the dorsal hood apparatus (see Figure 12-94). Occasionally, more than four lumbricals are found in one hand.[111]

During contraction, the lumbricals pull the FDP tendons distally, thus possessing the unique ability to relax their own antagonist.[112] They function to perform the motion of interphalangeal joint extension with the MCP joint held in extension and can assist in MCP flexion.[109]

The lumbrical muscles also serve an important role in the proprioception of the hand, providing feedback about the position and movement of the hand and finger joints.[112]

CLINICAL PEARL

In instances of lumbrical spasm or contracture, attempts to flex the fingers via the FDP result in transmission of force through the lumbricals into the extensor apparatus, producing extension rather than flexion.[112] A "lumbrical plus" deformity occurs if there is excessive lumbrical force, or if there is imbalance of opposing forces, which produces exaggerated lumbrical action (i.e., MCP joint flexion and interphalangeal joint extension).[112]

The lumbricals have dual innervation. Lumbricals I and II are innervated typically by the median nerve, whereas the third and fourth lumbricals are innervated by the ulnar nerve. The synergists for the lumbricals include the posterior interossei, flexor digitorum profundus and superficialis, abductor digiti minimi, flexor digiti minimi, opponens digiti minimi, extensor digitorum communis, extensor indices, and anterior interossei. The antagonists include the extensor digitorum communis, extensor indices, anterior interossei, and flexor digitorum profundus and superficialis.

To specifically test this muscle group, the patient is positioned in sitting or supine and is asked to place the hand into an intrinsic plus position (Figure 12-97) and to hold a piece of paper. Using one hand, the clinician tries to pull a sheet of

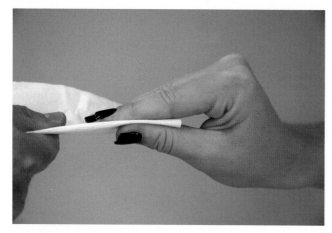

FIGURE 12-97 Test position for the lumbricals

paper from the patient's grasp. Pressure is thus applied in two distinct phases:

1. A flexion force is applied to the posterior surfaces of the distal and middle phalanges.
2. An extension force is applied to the anterior surfaces of the proximal phalanges.

MUSCLE TESTING OF THE HIP

The hip joint is surrounded by a large number of muscles that accelerate, decelerate, and stabilize the hip joint. Indeed, 21 muscles cross the hip, providing both triplanar movement and stability between the femur and acetabulum.[113] Consequently, abnormal performance of the hip muscles may alter the distribution of forces across the joint articular surfaces, potentially causing, or at least predisposing, degenerative changes in the articular cartilage, bone, and surrounding connective tissues.[113]

CLINICAL PEARL

Because the hip joint is able to move through a wide ROM, a muscle's line of pull may be altered with changing hip positions, which makes describing a muscles action difficult. For example, the orientation of the gluteus medius allows it to work as an internal rotator in hip flexion yet as a weak external rotator in hip extension.[114] Similarly, the tensor fasciae latae is a hip abductor and flexor, depending on position, while being a weak internal rotator in all positions.[75]

TABLE 12-6	Origin, Insertion, and Innervation of Muscles Acting across the Hip Joint		
Muscle	**Origin**	**Insertion**	**Innervation**
Adductor brevis	External aspect of the body and inferior ramus of the pubis.	The line from the greater trochanter of the linea aspera of the femur	Obturator nerve
Adductor longus	In angle between pubic crest and symphysis.	The middle third of the linea aspera of the femur	Obturator nerve
Adductor magnus	Inferior ramus of pubis, ramus of ischium, and the inferolateral aspect of the ischial tuberosity.	To the linea aspera and adductor tubercle of the femur	Obturator nerve and tibial portion of the sciatic nerve
Biceps femoris	Long head arises from the sacrotuberous ligament and posterior aspect of the ischial tuberosity. Short head does not act across the hip.	On the lateral aspect of the head of the fibula, the lateral condyle of the tibial tuberosity, the lateral collateral ligament, and the deep fascia of the leg	Tibial portion of the sciatic nerve, S1
Gemelli (superior and inferior)	Superior–posterior (dorsal) surface of the spine of the ischium and inferior-upper part of the tuberosity of the ischium.	Superior- and inferior-medial surface of the greater trochanter	Sacral plexus
Gluteus maximus	Posterior gluteal line of the ilium, iliac crest, aponeurosis of the erector spinae, posterior (dorsal) surface of the lower part of the sacrum, side of the coccyx, sacrotuberous ligament, and intermuscular fascia.	Iliotibial tract of the fasciae latae and gluteal tuberosity of the femur	Inferior gluteal nerve
Gluteus medius	Outer surface of the ilium between the iliac crest and the posterior gluteal line, anterior gluteal line, and fascia.	Lateral surface of the greater trochanter	Superior gluteal nerve
Gluteus minimus	Outer surface of the ilium between the anterior and inferior gluteal lines, and the margin of the greater sciatic notch.	On the anterior surface of the greater trochanter	Superior gluteal nerve
Gracilis	The body and inferior ramus of the pubis.	The superior medial surface of the proximal tibia, just proximal to the tendon of the semitendinosus	Obturator nerve

TABLE 12-6	Origin, Insertion, and Innervation of Muscles Acting across the Hip Joint (continued)		
Muscle	**Origin**	**Insertion**	**Innervation**
Iliacus	Superior two-thirds of the iliac fossa and upper surface of the lateral part of the sacrum.	Fibers converge with tendon of the psoas major to lesser trochanter.	Femoral nerve.
Obturator externus	Rami of the pubis, ramus of the ischium, and medial two-thirds of the outer surface of the obturator membrane.	Trochanteric fossa of the femur.	Obturator nerve.
Obturator internus	Internal surface of the anterolateral wall of the pelvis and obturator membrane.	Medial surface of the greater trochanter.	Sacral plexus.
Pectineus	Pectineal line.	Along a line extending from the lesser trochanter to the linea aspera.	Femoral or obturator or accessory obturator nerves.
Piriformis	Pelvic surface of the sacrum, gluteal surface of the ilium, capsule of the sacroiliac joint, and sacrotuberous ligament.	Upper border of the greater trochanter of femur.	Sacral plexus.
Psoas major	Transverse processes of all the lumbar vertebrae bodies and intervertebral disks of the lumbar vertebrae.	Lesser trochanter of the femur.	Lumbar plexus.
Quadratus femoris	Ischial body next to the ischial tuberosity.	Quadrate tubercle on femur.	Nerve to quadratus femoris.
Rectus femoris	By two heads, from the anterior–inferior iliac spine, and a reflected head from the groove above the acetabulum.	Upper border of the patella.	Femoral nerve.
Sartorius	Anterior–superior iliac spine and notch below it.	Upper part of the medial surface of the tibia in front of the gracilis.	Femoral nerve.
Semimembranosus	Ischial tuberosity.	The posterior-medial aspect of the medial condyle of the tibia.	Tibial nerve.
Semitendinosus	Ischial tuberosity.	Upper part of the medial surface of the tibia behind the attachment of the sartorius and below that of the gracilis.	Tibial nerve.
Tensor fascia latae	Anterior part of outer lip of the iliac crest and the lateral surface of the anterior superior iliac spine.	Iliotibial tract.	Superior gluteal nerve.

The hip muscles and their respective actions are outlined in Tables 12-6 and 12-7.

Iliopsoas. The iliopsoas muscle, formed by the iliacus and psoas major muscles (Figure 12-98), is the most powerful of the hip flexors. This muscle also functions as a weak adductor and external rotator of the hip. The iliopsoas attaches to the hip joint capsule, thereby affording it some support. Because the muscle spans both the axial and appendicular components of the skeleton, it also functions as a trunk flexor and affords an important element of vertical stability to the lumbar spine, especially when the hip is in full extension and passive tension is greatest in the muscle.[113,115] Theoretically, a sufficiently strong and isolated bilateral contraction of any hip flexor muscle will rotate the femur toward the pelvis, the pelvis (and possibly the trunk) toward the femur, or both actions simultaneously.[113] The synergists of this muscle include the sartorius, pectineus, tensor fasciae latae, adductor brevis and longus, adductor magnus (anterior portion), gluteus minimus, rectus femoris, gluteus medius, gluteus maximus, piriformis, biceps femoris (long head), and gracilis. The antagonists of this muscle include the erector spinae, gluteus maximus, adductor magnus (posterior portion), gluteus medius, hamstrings, gluteus minimus, tensor fasciae latae, and sartorius.

To specifically test this muscle, the patient is positioned in supine or sitting:

▶ *Supine.* The patient's lower extremity is positioned in knee extension, slight hip abduction, and flexion of the hip (Figure 12-99).

▶ *Sitting.* With the knee flexed, the patient flexes the hip (Figure 12-100).

With both positions, the clinician applies pressure on the distal femur in the direction of hip extension and abduction while the patient attempts to prevent the motion. Caution should be taken to ensure that the patient does not externally

TABLE 12-7	Hip Actions and Muscles If in Anatomic Position	
Hip Action	**Prime Movers**	**Assistant Movers**
Flexors	Iliopsoas Sartorius Tensor fasciae latae Rectus femoris Pectineus Adductor longus	Adductor brevis Gracilis Gluteus minimus (anterior fibers)
Extensors	Gluteus maximus Semitendinosus Semimembranosus Biceps femoris (long head) Adductor magnus (posterior head)	Gluteus medius (middle and posterior fibers) Adductor magnus (anterior head)
Abductors	Gluteus medius (all fibers) Gluteus minimus (all fibers) Tensor fasciae latae	Sartorius Rectus femoris Piriformis
Adductors	Adductor magnus (anterior and posterior heads) Adductor longus Adductor brevis Gracilis Pectineus	Biceps femoris (long head) Gluteus maximus (posterior fibers) Quadratus lumborum Obturator externus
External rotators	Gluteus maximus Gemellus inferior Gemellus superior Obturator internus Quadratus femoris Piriformis (at less than 60° hip flexion)	Gluteus medius (posterior fibers) Gluteus minimus (posterior fibers Biceps femoris (long head) Sartorius Obturator externus
Internal rotators	No prime movers	Semitendinosus Semimembranosus Gracilis Piriformis (at 90° hip flexion) Gluteus medius (anterior fibers) Adductor longus Adductor brevis Pectineus Adductor magnus (posterior head) Gluteus minimus (anterior fibers) Tensor fasciae latae

Data from Anderson LC: The anatomy and biomechanics of the hip joint. J Back Musculoskeletal Rehabil 4:145–153, 1994; and Neumann DA: Kinesiology of the hip: a focus on muscular actions. J Orthop Sports Phys Ther 40:82-94, 2010.

rotate the femur, as this will cause the hip adductors to contract. Substitution or trick motions can include hip abduction and external rotation, hip abduction and internal rotation, or assistance from the rectus femoris. The gravity-minimized/eliminated position for this muscle is with the patient positioned in sidelying with the extremity supported on a friction-free surface and the hip positioned in neutral rotation with the knee flexed to 90°.

Gluteus Maximus. The gluteus maximus (Figure 12-101) is the largest and most important hip extensor and external rotator of the hip. The muscle consists of a larger superficial and a deep portion. The inferior gluteal nerve, which innervates the muscle, is located on the deep portion.

The gluteus maximus is usually active only when the hip is in flexion, such as during stair climbing or cycling, or when extension of the hip is resisted.[116] The synergists for this muscle include the adductor magnus, gluteus medius, hamstrings, gluteus minimus, tensor fasciae latae, piriformis, sartorius, iliopsoas, adductor brevis and longus, pectineus, and gracilis. The antagonists of this muscle include the iliopsoas; pectineus; tensor fasciae latae; adductor magnus, brevis, and longus; gluteus medius and minimus; sartorius; rectus femoris; gracilis; and piriformis.

To specifically test this muscle, the patient is positioned in prone with the knee flexed to at least 90° (to eliminate hamstring activation) and the hip extended (Figure 12-102). The clinician applies a force over the distal femur in a direction of hip flexion while the patient attempts to prevent the motion. Substitution or trick motions can include assistance from the hamstrings or an increase in the lumbar lordosis. The gravity-minimized/eliminated position for this muscle is with the patient positioned in sidelying with the extremity supported, the hip flexed to 90°, and the knee flexed.

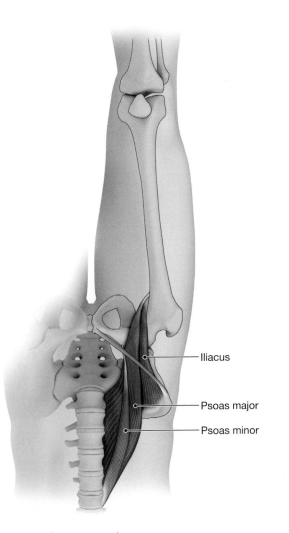

FIGURE 12-98 Iliopsoas muscle

Iliacus

Psoas major

Psoas minor

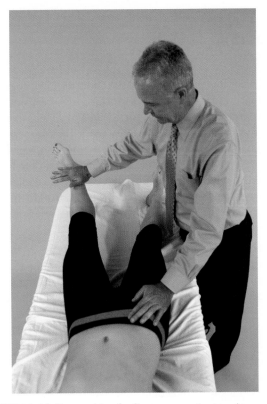

FIGURE 12-99 Test position for iliopsoas—patient supine

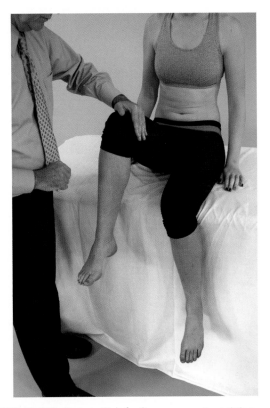

FIGURE 12-100 Test position for iliopsoas—patient sitting

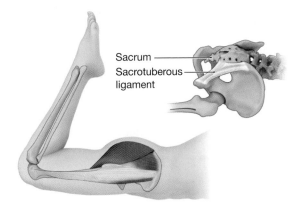

Sacrum

Sacrotuberous ligament

FIGURE 12-101 Gluteus maximus muscle

Gluteus Medius. The gluteus medius (Figure 12-103) is critical for balancing the pelvis in the frontal plane during one-leg stance,[117] which accounts for approximately 60% of the gait cycle.[118] During one-leg stance, approximately 3 times the body weight is transmitted to the hip joint with two-thirds of that being generated by the hip abductor mechanism.[118] In addition to its role as a stabilizer, the gluteus medius also functions as a decelerator of hip adduction.

Because of its shape, the gluteus medius is known as the deltoid of the hip. The muscle can be divided into two functional parts: an anterior portion and a posterior portion. The anterior portion works to flex, abduct, and internally rotate the hip. The posterior portion extends and externally rotates the hip. On the deep surface of this muscle is located the superior gluteal nerve and the superior and inferior gluteal vessels. The synergists of this muscle include the gluteus maximus and minimus, tensor fasciae latae, sartorius, iliopsoas,

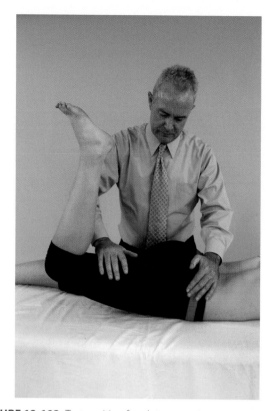

FIGURE 12-102 Test position for gluteus maximus

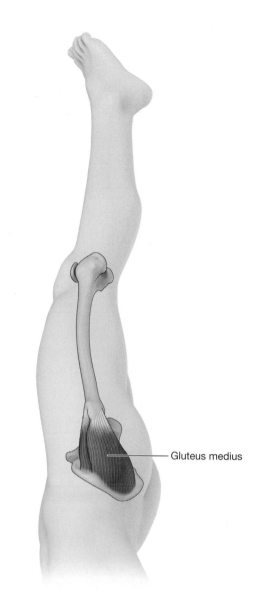

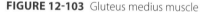

Gluteus medius

FIGURE 12-103 Gluteus medius muscle

rectus femoris, pectineus, adductor longus and brevis, adductor magnus, gracilis, hamstrings, and piriformis. The antagonists of the muscle include the tensor fasciae latae, sartorius, iliopsoas, rectus femoris, pectineus, adductor longus and brevis, adductor magnus, gracilis, hamstrings, gluteus maximus, piriformis, and gluteus minimus.

To specifically test this muscle the patient is positioned in sidelying with the tested leg uppermost. The patient hip is positioned in abduction, slight extension, and external rotation (Figure 12-104). While stabilizing the pelvis with one hand, the clinician applies a force of abduction and minimal flexion to the hip while the patient attempts to prevent the motion. Substitution or trick motions can include assistance from the quadratus lumborum and the lateral abdominals, which can tilt the pelvis laterally, giving the appearance of abduction; assistance from the gluteus maximus (superior fibers); or allowing the patient to roll slightly toward the supine position, which places the tensor fasciae latae in a more favorable position for hip abduction. The gravity-minimized/eliminated position for this muscle is with the patient positioned in supine with the extremity on a friction-free surface.

Gluteus Minimus. The gluteus minimus (Figure 12-105) is a rather thin muscle situated between the gluteus medius muscle and the external surface of the ilium. The muscle is the major internal rotator of the femur. It receives assistance from the tensor fasciae latae, semitendinosus, semimembranosus, and gluteus medius.[116] The gluteus minimus also abducts the thigh, as well as helping the gluteus medius with pelvic support. The synergists of this muscle include the gluteus medius, tensor fasciae latae, sartorius, iliopsoas, rectus femoris, pectineus, adductor longus and brevis, adductor magnus (anterior portion), gracilis, hamstrings, gluteus maximus, and piriformis. The an-

tagonists of this muscle include the adductor longus and brevis, adductor magnus, gracilis, sartorius, iliopsoas, hamstrings, gluteus maximus, piriformis, pectineus, and gluteus medius.

To specifically test this muscle, the patient is positioned in sidelying with the tested side uppermost. The patient is asked to abduct the hip while avoiding any rotation, flexion, or extension of the hip (Figure 12-106). While stabilizing the pelvis with one hand, the clinician applies an adduction and minimal extension force to the hip while the patient attempts to prevent the motion from occurring.

Tensor Fasciae Latae (TFL). The TFL (Figure 12-107) envelops the muscles of the thigh and seldom works alone. In addition to counteracting the backward pull of the gluteus maximus on the iliotibial band (ITB), the TFL also flexes, abducts, and externally rotates the hip. The trochanteric bursa is found deep to this muscle, as it passes over the greater trochanter, and is a common source of lateral thigh pain.[119] The attachment of the TFL via the ITB to the anterolateral tibia provides a flexion moment in knee flexion and an extension moment in knee extension.[79] The synergists of this muscle include the iliopsoas, sartorius, pectineus, gluteus medius

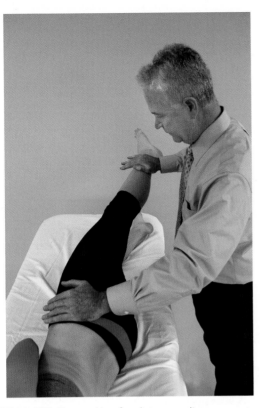

FIGURE 12-104 Test position for gluteus medius

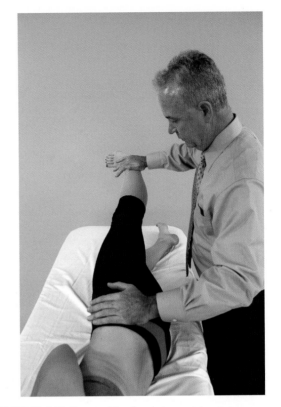

FIGURE 12-106 Test position for gluteus minimus

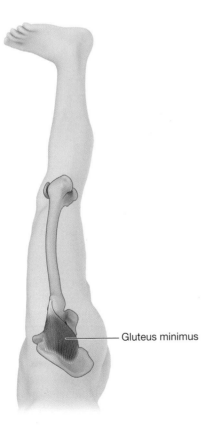

Gluteus minimus

FIGURE 12-105 Gluteus minimus muscle

adductor longus and brevis, pectineus, gracilis, gluteus maximus, piriformis, sartorius, iliopsoas, and piriformis.

To specifically test this muscle, the patient is positioned in supine with the knee extended. The patient is asked to abduct, flex, and internally rotate the hip and to hold the position (Figure 12-108) while the clinician applies resistance in a direction of hip extension and hip abduction (the rotational component is not resisted) on the distal tibia. Substitution or trick motions can include assistance from the hip flexors. The gravity-minimized/eliminated position for this muscle is with the patient positioned in long-sitting with the hips supported on the table, flexed to 45° and in neutral rotation, and the upper extremities supporting the trunk.

CLINICAL PEARL

The iliotibial band (ITB) or tract begins as a wide covering of the superior and lateral aspects of the pelvis and thigh in continuity with the fasciae latae (see Figure 12-101). It inserts distal and lateral to the patella at the tubercle of Gerdy on the lateral condyle of the tibia. Anteriorly, it attaches to the lateral border of the patella. Posteriorly, it is attached to the tendon of the biceps femoris. Laterally, it blends with an aponeurotic expansion from the vastus lateralis (see Muscles of the Knee).[120] Like the patella tendon, the ITB can be viewed as a ligament or a tendon. Its location adjacent to the center of rotation of the knee allows it to function as an anterolateral stabilizer of the knee in the frontal plane[121] and to both flex and extend the knee.[122,123] In knee flexion greater than 30°, the ITB becomes a weak knee flexor, as well as an external rotator of the tibia.

During static standing, the primary function of the ITB is to maintain knee and hip extension, providing the thigh

and minimus, gracilis, adductor longus and brevis, adductor magnus (anterior portion), gluteus maximus, piriformis, rectus femoris, and hamstrings. The antagonists of this muscle include the hamstrings, gluteus medius, adductor magnus,

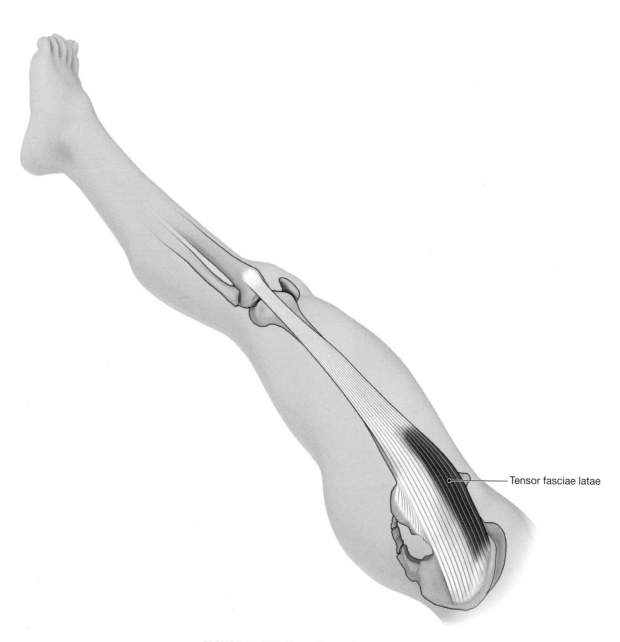

Tensor fasciae latae

FIGURE 12-107 Tensor fasciae latae muscle

muscles an opportunity to rest. While walking or running, the ITB helps maintain flexion of the hip and is a major support of the knee in squatting from full extension until 30° of flexion.

Rectus Femoris. The rectus femoris muscle (Figure 12-109), one of the four quadriceps muscles, is a two-joint muscle that arises from two tendons: one, the anterior or straight, from the anterior inferior iliac spine; the other, the posterior or reflected, from a groove above the brim of the acetabulum. The rectus femoris combines movements of flexion at the hip and extension at the knee. It functions more effectively as a hip flexor when the knee is flexed, such as when a person kicks a ball.[116] The specific test for this muscle is described in the section Muscle Testing of the Knee.

Hip External Rotators. The hip external rotators (Figure 12-110) include the piriformis, quadratus femoris, obturator internus, obturator externus, gemellus superior, and gemellus inferior.

▶ *Piriformis.* The piriformis (see Figure 12-110) is the most superior of the external rotators of the hip. The piriformis is an external rotator of the hip at less than 60° of hip flexion. At 90° of hip flexion, the piriformis reverses its muscle action, becoming an internal rotator and abductor of the hip.[124] The piriformis, with its close association with the sciatic nerve, can be a common source of buttock and leg pain.[125–128]

▶ *Quadratus femoris.* The quadratus femoris muscle (see Figure 12-110) is a flat, quadrilateral muscle, located between the inferior gemellus and the superior aspect of the adductor magnus.

▶ *Obturator internus.* The obturator internus (see Figure 12-110) is normally an external rotator of the hip and an internal rotator of the ilium but becomes an abductor of the hip at 90° of hip flexion.[129]

▶ *Obturator externus.* The obturator externus (see Figure 12-110), named for its location external to the pelvis, is an adductor and external rotator of the hip.[130]

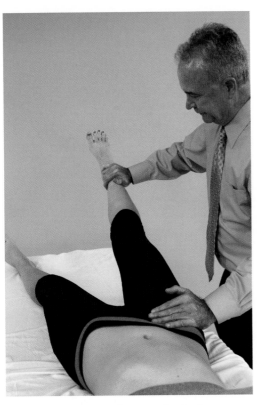

FIGURE 12-108 Test position for tensor fasciae latae

▶ *Superior and inferior gemelli muscles.* These muscles (see Figure 12-110) are considered accessories to the obturator internus tendon. The superior gemellus is the smaller of the two.[130]

The external rotators of the hip are tested as a group. The patient is positioned in sitting with the thigh supported on the table and the lower leg over the end of the table. The patient rotates the hip externally such that the foot moves toward the contralateral side (Figure 12-111). Using one hand, the clinician stabilizes the patient's thigh while with the other hand generating a force of internal rotation of the hip by applying pressure to the inner aspect of the leg (see Figure 12-111).

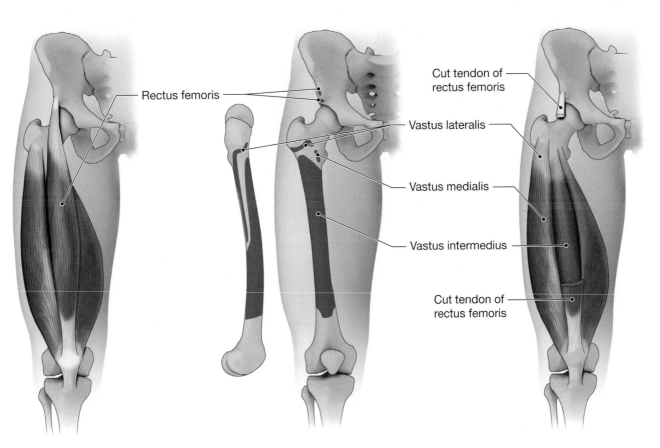

Rectus femoris

Cut tendon of rectus femoris

Vastus lateralis

Vastus medialis

Vastus intermedius

Cut tendon of rectus femoris

FIGURE 12-109 Quadriceps femoris muscle

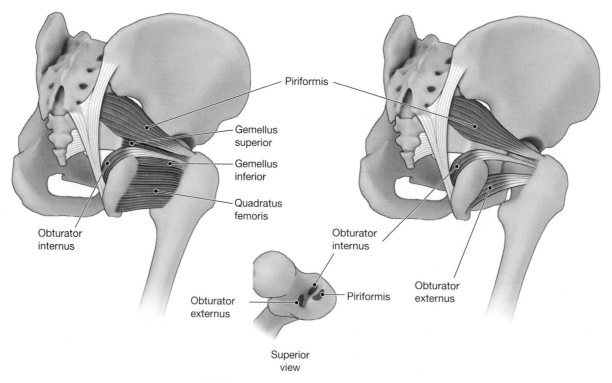

FIGURE 12-110 External rotators of the hip

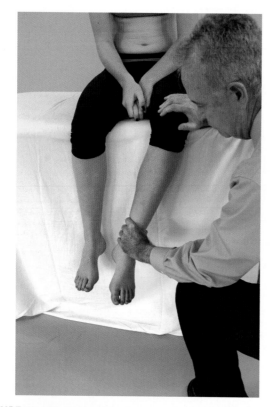

FIGURE 12-111 Test position for external rotators of the hip

by some surgeons necessarily cuts through at least part of the hip's posterior capsule, potentially disrupting several of the short external rotator tendons.[113] Studies have reported a significant reduction in the incidence of posterior hip dislocation when the surgeon carefully repairs the posterior capsule and external rotator tendons.[113,131,132]

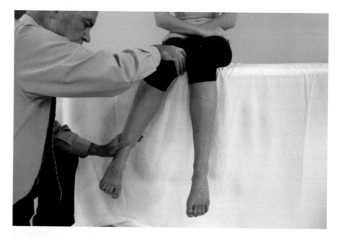

FIGURE 12-112 Test position for internal rotators of the hip

Hip Internal Rotators. The internal rotators of the hip consist of the tensor fasciae latae, gluteus minimus, and gluteus medius (anterior fibers). These muscles are tested as a group. The patient is positioned in sitting with the thigh supported on the table and the lower leg over the end of the table. The patient rotates the hip internally such that the foot moves away from the contralateral side. Using one hand, the clinician stabilizes the patient's thigh while with the other hand generating a force of external rotation of the hip by applying pressure to the outer aspect of the leg (Figure 12-112).

Hip Adductors. The adductors of the hip are found on the medial aspect of the joint (Figure 12-113). The main action of this muscle group is to adduct the thigh in the open kinetic chain and stabilize the lower extremity to perturbation in the closed kinetic chain. Each individual muscle can also provide assistance in hip flexion and rotation.[133]

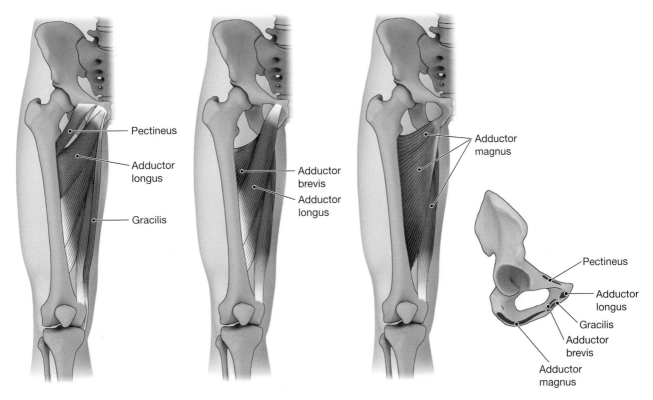

FIGURE 12-113 Hip adductor muscles

▶ *Adductor magnus.* The adductor magnus (see Figure 12-113) is the most powerful adductor, and it is active to varying degrees in all hip motions except abduction. The posterior portion of the adductor magnus is sometimes considered functionally as a hamstring because of its anatomic alignment. Because of its size, the adductor magnus is less likely to be injured than the other hip adductors.[134]

▶ *Adductor longus.* During resisted adduction, the adductor longus (see Figure 12-113) is the most prominent muscle of the adductors and forms the medial border of the femoral triangle. The adductor longus also assists with external rotation, in extension, and internal rotation in other positions. The adductor longus is the most commonly strained adductor muscle.[135]

▶ *Gracilis.* The gracilis (see Figure 12-113) is the most superficial and medial of the hip adductor muscles. It is also the longest. The gracilis functions to adduct and flex the thigh and flex and internally rotate the leg.

▶ *Pectineus.* The pectineus (see Figure 12-113) is an adductor, flexor, and internal rotator of the hip. Like the iliopsoas, the pectineus attaches to and supports the joint capsule of the hip.

The other adductors of the hip include the adductor brevis and obturator externus muscles.

The hip adductors are tested as a group. The patient is positioned in sidelying with the tested side closest to the table. The clinician supports the uppermost leg in hip abduction, and the patient is asked to adduct the lower leg off the table (Figure 12-114) while the clinician applies a downward force. The gravity-minimized/eliminated position for this muscle group is with the patient positioned in supine.

Sartorius. The sartorius muscle (see Figure 12-115) is the longest muscle in the body. The sartorius is responsible for flexion, abduction, and external rotation of the hip, and some degree of knee flexion.[136] Given its numerous actions, this muscle has numerous synergists and antagonists.

To specifically test this muscle, the patient is positioned in supine. The patient is asked to externally rotate, abduct, and flex the hip while also flexing the knee. The clinician places one hand on the outer aspect of the patient's knee and uses the other hand to cup the patient's ankle. The patient is asked to prevent any motion as the clinician applies an extension, internal rotation, and adduction force to the hip, while also applying an extension force to the knee (Figure 12-116).

Hamstrings. The hamstrings muscle group consists of the biceps femoris, the semimembranosus, and the semitendinosus.

▶ *Biceps femoris.* The long head of the biceps femoris (Figure 12-117) is the only portion that acts on the hip. It is active

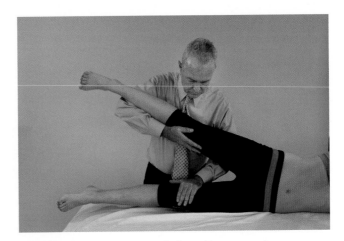

FIGURE 12-114 Test position for hip adductor muscle group

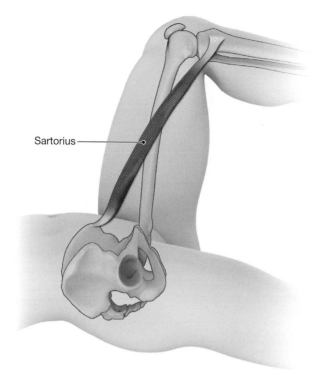

Sartorius

FIGURE 12-115 Sartorius muscle

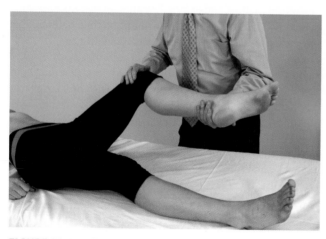

FIGURE 12-116 Test position for sartorius

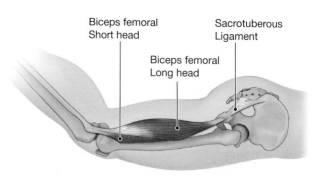

Biceps femoral
Short head

Sacrotuberous
Ligament

Biceps femoral
Long head

FIGURE 12-117 Biceps femoris muscle

during conditions that require lesser amounts of force, such as decelerating the limb at the end of the swing phase and during forceful hip extension.[137] As a whole, the biceps femoris extends the hip, flexes the knee, and externally rotates the tibia. The biceps femoris (53%) is the most commonly strained muscle of the hamstring complex.

▸ *Semimembranosus.* The semimembranosus (Figure 12-118), the most medial of the hamstrings, assists with hip extension, knee flexion, and internal rotation of the tibia.

▸ *Semitendinosus.* The semitendinosus (see Figure 12-118) has the longest tendinous insertion of the hamstrings. It assists with hip extension, knee flexion, and internal rotation of the tibia.

All three muscles of the hamstring complex (except for the short head of the biceps) work with the posterior adductor magnus and the gluteus maximus to extend the hip. In addition to the actions just listed, the hamstrings also weakly adduct the hip. When the hamstrings contract as a unit, their forces are exerted at the hip and knee joints simultaneously; functionally, however, they can actively mobilize only one of the two joints at the same time. Compared to walking and jogging, running is a stressful activity for the hamstrings and increases the high demands on their tendon attachments, especially during eccentric contractions. During running, the hamstrings have three main functions:

1. They decelerate knee extension at the end of the forward swing phase of the gait cycle. Through an eccentric contraction, the hamstrings decelerate the forward

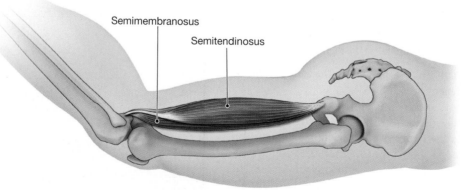

Semimembranosus

Semitendinosus

Right extrenity, posterolateral view

FIGURE 12-118 Semitendinosus and semimembranosus muscles

momentum (i.e., leg swing) at approximately 30° short of full knee extension. This action helps provide dynamic stabilization to the weight-bearing knee.

2. At foot strike, the hamstrings elongate to facilitate hip extension through an eccentric contraction, thus further stabilizing the leg for weight bearing.

3. The hamstrings assist the gastrocnemius in paradoxically extending the knee during the takeoff phase of the running cycle.

The specific tests for these muscles are described in the section Muscle Testing of the Knee.

MUSCLE TESTING OF THE KNEE

The major muscles that act on the knee joint complex are the quadriceps, the hamstrings (semimembranosus, semitendinosus, and biceps femoris), the gastrocnemius, the popliteus, and the hip adductors.

Quadriceps. The quadriceps muscles can act to extend the knee when the foot is off the ground, although more commonly, they work as decelerators, preventing the knee from buckling when the foot strikes the ground.[123,138] The four muscles that make up the quadriceps are the rectus femoris, the vastus intermedius, the vastus lateralis (VL), and the vastus medialis (see Figure 12-109). The quadriceps tendon represents the convergence of all four muscle tendon units, and it inserts at the anterior aspect of the superior pole of the patella. The quadriceps muscle group is innervated by the femoral nerve.

▶ *Rectus femoris.* The rectus femoris (see Figure 12-109) is the only quadriceps muscle that crosses the hip joint. It originates at the anterior inferior iliac spine. The other quadriceps muscles originate on the femoral shaft. This gives the hip joint considerable importance with respect to the knee extensor mechanism in the examination and intervention.[123] The line of pull of the rectus femoris, with respect to the patella, is at angle of about 5° with the femoral shaft.[123]

▶ *Vastus intermedius.* The vastus intermedius (see Figure 12-109) has its origin on the proximal part of the femur, and its line of action is directly in line with the femur.

▶ *Vastus lateralis.* The VL (see Figure 12-109) is composed of two functional parts: the VL and the vastus lateralis obliquus (VLO).[138] The VL has a line of pull of about 12–15° to the long axis of the femur in the frontal plane, whereas the VLO has a pull of 38–48°.[123]

▶ *Vastus medialis.* The vastus medialis (see Figure 12-109) is composed of two functional parts that are anatomically distinct[138]: the vastus medialis obliquus (VMO) and the vastus medialis proper, or longus (VML).[139]

■ *Vastus medialis obliquus.* The VMO (see Figure 12-109) arises from the adductor magnus tendon.[140] The insertion site of the normal VMO is the medial border of the patella, approximately one-third to one-half of the way down from the proximal pole. If the VMO remains proximal to the proximal pole of the patella and does not reach the patella, there is an increased potential for patellar malalignment.[141]

The vector of the VMO is medially directed, and it forms an angle of 50° to 55° with the mechanical axis of the leg.[138,140,142,143] The VMO is least active in the fully extended position[144-146] and plays little role in extending the knee, acting instead to realign the patella medially during the extension maneuver. It is active in this function throughout the whole range of extension.

According to Fox,[147] the vastus medialis is the weakest of the quadriceps group and appears to be the first muscle of the quadriceps group to atrophy and the last to rehabilitate.[148] The normal VMO/VL ratio of EMG activity in standing knee extension from 30° to 0° is 1:1,[149] but in patients who have patellofemoral pain, the activity in the VMO decreases significantly; instead of being tonically active, it becomes phasic in action.[150] The presence of swelling also inhibits the VMO, and it requires almost half of the volume of effusion to inhibit the VMO as it does to inhibit the rectus femoris and VL muscles.[151]

The VMO is frequently innervated independently from the rest of the quadriceps by a separate branch from the femoral nerve.[138]

■ *Vastus medialis longus.* The VML originates from the medial aspect of the upper femur and inserts anteriorly into the quadriceps tendon, giving it a line of action of approximately 15° to 17° off the long axis of the femur in the frontal plane.[123]

Because the quadriceps group is aligned anatomically with the shaft of the femur and not with the mechanical axis of the lower extremity, any quadriceps muscle contraction (regardless of knee flexion angle) results in compressive forces acting on the patellofemoral joint.[152] The quadriceps group is particularly important when climbing stairs, walking up inclines, or standing from a seated position.

The synergists of this muscle group include the gluteus maximus, tensor fasciae latae, iliopsoas, pectineus, gluteus minimus, gluteus medius, sartorius, adductor brevis and longus, and adductor magnus (anterior portion). The antagonists of this muscle group include the hamstrings, gracilis, sartorius, popliteus, gastrocnemius, tensor fasciae latae, gluteus maximus, adductor magnus (posterior portion), piriformis, and gluteus medius.

To specifically test this muscle group, the patient is positioned sitting at the edge of the table with the thigh supported and the leg hanging over the edge (Figure 12-119).

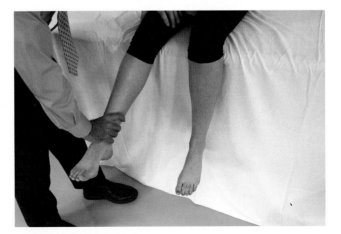

FIGURE 12-119 Test position for the quadriceps femoris group

The patient is asked to lean backward to relax the hamstrings and then to straighten the knee to just short of full extension. Using one hand, the clinician stabilizes the patient's thigh and places the other hand over the anterior surface of the distal leg just proximal to the ankle. The clinician applies a force into knee flexion with the hand just proximal to the ankle while asking the patient to resist the movement.

Hamstrings. As previously mentioned, the hamstrings primarily function to extend the hip and to flex the knee.

▶ *Semimembranosus.* At the knee, this muscle inserts on the posterior medial aspect of the medial condyle of the tibia and has an important expansion that reinforces the posteromedial corner of the knee capsule (see Figure 12-118). During knee flexion, the semimembranosus pulls the meniscus posteriorly and internally rotates the tibia on the femur.

▶ *Semitendinosus.* Passing over the MCL, the semitendinosus (see Figure 12-118) inserts into the medial surface of the tibia and deep fascia of the lower leg, distal to the attachment of the gracilis, and posterior to the attachment of the sartorius. These three structures are collectively called the *pes anserinus* ("goose's foot") at this point.

▶ *Biceps femoris.* The biceps femoris (see Figure 12-117) inserts on the lateral condyle of the tibia and the head of the fibula. The superficial layer of the common tendon has been identified as the major force creating external tibial rotation and controlling internal rotation of the femur.[153] The pull of the biceps on the tibia retracts the joint capsule and pulls the iliotibial tract posteriorly, keeping it taut throughout flexion.

The hamstrings are specifically tested based on their anatomy—the semimembranosus and semitendinosus are tested together, and the biceps femoris is tested separately. The gravity-minimized/eliminated position for this muscle group is with the patient positioned in sidelying with the tested leg on a friction-free surface.

▶ To specifically test the semimembranosus and semitendinosus, the patient is positioned in prone with the knee flexed to approximate 45° and the tibia internally rotated so that the toes are pointing inward (Figure 12-120). Using one hand to stabilize the patient's thigh, the clinician places the other hand just proximal to the ankle on the posterior aspect of the patient's leg and applies a force into

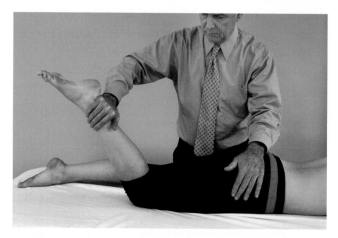

FIGURE 12-121 Test position for the semitendinosus and semi-membranosus

knee extension while asking the patient to prevent the motion (see Figure 12-120).

▶ To specifically test the biceps femoris, the patient is positioned in prone with the knee flexed to approximately 45° and the tibia in slight external rotation so that the toes are pointing outward (Figure 12-121). Using one hand to stabilize the patient's thigh, the clinician places the other hand just proximal to the ankle on the posterior aspect of the patient's leg and applies a force into knee extension while asking the patient to prevent the motion (see Figure 12-121).

Gastrocnemius. The gastrocnemius originates from above the knee by two heads, each head connected to a femoral condyle and to the joint capsule (Figure 12-122). Approximately halfway down the leg, the gastrocnemius muscles blend to form

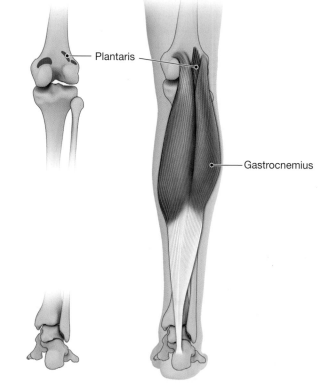

Plantaris

Gastrocnemius

FIGURE 12-122 Gastrocnemius and plantaris muscles

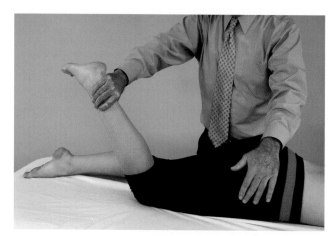

FIGURE 12-120 Test position for the biceps femoris

an aponeurosis. As the aponeurosis progressively contracts, it accepts the tendon of the soleus, a flat broad muscle deep to the gastrocnemius. The aponeurosis and the soleus tendon end in a flat tendon, called the *Achilles tendon,* which attaches to the posterior aspect of the calcaneus. The two heads of the gastrocnemius and the soleus are collectively known as the *triceps surae.*

At the knee, the gastrocnemius functions to flex or extend the knee, depending on whether the lower extremity is weight bearing or not. Kendall and colleagues[154] have proposed that a weakness of the gastrocnemius may cause knee hyperextension.

In addition, it has been proposed that the gastrocnemius acts as an antagonist of the anterior cruciate ligament, exerting an anteriorly directed pull on the tibia throughout the range of knee flexion–extension motion, particularly when the knee is near extension.[155,156]

The specific test for this muscle is described in the Muscles of the Leg and Foot section later.

Popliteus. The popliteus (Figure 12-123) originates from the lateral femoral condyle near the LCL. The muscle has several attachments, including the lateral aspect of the lateral femoral condyle, the posterior-medial aspect of the head of the fibula, and the posterior horn of the lateral meniscus.[157] The larger base of this triangular muscle inserts obliquely into the posterosuperior part of the tibia above the soleal line. The muscle has several important functions, including the reinforcement of the posterior third of the lateral capsular ligament[158] and the unlocking of the knee during flexion from terminal knee extension during gait. It performs this latter task by internally rotating the tibia on the femur, preventing impingement of the posterior horn of the lateral meniscus by drawing it posteriorly, and, with the posterior cruciate ligament, preventing a posterior glide of the tibia.[158-161] Because knee joint injury frequently involves some component of transverse plane rotation and the popliteus muscle has been described as an important, primary, dynamic, transverse plane, rotatory knee-joint stabilizer, an understanding of its function in relation to other posterolateral knee joint structures is important.[162] Attached to the popliteus tendon is the popliteofibular ligament, which forms a strong attachment between the popliteal tendon and the fibula. This ligament adds to posterolateral stability.[163-166]

> **CLINICAL PEARL**
>
> A medial portion of the popliteus penetrates the joint, becoming intracapsular with the lateral meniscus. This part of the popliteus tendon is pain sensitive, and an injury here can often mimic a meniscal injury on the lateral aspect of the joint line.[167] Differentiation between these two lesions can be elucidated with the reproduction of pain with resisted knee flexion in an extended and externally rotated position of the tibia if the popliteus is involved.

The popliteus muscle is innervated by the tibial nerve. The synergists of this muscle include the hamstrings, gracilis, sartorius, gastrocnemius, and tensor fasciae latae. The antagonists of this muscle include the biceps femoris and the quadriceps.

To specifically test this muscle, the patient is positioned in sitting with the knee flexed to 90°. The patient is asked to internally rotate the tibia (Figure 12-124). There is no resistance

Lateral view

Posterior view

FIGURE 12-123 Popliteus muscle

Popliteus

FIGURE 12-124 Testing the function of the popliteus

applied for this test—the test is used to determine whether the muscle is active and capable of internally rotating the tibia.

Tensor Fasciae Latae. In addition to its actions at the hip, the tensor fasciae latae (TFL) is also a weak extensor of the knee, but only when the knee is already extended. The specific test for this muscle is described in the Muscles of the Hip section.

MUSCLE TESTING OF THE LEG AND FOOT

Extrinsic Muscles of the Leg and Foot

The extrinsic muscles of the foot (Table 12-8) can be divided into anterior, posterior superficial, posterior deep, and lateral compartments.

Anterior Compartment

This compartment contains the dorsiflexors (extensors) of the foot. These include the tibialis anterior, extensor digitorum longus, extensor hallucis longus, and fibularis (peroneus) tertius.

Tibialis Anterior. The tibialis anterior originates from the upper two-thirds of the lateral surface of the tibia, interosseous membrane, and deep fascia and inserts into the medial and plantar surface of the medial cuneiform and base of the first metatarsal bone of the foot (Figure 12-125). The tibialis anterior muscle, which is the first large tendon palpated anterior to the medial malleolus, produces the motion of dorsiflexion and inversion.

The tibialis anterior is innervated by the deep fibular (peroneal) nerve. The synergists of this muscle include the extensor digitorum longus, extensor hallucis longus, fibularis tertius, tibialis posterior, flexor digitorum longus, flexor hallucis longus, gastrocnemius, and soleus. The antagonists for this muscle include the tibialis posterior, fibularis longus and brevis, gastrocnemius, soleus, flexor digitorum longus, flexor hallucis longus, fibularis tertius, and extensor digitorum longus.

To specifically test this muscle, the patient is positioned in supine or sitting, and the patient's foot is positioned in dorsiflexion and inversion, with the great toe pointing downward (to minimize activation of the extensor hallucis longus). The knee must remain flexed during the test to allow complete dorsiflexion. Using one hand, the leg is stabilized by the clinician, while resistance is applied to the medial posterior aspect of the forefoot in an inferior/lateral direction into plantarflexion and eversion (Figure 12-126).

Extensor Digitorum Longus. The extensor digitorum longus (EDL) arises from the lateral condyle of the tibia, the proximal three-fourths of the anterior surface of the body of the fibula, the proximal portion of the interosseous

TABLE 12-8	Extrinsic Muscle Attachments and Innervation		
Muscle	**Proximal**	**Distal**	**Innervation**
Gastrocnemius	Medial and lateral condyle of femur	Posterior surface of calcaneus through Achilles tendon	Tibial S2 (S1)
Plantaris	Lateral supracondylar line of femur	Posterior surface of calcaneus through Achilles tendon	Tibial S2 (S1)
Soleus	Head of fibula, proximal third of shaft, soleal line, and midshaft of posterior tibia	Posterior surface of calcaneus through Achilles tendon	Tibial S2 (S1)
Tibialis anterior	Distal to lateral tibial condyle, proximal half of lateral tibial shaft, and interosseous membrane	First cuneiform bone, medial and plantar surfaces, and base of first metatarsal	Deep peroneal L4 (L5)
Tibialis posterior	Posterior surface of tibia, proximal two-thirds posterior of fibula, and interosseous membrane	Tuberosity of navicular bone and tendinous expansion to other tarsals and metatarsals	Tibial L4 and L5
Fibularis (peroneus) longus	Lateral condyle of tibia, head and proximal two-thirds of fibula	Base of first metatarsal and first cuneiform, lateral side	Superficial peroneal L5 and S1 (S2)
Fibularis (peroneus) brevis	Distal two-thirds of lateral fibular shaft	Tuberosity of fifth metatarsal	Superficial peroneal L5 and S1 (S2)
Fibularis (peroneus) tertius	Lateral slip from extensor digitorum longus	Tuberosity of fifth metatarsal	Deep peroneal L5 and S1
Flexor hallucis longus	Posterior distal two-thirds fibula	Base of distal phalanx of great toe	Tibial S2 (S3)
Flexor digitorum longus	Middle three-fifths of posterior tibia	Base of distal phalanx of lateral four toes	Tibial S2 (S3)
Extensor hallucis longus	Middle half of anterior shaft of fibula	Base of distal phalanx of great toe	Deep peroneal L5 and S1
Extensor digitorum longus	Lateral condyle of tibia, proximal anterior surface of shaft of fibula	One tendon to each lateral four toes, to middle phalanx, and extending to distal phalanges	Deep peroneal L5 and S1

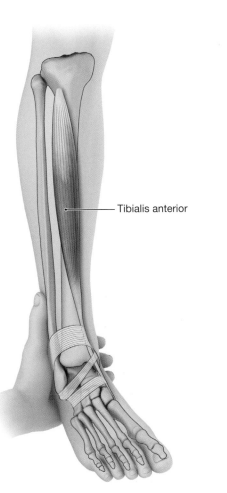

Tibialis anterior

FIGURE 12-125 Tibialis anterior muscle

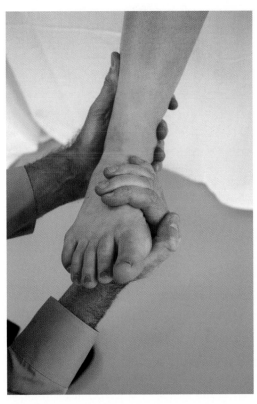

FIGURE 12-126 Testing position for tibialis anterior

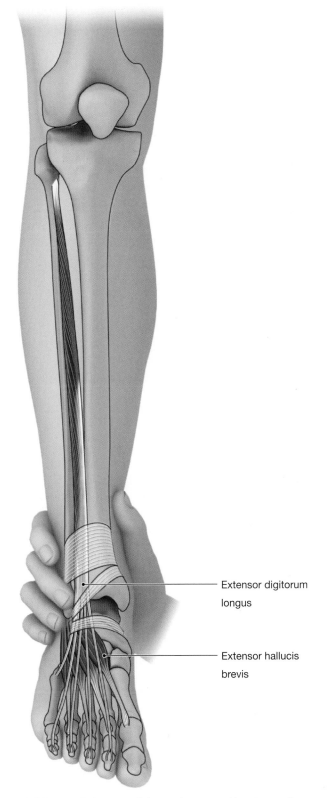

Extensor digitorum longus

Extensor hallucis brevis

FIGURE 12-127 Extensor digitorum longus and brevis muscles

membrane, the deep fascia, and the adjacent intermuscular septa (Figure 12-127). The muscle divides into four slips that insert into the middle and distal phalanges of the lateral four toes. The EDL functions to produce ankle dorsiflexion, foot eversion, and extension of the metatarsophalangeal (MTP), proximal, and DIP joints of the lateral four toes.

The EDL is innervated by the deep fibular (peroneal) nerve. The synergists of this muscle include the extensor digitorum

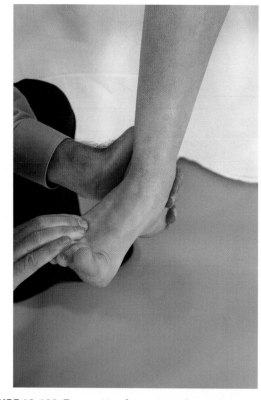

FIGURE 12-128 Test position for extensor digitorum longus

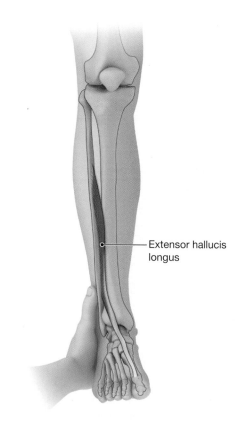

FIGURE 12-129 Extensor hallucis longus muscles

brevis, extensor hallucis longus, tibialis anterior, fibularis tertius, and fibularis longus and brevis. The antagonists of this muscle include the flexor digitorum longus, lumbricals, anterior interossei, posterior interossei, tibialis posterior, flexor digitorum brevis, gastrocnemius, soleus, flexor hallucis longus, fibularis longus and brevis, tibialis anterior, and extensor hallucis longus.

To specifically test this muscle, the patient is positioned sitting or supine, and the patient is asked to extend the toes. Using one hand to stabilize the metatarsals and keeping the foot in slight plantarflexion, the clinician uses the other hand to apply force against the proximal phalanges of toes 2 through 5 in the direction of toe flexion (Figure 12-128).

Extensor Hallucis Longus (EHL). The EHL arises from the anterior middle third of the surface of the fibula and interosseous membrane. As the muscle fibers descend, they become a tendon that inserts on the base of the distal phalanx of the great toe (Figure 12-129). The EHL functions to extend the great toe and dorsiflex the foot, and it assists with foot inversion.

The EHL is innervated by the deep fibular (peroneal) nerve. The synergists of this muscle include the extensor digitorum brevis, tibialis anterior, extensor digitorum longus, and fibularis tertius. The antagonists of this muscle include the flexor hallucis longus, gastrocnemius, soleus, tibialis posterior, flexor digitorum longus, flexor hallucis longus, fibularis longus and brevis, and abductor hallucis.

To specifically test this muscle, the patient is positioned in supine or sitting and the ankle is positioned in a neutral position. The patient is asked to extend the MTP and interphalangeal joints of the great toe and to hold a position while the clinician applies pressure on the distal phalanx in a plantarflexion direction (Figure 12-130).

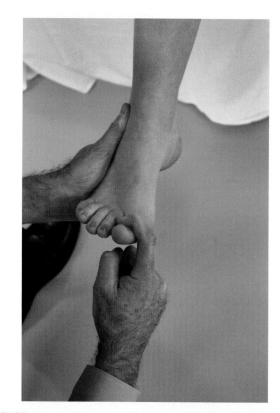

FIGURE 12-130 Test position for the extensor hallucis longus

Fibularis (Peroneus) Tertius. The fibularis tertius arises from the lower third of the anterior surface of the fibula, the lower part of the interosseous membrane, and the adjacent intermuscular septum (see Figure 12-127). Working alone,

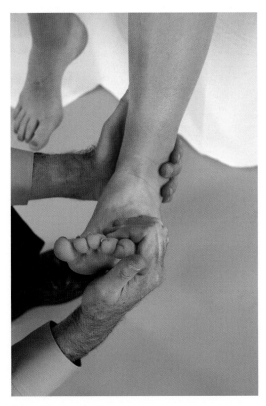

FIGURE 12-131 Test position for the peroneus tertius

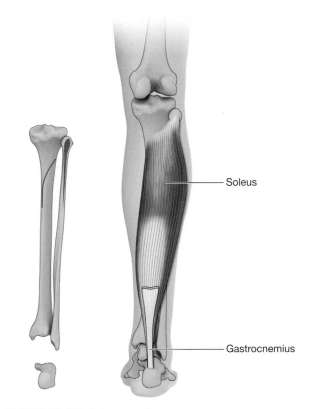

FIGURE 12-132 Soleus muscle

the muscle functions to provide ankle dorsiflexion and foot eversion.

The fibularis tertius is innervated by the deep fibular (peroneal) nerve. The synergists for this muscle include the extensor digitorum longus, extensor hallucis longus, tibialis anterior, and fibularis longus and brevis. The antagonist of this muscle include the flexor digitorum longus, tibialis posterior, gastrocnemius, soleus, flexor hallucis longus, fibularis longus and brevis, tibialis anterior, and extensor hallucis longus.

To specifically test this muscle, the patient is positioned sitting or supine, and the patient is asked to dorsiflex and then evert the foot (Figure 12-131). While using one hand to stabilize the patient's lower leg, the clinician uses the other hand to apply pressure along the dorsal and lateral aspects of the foot into a plantarflexion and inversion direction while asking the patient to prevent the motion.

Posterior Superficial Compartment

This compartment, located posterior to the interosseous membrane, contains the calf muscles that plantarflex the foot. These include the gastrocnemius, soleus (Figure 12-132), and plantaris muscles (see Figure 12-122).

Gastrocnemius. The two heads of the gastrocnemius arise from the posterior aspects of the distal femur (see Figure 12-122).[168] As the two muscles descend, they form the Achilles tendon along with the soleus muscle. The Achilles tendon courses distally to attach about three-quarters of an inch below the superior portion of the os calcis, on the medial aspect of the calcaneus. The medial head of the gastrocnemius is by far the largest component and, according to electromyographic studies, is the most active of the two during running.[169,170]

CLINICAL PEARL

The Achilles tendon is formed from the conjoint tendons of the gastrocnemius and soleus muscles. The fibers from the gastrocnemius and soleus interweave and twist as they descend, producing an area of high stress 2 to 6 cm above the distal tendon insertion.[171] A region of relative avascularity exists in the same area,[172] which correlates well with the site of some Achilles tendon injuries, including complete spontaneous rupture.[169,173,174] The Achilles tendon is the thickest, strongest tendon in the body.[168]

The gastrocnemius functions to provide ankle plantarflexion, knee flexion, and mild ankle inversion.

The gastrocnemius is innervated by the tibial nerve. The synergists of this muscle include the flexor digitorum longus, tibialis posterior, flexes hallucis longus, fibularis longus and brevis, soleus, hamstrings, gracilis, sartorius, tensor fasciae latae, popliteus, tibialis anterior, and extensor hallucis longus. The antagonists of this muscle include the extensor digitorum longus, extensor hallucis longus, tibialis anterior, fibularis tertius, quadriceps, and peroneus longus and brevis.

To specifically test the gastrocnemius, the patient is positioned in standing on one leg holding onto something for balance. Keeping the knee straight, the patient is asked to raise up on the toes (Figure 12-133). For a normal grading, the patient should be able to repeat this 10 times.

Soleus. The soleus muscle arises from the posterior proximal one third of the fibula and the middle third of the tibia (see Figure 12-132). It conjoins with the gastrocnemius tendon to form the Achilles tendon. The soleus muscle, which is innervated by the tibial nerve, produces ankle plantarflexion. The

MANUAL MUSCLE TESTING

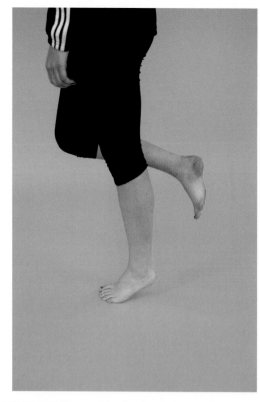

FIGURE 12-133 Test position for the gastrocnemius

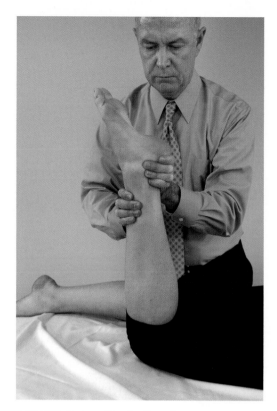

FIGURE 12-134 Test position for the soleus

synergists of this muscle include the flexor digitorum longus, tibialis posterior, flexor hallucis longus, fibularis longus and brevis, gastrocnemius, tibialis anterior, and extensor hallucis longus. The antagonists of this muscle include the extensor digitorum longus, extensor hallucis longus, tibialis anterior, fibularis tertius, and fibularis longus and brevis.

CLINICAL PEARL

The soleus, unlike the gastrocnemius, does not cross the knee joint and is subject to early disuse atrophy with undertraining and/or immobilization.[169]

To specifically test this muscle, the patient is positioned in prone with the knee flexed to 90°. Using one hand, the clinician stabilizes the distal leg of the patient by holding the proximal ankle. The patient is asked to plantarflex the ankle without inversion or eversion of the foot, and the clinician applies a dorsiflexion force to the posterior calcaneus (Figure 12-134).

Plantaris. The plantaris muscle originates from the distal portion of the lateral supracondylar line of the femur, the adjacent part of the popliteal surface, and the oblique popliteal ligament (see Figure 12-122). Its tendon inserts on the posterior calcaneus. The plantaris muscle, which has its own tendon and contributes no fibers to the Achilles tendon, works with the gastrocnemius to plantarflex the ankle and assists in flexion of the knee joint.[175] The plantaris muscle is tested using the specific test of the gastrocnemius.

Posterior Deep Compartment

This compartment contains the flexors of the foot. These muscles course behind the medial malleolus. They include

the posterior tibialis, flexor digitorum longus, and flexor hallucis longus.

Tibialis Posterior. The tibialis posterior arises from the majority of the interosseous membrane, lateral portion of the posterior aspect of the tibia, proximal two-thirds of the medial surface of the fibula, the adjacent intermuscular septa, and deep fascia (Figure 12-135). Its extensive insertions include the tuberosity of the navicular bone, by fibrous expansions to the sustentaculum tali, three cuneiforms, the cuboid, and bases of the second, third, and fourth metatarsal bones. The primary function of the tibialis posterior muscle is to invert and plantarflex the foot. It also provides support to the medial longitudinal arch.[176] The tibialis posterior is innervated by the tibial nerve. The synergists of this muscle include the flexor digitorum longus, flexor hallucis longus, fibularis longus and brevis, gastrocnemius, soleus, tibialis anterior, and extensor hallucis longus. The antagonists of this muscle include the fibularis longus and brevis, fibularis tertius, extensor digitorum longus, extensor hallucis longus, and tibialis anterior.

To specifically test this muscle, the patient is positioned supine or sitting with the foot and ankle plantarflexed and inverted. The patient is asked to sustain this position throughout the test. Using one hand, the clinician stabilizes the proximal to the patient's ankle, while using the other hand to apply an eversion and dorsiflexion force to the patient's foot and ankle (Figure 12-136).

Flexor Digitorum Longus (FDL). The FDL originates from the posterior aspect of the tibia and inserts on the distal phalanges of toes 2 to 5 (Figure 12-137). The FDL functions to flex the phalanges of the lateral four toes and assists with plantarflexion of the foot. The FDL is innervated by the tibial nerve. The synergists of this muscle include the lumbricals, anterior

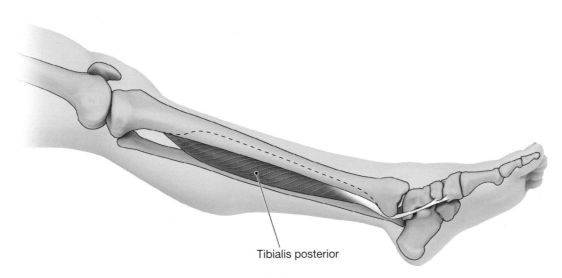

Tibialis posterior

FIGURE 12-135 Tibialis posterior muscle

interossei, posterior interossei, tibialis posterior, flexor hallucis longus, fibularis longus and brevis, gastrocnemius, soleus, tibialis anterior, and extensor hallucis longus. The antagonists of this muscle include the extensor digitorum longus, extensor hallucis longus, extensor digitorum brevis, tibialis anterior, fibularis tertius, and fibularis longus and brevis.

To specifically test this muscle, the patient is positioned supine or sitting. The patient is asked to flex the toes and to sustain the position throughout the test. Using one hand to stabilize the midfoot, the clinician applies an extension force to the toes (Figure 12-138).

Flexor Hallucis Longus (FHL). The FHL originates from the distal two-thirds of the fibula and inserts on the distal phalanx of the great toe (Figure 12-139). The FHL flexes the great toe and also assists with plantarflexion of the foot. The FHL is innervated by the tibial nerve. The synergists of this muscle include the abductor hallucis, flexor digitorum longus, tibialis posterior, fibularis longus and brevis, gastrocnemius, soleus, tibialis anterior, and extensor hallucis longus. The antagonists of this muscle include the extensor hallucis longus, extensor digitorum brevis, extensor digitorum longus, tibialis anterior, fibularis tertius, and fibularis longus and brevis.

To specifically test this muscle, the patient is positioned in supine or sitting and is asked to flex the great toe. It is impor-

tant to note that the patient may have difficulty isolating the motion of this toe from the other toes. Using one hand to stabilize the patient's ankle, the clinician uses the other hand to stabilize the metatarsals while applying an extension force of the great toe (Figure 12-140).

Lateral Compartment

This compartment contains the fibularis (peroneus) longus and brevis (Figure 12-141). The fibularis (peroneal) tendons

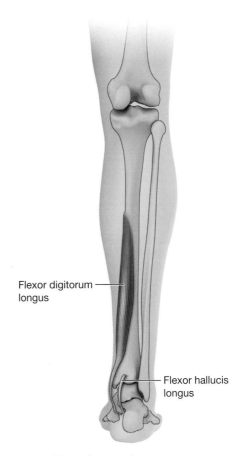

Flexor digitorum longus

Flexor hallucis longus

FIGURE 12-137 Flexor digitorum longus

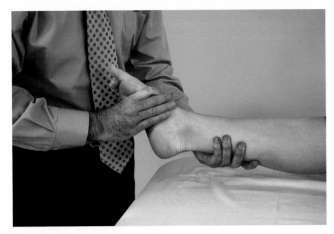

FIGURE 12-136 Test position for the tibialis posterior

391

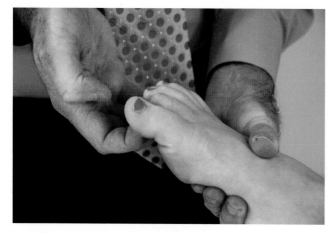

FIGURE 12-138 Test position for the flexor digitorum longus

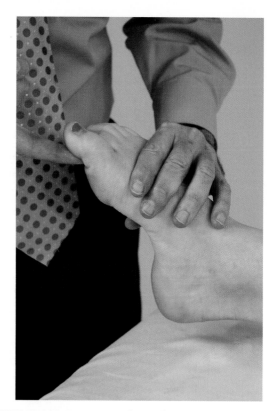

FIGURE 12-140 Test position for the flexor hallucis longus

lie behind the lateral malleolus in a fibro-osseous tunnel formed by a groove in the fibula and the superficial fibular (peroneal) retinaculum.

Fibularis (Peroneus) Longus and Brevis. The fibularis longus arises from the lateral condyle of the tibia, the proximal two-thirds of the fibula, and the adjacent intermuscular

septum and inserts at the base of the first metatarsal and the medial cuneiform bone. The fibularis brevis arises from the distal two-thirds of the fibula and the adjacent intermuscular septum and inserts on the tuberosity on the base of the fifth metatarsal. The two muscles work in combination to produce ankle plantarflexion, foot eversion, and first metatarsal depression (longus).

Both of the muscles are innervated by the superficial fibular (peroneal) nerve. The synergists to these two muscles include the fibularis tertius, flexor digitorum longus, tibialis posterior, flexor hallucis longus, gastrocnemius, soleus, and extensor digitorum longus. The antagonist of these two muscles include the tibialis anterior, tibialis posterior, flexor digitorum longus, flexor hallucis longus, extensor hallucis longus, extensor digitorum longus, fibularis tertius, gastrocnemius, and soleus.

CLINICAL PEARL

The fibularis (peroneal) muscles serve as both plantarflexors and evertors of the foot.[177,178] The fibularis (peroneus) longus also abducts the forefoot in the transverse plane, thereby serving as a support for the medial longitudinal arch.[179]

The fibularis longus and fibularis brevis are the only muscles innervated by the superficial fibular (peroneal) nerve.

Both of these muscles are tested together. The patient is positioned in sitting or supine, and is asked to plantarflex and evert the foot (Figure 12-142). Using one hand, the clinician stabilizes the distal leg and, using the other hand, applies a force on the lateral aspect of the foot into inversion and dorsiflexion.

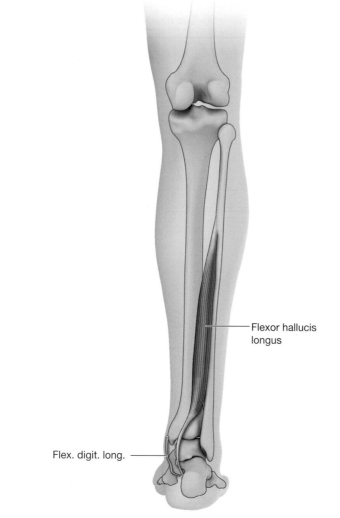

Flexor hallucis longus

Flex. digit. long.

FIGURE 12-139 Flexor hallucis longus muscle

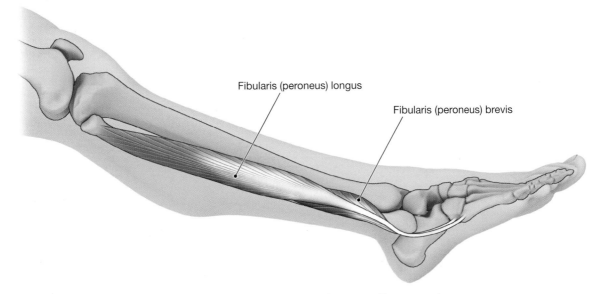

FIGURE 12-141 Fibularis (peroneus) longus and brevis muscles

Intrinsic Muscles of the Foot

Beneath the plantar aponeurosis–plantar fascia are the four muscular layers of the intrinsic muscles of the plantar foot (Table 12-9), as well as the plantar ligaments of the rear- and mid-foot. The intrinsic muscles provide support to the foot during propulsion.[180]

The intrinsic muscles of the foot include the following:

▶ *Abductor hallucis.* This muscle arises from the medial process of the calcaneal tuberosity and inserts into the medial side of the base of the proximal phalanx of the great toe (Figure 12-143). The muscle, which is innervated by the medial plantar nerve, functions to abduct the great toe and to stabilize the first metatarsal. The synergist of this muscle is the flexor hallucis longus. The antagonists of this muscle are the adductor hallucis, extensor hallucis longus, and extensor digitorum brevis.

To specifically test this muscle, the patient is positioned in supine or sitting. Using one hand, the clinician stabilizes the patient's foot while using the other hand to apply adduction force to the great toe and while asking the patient to prevent the motion (Figure 12-144). It is important to remember that this muscle is difficult for many people to isolate.

▶ *Abductor digiti minimi.* This muscle arises from the lateral process of the calcaneal tuberosity as well as the plantar aponeurosis and inserts into the lateral side of the base of the proximal phalanx of the little toe. The muscle functions to assist in flexion of the interphalangeal joint of the fifth digit and to stabilize the forefoot. The synergists of this muscle include the flexor digitorum longus and the fourth lumbrical. The antagonist to this muscle is the fifth anterior interossei.

▶ *Flexor digitorum brevis* (Figure 12-145). This muscle arises from the medial process of the calcaneal tuberosity, lateral to the abductor hallucis and deep to the central portion of the plantar fascia, and inserts into the middle phalanx of the lateral four toes. The flexor digitorum

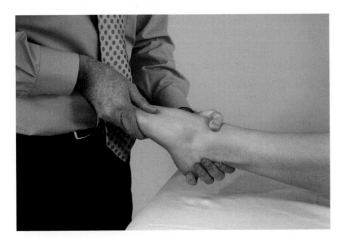

FIGURE 12-142 Test position for the longus and brevis fibularis

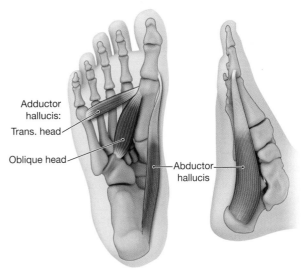

FIGURE 12-143 Abductor hallucis and adductor hallucis muscles

Adductor hallucis:
Trans. head
Oblique head
Abductor hallucis

393

TABLE 12-9   Intrinsic Muscles of the Foot

Muscle	Proximal	Distal	Innervation
Extensor digitorum brevis	Distal superior surface of calcaneus	Posterior (dorsal) surface of second through fourth toes and base of proximal phalanx	Deep peroneal S1 and S2
Flexor hallucis brevis	Plantar surface of cuboid and third cuneiform bones	Base of proximal phalanx of great toe	Medial plantar S3 (S2)
Flexor digitorum brevis	Tuberosity of calcaneus	One tendon slips into base of middle phalanx of each of the lateral four toes	Medial and lateral plantar S3 (S2)
Extensor hallucis brevis	Distal superior and lateral surfaces of calcaneus	Posterior (dorsal) surface of proximal phalanx	Deep peroneal S1 and S2
Abductor hallucis	Tuberosity of calcaneus and plantar aponeurosis	Base of proximal phalanx and medial side	Medial plantar L5 and
Adductor hallucis	Base of second, third, and fourth metatarsals and deep plantar ligaments	Proximal phalanx of first digit lateral side	Medial and lateral plantar S1 and S2
	Lumbricales medial and adjacent sides of flexor digitorum longus tendon to each lateral digit	Medial side of proximal phalanx and extensor hood	Medial and lateral plantar L5, S1, and S2 (L4)
Plantar interossei			
First	Base and medial side of third metatarsal	Base of proximal phalanx and extensor hood of third digit	
Second	Base and medial side of fourth metatarsal	Base of proximal phalanx and extensor hood of fourth digit	Medial and lateral plantar S1 and S2
Third	Base and medial side of fifth metatarsal	Base of proximal phalanx and extensor hood of fifth digit	
Posterior (dorsal) interossei			
First	First and second metatarsal bones	Proximal phalanx and extensor hood of second digit medially	
Second	Second and third metatarsal bones	Proximal phalanx and extensor hood of second digit laterally	Medial and lateral plantar S1 and S2
Third	Third and fourth metatarsal bones	Proximal phalanx and extensor hood of third digit laterally	
Fourth	Fourth and fifth metatarsal bones	Proximal phalanx and extensor hood of fourth digit laterally	
Abductor digiti minimi	Lateral side of fifth metatarsal bone	Proximal phalanx of fifth digit	Lateral plantar S1 and S2

brevis flexes the PIP joints and assists in flexion of the MTP joints of the second through fifth digits.

To specifically test this muscle, the patient is positioned in sitting or supine. Using one hand to stabilize the patient's midfoot, the clinician uses the other hand to apply pressure against the plantar surface of the PIP joints of the second through fifth digits (Figure 12-146).

▶ *Flexor digitorum accessorius (quadratus plantae; Figure 12-147).* This muscle arises from the calcaneal tuberosity via two heads. The medial head arises from the medial surface of the calcaneus and the medial border of the long plantar ligament, whereas the lateral head arises from the

lateral border of the plantar surface of the calcaneus and the lateral border of the long plantar ligament. The muscle terminates in tendinous slips, joining the long flexor tendons to the second, third, fourth, and occasionally fifth toes. This muscle modifies the line of pull of the flexor digitorum longus tendons and assists in flexion of the second through fifth digits. There is no specific test for this muscle.

▶ *Lumbricales.* There are four lumbricales (see Figure 12-148), all of which arise from the tendon of the flexor digitorum longus. The first arises from the medial side of the tendon of the second toe, the second from adjacent sides of the tendons

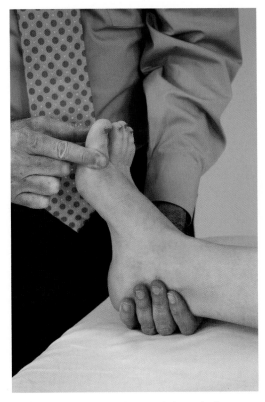

FIGURE 12-144 Test position for the abductor hallucis

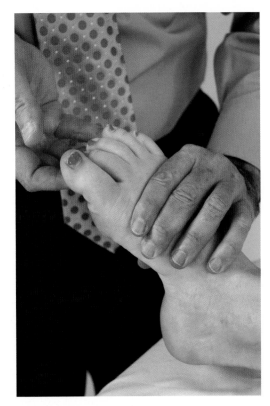

FIGURE 12-146 Test position for the flexor digitorum brevis

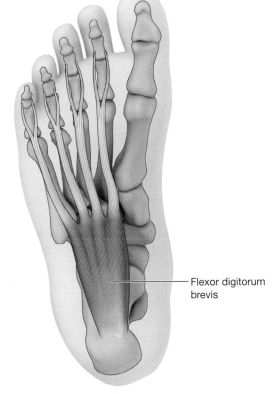

FIGURE 12-145 Flexor digitorum brevis muscle

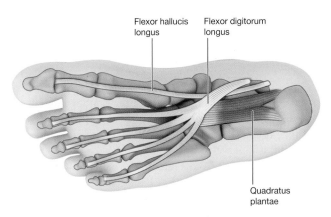

FIGURE 12-147 Quadratus plantae muscle

and interossei into the bases of the terminal phalanges of the four lateral toes. The function of the lumbricales is to flex the MTP joint and extend the PIP joint. The first lumbrical is innervated by the medial plantar nerve, whereas lumbricals two through four are innervated by the lateral plantar nerve. The synergist to these muscles is the flexor digitorum longus. The antagonists of this muscle group include the extensor digitorum longus and the extensor digitorum brevis.

To specifically test these muscles, the patient is positioned supine or sitting and is asked to flex the MTP joints of the feet. While using one hand to stabilize the patient's foot, the clinician uses the other hand to apply an extension force under the MTP joints of toes 2 through 4 (Figure 12-149).

▶ *Flexor hallucis brevis (Figure 12-150).* This muscle arises from the medial part of the plantar surface of the cuboid bone, the adjacent portion of the lateral cuneiform, and

for the second and third toes, the third from adjacent sides of the tendons for the third and fourth toes, and the fourth from adjacent sides of tendons for the fourth and fifth toes. They insert with the tendons of the extensor digitorum longus

395

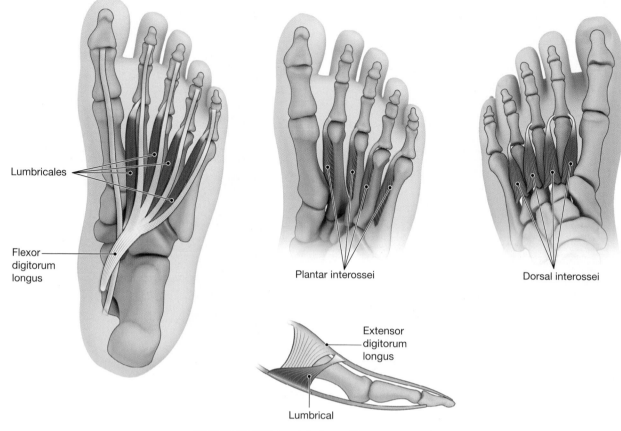

Lumbricales

Flexor digitorum longus

Plantar interossei

Dorsal interossei

Extensor digitorum longus

Lumbrical

FIGURE 12-148 Lumbricales and interossei muscles

the posterior tibialis tendon and inserts on the medial and lateral side of the proximal phalanx of the great toe. This muscle functions to flex the MTP joint of the great toe and is innervated by the tibial nerve.

To specifically test this muscle, the patient is positioned in supine or sitting. Using one hand to stabilize the foot proximal to the MTP joint and maintaining a neutral position of the foot and ankle, the clinician uses the other hand to apply an extension force at the MTP joints of the great toe (Figure 12-151).

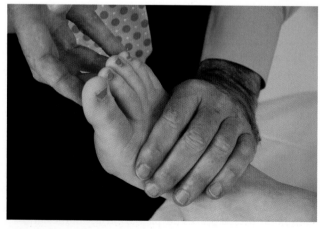

FIGURE 12-149 Test position for the lumbricales

▶ *Adductor hallucis (see Figure 12-143).* This muscle arises via two heads: an oblique and a transverse head. The oblique head arises from the bases of the second, third, and fourth metatarsal bones and the sheath of the fibularis (peroneus) longus. The transverse head arises from the joint capsules of the second, third, fourth, and fifth MTP heads and the deep transverse metatarsal ligament. The adductor hallucis inserts on the lateral side of the base of the proximal phalanx of the great toe. The adductor hallucis functions to adduct and assists in flexion of the MTP joint of the great toe and is innervated by the tibial nerve. There is no specific test for this muscle.

▶ *Posterior (dorsal) interossei (see Figure 12-148).* The four posterior (dorsal) interossei are bipennate, and they arise from adjacent sides of the metatarsal bones. The first inserts into the medial side of the proximal phalanx of the second toe. The second inserts into the lateral side of the proximal phalanx of the second toe. The third inserts into the lateral side of the proximal phalanx of the third toe, and the fourth inserts into the lateral side of the proximal phalanx of the fourth toe. The posterior (dorsal) interossei function to abduct the second, third, and fourth toes around an axis through the second metatarsal ray. The posterior interossei are innervated by the lateral plantar nerve. The synergists of these muscles include the flexor digitorum longus, flexor hallucis longus, and lumbricals

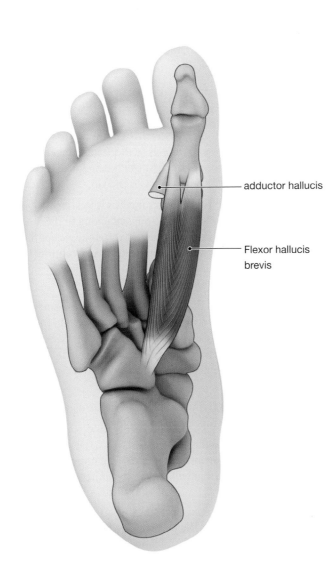

FIGURE 12-150 Flexor hallucis brevis muscle

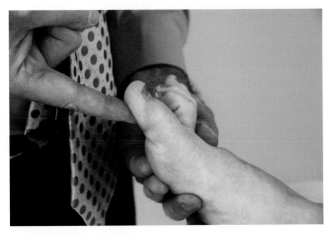

FIGURE 12-151 Test position for the flexor hallucis brevis

2 through 4. The antagonists of these muscles are the anterior interossei.

▶ *Plantar interossei (see Figure 12-148)*. The three plantar interossei are unipennate and arise from the bases and medial sides of the third, fourth, and fifth metatarsal bones. They insert into the medial sides of the bases of the proximal phalanges of the third, fourth, and fifth toes. The plantar interossei function to adduct the lateral three toes from

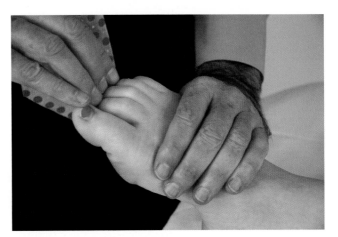

FIGURE 12-152 Test position for the interossei muscles

the midline and are innervated by the lateral plantar nerve. The synergists of this muscle include the flexor digitorum longus, flexor hallucis longus, and lumbricals 2 through 4. The antagonists of this muscle are the posterior interossei.

To specifically test these muscle groups, the patient is positioned in supine or sitting and is asked to extend the interphalangeal joints of the four lateral toes. The clinician stabilizes the MTP joints and places a finger on the posterior surface of the distal phalanges of each toe in the direction of flexion (Figure 12-152).

Posterior (Dorsal) Intrinsic Muscles

The posterior (dorsal) intrinsic muscles of the foot are the extensor hallucis brevis (EHB) and extensor digitorum brevis (EDB).

Extensor Hallucis Brevis. The EHB inserts into the base of the proximal phalanx of the great toe. The muscle is innervated by the lateral terminal branch of the deep fibular (peroneal) nerve. The extensor hallucis brevis is tested along with the extensor hallucis longus. Unless innervation to the extensor hallucis longus is absent, a weakness of the extensor digitorum brevis cannot be determined accurately.

Extensor Digitorum Brevis. The EDB originates from the superior lateral aspect of the calcaneus and inserts into the base of the second, third, and fourth proximal phalanges (see Figure 12-127). The EDB functions to extend the MTP joints of toes 1 through 4.

The EDB is innervated by the lateral terminal branch of the deep fibular (peroneal) nerve. The synergists of this muscle include the extensor hallucis longus and the extensor digitorum longus. The antagonist of this muscle include the flexor digitorum longus, flexor hallucis longus, abductor hallucis, lumbricals, anterior interossei, and dorsal interossei.

The EDB is tested together with the extensor digitorum longus (see Figure 12-128).

MUSCLE TESTING OF THE TRUNK

Various manual muscle testing methods have been used to assess adult abdominal strength clinically:

▶ Kendall and colleagues[37] have proposed two different procedures to measure abdominal muscle strength.

1. An assessment of a person's ability to keep the lumbar spine flat against the table while lowering both legs, with knees extended, from an initial position of 90° of hip flexion. The point in the range of motion at which the lumbar spine begins to demonstrate lordosis determines the muscle grade.

2. An assessment of strength based on the ability to flex the vertebral column and come to a sitting position while the legs remain stabilized in extension.

▶ Daniels and Worthingham[181] assign grades of trunk flexor muscle strength by having the person clear the scapulae from the table during trunk flexion. The lower extremities are stabilized in extension during their Normal (Grade 5), Good (Grade 4), and Fair (Grade 3) muscle test positions.

▶ Harvey and Scott[182] used a timed curl-down (reverse sit-up) test to measure abdominal muscle strength in young women.

The Specific Tests

Neck Flexors. The neck flexors include the following muscles:

▶ *Sternocleidomastoid (SCM).* The SCM is the largest muscle in the anterior neck. It is attached inferiorly by two heads, arising from the posterior aspect of the medial third of the clavicle and the manubrium of the sternum. From here, it passes superiorly and posteriorly to attach on the mastoid process of the temporal bone. The motor supply for this muscle is from the accessory nerve (CN XI), whereas the sensory innervation is supplied from the anterior (ventral) rami of C2 and C3.[183]

▶ *Prevertebral muscles* (longus colli, longus capitis, rectus capitis anterior, and rectus capitis lateralis).

■ *Longus colli.* The longus colli consists of a vertical portion that originates from the bodies of the first three thoracic and last three cervical vertebrae, an inferior oblique portion that originates from the bodies of the first three thoracic vertebrae, and the superior oblique portion that originates from anterior tubercles of the transverse processes of C3-5. The various portions of the longus colli insert into the bodies of C2-4, the anterior tubercles of the transverse processes of C5-6, and the anterior tubercle of the atlas. The longus colli is innervated by branches of the anterior primary rami of C2-8.

■ *Longus capitis.* The longus capitis originates from the anterior tubercles of the transverse processes of C3-6 and inserts onto the inferior surface of the basilar part of the occipital bone. The longus capitis is innervated by the muscular branches of C1-4.

■ *Rectus capitis anterior (RCA).* The RCA originates from the lateral mass of the atlas and inserts onto the base of the occipital bone in front of the foramen magnum. The RCA is innervated by the muscular branches of C1-2.

■ *Rectus capitis lateralis (RCL).* The RCL originates from the upper surface of the transverse process of the atlas and inserts onto the inferior surface of the jugular process of the occipital bone. The RCL is innervated by branches of the anterior rami of C1-2.

▶ *Scalenus anterior, medius, and posterior.* The scalenes extend obliquely like ladders (*scala* means ladder in Latin).

■ *Scalenus anterior.* The scalenus anterior runs vertically, behind the SCM on the lateral aspect of the neck. Arising from the anterior tubercles of the C3-6 transverse processes, it travels to the scalene tubercle on the inner border of the first rib. It is supplied by the anterior (ventral) rami of C4, C5, and C6.

■ *Scalenus medius.* The scalenus medius is the largest and longest of the scalenus group, attaching to the transverse processes of all cervical vertebrae except the atlas (although it often attaches to this) and running to the upper border of the first rib. It is innervated by the anterior (ventral) rami of C3-8.

■ *Scalenus posterior.* The scalenus posterior is the smallest and deepest of the scalenus group, running from the posterior tubercles of the C4-6 transverse processes to attach to the outer aspect of the second rib. It is innervated by the anterior (ventral) rami of C5, C6, and C7.

▶ *Suprahyoid.* The suprahyoid muscles include digastric, stylohyoid, geniohyoid, and mylohyoid.

▶ *Geniohyoid.* The geniohyoid muscle is a narrow muscle situated under the mylohyoid muscle. The muscle functions to elevate the hyoid bone. It is innervated by C1 through CN XII.

▶ *Digastric.* As its name suggests, the digastric muscle consists of two bellies. The posterior belly arises from the mastoid notch of the temporal bone, whereas the anterior belly arises from the digastric fossa of the mandible. The posterior belly is innervated by a branch from the facial nerve. The anterior belly is innervated by the inferior alveolar branch of the trigeminal nerve.

▶ *Mylohyoid.* This flat, triangular muscle arises from the whole length of the mylohyoid line of the mandible. The posterior fibers pass inferomedially to insert into the body of the hyoid bone. The middle and anterior fibers insert into a median fibrous raphe extending from the symphysis menti to the hyoid bone, where they joint at an angle with the fibers of the opposite muscle. The mylohyoid muscle is innervated by the mylohyoid nerve, a branch of the inferior alveolar nerve, which is a branch of the mandibular nerve, a division of the trigeminal nerve.

▶ *Stylohyoid.* The stylohyoid muscle arises from the posterior and lateral surface of the styloid process of the temporal bone, near the base, and, passing inferiorly and anteriorly, inserts into the body of the hyoid bone at its junction with the greater cornu and just superior the omohyoid muscle. It is innervated by the facial nerve (CN VII).

▶ *Infrahyoid.* The infrahyoid muscles comprise the sternohyoid, omohyoid, sternothyroid, and thyrohyoid muscles.

■ *Sternohyoid.* The sternohyoid muscle is a straplike muscle that originates from the sternum and inserts on the hyoid bone.

- *Omohyoid.* The omohyoid muscle, situated lateral to the sternohyoid, consists of two bellies. The superior belly arises from the intermediate tendon and inserts on the hyoid bone, whereas the inferior belly arises from the superior border of the scapular and inserts on the intermediate tendon.
- *Sternothyroid.* The sternothyroid muscle arises from the sternum and inserts on the thyroid cartilage.
- *Thyrohyoid.* The thyrohyoid muscle arises from the thyroid cartilage and inserts on the hyoid bone.

  These infrahyoid muscles are innervated by fibers from the upper cervical nerves. The nerves to the lower part of these muscles are given off from a loop, the ansa cervicalis.

To specifically test this muscle group, the patient is positioned in supine with the head in the anatomic position. The patient is asked to lift the head of the treatment table while keeping the chin tucked. Grading can be done as follows[184]:

- ▶ 10   N   5/5: five repetitions
- ▶ 5   F   3/5: 3 to 4 repetitions
- ▶ 2   P   2/5: 1 to 2 repetitions
- ▶ 0   Zero   0/5: zero repetitions

Neck Extensors. The neck extensors include the following muscles:

- *Upper trapezius.* See Muscle Testing of the Shoulder.
- *Splenius capitis.* The splenius capitis extends upward and laterally, from the posterior (dorsal) edge of the nuchal ligament and the spinous processes of the lower cervical and upper thoracic vertebrae (T4-C7) to the mastoid process of the occipital bone just inferior to the superior nuchal line and deep to the SCM muscle. This muscle is segmentally innervated by the lateral branches of the posterior (dorsal) rami of the spinal nerves.
- *Splenius cervicis.* The splenius cervicis is just inferior and appears continuous with the capitis, extending from the spines of the third to the sixth thoracic vertebrae to the posterior tubercles of the transverse processes of the upper cervical vertebrae. This muscle is segmentally innervated by the lateral branches of the posterior (dorsal) rami of the spinal nerves.
- *Erector spinae (cervical).* The erector spinae complex spans multiple segments, forming a large musculotendinous mass consisting of the iliocostalis, longissimus, and spinalis muscles. This muscle group is segmentally innervated by the lateral branches of the posterior (dorsal) rami of the spinal nerves.
- *Transversospinalis.* The transversospinalis muscles are a group of muscles that include the semispinalis, the multifidus, and the rotatores. This muscle group is segmentally innervated by the posterior (dorsal) rami of the spinal nerves.

To specifically test this muscle group, the patient is positioned in prone with the head in the anatomic position. The patient is asked to lift the head of the treatment table and to hold it against gravity. Grading can be done as follows[184]:

- ▶ 10   N   5/5: 20 seconds
- ▶ 5   F   3/5: 10 to 19 seconds
- ▶ 2   P   2/5: 1 to 9 seconds
- ▶ 0   Zero   0/5: zero seconds.

Anterior Trunk (Upper Abdominal) Flexors. The anterior trunk flexors include the rectus abdominis, transversus abdominis, and internal and external abdominal obliques.

- *Rectus abdominis.* The rectus abdominis originates from the cartilaginous ends of the fifth through seventh ribs and xiphoid and inserts on the superior aspect of the pubic bone.
- *Transversus abdominis.* The transverse abdominis muscle originates from the lateral one-third of the inguinal ligament, the anterior two-thirds of the inner lip of the iliac crest, the lateral raphe of the thoracolumbar fascia, and the internal aspects of the lower six costal cartilages, where it interdigitates with the diaphragm.[185] Its upper and middle fibers run transversely around the trunk and blend with the fascial envelope of the rectus abdominis muscle, while the lower fibers blend with the insertion of the internal oblique muscle on the pubic crest.
- *Internal oblique.* The internal oblique, which forms the middle layer of the lateral abdominal wall, is located between the transversus abdominis and the external oblique muscles.[186] It has multiple attachments to the inguinal ligament, lateral raphe, iliac crest, pubic crest, transverse abdominis, and costal cartilages of the seventh through ninth costal cartilages.
- *External oblique.* The external oblique originates from the lateral aspect of the 5th through 12th ribs and through interdigitations with the serratus anterior and latissimus dorsi. The muscle travels obliquely, medially, and inferiorly to insert into the linea alba, inguinal ligament, anterior–superior iliac spine, iliac crest, and pubic tubercle.

To specifically test this muscle group, the patient is positioned in the supine with the hips and knees flexed, the feet flat on the table, and the shoulder joints flexed to 90°. The patient is asked to assume a sitting position without using the upper extremities. Grading can be done as follows:

10	N	5/5: Able to correctly complete test movement (flex the vertebral column and keep it flexed while entering the hip-flexion phase and coming to a sitting position) with the hands clasped behind the head
9	G+	4+/5: Able to correctly complete test movement with hands at shoulders
8	G	4/5: Able to correctly complete test movement with arms crossed at the chest
7	G−	4−/5: Able to correctly complete test movement with arms crossed at the abdomen
6	F+	3+/5: Able to correctly complete test movement with arms extended forward
5	F	3/5: Able to correctly perform posterior pelvic tilt and flex the vertebral column with arms extended forward, but is unable to maintain the trunk flexion when attempting to enter the hip-flexion phase of the test movement

4   F–   3–/5: Able to tilt the pelvis posteriorly and keep the pelvis and thorax approximated as the head is raised from the table

2   P   2/5: Same position as 3–/5 grade: able to tilt the pelvis posteriorly but unable to maintain it as head is raised from the table

1   T   1/5: Same position as 3-/5 grade: When patient attempts to depress the chest or tilt the pelvis posteriorly, a contraction can be felt in the anterior abdominal muscles, but there is no approximation of the pelvis and thorax

0   Zero   0/5: No palpable muscle contraction

Lateral Trunk Flexors. The lateral trunk flexors include the erector spinae and the abdominals on the same side as the direction of side flexion. To specifically test this muscle group, the patient is positioned in sidelying with the leg straight and a pillow between the legs. The clinician stabilizes the legs and, while maintaining the upper arm along the side and the other arm across the chest, the patient is asked to lift the body off the floor toward the ceiling. This test can be graded as follows:

▶ *Normal:* able to fully lift and bend the back sideways

▶ *Good:* able to lift and then the back sideways with the shoulder 4 inches from the floor

▶ *Fair:* able to lift and bend the back sideways with the shoulder 2 inches from the floor

▶ *Poor:* unable to lift and bend the back sideways

Anterior Trunk (Lower Abdominals) Flexors. To specifically test this muscle group, the patient is positioned in supine with both of the legs straight and the arms folded across the chest. The patient is asked to raise the legs to a vertical position one at a time while keeping the back flat on the floor and then to slowly lower the legs together to the floor. This test can be graded based on the height at which the patient is unable to maintain the low back flat on the floor, as follows:

10   N   5/5   Able to perform posterior pelvic tilt and hold low back flat on table while lowering the legs to the fully extended position 0° to 15° (table level)

9   G+   4+/5   Able to perform posterior pelvic tilt and hold low back flat on table while lowering the legs to an angle of 15° to 30° with the table

8   G   4/5   Able to perform posterior pelvic tilt and hold low back flat on table while lowering the legs to an angle of 30° to 45° with the table

7   G–   4–/5   Able to perform posterior pelvic tilt and hold low back flat on table while lowering the legs to an angle of 45° to 60° with the table

6   F+   3+/5   Able to perform posterior pelvic tilt and hold low back flat on table while lowering the legs to an angle of 60° to 75° with the table

5   F   3/5   Able to perform posterior pelvic tilt and hold low back flat on table while lowering the legs to an angle of >75° with the table

4   F–   3–/5   and lower: The leg lowering test is not performed

The clinician should note if the patient exhibits any of the following faulty movement patterns:

▶ Excessive participation of the rectus abdominis throughout leg lowering

▶ Excessive participation of head and neck for stabilization

▶ Increased intra-abdominal pressure to stabilize lumbar spine (holding breath)

Back Extensors. The muscles that provide back extension are numerous and very difficult to isolate. To specifically test this muscle group, the patient is positioned in prone with the hands clasped behind the back. The patient is asked to raise the trunk off the floor. According to Kendall and colleagues,[37] back extensor strength is best graded as slight, moderate, or marked, based on the judgment of the examiner. For example:

▶ *Slight:* Able to complete test movement with hands behind the head

▶ *Moderate:* Able to complete test movement with hands clasped behind the back

▶ *Marked:* Able to partially complete the test movement to the point where the xiphoid process is raised slightly, with the hands clasped behind the back

McGill and colleagues[187,188] have published normative data for the lateral, flexor, and extensor tests for young (mean age 21 years), healthy individuals (Table 12-10).

The following tests can be used to assess the strength of the lumbar stabilizers.

Lower Abdominal Hollowing. The abdominal hollowing exercise tests the ability of the multifidus and transverse abdominis to co-contract.[189,190] These muscles are important for the provision of segmental control to the spine, because they provide an important stiffening effect on the lumbar spine, thereby enhancing dynamic stability.[191]

The patient is positioned supine. The patient is instructed to contract the deep abdominal muscles and to draw the navel up toward the chest and in toward the spine, so as to hollow the abdomen. When the muscle contracts properly, an increase in tension can be felt at a point 2 cm medial and inferior to the anterior superior iliac spine. If a bulging is felt at this point, the internal oblique is contracting rather than the transverse abdominis.[189,190] The multifidus is palpated simultaneously and should be felt to swell at a point just lateral to the spinous process.[189,190] The patient's head and upper trunk must remain stable, and he or she is not permitted to flex forward, push through the feet, or tilt the pelvis.

Spine Rotators and Multifidus Test. This test is designed to assess the ability of the spinal rotators and multifidus to stabilize the trunk during dynamic extremity movements.[192] The patient is positioned in the quadruped position, with the pelvis positioned in neutral using muscular control. The patient is then asked to perform the following maneuvers: (1) single straight arm and hold, (2) single straight leg lift and hold, and (3) contralateral straight arm and straight leg lift and hold. The scoring for this test is as follows[192]:

Normal (5) =   able to perform contralateral arm and leg lift, both sides, while maintaining neutral pelvis (20- to 30-second hold)

TABLE 12-10	Endurance Times and Flexion/Extension Ratios for the Flexor Endurance Test, Lateral Endurance Test, and Extensor Endurance Test		
Test	**Men (mean age 21 years)**	**Women (mean age 21 years)**	**Men (mean age 34 years)**
Extension	162 seconds	185 seconds	103
Flexion	136 seconds	134 seconds	66
Right lateral endurance (SB) test	95 seconds	75 seconds	54
Left lateral endurance (SB) test	99 seconds	78 seconds	54
Flexion/extension ratio	0.84	0.72	0.71
RSB/LSB ratio	0.96	0.96	1.05
RSB/extension ratio	0.58	0.40	0.57
LSB/extension ratio	0.61	0.42	0.58

Good (4) = able to maintain neutral pelvis while performing single leg lift, but not able to hold pelvis in neutral when doing contralateral arm and leg lift (15- to 20-second hold)

Fair (3) = Able to do single arm lift and maintain neutral pelvis (15- to 20-second hold)

Poor (2) = Unable to maintain neutral pelvis while doing single arm lift

Trace (1) = Unable to raise arm or leg off the table to the straight position

Abdominal Endurance Test. This test measures the endurance of the abdominals. The patient is positioned supine, with the hips flexed to approximately 45°, the feet flat on the bed, and the arms by the side. A line is drawn 8 cm (for patients 40 years and older) or 12 cm (for patients younger than 40 years of age) distal to the fingers.[193] The patient is asked to tuck in the chin and to curl the trunk and touch the line with the fingers. The patient holds this position for as long as possible. The test is graded as follows[154,194]:

Normal (5) = 20- to 30-second hold

Good (4) = 15- to 20-second hold

Fair (3) = 10- to 15-second hold

Poor (2) = 1- to 10-second hold

Trace (1) = Unable to raise more than the head off the table

Side Support or Side Bridge Test. The so-called side support or side bridge position has been identified as optimizing the challenge to the quadratus lumborum while minimizing the load on the lumbar spine.[187] The patient is in the sidelying position, with the knees flexed to 90° and resting the upper body on the elbow. The test can be made more difficult by having the knees extended so that the legs are straight. The patient is asked to lift the pelvis off the table and to straighten the curve of the spine without rolling forward or backward. This position is then held. The test is graded as follows:

Normal (5) = Able to lift pelvis off the table and hold spine straight for a 20- to 30-second hold

Good (4) = Able to lift pelvis off the table but has difficulty holding spine straight for a 15- to 20-second hold

Fair (3) = Able to lift pelvis off the table but has difficulty holding spine straight for a 10- to 15-second hold

Poor (2) = Able to lift pelvis off the table but cannot hold spine straight for a 1- to 10-second hold

Trace (1) = Unable to lift pelvis off the table

Double Straight Leg Lowering Test. The straight leg lowering test can be used to assess core strength.[189,195-201] The patient is in the supine hooklying position, with the hips flexed to 90° and with a pressure cuff placed under the lumbar spine at the level of L4 to L5. The cuff is inflated to 40 mm Hg. The clinician raises the patient's legs until the pelvis is seen to posteriorly rotate, and the needle on the pressure monitor begins to move. The patient is asked to perform the lower abdominal hollowing maneuver so as to prevent further pelvic motion, and is then asked to lower the legs toward the bed while maintaining the lower abdominal hollowing. At the point when the cuff pressure is seen to increase or decrease, or when the pelvis anteriorly rotates, the test is over, and the hip angle at which this occurs is measured. This test may also be graded using the following scoring[194]:

Normal (5) = Able to reach 0 to 15° from the table before pelvis tilts

Good (4) = Able to reach 16 to 45° from the table before pelvis tilts

Fair (3) = Able to reach 46 to 75° from the table before pelvis tilts

Poor (2) = Able to reach 75 to 90° from the table before pelvis tilts

Trace (1) = Unable to hold pelvis in neutral

A study by Youdas and colleagues[201] found that the odds of a patient having chronic low back pain is increased if the score on the leg lowering test for the abdominal muscles exceeds 50° for men and 60° for women. Another study[202] found that there is a natural tendency for the pelvis to rotate anteriorly from very early on during this test, and that, as healthy young subjects were unable to prevent the tilting, the preceding scoring system may be questionable.

The Bent Knee Lowering Test. The lower abdominal musculature can be assessed in a similar fashion.[195,196,199] The patient is positioned supine with the knees and hips flexed to approximately 90°. A pressure cuff, inflated to 40 mm Hg, is placed under the L4 to L5 segment. The patient is asked to perform the abdominal hollowing maneuver, and then to slowly lower the legs to the bed until the pressure on the monitor is seen to decrease. The hip angle is again measured at the point where there is a change in the pressure cuff reading, or where the anterior tilt of the pelvis occurred.

Normal (5) = Able to reach 0 to 15° from the table before pelvis tilts

Good (4) = Able to reach 16 to 45° from the table before pelvis tilts

Fair (3) = Able to reach 46 to 75° from the table before pelvis tilts

Poor (2) = Able to reach 75 to 90° from the table before pelvis tilts

Trace (1) = Unable to hold pelvis in neutral

Trunk Raise. The trunk raise test can be used to assess the endurance of the iliocostalis lumborum (erector spinae) and the multifidus.[195,199,203,204] The patient is positioned prone, with the hands behind the back, or by the sides. The patient is instructed to extend at the lumbar spine by raising the chest off the bed to approximately 30° (the axilla can be used as the reference for the axis if a goniometer is used) and to hold the position for as long as possible. The clinician times the test[195]:

Normal (5) = 20- to 30-second hold

Good (4) = 15- to 20-second hold

Fair (3) = 10- to 15-second hold

Poor (2) = 1- to 10-second hold

Trace (1) = Unable to raise more than the head off the table

Lunge. The patient is asked to perform a lunge. The clinician notes the quality and quantity of the motion, as well as the ability of the patient to sustain the position for 30 seconds.[205] Excessive shaking of the legs with this maneuver may indicate weakness of the lumbopelvic stabilizers or poor balance and proprioception.

Muscle Testing the Trunk in the Athletic Population

According to McGill and colleagues,[188,189] the torso flexors, extensors, and lateral musculature are involved in spine stability during virtually any task, and therefore the endurance of each of these muscles groups should be measured. The following tests are recommended:

▶ *Flexor endurance test.* The patient is positioned in sitting with the back supported at an angle of approximately 60° from the floor (Figure 12-153), with both knees and hips flexed to 90° and the arms folded across the chest. The patient's foot can be stabilized manually or by using a belt

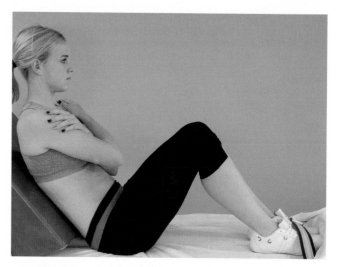

FIGURE 12-153 Flexor endurance test—start position

(see Figure 12-153). Once the patient is ready, the support is removed from the back (Figure 12-154), and the patient attempts to maintain the isometric posture for as long as possible. Failure occurs when the patient is no longer able to maintain the position.

▶ *Lateral endurance test.* The patient is positioned in the full side bridge position (Figure 12-155). The patient attempts to maintain this position for as long as possible. Failure occurs when the patient loses the straight-backed posture and the hip returns to the table. The test is then repeated on the other side.

▶ *Extensor endurance test.* The patient is positioned in prone with the lower extremity supported so that the trunk and upper extremities are over the edge of the table (Figure 12-156). The upper extremities are held across the chest. Failure occurs when the upper body drops from the horizontal position.

McGill used these tests on young, healthy individuals (92 men and 137 women with a mean age of 21 years), and with a group of men with a mean age of 34 years with no history of back trouble. The results are depicted in Table 12-10. According to McGill, the interpretation of absolute endurance should be secondary to interpreting the imbalance among the three muscle groups, and the discrepancies outlined in Table 12-11

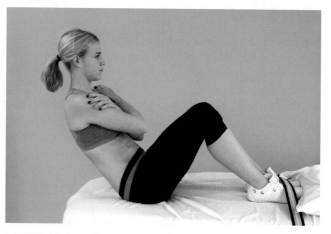

FIGURE 12-154 Flexor endurance test—support removed

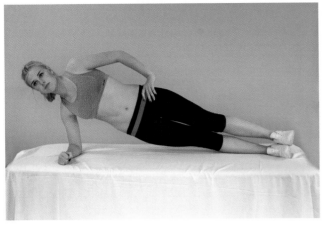

FIGURE 12-155 Lateral endurance test

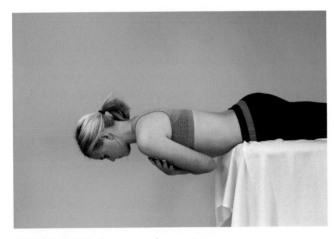

FIGURE 12-156 Extensor endurance test

suggest unbalanced endurance, which increases the potential for injury and should thus be the focus of the intervention.

USING SPECIFIC MUSCLE TESTING FOR DIAGNOSIS

Specific muscle testing can provide the clinician with valuable information in addition to the strength grade of the muscle. Cyriax reasoned that if the clinician isolates and then applies tension to a structure, he or she could make a conclusion as to the integrity of that structure.[206] According to Cyriax, pain with

TABLE 12-11	Asymmetrical Unbalances
Right side bridge/left side bridge endurance	>0.05
Flexion/extension endurance	>1.0
Side bridge (either side)/extension endurance	>0.75
Extensor strength (N. m)/extensor endurance (seconds)—strength to endurance ratio	>4.0

a contraction generally indicates an injury to the muscle or a capsular structure.[206] This suspicion can be confirmed by combining the findings from the isometric test with the findings of the passive motion and the joint distraction and compression tests (Table 12-12). Pain that occurs consistently with resistance, whatever the length of the muscle, may indicate a tear of the muscle belly. Pain with muscle testing may indicate a muscle injury, a joint injury, or a combination of both. Pain that does not occur during the test, but occurs on the release of the contraction, is thought to have an articular source, produced by the joint glide that occurs following the release of tension.

CLINICAL PEARL

Pain that occurs with resistance, accompanied by pain at the opposite end of passive range, indicates muscle impairment.

Cyriax also introduced the concept of tissue reactivity. Tissue reactivity is the manner in which different stresses and movements can alter the clinical signs and symptoms. This knowledge can be used to gauge any subtle changes to the patient's condition.[207]

Strength testing may also be used to examine the neurologic integrity of muscles. Weakness in muscle testing must be differentiated between weakness throughout the range of motion (pathologic weakness) and weakness that only occurs in certain positions (positional weakness).

Thus, strength testing can provide the clinician with the following findings[154]:

▶ A weak and painless contraction may indicate palsy or a complete rupture of the muscle–tendon unit. The motor disorder of peripheral neuropathy is first manifested by weakness and diminished or absent tendon reflex.[208]

▶ A strong and painless contraction indicates a normal finding.

TABLE 12-12	Differential Diagnosis of Contractile, Inert, and Neural Tissue Injury		
	Contractile Tissue	**Inert Tissue**	**Neural Tissue**
Pain	Cramping, dull, and ache	Dull–sharp	Burning and lancinating
Paresthesia	No	No	Yes
Duration	Intermittent	Intermittent	Intermittent–constant
Dermatomal distribution	No	No	Yes
Peripheral nerve sensory distribution	No	No	Yes (if peripheral nerve involved)
End-feel	Muscle spasm	Boggy and hard capsular	Stretch

► A weak and painful contraction: A study by Franklin and colleagues[209] indicated that the conditions related to this finding need to be expanded to include not only serious pathology, such as a significant muscle tear or tumor, but relatively minor muscle damage and inflammation such as that induced by eccentric isokinetic exercise.[4]

► A strong and painful contraction indicates a grade I contractile lesion.

The degree of certainty regarding the findings just described depends on a combination of the length of the muscle tested and the force applied. To fully test the integrity of the muscle–tendon unit, a maximum contraction must be performed in the fully lengthened position of the muscle–tendon unit. Although this position fully tests the muscle–tendon unit, there are some problems with testing in this manner:

► The joint and its surrounding inert tissues are in a more vulnerable position and could be the source of the pain.

► It is difficult to differentiate among damage to the contractile tissue of varying severity. The degree of significance with the findings in resistive testing depends on the position of the muscle and the force applied (Table 12-13). For example, pain reproduced with a minimal contraction in the rest position for the muscle is more strongly suggestive of a contractile lesion than pain reproduced with a maximal contraction in the lengthened position for the muscle.

► As a muscle lengthens, it reaches a point of passive insufficiency, where it is not capable of generating its maximum force output.

TABLE 12-13	Strength Testing Related to Joint Position and Muscle Length
Muscle Length	**Rationale**
Fully lengthened	Muscle in position of passive insufficiency
	Tightens the inert component of the muscle
	Tests for muscle tears (tenoperiosteal tears) while using minimal force
Midrange	Muscle in strongest position
	Tests overall power of muscle
Fully shortened	Muscle in its weakest position
	Used for the detection of palsies, especially if coupled with an eccentric contraction

If the same muscle is tested on the opposite side, using the same testing procedure, the concern about the length of the muscle is removed, because the focus of the test is to provide a comparison with same muscle on the opposite side, rather than to assess the absolute force output.

CLINICAL PEARL

To avoid confusion when interpreting the results from specific muscle testing, the clinician must always ascertain which grading system is being used and the various definitions for each of the grades (Table 12-14).

TABLE 12-14	Comparison of MMT Grades[a]			
Medical Research Council[b]	**Worthingham[c]**	**McCreary[d]**		**Explanation**
5	Normal (N)	100%		Holds test position against maximal resistance
4+	Good + (G+)			Holds test position against moderate to strong pressure
4	Good (G)	80%		Holds test position against moderate resistance
4−	Good − (G−)			Holds test position against slight to moderate pressure
3+	Fair + (F+)			Holds test position against slight resistance
3	Fair (F)	50%		Holds test position against gravity
3−	Fair − (F−)			Gradual release from test position
2+	Poor + (P+)			Moves through partial ROM against gravity OR Moves through complete ROM, gravity eliminated, and holds against pressure
2	Poor (P)	20%		Able to move through full ROM, gravity eliminated

TABLE 12-14 **Comparison of MMT Grades[a] (continued)**

Medical Research Council[b]	Worthingham[c]	McCreary[d]	Explanation
2–	Poor – (P–)		Moves through partial ROM, gravity eliminated
1	Trace (T)	5%	No visible movement; palpable or observable tendon prominence/flicker contraction
0	0	0%	No palpable or observable muscle contraction
The grades of 0, 1, and 2 are tested in the gravity-minimized position (contraction is perpendicular to the gravitational force). All other grades are tested in the antigravity position.	The more functional of the three grading systems because it tests a motion that utilizes all of the agonists and synergists involved in the motion.[a]	Designed to test a specific muscle rather than the motion. Requires both selective recruitment of a muscle by the patient and a sound knowledge of anatomy and kinesiology on the part of the clinician to determine the correct alignment of the muscle fibers.[a]	

[a]Palmer ML, Epler M: Principles of examination techniques, in Palmer ML, Epler M (eds): Clinical Assessment Procedures in Physical Therapy. Philadelphia, JB Lippincott, 1990, pp 8-36.

[b]Frese E, Brown M, Norton B: Clinical reliability of manual muscle testing: middle trapezius and gluteus medius muscles. Phys Ther 67:1072-1076, 1987.

[c]Daniels K, Worthingham C: Muscle Testing Techniques of Manual Examination (ed 5). Philadelphia, WB Saunders, 1986.

[d]Kendall FP, McCreary EK, Provance PG: Muscles: Testing and Function. Baltimore, Williams & Wilkins, 1993.

REFERENCES

1. American Medical Association: Guides to the Evaluation of Permanent Impairment (ed 5). Chicago, American Medical Association, 2001.
2. Beasley WC: Quantitative muscle testing: principles and applications to research and clinical services. Arch Phys Med Rehabil 42:398-425, 1961.
3. MacConnail MA, Basmajian JV: Muscles and Movements: A Basis for Human Kinesiology. New York, Robert Krieger, 1977.
4. White DJ: Musculoskeletal examination, in O'Sullivan SB, Schmitz TJ (eds): Physical Rehabilitation (ed 5). Philadelphia, FA Davis, 2007, pp 159-192.
5. Florence JM, Pandya S, King WM, et al: Intrarater reliability of manual muscle test (Medical Research Council scale) grades in Duchenne's muscular dystrophy. Phys Ther 72:115-122; discussion 122-126, 1992.
6. Barr AE, Diamond BE, Wade CK, et al: Reliability of testing measures in Duchenne or Becker muscular dystrophy. Arch Phys Med Rehabil 72:315-9, 1991.
7. Nadler SF, Rigolosi L, Kim D, et al: Sensory, motor, and reflex examination, in Malanga GA, Nadler SF (eds): Musculoskeletal Physical Examination—An Evidence-Based Approach. Philadelphia, Mosby, 2006, pp 15-32.
8. Bohannon RW: Make tests and break tests of elbow flexor muscle strength. Phys Ther 68:193-194, 1988.
9. Stratford PW, Balsor BE: A comparison of make and break tests using a hand-held dynamometer and the Kin-Com. J Orthop Sports Phys Ther 19:28-32, 1994.
10. Andrews AW, Thomas MW, Bohannon RW: Normative values for isometric muscle force measurements obtained with hand-held dynamometers. Phys Ther 76:248-259, 1996.
11. Sapega AA: Muscle performance evaluation in orthopedic practice. J Bone Joint Surg 72A:1562-1574, 1990.
12. Iddings DM, Smith LK, Spencer WA: Muscle testing: part 2. Reliability in clinical use. Phys Ther Rev 41:249-256, 1961.
13. Silver M, McElroy A, Morrow L, et al: Further standardization of manual muscle test for clinical study: applied in chronic renal disease. Phys Ther 50:1456-1465, 1970.
14. Marx RG, Bombardier C, Wright JG: What we know about the reliability and validity of physical examination tests used to examine the upper extremity. J Hand Surg 24A:185-193, 1999.
15. Astrand PO, Rodahl K: Textbook of Work Physiology. New York, McGraw-Hill, 1973.
16. Astrand PO, Rodahl K: The Muscle and Its Contraction: Textbook of Work Physiology. New York, McGraw-Hill, 1986.
17. Muller EA: Influences of training and inactivity of muscle strength. Arch Phys Med Rehabil 51:449-462, 1970.
18. Phillips BA, Lo SK, Mastaglia FL: Muscle force measured using "break" testing with a hand-held myometer in normal subjects aged 20 to 69 years. Arch Phys Med Rehabil 81:653-661, 2000.
19. Beck M, Giess R, Wurffel W, et al: Comparison of maximal voluntary isometric contraction and Drachman's hand-held dynamometry in evaluating patients with amyotrophic lateral sclerosis. Muscle Nerve 22:1265-1270, 1999.
20. Roy MA, Doherty TJ: Reliability of hand-held dynamometry in assessment of knee extensor strength after hip fracture. Am J Phys Med Rehabil 83:813-818, 2004.
21. Hutten MM, Hermens HJ: Reliability of lumbar dynamometry measurements in patients with chronic low back pain with test–retest measurements on different days. Eur Spine J 6:54-62, 1997.
22. Stokes HM, Landrieu KW, Domangue B, et al: Identification of low effort patients through dynamometry. J Hand Surg 20A:1047-1056, 1995.
23. Bohannon RW: Hand-held compared with isokinetic dynamometry for measurement of static knee extension torque (parallel reliability of dynamometers). Clin Phys Physiol Meas 11:217-222, 1990.
24. Hartsell HD, Forwell L: Postoperative eccentric and concentric isokinetic strength for the shoulder rotators in the scapular and neutral planes. J Orthop Sports Phys Ther 25:19-25, 1997.
25. Hartsell HD, Spaulding SJ: Eccentric/concentric ratios at selected velocities for the invertor and evertor muscles of the chronically unstable ankle. Br J Sports Med 33:255-258, 1999.
26. Griffin JW: Differences in elbow flexion torque measured concentrically, eccentrically and isometrically. Phys Ther 67:1205-1208, 1987.
27. Hortobagyi T, Katch FI: Eccentric and concentric torque-velocity relationships during arm flexion and extension. J Appl Physiol 60:395-401, 1995.
28. Trudelle-Jackson E, Meske N, Highenboten C, et al: Eccentric/concentric torque deficits in the quadriceps muscle. J Orthop Sports Phys Ther 11:142-145, 1989.

29. Rothstein JM, Lamb RL, Mayhew TP: Clinical uses of isokinetic measurements. Critical issues. Phys Ther 67:1840-1844, 1987.

30. Bohannon RW: Manual muscle test scores and dynamometer test scores of knee extension strength. Arch Phys Med Rehabil 67:390-392, 1986.

31. Mulroy SJ, Lassen KD, Chambers SH, et al: The ability of male and female clinicians to effectively test knee extension strength using manual muscle testing. J Orthop Sports Phys Ther 26:192-199, 1997.

32. Jobe FW, Pink M: Classification and treatment of shoulder dysfunction in the overhead athlete. J Orthop Sports Phys Ther 18:427-431, 1993.

33. Haymaker W, Woodhall B: Peripheral Nerve Injuries. Principles of Diagnosis. London, WB Saunders, 1953.

34. Brodal A: Neurological Anatomy. London, Oxford University Press, 1981.

35. Mercer S, Campbell AH: Motor innervation of the trapezius. J Man Manip Ther 8:18-20, 2000.

36. Ayub E: Posture and the upper quarter, in Donatelli RA (ed): Physical Therapy of the Shoulder (ed 2). New York, Churchill Livingstone, 1991, pp 81-90.

37. Kendall FP, McCreary EK, Provance PG, et al: Muscles: Testing and Function, with Posture and Pain. Baltimore, Williams & Wilkins, 2005.

38. Neumann DA: Shoulder complex, in Neumann DA (ed): Kinesiology of the Musculoskeletal System: Foundations for Physical Rehabilitation. St Louis, Mosby, 2002, pp 91-132.

39. White SM, Witten CM: Long thoracic nerve palsy in a professional ballet dancer. Am J Sports Med 21:626-629, 1993.

40. Jobe CM: Gross anatomy of the shoulder, in Rockwood CA, Matsen FA (eds): The Shoulder (ed 2). Philadelphia, WB Saunders, 1998, pp 35-97.

41. Connor PM, Yamaguchi K, Manifold SG, et al: Split pectoralis major transfer for serratus anterior palsy. Clin Orthop 341:134-142, 1997.

42. Schultz JS, Leonard JA: Long thoracic neuropathy from athletic activity. Arch Phys Med Rehabil 73:87-90, 1992.

43. Gregg JR, Labosky D, Hearty M, et al: Serratus anterior paralysis in the young athlete. J Bone Joint Surg 61A:825-832, 1979.

44. Marks PH, Warner JJP, Irrgang JJ: Rotator cuff disorders of the shoulder. J Hand Ther 7:90-98, 1994.

45. Warner JJ, Navarro RA: Serratus anterior dysfunction. Recognition and treatment. Clin Orthop Rel Res 349:139-48, 1998.

46. Leffert RD: Neurological problems, in Rockwood CA, Jr, Matsen FR III (eds): The Shoulder. Philadelphia, WB Saunders, 1990, pp 750-773.

47. Perry J: Biomechanics of the shoulder, in Rowe CR (ed): The Shoulder. New York, Churchill Livingstone, 1988, pp 1-15.

48. Warner JJP, Micheli LJ, Arslanian LE, et al: Scapulothoracic motion in normal shoulders and shoulders with glenohumeral instability and impingement syndrome. A study using Moire topographic analysis. Clin Orthop 285:191-199, 1992.

49. Post M: Pectoralis major transfer for winging of the scapula. J Shoulder Elbow Surg 4:1-9, 1995.

50. Kapandji IA: The Physiology of Joints. New York, Churchill Livingstone, 1974.

51. Dunleavy K: Relationship between the shoulder and the cervicothoracic spine. La Crosse, Wisc, Orthopedic Section, APTA, 2001.

52. Porterfield, J, De Rosa C: Mechanical Neck Pain: Perspectives in Functional Anatomy. Philadelphia, WB Saunders, 1995.

53. Murray MP, Gore DR, Gardner GM, et al: Shoulder motion and muscle strength of normal men and women in two age groups. Clin Orthop Rel Res 192:268-273, 1985.

54. Mikesky AE, Edwards JE, Wigglesworth JK, et al: Eccentric and concentric strength of the shoulder and arm musculature in collegiate baseball pitchers. Am J Sports Med 23:638-42, 1995.

55. Perry J: Muscle Control of the Shoulder, in Rowe CR (ed): The Shoulder. New York, Churchill Livingstone, 1988, pp 17-34.

56. Culham E, Peat M: Functional anatomy of the shoulder complex. J Orthop Sports Phys Ther 18:342-350, 1993.

57. Blackburn TA, McLeod WD, White B, et al: EMG analysis of posterior rotator cuff exercises. Athl Training 25:40-45, 1990.

58. Bradley JP, Tibone JE: Electromyographic analysis of muscle action about the shoulder. Clin Sports Med 4:789-805, 1991.

59. Perry J, Glousman RE: Biomechanics of throwing, in Nicholas JA, Hershman EB (eds): The Upper Extremity in Sports Medicine. St Louis, CV Mosby, 1990, pp 727-751.

60. Sharkey NA, Marder RA: The rotator cuff opposes superior translation of the humeral head. Am J Sports Med 23:270-275, 1995.

61. Sharkey NA, Marder RA, Hanson PB: The role of the rotator cuff in elevation of the arm. Trans Orthop Res Soc 18:137, 1993.

62. Turkel SJ, Panio MW, Marshall JL, et al: Stabilizing mechanisms preventing anterior dislocation of the glenohumeral joint. J Bone Joint Surg [Am] 63:1208-1217, 1981.

63. Chepeha JC: Shoulder trauma and hypomobility, in Magee DJ, Zachazewski JE, Quillen WS (eds): Pathology and Intervention in Musculoskeletal Rehabilitation. St Louis, Saunders, 2009, pp 92-124.

64. Vangsness CT, Jr, Jorgenson SS, Watson T, et al: The origin of the long head of the biceps from the scapula and glenoid labrum. An anatomical study of 100 shoulders. 95J Bone Joint Surg [Br] 76:951-4, 1994.

65. Altchek D, Wolf B: Disorders of the biceps tendon, in Krishnan S, Hawkins R, Warren R (eds): The Shoulder and the Overhead Athlete. Philadelphia, PA, Lippincott, Williams & Wilkins, 2004, pp 196-208.

66. Habermeyer P, Magosch P, Pritsch M, et al: Anterosuperior impingement of the shoulder as a result of pulley lesions: a prospective arthroscopic study. J Shoulder Elbow Surg 13:5-12, 2004.

67. Krupp RJ, Kevern MA, Gaines MD, et al: Long head of the biceps tendon pain: differential diagnosis and treatment. J Orthop Sports Phys Ther 39:55-70, 2009.

68. Mathes SJ, Nahai F: Biceps brachii, in Mathes SJ, Nahai F (eds): Clinical Atlas of Muscle and Musculocutaneous Flaps. St Louis, Mosby, 1979, pp 426-432.

69. Matsen FA, III, Arntz CT: Subacromial impingement, in Rockwood CA, Jr, Matsen FA III (eds): The Shoulder. Philadelphia, WB Saunders, 1990, pp 623-648.

70. Neer CS II: Anterior acromioplasty for the chronic impingement syndrome in the shoulder: a preliminary report. J Bone Joint Surg [Am] 54:41-50, 1972.

71. Neer C: Impingement lesions. Clin Orthop 173:71-77, 1983.

72. Lucas DB: Biomechanics of the shoulder joint. Arch Surg 107:425-432, 1973.

73. Levy AS, Kelly BT, Lintner SA, et al: Function of the long head of the biceps at the shoulder: electromyographic analysis. J Shoulder Elbow Surg 10:250-255, 2001.

74. Andrews JR, Carson WG, McLeod WD: Glenoid labrum tears related to the long head of the biceps. Am J Sports Med 13:337-341, 1985.

75. Basmajian JV, Deluca CJ: Muscles Alive: Their Functions Revealed by Electromyography. Baltimore, Williams & Wilkins, 1985.

76. Basmajian JV, Bazant FJ: Factors preventing downward dislocation of the adducted shoulder joint: an electromyographic and morphological study. J Bone Joint Surg 41A:1182-1186, 1959.

77. Itoi E, Kuechle DK, Newman SR, et al: Stabilising function of the biceps in stable and unstable shoulders. J Bone Joint Surg [Am] 75B:546-550, 1993.

78. Rodosky MW, Harner CD, Fu FH: The role of the long head of the biceps muscle and superior glenoid labrum in anterior stability of the shoulder. Am J Sports Med 22:121-130, 1994.

79. Norkin C, Levangie P: Joint Structure and Function: A Comprehensive Analysis. Philadelphia, FA Davis, 1992.

80. Pagnani M, Deng X-H, Warren RF, et al: Effect of lesions of the superior portion of the glenoid labrum on glenohumeral translation. J Bone Joint Surg 77A:1002-1010, 1995.

81. Payne LZ, Deng X, Craig EV, et al: The combined dynamic and static contributions to subacromial impingement. Am J Sports Med 25:801-808, 1997.

82. Warner JJP, McMahon PJ: The role of the long head of the biceps brachii in superior stability of the glenohumeral joint. J Bone Joint Surg 77A:366-372, 1995.

83. Kido T, Itoi E, Konno N, et al: The depressor function of biceps on the head of the humerus in shoulders with tears of the rotator cuff. J Bone Joint Surg 82B:416-419, 2000.

84. Itoi E, Hsu HC, Carmichael SW, et al: Morphology of the torn rotator cuff. J Anat 186:429-434, 1995.

85. Jobe FW, Nuber G: Throwing injuries of the elbow. Clin Sports Med 5:621, 1986.

86. Ryan J: Elbow, in Wadsworth C (ed): Current Concepts of Orthopedic Physical Therapy—Home Study Course. La Crosse, Wisc, Orthopaedic Section, APTA, 2001.

87. Neumann DA: Elbow and forearm complex, in Neumann DA (ed): Kinesiology of the Musculoskeletal System: Foundations for Physical Rehabilitation. St Louis, Mosby, 2002, pp 133-171.

88. Schuind F, Garcia-Elias M, Cooney WP, et al: Flexor tendon forces: In vivo measurements. J Hand Surg 17A:291-298, 1992.

89. Schuind FA, Goldschmidt D, Bastin C, et al: A biomechanical study of the ulnar nerve at the elbow. J Hand Surg [Br] 20:623-627, 1995.

90. Jackson-Manfield P, Neumann DA: Structure and function of the elbow and forearm complex, in Jackson-Manfield P, Neumann DA (eds):

Essentials of Kinesiology for the Physical Therapist Assistant. St Louis, MO, Mosby Elsevier, 2009, pp 91-122.

91. Pauly JE, Rushing JL, Schering LE: An electromyographic study of some muscles crossing the elbow joint. Anat Rec 1:42, 1967.

92. Basmajian JV, Latif A: Integrated actions and functions of the chief flexors of the elbow: a detailed electromyographic analysis. J Bone Joint Surg 39A:1106-1118, 1957.

93. Funk DA, An KA, Morrey BF, et al: Electromyographic analysis of muscles across the elbow joint. J Orthop Res 5:529-538, 1987.

94. Basmajian JV, Deluca CJ: Muscles Alive (ed 5). Baltimore, Williams & Wilkins, 1985, pp 268-269.

95. Thepaut-Mathieu C, Maton B: The flexor function of the muscle pronator teres in man: a quantitative electromyographic study. Eur J Appl Physiol 54:116-121, 1985.

96. An KN, Morrey BF: Biomechanics of the elbow, in Morrey BF (ed): The Elbow and Its Disorders (ed 2). Philadelphia, WB Saunders, 1993, pp 53-73.

97. An KN, Hui FC, Morrey BF, et al: Muscles across the elbow joint: a biomechanical analysis. J Biomech 14:659-669, 1981.

98. Davidson PA, Pink M, Perry J, et al: Functional anatomy of the flexor pronator muscle group in relation to the medial collateral ligament of the elbow. Am J Sports Med 23:245-250, 1995.

99. Reid DC: Functional Anatomy and Joint Mobilization (ed 2). Edmonton, University of Alberta Press, 1975.

100. Hirasawa Y, Sawamura H, Sakakida K: Entrapment neuropathy due to bilateral epitrochlearis muscles: a case report. J Hand Surg Am 4:181-184, 1979.

101. Onieal M-E: Common wrist and elbow injuries in primary care. Lippincotts Prim Care Pract 3:441-450, 1999.

102. Brand PW, Hollister AM, Agee JM: Transmission, in Brand PW, Hollister AM (eds): Clinical Mechanics of the Hand. St Louis, Mosby, 1999, pp 61-99.

103. Wadsworth C: Wrist and hand, in Wadsworth C (ed): Current Concepts of Orthopedic Physical Therapy—Home Study Course. La Crosse, Wisc, Orthopaedic Section, APTA, 2001.

104. Kaplan EB: Anatomy and kinesiology of the hand, in Flynn JE (ed): Hand Surgery (ed 2). Baltimore, Williams & Wilkins, 1975.

105. Holtzhausen L-M, Noakes TD: Elbow, forearm, wrist, and hand injuries among sport rock climbers. Clin J Sports Med 6:196-203, 1996.

106. Linburg RM, Conmstock BE: Anomalous tendon slips from the pollicis longus to the flexor digitorum profundus. J Hand Surg 4:79-83, 1979.

107. Rennie WRJ, Muller H: Linburg syndrome. Can J Surg 41:306-308, 1998.

108. Brand PW: Clinical Mechanics of the Hand. St Louis, Mosby, 1985.

109. Tubiana R, Thomine J-M, Mackin E: Examination of the Hand and Wrist. London, Mosby, 1996.

110. Ketchum LD, Thompson DE: An experimental investigation into the forces internal to the human hand, in Brand PW (ed): Clinical Mechanics of the Hand. St Louis, CV Mosby, 1985.

111. Hollinshead WH: Anatomy for Surgeons (ed 2). New York, Harper & Row, 1969.

112. Wadsworth CT: Anatomy of the Hand and Wrist, Manual Examination and Treatment of the Spine and Extremities. Baltimore, Williams & Wilkins, 1988, pp 128-138.

113. Neumann DA: Kinesiology of the hip: a focus on muscular actions. J Orthop Sports Phys Ther 40:82-94, 2010.

114. Delp SL, Hess WE, Hungerford DS, et al: Variation of rotation moment arms with hip flexion. J Biomech 32:493-501, 1999.

115. Yoshio M, Murakami G, Sato T, et al: The function of the psoas major muscle: passive kinetics and morphological studies using donated cadavers. J Orthop Sci 7:199-207, 2002.

116. Hall SJ: The biomechanics of the human lower extremity, in Basic Biomechanics (ed 3). New York, McGraw-Hill, 1999, pp 234-281.

117. Janda V: On the concept of postural muscles and posture in man. Aust J Physiother 29:83-84, 1983.

118. Fagerson TL: Hip pathologies: diagnosis and intervention, in Magee DJ, Zachazewski JE, Quillen WS (eds): Pathology and Intervention in Musculoskeletal Rehabilitation. St Louis, Saunders, 2009, pp 497-527.

119. Gordon EJ: Trochanteric bursitis and tendinitis. Clin Orthop 20:193-202, 1961.

120. Renne JW: The iliotibial band friction syndrome. J Bone Joint Surg 57:1110-1111, 1975.

121. Evans P: The postural function of the iliotibial tract. Ann R Coll Surg Engl 61:271-280, 1979.

122. Pease BJ, Cortese M: Anterior knee pain: differential diagnosis and physical therapy management, Orthopaedic Physical Therapy Home Study Course 92-1. La Crosse, Wisc, Orthopaedic Section, APTA, 1992.

123. Grelsamer RP, McConnell J: Normal and abnormal anatomy of the extensor mechanism, In The Patella: A Team Approach. Austin, Texas, PRO-ED, 1998, pp 11-24.

124. Kapandji IA: The Physiology of the Joints, Lower Limb. New York, Churchill Livingstone, 1991.

125. Durrani Z, Winnie AP: Piriformis muscle syndrome: an underdiagnosed cause of sciatica. J Pain Symptom Manage 6:374-379, 1991.

126. Julsrud ME: Piriformis syndrome. J Am Podiatr Med Assoc 79:128-131, 1989.

127. Pace JB, Nagle D: Piriformis syndrome. West J Med 124:435-439, 1976.

128. Steiner C, Staubs C, Ganon M, et al: Piriformis syndrome: pathogenesis, diagnosis, and treatment. J Am Osteopath Assoc 87:318-323, 1987.

129. Harvey G, Bell S: Obturator neuropathy. An anatomic perspective. Clin Orthop Rel Res 363:203-11, 1999.

130. Williams PL, Warwick R, Dyson M, et al: Gray's Anatomy (ed 37). London, Churchill Livingstone, 1989.

131. Dixon MC, Scott RD, Schai PA, et al: A simple capsulorrhaphy in a posterior approach for total hip arthroplasty. J Arthroplasty 19:373-376, 2004.

132. Mihalko WM, Whiteside LA: Hip mechanics after posterior structure repair in total hip arthroplasty. Clin Orthop Rel Res 420:194-198, 2004.

133. Lynch SA, Renstrom PA: Groin injuries in sport: treatment strategies. Sports Med 28:137-144, 1999.

134. Holmich P: Adductor related groin pain in athletes. Sports Med Arth Rev 5:285-291, 1998.

135. Hasselman CT, Best TM, Garrett WE: When groin pain signals an adductor strain. Physician Sports Med 23:53-60, 1995.

136. Johnson CE, Basmajian JV, Dasher W: Electromyography of the sartorius muscle. Anat Rec 173:127-130, 1972.

137. Anderson MA, Gieck JH, Perrin D, et al: The relationship among isokinetic, isotonic, and isokinetic concentric and eccentric quadriceps and hamstrings force and three components of athletic performance. J Orthop Sports Phys Ther 14:114-120, 1991.

138. Lieb F, Perry J: Quadriceps function. J Bone Joint Surg [Am] 50:1535, 1968.

139. Hallisey MJ, Doherty N, Bennett WF, et al: Anatomy of the junction of the vastus lateralis tendon and the patella. J Bone Joint Surg [Am] 69:545-549, 1987.

140. Bose K, Kanagasuntheram R, Osman MBH: Vastus medialis oblique: an anatomic and physiologic study. Orthopedics 3:880-883, 1980.

141. Grelsamer RP: Patellar Malalignment. J Bone Joint Surg [Am] 82A:1639-1650, 2000.

142. Koskinen SK, Kujala UM: Patellofemoral relationships and distal insertion of the vastus medialis muscle: a magnetic resonance imaging study in nonsymptomatic subjects and in patients with patellar dislocation. Arthroscopy 8:465-468, 1992.

143. Raimondo RA, Ahmad CS, Blankevoort L, et al: Patellar stabilization: a quantitative evaluation of the vastus medialis obliquus muscle. Orthopedics 21:791-795, 1998.

144. Nakamura Y, Ohmichi H, Miyashita M: EMG relationship during maximum voluntary contraction of the quadriceps, IX Congress of the International Society of Biomechanics. Waterloo, Ontario, 1983.

145. Knight KL, Martin JA, Londeree BR: EMG comparison of quadriceps femoris activity during knee extensions and straight leg raises. Am J Phys Med 58:57-69, 1979.

146. Brownstein BA, Lamb RL, Mangine RE: Quadriceps torque and integrated electromyography. J Orthop Sports Phys Ther 6:309-314, 1985.

147. Fox TA: Dysplasia of the quadriceps mechanism: hypoplasia of the vastus medialis muscle as related to the hypermobile patella syndrome. Surg Clin North Am 55:199-226, 1975.

148. Tria AJ, Palumbo RC, Alicia JA: Conservative care for patellofemoral pain. Orthop Clin North Am 23:545-554, 1992.

149. Reynolds L, Levin TA, Medeiros JM, et al: EMG activity of the vastus medialis oblique and the vastus lateralis in their role in patellar alignment. Am J Sports Med 62:62-70, 1983.

150. Moller BN, Krebs B, Tideman-Dal C, et al: Isometric contractions in the patellofemoral pain syndrome. Arch Orthop Trauma Surg 105:24, 1986.

151. Reid DC: Anterior knee pain and the patellofemoral pain syndrome, in Sports Injury Assessment and Rehabilitation. New York, Churchill Livingstone, 1992, pp 345-398.

152. Larson RL, Jones DC: Dislocations and ligamentous injuries of the knee, in Rockwood CA, Green DP (eds): Fractures in Adults (ed 2). Philadelphia, JB Lippincott, 1984, pp 1480-1591.

153. Gill DM, Corbacio EJ, Lauchle LE: Anatomy of the knee, in Engle RP (ed): Knee Ligament Rehabilitation. New York, Churchill Livingstone, 1991, pp 1-15.

154. Kendall FP, McCreary EK, Provance PG: Muscles: Testing and Function. Baltimore, Williams & Wilkins, 1993.

155. O'Connor JJ: Can muscle co-contraction protect knee ligaments after injury or repair? J Bone Joint Surg 75-B:41-48, 1993.

156. Fleming BC, Renstrom PA, Goran O, et al: The gastrocnemius muscle is an antagonist of the anterior cruciate ligament. J Orthop Res 19:1178-1184, 2001.

157. Timm KE: Knee, in Richardson JK, Iglarsh ZA (eds): Clinical Orthopaedic Physical Therapy. Philadelphia, WB Saunders, 1994, pp 399-482.

158. Sudasna S, Harnsiriwattanagit K: The ligamentous structures of the posterolateral aspect of the knee. Bull Hosp Joint Dis Orthop Institute 50:35-40, 1990.

159. Brownstein B, Noyes FR, Mangine RE, et al: Anatomy and biomechanics, in Mangine RE (ed): Physical Therapy of the Knee. New York, Churchill Livingstone, 1988, pp 1-30.

160. Magee DJ: Orthopedic Physical Assessment (ed 2). Philadelphia, WB Saunders, 1992.

161. Reid DC: Knee ligament injuries, anatomy, classification, and examination, in Reid DC (ed): Sports Injury Assessment and Rehabilitation. New York, Churchill Livingstone, 1992, pp 437-493.

162. Nyland J, Lachman N, Kocabey Y, et al: Anatomy, function, and rehabilitation of the popliteus musculotendinous complex. J Orthop Sports Phys Ther 35:165-179, 2005.

163. Veltri DM, Deng XH, Torzilli PA, et al: The role of the cruciate and posterolateral ligaments in stability of the knee. A biomechanical study. Am J Sports Med 23:436-443, 1995.

164. Veltri DM, Deng XH, Torzilli PA, et al: The role of the popliteofibular ligament in stability of the human knee. A biomechanical study. Am J Sports Med 24:19-27, 1996.

165. Maynard MJ, Deng XH, Wickiewicz TL, et al: The popliteofibular ligament. Rediscovery of a key element in posterolateral stability. Am J Sports Med 24:311-316, 1996.

166. Veltri DM, Warren RF, Wickiewicz TL, et al: Current status of allographic meniscal transplantation. Clin Orthop 306:155-162, 1994.

167. Last RJ: The popliteus muscle and the lateral meniscus. J Bone Joint Surg 32B:93-99, 1950.

168. Scioli MW: Achilles tendinitis. Orthop Clin North Am 25:177-182, 1994.

169. Soma CA, Mandelbaum BR: Achilles tendon disorders. Clin Sports Med 13:811-23, 1994.

170. Gerdes MH, Brown TW, Bell A, et al: A flap augmentation technique for Achilles tendon repair. Postoperative strength and functional outcome. Clin Orthop 280:241-246, 1992.

171. Reynolds NL, Worrell TW: Chronic Achilles peritendinitis: etiology, pathophysiology, and treatment. J Orthop Sports Phys Ther 13:171-176, 1991.

172. Carr AJ, Norris SH: The blood supply of the calcaneal tendon. J Bone Joint Surg 71B:100-101, 1989.

173. Lagergren C, Lindholm A: Vascular distribution in the Achilles tendon: an angiographic and microangiographic study. Acta Chir Scand 116:491-495, 1958.

174. Nelen G, Martens M, Bursens A: Surgical treatment of chronic Achilles tendinitis. Am J Sports Med 17:754-759, 1989.

175. Nichols AW: Achilles tendinitis in running athletes. J Am Board Fam Pract 2:196-203, 1989.

176. Conti SF: Posterior tibial tendon problems in athletes. Orthop Clin North Am 25:109-121, 1994.

177. Clarke HD, Kitaoka HB, Ehman RL: Peroneal tendon injuries. Foot Ankle 19:280-288, 1998.

178. Brage ME, Hansen ST: Traumatic subluxation/dislocation of the peroneal tendons. Foot Ankle 13:423-431, 1992.

179. Thordarson DB, Schotzer H, Chon J, et al: Dynamic support of the human longitudinal arch. Clin Orthop 316:165-172, 1995.

180. Mann R, Inman V: Phasic activity of intrinsic muscles of the foot. J Bone Joint Surg 46A:469-480, 1964.

181. Daniels K, Worthingham C: Muscle Testing Techniques of Manual Examination (ed 5). Philadelphia, WB Saunders, 1986.

182. Harvey VP, Scott GD: An investigation of the curl-down test as a measure of abdominal strength. Res Q 38:22-27, 1967.

183. Fitzgerald MJT, Comerford PT, Tuffery AR: Sources of innervation of the neuromuscular spindles in sternomastoid and trapezius. J Anat 134:471-490, 1982.

184. Palmer ML, Epler M: Clinical Assessment Procedures in Physical Therapy. Philadelphia, JB Lippincott, 1990.

185. Huijbregts PA: Lumbopelvic region: anatomy and biomechanics, in Wadsworth C (ed): Current Concepts of Orthopaedic Physical Therapy—Home Study Course. La Crosse, Wisc, Orthopaedic Section, APTA, 2001.

186. Lee DG: The Pelvic Girdle: An Approach to the Examination and Treatment of the Lumbo-Pelvic-Hip Region (ed 2). Edinburgh, Churchill Livingstone, 1999.

187. McGill SM, Childs A, Liebenson C: Endurance times for low back stabilization exercises: clinical targets for testing and training from a normal database. Arch Phys Med Rehabil 80:941-944, 1999.

188. Green JP, Grenier SG, McGill SM: Low-back stiffness is altered with warm-up and bench rest: implications for athletes. Med Sci Sports Exerc 34:1076-1081, 2002.

189. Jull G, Richardson CA, Hamilton C, et al: Towards the Validation of a Clinical Test for the Deep Abdominal Muscles in Back Pain Patients, Manipulative Physiotherapists Association of Australia, 1995.

190. Richardson CA, Jull GA, Hodges P, et al: Therapeutic Exercise for Spinal Segmental Stabilization in Low Back Pain. London, Churchill Livingstone, 1999.

191. Aspden RM: Review of the functional anatomy of the spinal ligaments and the lumbar erector spinae muscles. Clin Anat 5:372-387, 1992.

192. Magee DJ: Lumbar Spine, in Magee DJ (ed): Orthopedic Physical Assessment (ed 4). Philadelphia, WB Saunders, 2002, pp 467-566.

193. Moreland J, Finch E, Stratford P, et al: Interrater reliability of six tests of trunk muscle function and endurance. J Orthop Sports Phys Ther 26:200-208, 1997.

194. Reese NB: Muscle and Sensory Testing. Philadelphia, WB Saunders, 1999.

195. Ashmen KJ, Swanik CB, Lephart SM: Strength and flexibility characteristics of athletes with chronic low back pain. J Sport Rehabil 5:372-387, 1996.

196. Hodges P, Richardson C, Jull G: Evaluation of the relationship between laboratory and clinical tests of transversus abdominis function. Physiother Res Int 1:30-40, 1996.

197. O'Sullivan P, Twomey L, Allison G: Evaluation of specific stabilizing exercise in the treatment of chronic low back pain with radiologic diagnosis of spondylolysis or spondylolisthesis. Spine 22:2959-2967, 1997.

198. O'Sullivan P, Twomey L, Allison G: Altered patterns of abdominal muscle activation in chronic back pain patients. Aust J Physiother 43:91-98, 1997.

199. Clark MA: Integrated Training for the New Millennium. Thousand Oaks, Calif, National Academy of Sports Medicine, 2001.

200. Clarkson HM: Musculoskeletal Assessment (ed 2). Philadelphia, Lippincott Williams & Wilkins, 2000.

201. Youdas JW, Garrett TR, Egan KS, et al: Lumbar lordosis and pelvic inclination in adults with chronic low back pain. Phys Ther 80:261-275, 2000.

202. Zannotti CM, Bohannon RW, Tiberio D, et al: Kinematics of the double-leg-lowering test for abdominal muscle strength. J Orthop Sports Phys Ther 32:432-436, 2002.

203. Gracovetsky S, Farfan HF: The optimum spine. Spine 11:543, 1986.

204. Gracovetsky S, Farfan HF, Helleur C: The abdominal mechanism. Spine 10:317-324, 1985.

205. Hyman J, Liebenson C: Spinal stabilization exercise program, in Liebenson C (ed): Rehabilitation of the Spine: A Practitioner's Manual. Baltimore, Lippincott Williams & Wilkins, 1996, pp 293-317.

206. Cyriax J: Textbook of Orthopaedic Medicine, Diagnosis of Soft Tissue Lesions (ed 8). London, Bailliere Tindall, 1982.

207. Tovin BJ, Greenfield BH: Impairment-based diagnosis for the shoulder girdle, in Evaluation and Treatment of the Shoulder: An Integration of the Guide to Physical Therapist Practice. Philadelphia, FA Davis, 2001, pp 55-74.

208. Rowland LP: Diseases of the motor unit, in Kandel ER, Schwartz JH, Jessell TM (eds): Principles of Neural Science (ed 4). New York, McGraw-Hill, 2000, pp 695-712.

209. Franklin ME: Assessment of exercise induced minor lesions: the accuracy of Cyriax's diagnosis by selective tissue tension paradigm. J Orthop Sports Phys Ther 24:122, 1996.

CHAPTER 13

Patient Transfers and Mobility

CHAPTER OBJECTIVES

At the completion of this chapter,
the reader will be able to:

1. Understand the importance of choosing the most efficient and safest method of transfer and mobility task

2. Determine the best transfer or mobility procedure based on the level of patient dependence or independence

3. Discuss the importance of patient safety during transfers and mobility tasks

4. Discuss the importance of clinician safety during transfers and mobility tasks

5. Transfer a patient to and from a number of different types of surfaces

6. Perform a variety of mobility tasks

7. Describe the various wheelchair components and their functions

8. Measure a patient for a wheelchair

9. Train a patient in how to use a wheelchair

OVERVIEW

A transfer can be viewed as the safe movement of a person from one place or surface to another, and as an opportunity to train an individual to enhance independent function. In both cases the clinician must choose the most efficient and safest method.

Controlling a patient's movement, while moving the patient from one position, or surface, to another, or preventing a patient falling requires that the clinician be close to the center of motion (COM) of the patient, which is typically located between the shoulders and the pelvis. When these points of control are used, patient transfers are more efficient and patient safety is enhanced. The most efficient way to enhance the movement of the patient (unless he or she is totally dependent)

is to encourage movement of the distal component of the body—the part of the body that is farthest from the trunk. For example, when assisting a patient to stand from a seated position, a common verbal cue is to ask the patient to lean his or her trunk forward. In addition, it is also important to have the patient look in the direction of the transfer's destination to encourage correct head turning.

PATIENT TRANSFERS

One of the purposes of transfers is to permit a patient to function in different environments and to increase the level of independence of the patient. Because of advancements in recent years, a number of moving and lifting devices (total body lifts and sit-to-stand lifts) have been designed and incorporated into the healthcare system. However, because of the expense and sometimes the inconvenience of these devices, manual transfers continue to be commonly used. In these cases, the best body mechanics possible should be used to maximize the ability to encompass a task with minimal effort and maximum safety (see Chapter 10). It is important to note that certain transfers increase the risk for injury (Table 13-1), necessitating additional care and attention. Depending on the functional ability of the patient, a transfer may be performed independently by the patient, with assistance from the clinician (minimal, moderate, maximal, or standby supervision), or dependently (Table 13-2).

CLINICAL PEARL

During a sit-to-stand transfer, a number of forces occur. These include:

▶ Gravity.

▶ The combined weight of the clinician's trunk, arms, and head (TAH), which is approximately 65% of the total weight of the body. The moment arm (MA) for TAH (TAH_{MA}) is the perpendicular distance between gravity's line of action acting on the TAH to the axis.

▶ The force required to extend the clinician's trunk, which is borne by the erector spinae muscles (Mu). The moment arm for Mu is the perpendicular distance between the line of action of Mu and the axis (MA_{Mu}).

▶ The weight of the patient (depends on the level of assistance required).

There are two options for the lower extremities:

▶ Keeping the knees extended

▶ Flexing the knees

To calculate the difference in forces that the erector spinae muscles of the trunk of an individual weighing 160 pounds (712 N) must generate between the two lower extremity positions (excluding the weight of the patient), a few simple mathematical equations can be used:

Knees extended:

$$TAH = 712 \times 0.65 = 463 \text{ N}$$

$$MA_{TAH} = 0.5 \text{ m}; MA_{Mu} = 0.04 \text{ m}$$

$$Mu = (TAH \times MA_{TAH})/MA_{Mu} = (463 \text{ N} \times 0.5 \text{ m})/0.04 \text{ m} = 5782 \text{ N}$$
(approximately 1300 pounds)

Knees flexed:

$$TAH = 712 \times 0.65 = 463 \text{ N}$$

$$MA_{TAH} = 0.25 \text{ m}; MA_{Mu} = 0.04 \text{ m}$$

$$Mu = (TAH \times MA_{TAH})/MA_{Mu} = (463 \text{ N} \times 0.25 \text{ m})/0.04 \text{ m} = 2894 \text{ N}$$
(approximately 650 pounds)

A number of factors influence the decision as to how a transfer is to be performed and how many helpers are needed (Table 13-3). In addition to the factors listed in Table 13-3, the clinician should consider the following before performing a transfer:

TABLE 13-1	Transfer Techniques and Their Risk for Injury from the Least to Most Stressful
Transferring a patient from bathtub to chair	
Transferring a patient from bed to chair	
Transferring a patient from chair to bed	
Transferring a patient from chair to toilet	
Transferring a patient from toilet to chair	

Data from Garg A, Owen BD, Carlson B: An ergonomic evaluation of nursing assistants' job in a nursing home. Ergonomics 35:979-995, 1992.

▶ The patient's level of cognition, emotional capability, and physical ability.

▶ How much assistance the clinician requires. When in doubt, a second person should be used.

▶ The appropriate equipment should be arranged before the transfer.

▶ Correct positioning of both the patient and the clinician. The clinician should maintain a large base of support (BOS) and use proper body mechanics throughout the transfer.

A patient's medical or physical condition may require modification to a transfer technique. For example, range of motion restrictions, decreased muscle control, and poor balance may require an adaptation to the transfer technique. In the case of decreased muscle control, it is generally easier for the patient to transfer toward the stronger side.

Before meeting the patient, the clinician should review the medical record to determine the patient's limitations and

TABLE 13-2	Levels of Physical Dependence and Recommended Assists	
Level of Dependence	**Definition**	**Recommended Assist**
Independent	The patient does not require any assistance to complete the task safely and in an acceptable time frame.	None
Modified independent assisted	The patient uses adaptive or assistive equipment (furniture, bed rail, grab bars, transfer board)	Gait or transfer belt Assistive device
Assisted	The patient requires assistance (oral or tactile cues) from another person to perform the activity safely and in an acceptable time frame	Gait or transfer belt Assistive device
Standby (supervision)	The patient requires oral or tactile cues from another person position close to, but not touching, the person to perform the activity safely and in an acceptable time frame.	Gait or transfer belt Assistive device
Contact guard	The patient requires the clinician to maintain contact with the patient or safety belt to complete the task. Contact guard is usually needed to assist if there is a loss of balance.	Gait or transfer belt Assistive device
Minimal assist	The patient requires 25% assist from the clinician to complete the task.	Stand-assist lift Transfer board Gait or transfer belt
Moderate assist	The patient requires 50% assist from the clinician to complete the task.	Stand-assist lift
Maximal assist	The patient requires 75% assist from the therapist to complete the task.	Mechanical lift with full sling Stand-assist lift
Dependent	The patient is unable to participate, and the clinician must provide all of the effort to perform the task.	Mechanical lift with full sling Transfer chair that can be converted into a stretcher

TABLE 13-3	Factors That Influence Decision Making for Transfers	
Factor	**Example**	**Influences on Decision**
Patient	Weight, cooperation, level of fear, physical capabilities, movement precautions, head control, pain level, and any external device	Small movements generally allow for greater control over both the movement and any equipment. More assistance generally allows for greater control and support.
Environment	The proximity of the transfer surfaces, the height differences between the two surfaces, and the width of the two transfer surfaces	The two transfer surfaces should be arranged so that the clinician can maintain an upright position that minimizes trunk flexion, can achieve good trunk stability, and can perform the transfer with an unobstructed path.
Task	The type of transfer and the objective of the transfer	The type of transfer is largely determined by the patient's capabilities so that the patient can assist as much as possible.

abilities. In addition, when appropriate, the clinician should interview the patient's family for information as to their abilities. Physical abilities to consider include gross motor strength and control, joint and soft tissue flexibility, sitting and standing endurance, and sitting and standing balance. The major muscle groups involved with transfers include the elbow extensors and flexors, the shoulder extensors and flexors, and the hip and knee extensors. Having reviewed the medical record and talked to the patient's family, and with consideration of the goals of the treatment, the clinician must determine whether mechanical or human assistance will be needed. The types of equipment that can be used in transfers include but are not limited to a trapeze bar, a transfer board, a transfer/gait belt, and a hydraulic or pneumatic lift/hoist.

▶ *Trapeze bar.* Consists of a metal triangle, a chain, and clamps and is used to assist patients to maneuver in bed by pulling with one or both upper extremities.

▶ *Transfer boards.* These items, which come in a variety of shapes and sizes, are most commonly used for horizontal transfers such as when transferring from the bed to a wheelchair, or a wheelchair to a mat table.

▶ *Transfer/gait belt.* As a patient's activities advance to those tasks requiring a higher COM, a smaller BOS, and an increased demand in dynamic stability, the risk of falling increases. These belts provide an alternative method of providing a control point near the center of the patient's body during transfers in situations when direct manual contacts cannot be safely maintained. In some settings, transfer belts may be required equipment.

▶ *Hydraulic or pneumatic lift/hoist.* These pieces of equipment (Figure 13-1), which are commonly referred to as Hoyer lifts, are designed for a number of uses such as to help transport patients from a bed to a chair, wheelchair, or toilet, or to assist a patient to stand from a seated position. Their operation can be manual, through the use of a pump handle, or electric. Each lift is fitted with caster wheels to aid in positioning and maneuvering, and the base of the lift can be widened to fit around a wheelchair or other equipment. In addition, each lift has a sling made of a variety of fabrics and designs on which the patient rests. The sling is attached to a spreader bar on the lift by two chains with hooks, and the length of the chain can be adjusted to accommodate the height of the patient.

CLINICAL PEARL

Documentation with regard to a transfer must include the equipment or devices used, the amount or type of assistance a patient requires to perform the transfer, the amount of time to complete it, the level of safety demonstrated, and the level of consistency of the performance.

Transfers require movements that move the center of gravity (COG) away from the center of the BOS for both the patient and the clinician. These movements have the potential of causing a loss of balance. After the introduction to the patient, it is important to inform the patient of what transfer is to occur and why.

CLINICAL PEARL

The primary responsibility of the clinician during a transfer is to avoid patient injury or injury to himself or herself.

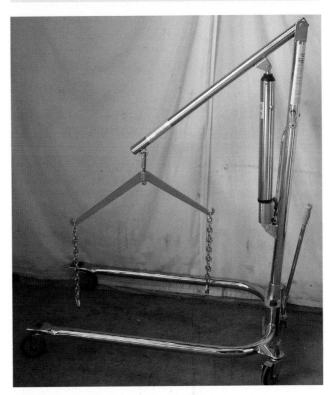

FIGURE 13-1 Hydraulic or pneumatic lift/hoist

Setting the feet in stride and slightly apart provides a larger BOS. The clinician's feet should also be unencumbered to move as the situation requires, always allowing the BOS to be reestablished under the moving COG. Crossing of the clinician's legs during movement should be avoided because it decreases the size of the BOS and constrains freedom of foot movement.

Patients must know what they are to do and when they are to do it during transfers to participate effectively. Any instructions must be kept simple, informative, and in a terminology that the patient can understand. Medical terms should be used only when the patient readily understands them. Verbal explanation and demonstration should be used to highlight the expectations and transfer sequence. Having the patient repeat the instructions ensures that the patient understands them. If necessary, instruct the patient in smaller segments of the transfer before performing the entire transfer. Manual contacts can be used with the patient to direct his or her participation during the transfer.

Commands and counts can be used to help synchronize the various components of the transfer. The typical command and count used is "one, two, three, lift." It is important to remember that a transfer is not considered complete until the patient is safe in the new position, at which point the transfer team can release control of the patient.

The most common transfers are described in this chapter.

Transfer from Bed to Wheeled Stretcher—Sliding Method

The clinician informs the patient about what is to take place and then positions the wheeled stretcher parallel to, against, and at approximately the same height as the bed. Whenever possible, the surface to which the patient is being transferred should be made a little lower than the surface the patient is being transferred from. It is also important to ensure that the height of the transfer surface is appropriate for the people performing the transfer. As a general rule, this is at waist level. The cart is positioned on the patient's uninvolved side. The bed rails and stretcher rails are lowered and both the bed and the stretcher are secured using wheel locks or other appropriate devices. If the patient can move without assistance, the stretcher is stabilized and the clinician merely provides verbal assistance. If the patient is unable to assist in the transfer, three or more able-bodied individuals are needed to perform the transfer using a draw sheet. The draw sheet is placed under the patient and is then rolled and grasped close to the patient by each clinician (Figure 13-2). The three clinicians are positioned so that two of them are on the side to which the patient is moving, which is the same side as the wheeled stretcher (see Figure 13-2), and the other clinician, whose main function is to help guide the direction of the transfer, is on the other side of the bed (VIDEO 13-1). When all three clinicians are positioned correctly, the clinician at the head of the bed takes responsibility for coordinating the transfer and issuing the various commands. During the first lift, the patient is pulled toward the edge of the side of the bed in the direction of the transfer (Figure 13-3), then to the edge of the bed (Figure 13-4), and finally onto the cart (Figure 13-5).

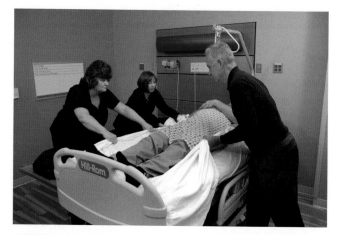

FIGURE 13-2 Clinician positioning in preparation for sliding transfer

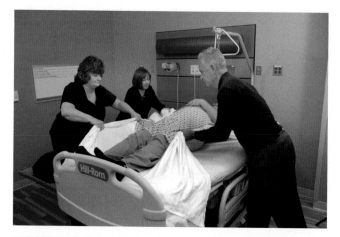

FIGURE 13-3 Patient is moved toward the wheeled stretcher

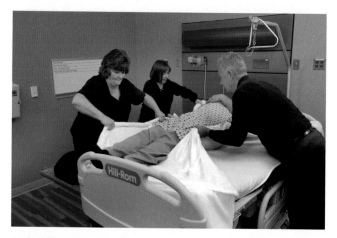

FIGURE 13-4 Patient is moved to the edge of the bed

Video Description

Note how the clinicians roll the edges of the sheet to form a handle. One clinician is designated to coordinate the transfer. Whenever there are an odd number of helpers, the majority of the helpers are positioned on the side toward which the patient is being moved. Depending on the width of the bed and stretcher, and the size of the patient,

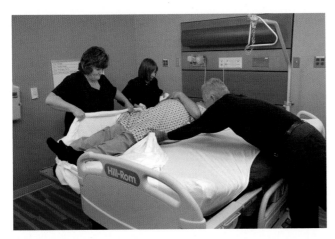

FIGURE 13-5 Patient is moved onto the wheeled stretcher

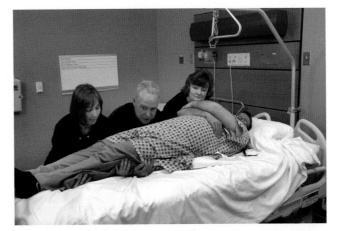

FIGURE 13-6 Clinician positioning for three-person carry

it may be necessary for one or more of the clinicians to assume a kneeling position on one of the transfer surfaces. Note how the clinician on the side opposite the direction of the transfer leans forward over the transfer surface while securing the thighs against the side of the bed so as to maintain good trunk stability and enhance leverage.

A number of devices have recently been introduced that minimize the level of physical assistance by the clinician. These include:

▶ *Rigid or semirigid transfer boards.* These friction-reducing devices are made of a variety of materials and have handles along the edge of the board in the form of openings.

▶ *Patient roller.* This is a mechanical device that consists of multiple rollers placed within a rigid frame and enclosed in a cover. This device is commonly used to transfer patients from wheel stretchers to surgical tables.

▶ *Slippery sheet.* This is essentially a nylon flat sheet, coated with a low-friction solution, with handles on the sides.

▶ *Air assistive device.* This device consists of an upper and a lower air chamber, both of which are mechanically inflated to create a cushioned film of air underneath the patient, thereby reducing friction.

Transfer from Bed to Wheeled Stretcher—Three-Person Carry

This technique is used when the bed and wheeled stretcher cannot be arranged either parallel to each other or at a safe height distance. The clinicians involved in the transfer must remove all jewelry to prevent scratching the patient. One of the three clinicians positions the cart perpendicular to the bed with the head of the cart at the foot end of the bed. Alternatively, the cart can be positioned perpendicular to the bed with the foot of the cart at the head of the bed. The three clinicians stand on the same side of the bed and are positioned in such a way that one can support the head and upper trunk of the patient, one can support the midsection of the patient, and one can support the lower extremities (Figure 13-6). Ideally, the strongest clinician is in the middle position or at the head. The clinician at the head of the bed takes responsibility for coordinating the

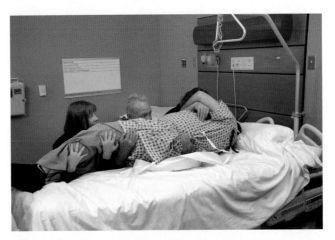

FIGURE 13-7 Patient is cradled in clinicians' arms

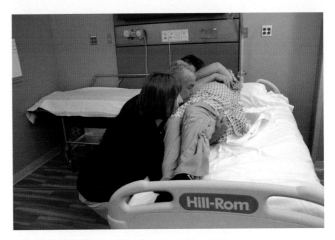

FIGURE 13-8 Patient is rolled toward the clinicians

transfer and issuing the various commands. When the three clinicians are positioned correctly, each of them slides both arms under the patient so that the elbows rest on the treatment table and the patient is cradled from head to foot (Figure 13-7). Each clinician places one foot in front of the other and, on the first lift command, the patient is moved to the edge of the bed. Then, by flexing the elbows, the clinicians roll the patient onto his or her side as in a log roll, so that the patient is now cradled in the bend of the clinicians' elbows, which brings the weight of the patient closer to the center of the clinicians' BOS (Figure 13-8). On the second lift command, the clinicians simultaneously stand and lift the patient. On the command to pivot, the clinicians pivot and line up parallel to the cart, moving forward in a straight line until all three clinicians feel the edge of the wheeled stretcher against their thighs. Again each clinician places one foot in front of the other and, on the command to lower the patient, the clinicians bend their legs until the elbows rest on the edge of the stretcher (Figure 13-9) and then slowly uncradle the patient onto the center of the wheeled stretcher (Figure 13-10). Once the patient is positioned correctly, the clinicians remove their arms from under the patient, and the rails of the stretcher are raised (Figure 13-11).

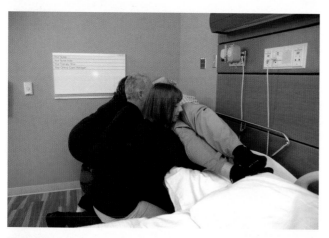

FIGURE 13-9 Patient is lowered onto the wheeled stretcher

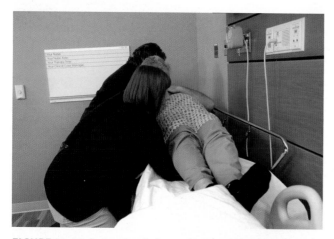

FIGURE 13-10 Patient is rolled onto the wheeled stretcher

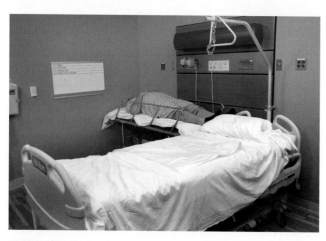

FIGURE 13-11 Patient position after transfer with side rails raised

Transfer from Bed to Chair Using Hydraulic/Pneumatic Lift

The clinician moves the lift close to the patient and detaches the sling. The clinician first places a rolled sling under the patient by rolling the patient onto one side. The sling is positioned so that the seams are on the outside, away from the patient, to avoid pressure areas. Once the rolled sling is positioned correctly, the patient is then rolled to the other side, and the sling is unrolled. The clinician positions the lift so that the spreader bar is across the patient, and both ends of the chain are then attached to their respective sides of the sling. The shorter segment of each chain is attached to the upper part of the sling, which is the part that supports the patient's back. The longer segment of each chain is attached to the lower part of the sling, which is the part that supports the patient's lower extremities. The chain hooks are attached from inside the sling to the outside to reduce the likelihood of patient injury by the hook. Once the chains have been attached, the clinician begins the operation of lifting the patient, using the lift to move the patient into a sitting position. Once the patient is secured in the sitting position, the clinician uses one arm under the patient's lower extremities to assist the patient's lower extremities off the bed so that the patient is fully suspended by the lift. While the clinician prevents the patient from swaying excessively, the patient is moved to a locked wheelchair, the base of the lift is placed in the wide position, and the lift is maneuvered so that the patient is over the seat of the locked wheelchair. The clinician then operates the lift to slowly lower the patient into the wheelchair while applying a slight pressure in the horizontal plane at the patient's knees or thighs to place the patient into the wheelchair correctly so that the patient's back is resting firmly against the back of the wheelchair. Once the patient is correctly and safely seated in the wheelchair, the chains are removed from the sling and, after checking that the patient is capable of sitting without assistance, the clinician moves the hydraulic lift safely away from the patient. Depending on when the next transfer is to take place, the sling may be left in situ depending on the design of the sling. One-piece slings are left in place under the patient, whereas the portion behind the patient's back in a two-piece sling can be removed.

WHEELCHAIR MOBILITY

A wheelchair is a medical device in the form of a postural support system on wheels that is used by people for whom walking is difficult or impossible because of illness or disability. Whenever possible, every attempt should be made to design the wheelchair to provide the patient with maximum function, comfort, stability, safety, and protection while also reducing the amount of force required to propel the wheelchair. Fortunately, wheelchairs are now available in a variety of sizes and styles, and wheelchair design continues to improve in both safety and construction.

Wheelchairs can be grouped into several classes: indoor (small wheelbase to allow maneuvering in confined spaces, but lacks the ability or power to negotiate obstacles), indoor/outdoor (provides mobility for those who stay on finished surfaces, such as sidewalks, driveways, and flooring), and active indoor/outdoor (provides the ability to travel long distances, move fast, and drive over unstructured environments such as grass, gravel, and uneven terrain). Wheelchair fitting is highly individualized and requires a team effort among the physiatrist, neurologist, or orthopedist; occupational or physical therapist; the specialist in assistive technology and driver training; and rehabilitation technology providers. When helping choose a wheelchair, a few considerations must be taken into account. These considerations are both patient and design based. The patient considerations include:

▶ *Patient needs.* These needs can include recreational, social, or vocational needs. Depending on the patient's age, peer acceptance may be a patient need. An individual's needs can change with time, so it is well worth asking questions about any anticipated future needs, prognosis, or change.

▶ *Mobility needs.* It is important for the clinician to take time to observe the patient and the current wheelchair to determine how well the wheelchair is serving the patient's mobility needs. Questions should be asked about locomotion requirements for the home and community.

▶ *Physical abilities.* Manual wheelchairs require a significant amount of strength and endurance to operate, so it is important for the clinician to help choose a wheelchair that will not hinder mobility because of a patient's physical limitations. It is also important to determine the patient's ability to alter his or her own position, especially over bony prominences.

▶ *Sensory awareness.* The clinician must determine whether the patient has any impaired peripheral circulation, abnormal skin integrity, or neurologic dysfunction.

▶ *Dexterity and coordination.* Many of the components of the wheelchair, such as the brakes and seatbelt on a standard wheelchair, require a fair degree of dexterity and coordination on the part of the patient.

▶ *Anthropometric characteristics.* Of particular importance are the patient's height and weight (see Wheelchair Measurements, later).

The design considerations (see Wheelchair Components, later) include:

▶ Wheelchair weight
▶ Seating system
▶ Armrest style
▶ Front rigging (leg rests and footplates)
▶ Frame
▶ Drive wheels
▶ Tires
▶ Casters
▶ Manual versus power source
▶ Expected use of the chair
▶ Length of time the chair will be used—temporary or permanent

When combined, all of the listed design components add to the overall weight of a wheelchair. The more popular

wheelchairs range in weight from 25 pounds (ultralight) to 45 pounds (standard).

All wheelchairs should be kept in good working order to ensure patient safety, ease of use, control of repair costs, and extended life of the chair. This may include regular lubrication, tire care, spoke maintenance, and lock maintenance. The owner's manual is an important resource and provides information about which parts of the wheelchair have a warranty, how to take care of the wheelchair, and where to buy replacements or accessories.

Wheelchair Components

The choice of which of the various wheelchair components should be used is based on the patient's needs and abilities. With each choice there are positives and negatives. For example, the clinician often has to choose between stability and mobility, or between size and maneuverability. It is therefore important for the clinician to make the patient aware not only of the available options but also of the advantages and disadvantages of each.

Frame

Stainless steel tubing used to be the only frame material available and made the wheelchair very heavy. However, wheelchair users today have their choice of aluminum, airplane steel, aluminum, and titanium. A standard wheelchair (Figure 13-12) with a fixed box frame can be designed to support up to 1000 pounds. However, because the frame is fixed, it results in less shock absorption. Next in terms of durability are wheelchairs with folding frames, which are constructed with a cross-brace design. This design allows the right and left sides of the chair to be brought together for ease in transportation and compact storage. Although the folding-frame wheelchair provides better suspension than a fixed box-frame wheelchair, it requires more energy to propel than the rigid frame design ones.

CLINICAL PEARL

Integrated standing wheelchairs are designed to allow a patient to move between sitting and standing while being supported by the chair.

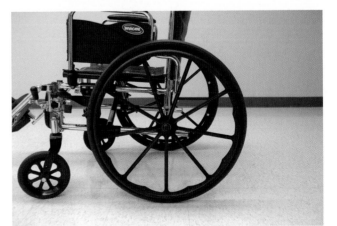

FIGURE 13-12 Standard wheelchair frame

In general, the lighter the weight of the frame, the greater the ease of use, but the lesser the structural strength provided. The level of expected activity and the environment where the wheelchair will be used should be taken into account when deciding on frame construction.

CLINICAL PEARL

An antitipping device can be attached to the frame of the wheelchair. These devices are posterior extensions attached to the low horizontal supports. They prevent the chair from tipping backward, which limits going over curbs or over doorsills.

Items such as a headrest, lateral trunk support, back panel, armrest trough, and lower extremity supports can be added to a chair to accomplish specific goals. The clinician should observe the position of the head, trunk, pelvis, knees, and feet of the patient in the wheelchair, in addition to determining the patient's sitting balance, stability, reaching ability, ability to change positions, transferability, and preferred method of propulsion.

Upholstery

Upholstery for wheelchairs must withstand daily use in all kinds of weather. Consequently, manufacturers provide a variety of options to users, ranging from cloth to new synthetic fabrics to leather. Many manufacturers also offer a selection of upholstery colors, ranging from black to neon, to allow for individual selection and differing tastes among consumers.

Seating System

Most standard wheelchairs come with a rigid or sling seat. However, as it is the seat that provides postural support to the patient, the seating system is considered to be one of the most important of the wheelchair components. For example, a sling seat encourages a forward head posture, the hips to slide forward, the thighs to adduct and internally rotate, and the patient to sit asymmetrically, which reinforces poor pelvic position. The aim of proper seating and positioning is to promote function, prevent secondary complications, prevent deformity, improve body alignment, and prevent tissue damage.

CLINICAL PEARL

It is very important to remember that no design of cushion will prevent skin breakdown without frequent repositioning by the patient or caregiver.

Whenever possible, seating must be customized on an individual basis, and in most cases seating surfaces are purchased separately from the wheelchairs themselves. Generally speaking, there are two types of cushions:

▶ *Uniform cushions.* These cushions are fabricated from wood or plastic and padded with foam. They create a stable firm sitting surface, improve pelvic position, and reduce the tendency for the patient to slide forward or sit with a posterior pelvic tilt. Foam cushions are lighter but can also be bulky.

▶ *Contoured cushions.* These cushions, which can be inflatable or made from a gel-like substance, function to distribute weight bearing-pressures, which assists in preventing decubitus ulcers in patients with decreased sensation, prolongs wheelchair sitting times, and accommodates moderate to severe postural deformities. The inflatable cushions are light, whereas the gel cushions are heavy, more expensive, and require continuous maintenance. However, gel cushions can be custom molded, are designed to accommodate moderate to severe postural deformity, and make it easy for caregivers to reposition the patient.

CLINICAL PEARL

The depth of the cushion is an important consideration. One that is too deep may interfere with slide board transfers.

Backrest

As with seat cushion systems, backrests come in rigid and sling varieties. The standard-height backrest provides support to the mid-scapula region. A number of modifications can be made to suit the user:

▶ A lower back height may increase functional mobility—typically seen in sports chairs—but may also increase back strain.

▶ *Lateral trunk supports:* improve trunk alignment for patients with scoliosis or poor stability.

▶ *Insert or contour backs:* improve trunk extension and overall upright alignment.

▶ A high back height may be necessary for patients with poor trunk stability or with extensor spasms.

▶ *Reclining wheelchairs.* These are designed with an extended back and typically with elevating leg rests. The angle of the back is adjusted by releasing knobs on the side of the wheelchair. A head support is required on a reclining back wheelchair. A bar across the back of the reclining wheelchair provides support and stability. The purpose of the reclining wheelchair is to allow intermittent or constant reclined positioning. Reclining wheelchairs are indicated for patients who are unable to independently maintain an upright sitting position. The chairs can be controlled either manually or electrically (if the patient cannot do active push-ups or pressure relief maneuvers).

▶ *Tilt in space.* A chair that is designed to allow for a reclining position without losing the required 90° of hip flexion and 90° of knee flexion. This type of chair is indicated for patients with extensor spasms that may throw the patient out of the chair, or for pressure relief.

Armrests

In addition to providing a place to rest the arms and to support the upper body, correctly positioned armrests also decrease the weight on the buttocks. Armrests are available in several styles depending on the patient's needs, from the standard armrest to the desk length, full length, or wraparound.

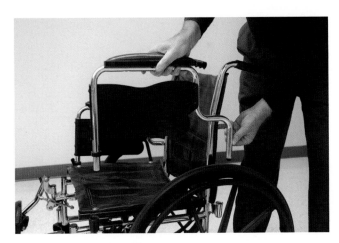

FIGURE 13-13 Removable armrest

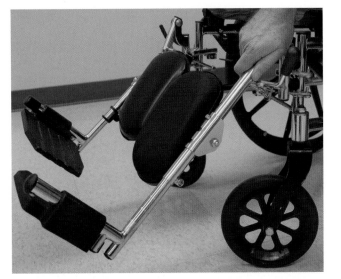

FIGURE 13-14 Front rigging of a wheelchair

▶ *Desk length.* This design, in which one portion of the armrest's length is lower than the remaining portion to allow the user closer access to desks and tables, also allows the patient to remove and reverse the armrest so that the higher part is closer to the front edge in order to aid in pushing to standing. The disadvantage of this type of armrest is that they provide less forearm support and are generally more expensive.

▶ *Full length.* These are designed to support the entire length of the forearm and are usually preferable if the patient weighs over 250 pounds.

▶ *Wraparound (space saver).* This design reduces the overall width of the chair by 1½″. The height of the armrests can also be adjustable.

Armrests are usually designed to be fixed or removable. Fixed armrests usually result in a lighter and narrower wheelchair, whereas removable armrests are important for patients who will be performing lateral transfers in and out of a wheelchair or for those who wish to sit closer to a table or desk. The removable armrests (Figure 13-13) are typically released using a lever, latch, or pushbutton.

> **CLINICAL PEARL**
>
> The choice of armrest height may be determined by the need for attachments. For example, armrests can be fitted with upper extremity support surface trays or troughs, which are helpful if the user has difficulty with upper body balance or decreased use of the upper extremities.

Many lightweight manual chairs are designed without armrests, which makes it easier for the user to roll up to a desk or table and to perform transfers, in addition to providing a streamlined look. In general, armrests increase the overall width of a wheelchair and decrease the mechanical advantage of the patient's arm position for propelling.

Front Rigging

The front rigging of a wheelchair (Figure 13-14), which consists of a footplate attached to either a foot rest or and elevating leg rest, provides support for the lower extremities.

▶ *Footplate.* A footplate (Figure 13-15) is standard equipment on a wheelchair. For rigid-frame chairs, the footplates are usually incorporated into the frame of the chair as part of the design. Cross-brace folding chairs often have footplates that swivel, flip up (Figure 13-16), and/or can be removed. Footplates can be adjusted to accommodate the patient's foot and provide a resting base for the feet, so that the feet are in neutral with a knee flexed to 90°. The angle of the footplate can be customized depending on a patient's needs. For example, wheelchair athletes prefer to have a slight inward angle for increased maneuverability. Heel loops can be fitted to help maintain

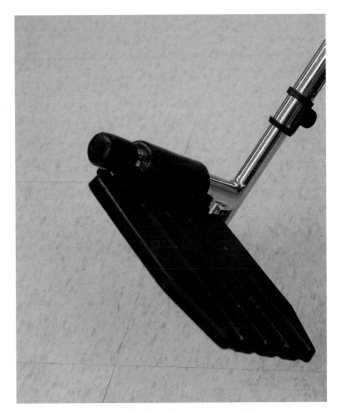

FIGURE 13-15 Wheelchair footplate

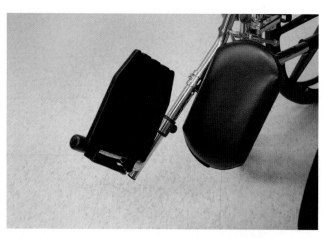

FIGURE 13-16 Wheelchair footplate flipped up

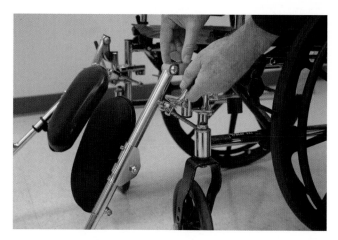

FIGURE 13-18 Elevating leg rest

the foot position and prevent posterior sliding of the foot. Ankle and calf straps can be added to stabilize the feet onto the footplates. Toe loops may also be used when the patient has difficulty maintaining the foot on the footplate in a forward direction.

▶ *Leg rests.* The standard leg rest positions the lower extremities at an angle of 70° from the horizontal plane. As with other wheelchair components, leg rests also come in a variety of designs including swing away, removable, and elevating.

▶ *Swing away (Figure 13-17).* This design facilitates in transfers and a clear front approach to the wheelchair when ambulating. The leg rests are snapped into place during wheelchair mobility. The disadvantage of this type of leg rest is that the leg rests are not lockable in the away position, which may allow the leg rest to swing back against the leg.

▶ *Removable.* These can be fully detached from the wheelchair, which can enable the patient to maneuver in smaller spaces and makes the wheelchair easier to transport. The disadvantage of this type of leg rest is that they may be lost.

▶ *Elevating (Figure 13-18).* This design can be used when the patient is unable to flex the knee, for postural support, or when a dependent leg contributes to lower extremity edema. The position of the leg rest, which can be raised and fixed at any angle from 90° to 0°, is adjusted

by pushing down on a lever on the side of the chair. Articulating leg rests allow the length of the leg rest to be adjusted to accommodate the full length of the patient's leg and to provide a padded calf support. This type of leg rest is suitable for patients with an arthrodesis of the knee, orthostatic hypotension, or a leg cast. Elevating leg rests can typically be released from the wheelchair or pivoted to one side during transfers. Elevated leg rests are contraindicated for patients with hypertonicity or adaptive shortening of the hamstrings. One of the disadvantages of this type of leg rest is that it increases the wheelchair's overall length and weight, which can have a negative impact on maneuverability and transportability.

Wheels

Most wheelchairs use four wheels: two large drive wheels (standard spokes or spokeless) at the back (fitted with an outer rim that allows for hand grip and propulsion) and two smaller ones (casters) at the front (Figure 13-19).

CLINICAL PEARL

Spoked wheels, although they require maintenance, are lightweight, and the spokes can be individually adjusted to keep the wheel perfectly round. The mag wheel is a type of spoked wheel that has six to eight broad struts connecting the hub to the outer rim of the wheel.

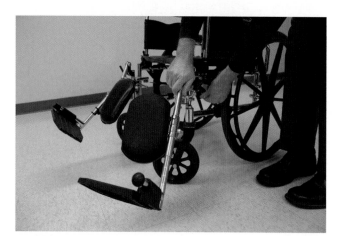

FIGURE 13-17 Swing-away leg rest

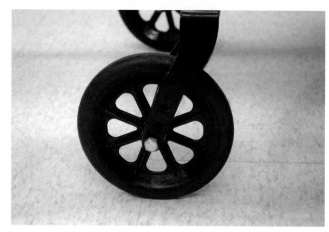

FIGURE 13-19 Wheelchair caster

The standard sizes for the drive wheel of a manual wheelchair are 22, 24, and 26 inches. However, smaller and larger wheel sizes are also available. For example, powered wheelchairs often incorporate a 10-inch wheel drive design.

Wheels that are fitted with an outer rim, referred to as a pushrim or handrim, enable patients to propel themselves without having to place their hands directly on the tires. For patients with only one functional arm, two outer rims can be fitted on one wheel so that arm drive achieves both forward and backward propulsion.

Projections (vertical, oblique, or horizontal) can be attached to the rims to facilitate with propulsion for patients with poor handgrip. However, the horizontal and oblique extensions add to the overall width of the chair and may reduce maneuverability.

The drive wheels are positioned nearly perpendicular to the floor in a standard wheelchair, but in chairs requiring more stability and agility, the wheels are often angled in.

> **CLINICAL PEARL**
>
> The inward angle of the wheel relative to the vertical position is referred to as the camber. Although a greater camber provides increased stability, the wider position of the wheels near the floor can limit the wheelchair's ability to pass through narrow spaces.

Tires

The tires used for the rear wheels may be solid hard rubber, pneumatic inflatable, semi-pneumatic, or radial. In general, solid tires are well suited for indoor use and require less energy to propel. The pneumatic tires provide a smoother ride and increased shock absorption and, if fitted with treads, can allow a patient to traverse uneven terrain. However, pneumatic tires require correct inflation for efficient propulsion and effective application of wheelchair locks. In addition, pneumatic tires are subject to blowouts, although newer designs have solid inserts that make them puncture proof and help to maintain inflation at the expense of being heavier.

Casters

Casters, the smaller wheels at the front of the wheelchair, vary in size (ranging from 2 to 8 inches in diameter) and composition (pneumatic, solid rubber, plastic, or a combination of these). The function of the casters is to allow changes in direction. Large casters create more stability, whereas small casters increase maneuverability. Caster locks can be added to facilitate wheelchair stability during transfers.

Wheel Locks

Wheel locks or brakes (Figure 13-20) are an important safety feature and must be engaged for all transfers in and out of the chair. The majority of wheel locks consist of a lever system with a cam, or a ratchet. Extensions may be added to increase the ease of both locking and unlocking. When a wheelchair has a reclining back, an additional brake is necessary. A hill holder is a mechanical brake that allows the chair to go forward, but automatically applies the brakes when the chair goes into reverse.

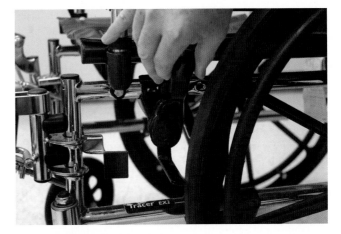

FIGURE 13-20 Wheelchair lock

Axle

The position of the axle affects the stability and maneuverability of the wheelchair as it determines the drive wheel position. For example, if the front and back wheels are closer together, the wheelchair is more nimble but also more challenging to control. The more recent wheelchair models have adjustable axles.

> **CLINICAL PEARL**
>
> Most modern standard wheelchairs have "dual axle" adjustments for the rear wheel and three placements to adjust the front caster. This allows the chair seat to be lowered or raised 2 inches.

Seatbelts

Seatbelts can be used for safety or for positioning:

▸ Restraining belts are used to prevent patients from falling out of the wheelchair.

▸ Seatbelts can be fitted to grasp over the pelvis at a 45° angle to the seat to help position the pelvis. An additional belt can also be added to provide lateral or medial support at the hip and knee to maintain alignment of the lower extremities and/or control spasticity.

Powered Chairs

This type of chair, which uses a power source (battery) that propels the wheelchair, is usually prescribed for patients who are not capable of self-propulsion or who have very low endurance. The battery is stored on the chair. Microprocessors allow the control of the wheelchair to be adapted to various controls (joystick, head, breath). Recent changes in the power bases have allowed for such innovations as power seat functions (power tilt, recline, elevating leg rest, seat elevator), and control interfaces (mini joysticks, head controls). Power wheelchair bases can be classified in one of three categories, based on the drive wheel location relative to the system's center of gravity:

▸ *Rear-wheel drive.* In this base design, the drive wheels are located behind the user's COG, and the casters are located in the front, providing predictable drive characteristics and stability. In general, a rear-wheel drive allows a chair to move more rapidly than a front-wheel drive wheelchair.

▶ *Mid-wheel drive.* In this design, the drive wheels are directly below the user's COG and the chair generally has a set of casters or antitippers in the front and rear of the drive wheels. The advantage of this system is a smaller turning radius. The disadvantage is a tendency to rock or pitch forward, especially with sudden stops or fast turns. In addition, this type of design can get stuck going over obstacles.

▶ *Front-wheel drive.* In this design, the drive wheels are located in front of the user's COG. This design provides stability and a tight turning radius, and the ability to climb obstacles or curbs more easily than a chair with a rear-wheel drive. One of the disadvantages of this design is its rearward COG, which makes it difficult to drive in a straight line, especially on uneven surfaces.

The disadvantages of power wheelchairs are that they:

▶ Are more expensive
▶ Are difficult to transport
▶ Have a battery that requires charging
▶ Require protection from wet weather

> ### CLINICAL PEARL
>
> ▶ Power chairs are more expensive than manual chairs. Power chairs have inherent safety concerns and create issues surrounding transportation and home accessibility.
>
> ▶ Manual wheelchairs are easier to transport and lift into a nonaccessible home.

Pediatric Wheelchairs

Children with cerebral palsy, spina bifida, or osteogenesis imperfecta may be candidates for either manual or power wheelchairs, depending on upper extremity strength, rate of fatigue, cognitive abilities, and family circumstances. Those with spinal muscular dystrophy, arthrogryposis, or high-level spinal cord injuries and those with progressively worsening Duchenne's muscular dystrophy are typically immediate candidates for powered mobility. Key decisions concerning wheelchair design must be a team effort.

A pediatric wheelchair must have approximately 4 inches of available space in the frame to accommodate growth. In addition, the seating system should be flexible enough to accommodate tonal or postural changes. Examples of flexibility in the system involve the placement of laterals, which are often attached to tracks, or the backrest can include T-nuts placed throughout the back to allow easy hardware mounting. Pediatric chairs often employ linear seating systems (to accommodate the delicate balance between providing contours in the system and accommodating growth) versus molded seats, which are more difficult to increase in size. Similarly, a contoured backrest is more accommodating and provides more contact surface and thus more comfort. Caregivers should be made aware of the proper use of all accessories, including head supports and upper chest supports.

One must also always consider the aesthetic appeal of the wheelchair. Where possible, the wheelchair should reflect the patient's individuality and personality.

Wheelchair Measurements

A correctly sized wheelchair contributes to the patient's overall function and well-being by preventing complications, enhancing posture, and optimizing mobility. The range of available pelvic and hip movements as they relate to spinal and pelvic alignment should be determined. To measure the patient for a wheelchair, the patient should be positioned supine on a firm surface in the 90-90-90 position (90° of hip flexion, 90° to 100° of knee flexion, and neutral 90° ankle position) (Table 13-4). The lower extremities must be well supported by the clinician in this position. It is important that the clinician maintain the tape measure in a straight line from one endpoint to the other, rather than allowing the tape to follow the contours of the patient's body, as the latter method will distort the results. The degree of knee flexion must be determined so that the influence of the hamstring muscle group is eliminated.[1] Range of motion measurements should include hip flexion, abduction, adduction, and internal and external rotation; their effect on pelvic position and general body alignment should be noted as well.

> ### CLINICAL PEARL
>
> Along with seat depth, seat width is the most important wheelchair measurement because of the effect the wheelchair's width has on the position of the arms for propelling the wheelchair.

Once range of motion is documented, a linear measurement of seat depth should be determined.

Once examination in the supine position is completed, the patient should be placed in a supported sitting position with the knees flexed to 100° or more to eliminate the influence of the hamstring muscle group. Ideally, seated examination should be done on a simulator, a chair specifically designed for planar seated examinations. If a simulator is not available, the measurement can be done on the mat table with a thin front edge to allow 100° of knee flexion. The clinician should confirm the fit of a new or existing wheelchair by observation, questioning the patient, and physical assessment of the patient's posture and mobility. For example, the thighs should be parallel to the floor, the knees should be at the same height as the hips, and the feet should be flat on the floor or the footplate.

> ### CLINICAL PEARL
>
> Many patients sacral sit—sit with the pelvis posteriorly rotated and the trunk resting on the sacrum rather than on the ischial tuberosities. Taking measurements when the patient is in this position will result in errors (see Table 13-4). As a quick check, measurements of the upper leg (from the popliteal fold to the most posterior point of the body) and lower leg (from the sole of the foot to the popliteal fold) should be within 1 inch of each other if the patient is sitting correctly.

TABLE 13-4	**Wheelchair Measurements**	
Dimension	**Guidelines**	**Average Size**
Seat height	The seat-to-floor height affects many functional activities, including the ability to eat and work at standard height tables and desks and the ability to use the lower extremities to propel the wheelchair. The measurement is taken from the sole of the patient's usual footwear to the popliteal fold. If the wheelchair will be propelled, this distance will be used as a seat height. However, if the patient will not be using the feet to propel the wheelchair, 2 inches is added to this measurement to allow clearance between the footplate and the floor. If the patient will be sitting on a cushion, the thickness of the cushion needs to be considered in the measurement, bearing in mind that a 3-inch-thick cushion may compress to 1 inch under the patient's body weight.	Bariatric: 19.5–20.5 inches Adult: 18–20.5 inches. Sports: Front, 16–22 inches; rear, 13–23 inches Pediatric: 15–21 inches Hemi/low seat: 15.5–17.5 inches. Reclining: 19.5–19.75 inches
Seat depth	This is the most critical measurement for pelvic position and is also the most common measurement for error because the upper leg length varies according to how the patient is sitting. If the patient is allowed to sacral sit during the measurement, the upper leg measurement will be falsely high; this is why this measurement should be made with the patient positioned in supine. The measurement is taken from the patient's posterior buttock/mat surface along the lateral thigh to the popliteal fold. Approximately 2 inches are subtracted from this measurement to avoid pressure from the edge of the seat against the popliteal space.	Bariatric: 15.75–17.5 inches Adult: 16–18 inches Sports: 10–20 inches Pediatric: 8–18 inches Hemi/low seat: 15.5–17.5 inches Reclining: 16–18 inches
Seat width	Measurement taken of the widest aspect of the patient's buttocks, hips or thighs, while taking into account the patient's customary clothing. 1–2 inches is added to this measurement so as to provide space for bulky clothing, orthoses, or clearance of the trochanters from the armrest side panel. It is important to remember that the greater the seat width, the more difficult it is to propel the chair and to navigate it through small spaces. To improve the accuracy of this measurement, a book can be placed gently against each of the patient's hips and a measurement taken between the inner edges of the books.	Bariatric: 16–30 inches Adult: 14–18 inches Sports: 12–20 inches Pediatric: 10–16 inches Hemi/low seat: 16–30 inches Reclining: 14–22 inches
Seat-back height	The height of the seat back determines the level of postural support provided to the patient. For a medium-height back, the measurement is taken from the seat of the chair to the floor of the axilla with the patient's shoulder flexed to 90°. 4 inches is subtracted from this measurement to allow the final back height to be below the inferior angles of the scapulae. NB: This measurement will be affected if a seat cushion is to be used—the patient should be measured while seated on the seat cushion, or the thickness of the cushion must be considered by adding that value to the actual measurement.	Bariatric: 16 inches Adult: As required Sports: 9–20 inches Pediatric: 8–16 inches Hemi/low seat: 16 inches Reclining: 22–24 inches
Armrest height	Measurement taken from the seat of the chair to the olecranon process with the patient's elbow flexed to 90°. 1 inch is added to this measurement. NB: This measurement will be affected if a seat cushion is to be used—the patient should be measured while seated on the seat cushion, or the thickness of the cushion must be considered by adding that value to the actual measurement.	Bariatric: As required Adult: 5–12 inches Sports: None Pediatric: 4.5–6.75 inches Hemi/low seat: 5–12 inches Reclining: 5–12 inches

Data from Dreeben, O: Physical Therapy Clinical Handbook for PTAs. London, Jones & Bartlett, 2008.

The two-finger rule can be used to check for the approximate fit of a standard wheelchair:

▶ *Seat depth:* Leave no more or less than two finger-widths of space behind the back of the calf and the front edge of the wheelchair.

▶ *Seat width:* Leave no more or less than two finger-widths of space between the hip and the inside of the wheelchair arm.

▶ *Seat height:* Leave no more or less than two finger-widths of space between the floor and floor plates.

▶ *Seat back height:* Leave no more or less than two finger-widths of space between the top of the wheelchair back and the patient's axilla.

▶ *Armrest height:* Leave no more or less than two finger-widths of space between the top of the drive wheel and the underside of the patient's forearm.

It is important for the patient to maintain good posture in the wheelchair. He or she should be seated well back in the chair, with the lower extremities on the foot rests or leg rests. Wheelchair users are susceptible to muscle imbalances. Nearly every motion and/or repetitive motion is forward, working such areas as the shoulder flexors (pectoralis major, and anterior deltoid) and shoulder internal rotators. These

CLINICAL PEARL

A lower seat height allows for greater upper extremity motions.

anterior muscles can become adaptively shortened, while the upper back muscles become weak and elongated. The typical posture of the wheelchair user is rounded shoulders with mild thoracic kyphosis and a forward head. This posture can result in impingement of the soft tissue structures of the acromiohumeral space. The patient should be able to maintain a seated position when his or her balance is challenged.

Wheelchair Tasks

A number of wheelchair transfers can be made easier with the following tasks:

▶ *Forward hip slide.* Most of the transfers from a wheelchair require that the patient be able to maneuver to the front edge of the seat, thereby placing their center of mass (COM) over his or her BOS (VIDEO 13-2). To do this, the patient can use one of the following methods:

- *Upward and forward lift.* The patient pushes down through the arms and/or legs, lifts the hips up above the seating surface, and then moves the buttocks forward.

- *Weight shift.* The patient leans the upper body to one side and then to the other, each time lifting the contralateral hip up and forward until the correct position is attained.

- *Forward hip slide.* The patient leans back in the chair and, by extending the trunk, slides the hips to the front edge of the seat before grasping the arms of the chair and pulling the trunk forward into an upright position.

  If the patient is unable to perform this movement independently, the clinician can assist by squatting or half kneeling in front of the patient and placing his or her hands behind patient's hip with the fingers or fingertips over the sacroiliac joints. From this position, the clinician pulls the patient's hips forward simultaneously, or alternating side to side, with the patient participating as much as possible. At the end of this technique, depending on the level of trunk control that the patient possesses, the clinician may need to place his or her hands behind the patient's shoulders and assist the patient in moving the shoulders forward over the pelvis into an erect sitting position.

▶ *Sitting push-up.* This technique, which requires the patient to form a series of sitting push-ups, can be used to assist the patient to the front edge of the seat. After each sitting push-up, the patient lowers himself or herself closer to the front edge of the wheelchair seat. The clinician may assist by lifting under the patient's buttocks, or by guarding at the shoulders. The sitting push-up can also be used to relieve pressure on the buttocks and posterior thighs (VIDEO 13-3).

▶ *Weight shifting side to side.* This technique can be used to assist the patient to the front edge of the seat. The clinician places one arm around the patient's shoulders from one side, and the other arm under the thigh at the opposite lower extremity. The patient's weight can then be shifted to one side. For example, if the clinician places his or her left arm around the patient's right shoulder, and the right hand is placed under the patient's left side, the patient's weight can be shifted to the right, which unweights the patient's left buttock, and then the clinician assists the patient in moving the left thigh forward. Once the left lower extremity is lowered to the supporting surface, the patient is returned to an erect sitting position and the technique is performed to the other side. This sequence is repeated until the patient reaches the front edge of the seat.

▶ *Foot position.* Once the patient's hips are moved to the front edge of the wheelchair seat, the patient's feet must be positioned posteriorly and approximately shoulder width apart (closer if both knees will be blocked during the transfer), so that the BOS is directly under the patient's new COM. If the patient is unable to position his or her feet independently, assistance is provided by the clinician. In certain circumstances, such as a weight-bearing restriction on one of the lower extremities, only one foot is positioned posteriorly, leaving the other extended out in front of the patient.

▶ *Trunk flexion.* As the mass of the trunk is moved forward over the BOS, so that the nose is over the toes, the patient is able to use the large muscles of the lower extremities more effectively. However, it is important to remember that a patient who has undergone a total hip arthroplasty (posterolateral approach) must limit trunk flexion by maintaining an upright position or lean somewhat posteriorly.

▶ *Hand positioning.* The position of the hands varies greatly depending on the patient's level of independence. If hand positioning can be performed independently, the patient positions the hands posterior to the flexed trunk before initiating a push-off from the armrests. Occasionally, the clinician may ask the patient to hold onto the clinician's forearm or hips. If the patient is unable to perform hand positioning independently, the clinician must position the hands and arms inside the armrests, in the patient's lap.

▶ *Moving backward.* The patient is asked to lean forward by flexing the trunk and then to place the hands on the armrests posterior to the shoulder. The feet are then placed as far posteriorly as possible while maintaining contact with the floor. The patient is asked to push down through the arms and legs and lift the hips up and back. This sequence is repeated as often as needed to achieve the correct position.

Wheelchair Transfers

A number of areas need to be addressed when training a patient on how to be as functionally independent as possible with a wheelchair. The various components of the wheelchair should be reviewed with the patient, and the patient should perform all of the necessary tasks while being supervised by the clinician.

Transfer from Wheelchair to Floor—Two-Person Lift

The two-person lift is used when the patient has some trunk control and upper extremity strength. It is important to ensure that the wheelchair is locked and that the foot rests are removed or swung out of the way. The armrest on the side of the wheelchair to which the patient will be transferred is also removed. One of the clinicians is positioned behind the patient, while the other clinician is in front of the patient. The patient is asked to hug himself or herself. The clinician behind the patient reaches under the patient's upper extremities and grasps the opposite wrist of the patient (right arm on left and left on right) to prevent the patient from abducting his or her arms during the lift. The clinician in front of the patient cradles the patient's thighs with one hand and the lower legs with the other hand. On the command from the clinician behind the patient, the patient is lifted by both clinicians to a height that clears all parts of the wheelchair and then, as a unit, the two clinicians step in the required direction before lowering the patient to the floor. Once the patient is correctly and safely positioned, he or she is released.

Transfer from Floor to Wheelchair—Two-Person Lift

The transfer of the patient back from the floor to the wheelchair is essentially the reverse of the previous procedure. The wheelchair is prepared—the brakes are secured and the armrests and foot rests are removed. The patient is positioned in long sitting. Both clinicians squat down, and then both use the same holding techniques as in the previous transfer. On the command from the clinician at the head of the patient, the patient is lifted to a height that will clear all parts of the wheelchair. Then, as a unit, the two clinicians transfer the patient onto the seat of the wheelchair. Both clinicians ensure that the patient assumes proper sitting posture before replacing the armrests and foot rests, and placing the patient's feet on the foot rests.

Transfer from Wheelchair to Treatment Table—Squat-Pivot Transfer

The squat-pivot transfer is used in those cases where a patient is able to bear weight but has insufficient strength or control of the lower extremities to stand upright. This is a physically demanding transfer for the clinician, who must decide whether extra assistance is required. Before the transfer can begin, the clinician must position the wheelchair near parallel to the treatment table, lock the wheels, and remove the wheelchair armrest on the side toward which the patient is moving. The clinician then removes or swings away the foot rests so that the patient's feet can be placed on the floor. The patient is fitted with a transfer belt. If the patient is unable to slide his or her hips forward in the wheelchair, the clinician uses one of the methods described under wheelchair tasks, or reaches around the back of the patient's pelvis and slides the patient forward in the seat of the wheelchair (VIDEO 13-4). When possible, the patient's feet should be positioned under the COM and slightly apart to maximize the BOS. If feasible, the patient should place each hand on an armrest with the forearms in a near vertical position so that the pushing force will be vertical. Once the patient is positioned correctly, the clinician places each foot and knee outside of the patient's feet and knees in preparation for blocking both of the patient's lower extremities by directing the force at the patient's proximal tibia (squeezing the patient's knees together is not recommended).

Throughout the transfer, the patient's lower extremities are not fully extended at any time. If applicable, the patient is asked to push down on the remaining armrest as the transfer is initiated. The clinician simultaneously pivots on the balls of the feet as the patient is lifted and shifts the COM laterally until the patient's hips are above the treatment table. The clinician then lowers the patient's hips to the table in a controlled manner, and then adjusts the patient's position as needed. The transfer from the treatment table back to the wheelchair is essentially the reverse.

Transfer from Wheelchair to Treatment Table—Standing Pivot

This technique is used for patients who are unable to stand independently, but are able to bear some weight through one or both of the lower extremities. Before the transfer can begin, the clinician must position the wheelchair parallel to the treatment table and then lock the wheels. The clinician then removes or swings away the foot rests so that the patient's feet can be placed on the floor. If the patient is unable to slide his or her hips forward in the wheelchair, the clinician uses one of the methods described under wheelchair tasks, or reaches around the back of the patient's pelvis and slides the patient forward in the seat of the wheelchair. Once the patient is positioned correctly, the clinician places each foot and knee outside of the patient's feet and knees in preparation for blocking one or both of the patient's lower extremities (VIDEO 13-5). Determining how much blocking will be required is a matter of clinical judgment. Patients who are progressing from dependent pivot transfers to assisted pivot transfers may require blocking of both knees, whereas patients transitioning from assisted pivot transfers may require only one or neither knee to be blocked.

▶ *Blocking one knee:* the clinician flexes his or her hips and knees to position his or her proximal tibia against the patient's tibia just inferior and central to the patient's tibial tuberosity. The clinician can also use both of his or her knees to block one of the patient's knees by placing the medial aspect of both knees on either side of the patient's tibial tuberosity.

▶ *Blocking both knees:* the clinician positions the patient's feet together and slightly staggered, and then places the medial aspect of both his or her knees against the anterolateral aspects of the patient's knees.

The blocking technique produces a counterforce that is necessary once the patient is upright to counteract the effect of gravity, which creates a flexion moment at the patient's hips and knees. By placing the feet outside of the patient's feet, the clinician creates a wide BOS, which is designed to help support the dynamic weight of two people once the patient is upright. To assist with the pivot, the patient's foot nearer the target surface should be moved slightly forward relative to the other foot. The clinician's foot placement mimics the patient's—on the side toward which the patient is turning, the clinician places that foot slightly posteriorly, and the other slightly anteriorly. Having the patient come to a standing position can occur in a number of ways:

▶ The clinician places both hands under the patient's buttocks, and the patient is asked to place both of his or her arms around the clinician's upper back (not the neck!) (VIDEO 13-6). On the clinician's count and command, the clinician initiates a rocking motion in time to the counts. On the command "up," the clinician straightens his or her legs and lifts the patient from the wheelchair to a height that is sufficient to clear the wheelchair and any height difference between the wheelchair and the treatment table.

▶ The patient places both hands on the wheelchair armrests and, on the clinician's count and command, pushes down on the armrests to bring himself or herself to the standing position while the clinician guards the patient. If a patient has undergone a total hip arthroplasty (posterolateral approach), pushing to a standing position can prove difficult: the patient must maintain his or her trunk position in an upright or slightly backward position during the transfer, which places the COM posterior to the feet, increasing the potential for falling backward. In addition, the clinician must monitor the amount of internal rotation of the patient's involved hip during the transfer. Having the patient transfer toward the uninvolved side creates less risk of hip internal rotation, although it is important that the patient be able to transfer toward both sides.

As the patient rises, the clinician leans posteriorly to accommodate the patient's anteriorly moving COM, while simultaneously guarding the patient against a fall. Once the patient's trunk is high enough to clear the chair, the clinician and patient begin to pivot toward the treatment table. The actual pivot may need to be performed in a series of small movements for the first few attempts. At the end of the pivot, the patient should be in the correct position for sitting on the table, and as the patient is lowered, he or she should reach back for the target surface. During the lowering process, the patient should be encouraged to maintain trunk flexion so that the patient's COM does not move too quickly in a posterior direction and so that the descent can be performed in a controlled manner. Once the patient is correctly and safely positioned, he or she can be released. The transfer from the treatment table back to the wheelchair is essentially the reverse.

CLINICAL PEARL

The standing pivot transfer can be used in cases of unilateral non–weight bearing by positioning the non–weight-bearing extremity forward rather than placing it under the patient's COM.

Transfer from Bed to Wheelchair— Assisted Standing Pivot

The assisted standing pivot transfer is similar to the standing pivot transfer, except that the clinician provides less assistance to the patient (VIDEO 13-7). The decision to use this transfer instead of the standing pivot transfer is based on the patient's level of independence. The assisted standing pivot can be used when a patient can bear some weight on the lower extremities but has weakness that necessitates some assistance. The planned transfer is typically set up so that the patient can move toward the uninvolved side during the transfer. The clinician assists the patient by controlling the patient's pelvis. This is accomplished by placing a hand posterior to the pelvis, on the side of the pelvis, or on the anterior aspect of the pelvis, depending on where the assistance is needed. The other hand is placed on the posterior aspect of the patient's opposite shoulder. Stability is provided by guarding or blocking the patient's uninvolved lower extremity using the same lower extremity (the patient's right knee is guarded with the clinician's right knee). On the clinician's command, the patient pushes to the standing position. Once in the full upright position and under control, the patient pivots or reaches for the wheelchair before lowering himself or herself with assistance as appropriate. Once the patient is correctly and safely positioned, he or she can be released. The transfer from the wheelchair back to the bed is essentially the reverse.

Transfer from Wheelchair to Treatment Table—Sliding Board

A sliding board transfer allows a patient to transfer between numerous sitting surfaces using a series of small shifts of the trunk without having to bear weight through the lower extremities. However, such transfers require high levels of trunk and upper body strength and sitting balance. Ideally, the transfer should occur between two surfaces that are the same height as each other, or from a slightly higher surface to a slightly lower one. Before the transfer is attempted, the clinician or the patient positions the wheelchair parallel to or at a slight angle to the treatment table, and locks the wheels. The foot rests are then removed or swung away, and the patient's feet are placed on the floor. The patient is asked to move forward on the seat of the wheelchair, and the armrest of the wheelchair on the side nearest the treatment table is removed. The patient is asked to lean away from the treatment table, and the sliding board is positioned well under the patient's buttocks before the patient returns to an upright position. The patient is instructed not to grasp the edge of the sliding board to prevent the fingers from being pinched during the technique. The technique for this transfer involves a series of seated push-ups—straightening the upper extremities, depressing the shoulders, and lifting the body up and across the sliding board toward the treatment table. If the patient's wrists are unable to weight bear sufficiently, the patient can use the outside of the fists. After each push-up and slide, the patient repositions his or her hands and the sequence is repeated until the patient is on the treatment table with only one buttock remaining on the sliding board. At this point, the patient leans away from the wheelchair to remove the sliding board, and the clinician ensures that the patient is in a position that can be maintained independently. During the initial attempts to use this technique, the clinician provides as much assistance as necessary. This assistance can vary from standing in front of the patient, observing, to blocking the patient's knees to prevent the patient from sliding off the sliding board. In addition, the patient may require assistance from the clinician to lift up the buttocks to assist with the sliding technique. The transfer from the treatment table back to the wheelchair is essentially the reverse.

Video Description

VIDEO 10-8 shows a transfer from a hospital bed to a wheelchair using a sliding board. The principles remain the same. Notice in the video how the clinician teaches the patient to position the board and reminds the patient to avoid pinching the fingers under the board during the transfer. Independent sliding board transfers require a high level of trunk and upper body strength and motor control.

Transfer from Wheelchair to Treatment Table—Push-Up

A push-up transfer is similar to the sliding board transfers except that the patient is permitted to bear weight through the lower extremities. Before the transfer is attempted, the clinician or the patient positions the wheelchair parallel to or at a slight angle to the treatment table, and locks the wheels. The foot rests are then removed or swung away, and the patient's feet are placed on the floor. The patient is asked to move forward on the seat of the wheelchair, and the armrest of the wheelchair on the side nearest the treatment table is removed. The patient is asked to place one hand on the treatment table and the other hand on the remaining armrest of the wheelchair. The patient pushes down on both arms and, while maintaining the hand on the treatment table, moves the

hand on the armrest to the seat of the wheelchair while pivoting toward the treatment table so that the back of the thighs touch the treatment table. The patient then lowers himself or herself onto the table. The transfer from the treatment table back to the wheelchair is essentially the reverse.

Transfer from Floor to Wheelchair— One-Person Dependent

On occasion, a patient can inadvertently fall out of or tip over a wheelchair and be unable to get back into the wheelchair. Depending on the size of the patient, and the physical capability of the clinician, another clinician may be needed for assistance. The following description is for a one-person transfer. The clinician positions the wheelchair on its back and at the patient's feet. Using one arm, the clinician places it under the patient's lower extremities and uses the other arm to wrap around the patient's upper back in such a way that the patient's lower extremities are flexed at the hips and knees. Maintaining good body mechanics, the clinician moves the patient so that the patient's ankles are over the front edge of the wheelchair seat, and then uses a series of short lifting and sliding movements to negotiate the patient into the wheelchair. Once the patient is positioned in the wheelchair, the clinician grasps both handles of the wheelchair while maintaining contact with the patient's upper trunk (or one handle of the wheelchair with one hand while supporting the patient's trunk with the other hand), and then lifts the patient and wheelchair as a unit toward the upright position. As the wheelchair and patient approach the upright position, the clinician uses one arm on the anterior aspect of the patient's upper trunk to prevent the patient from falling forward.

Transfer from Wheelchair to Floor—Independent

A variety of methods can be used by patients to transfer from the floor to a wheelchair. The transfer selected depends on the strength, agility, confidence, and range of motion of the patient. The most important strength components for the patient are the strength of the elbow extensors and shoulder extensors. During the initial training sessions, the patient must be guarded and occasionally assisted. In preparation for the transfer, the wheelchair casters are turned forward to prevent the wheelchair from tipping forward, and then the wheelchair is locked.

Anterior Approach

The patient's feet are placed on the floor, the footplates are raised, and the foot rests are removed or swung out of the way. The patient moves to the front of the wheelchair seat, and the lower extremities are positioned in extension. Using one hand, the patient positions it on the side, and toward the front edge of the wheelchair seat, while the other hand is placed on the caster or floor. The patient then lowers himself or herself to the floor. To independently return from the floor to the wheelchair, the procedure is reversed.

Posterior Approach

The patient assumes the quadruped position in front of the wheelchair, with the head closest to the seat (**VIDEO 13-9**). The patient places one hand on the seat toward the front edge, and places the other hand in the same position on the opposite side of the wheelchair seat. The patient then moves into a kneeling position by extending the elbows. One hand of the patient is then moved to the top of the armrest while the other remains on the wheelchair seat. Using a combination of upper extremity extension and shoulder girdle depression, the patient lifts himself or herself and starts to turn. The turn is continued until the patient is able to lower himself or herself onto the seat of the wheelchair. Using a hand on each armrest, the patient pushes down on the armrests and positions himself or herself properly in the wheelchair. To independently return to the floor from the wheelchair, the procedure is reversed (VIDEO 13-10).

Dependent Propulsion

To transport a patient in a wheelchair, the clinician must ensure that the patient is seated safely, which includes sitting well back in the seat, the arms resting on the armrests or in the patient's lap, and the lower extremities supported by the footplates or leg rests. After unlocking the brakes, the clinician should move the wheelchair as smoothly as possible while maintaining good body mechanics and at a speed that is comfortable and safe for the patient. Maneuvering a wheelchair over a smooth surface is much easier than maneuvering a wheelchair on uneven or yielding surfaces such as gravel, sand, grass, and carpet. In such instances, it is recommended that the wheelchair be tipped back to lift the casters off the ground, or to pull the wheelchair rather than push it.

Once a clinician has mastered how to maneuver a patient in a wheelchair in a variety of indoor environments and surfaces, further complexities can be added. Although a wide variety of methods can be used for the following tasks, only the safest ones are presented.

- *Assisted navigation through doorways.* The clinician determines that the patient is sitting safely and then determines the type of door (automatic or manual), and in which direction the door opens (away or toward). If the door is automatic, the clinician must ensure that the wheelchair is clear of the door's path before engaging the door opener, and must also be prepared to block the closing door if necessary to prevent the wheelchair or patient from being struck by the door. If the door is manual, the method used will depend on which direction the door opens:
  - *Door opens away from the patient.* In this scenario, the clinician releases the door latch with his or her back to the doorway, backs the wheelchair through the doorway while keeping the door open with his or her foot or shoulder, and then turns the wheelchair to face the desired direction once the wheelchair has cleared the doorway.
  - *Door opens toward the patient.* In this scenario, the clinician positions the wheelchair on the handle or left side of the door and then uses one hand to open the door while holding one push handle of the wheelchair with the other hand. As soon as the door is open, the clinician locks the door with his or her foot and pushes the wheelchair forward through the doorway. Once the wheelchair has passed completely to the doorway, the clinician releases the door and moves the wheelchair forward.

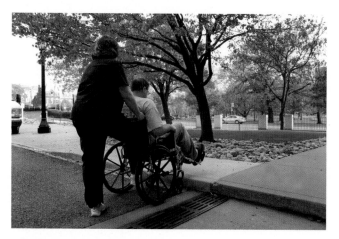

FIGURE 13-21 Wheelchair position to ascend curb

- *Assisted navigation on ascending an incline.* The most efficient way to propel the wheelchair up an incline is to push it forward up the incline with all four wheels in contact with the ground. For very steep slopes, zigzagging may be necessary. If appropriate, the patient can be asked to move the hips forward in the wheelchair, lean the trunk forward, and push equally on both handrims.

- *Assisted navigation on descending an incline.* The safest way to descend an incline is to roll the wheelchair backward down the slope with all four wheels in contact with the ground and while glancing back periodically to be sure the pathway is clear. If appropriate, the patient can be asked to position the hips to the rear of the seat and maintain the trunk erect.

- *Assisted navigation up a curb moving forward.* The wheelchair is positioned facing the curb (Figure 13-21). The clinician tips the chair back, raising the casters above the level of the curb, and then rolls the wheelchair forward until the casters are well over the sidewalk, before lowering the casters gently onto the sidewalk (Figure 13-22). At this point, if appropriate, the patient can be asked to lean the trunk forward and to push forward on the pushrims on the clinician's command. The wheelchair is then rolled forward until the drive wheels are resting against the curb, at which point the clinician gives the patient the command to push forward on the pushrims (if appropriate), and then rolls the drive wheels up onto the sidewalk by lifting on the push handles of the wheelchair using the power

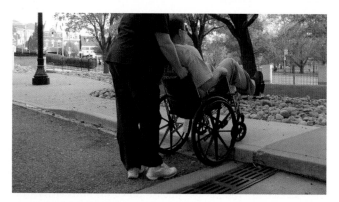

FIGURE 13-22 Casters resting on curb

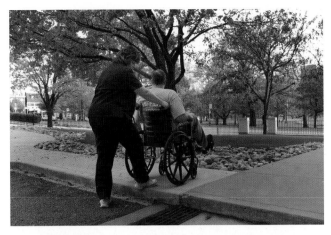

FIGURE 13-23 Wheelchair on top of curb

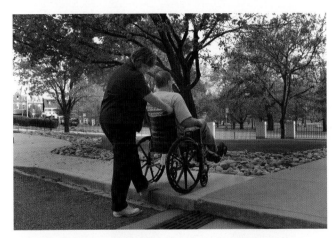

FIGURE 13-24 Wheelchair backed up to edge of curb

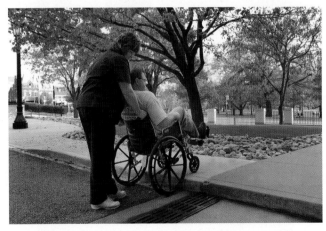

FIGURE 13-25 Drive wheels at bottom of curb

from the legs, and keeping the drive wheels in contact with the curb (Figure 13-23).

▶ *Assisted navigation down a curb moving backward.* The back of the wheelchair is positioned close to the edge of the curb (Figure 13-24). The clinician then steps off the edge of the curb while holding the push handles of the wheelchair. Maintaining the thigh against the back of the wheelchair, and while gripping the push handles, the clinician slowly rolls the drive wheels down over the curb, making sure that the tires maintain contact with the curb (Figure 13-25). If appropriate, the patient can assist by

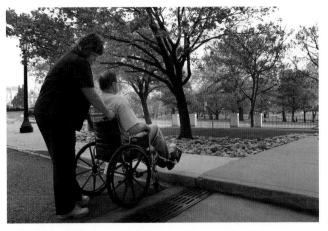

FIGURE 13-26 Wheelchair at bottom of curb

leaning the trunk forward as the chair rolls over and down the curb. Once the drive wheels are resting on the lower surface, the clinician tips the wheelchair back and rolls it backward until the casters and footplates fully clear the curb before gently lowering the front casters to the ground in a controlled fashion (Figure 13-26).

▶ *Assisted navigation up a curb moving backward.* The back of the drive wheels of the wheelchair are positioned up against the curb. The clinician stands up on the curb behind the wheelchair, grasps the push handles, and tips the wheelchair backward into a wheelie position. The clinician then pulls the wheelchair back, rolling it up onto the curb while maintaining the wheelie position. The clinician continues to roll the wheelchair back on the sidewalk until the casters are clearly over the sidewalk, before slowly lowering the casters to the ground in a controlled manner.

▶ *Assisted navigation ascending steps moving backward.* This task requires two to three transporters and should only be attempted when absolutely necessary. Normally, the strongest clinician is positioned behind the wheelchair and leads the activity while the other assistants help from the sides by grasping the frame of the chair. However, if the assistants are both strong, having the strongest clinician behind the wheelchair is not as critical. Once the clinician and assistants are in position, the wheelchair locks are disengaged and the wheelchair is backed to the bottom of the stairs until the drive wheels make contact with the bottom step (Figure 13-27). The clinician grasps the push handles and tips the wheelchair backward into a wheelie position so that the caster wheels are elevated (Figure 13-28). This tipped position is maintained throughout the task. On the count of "three," the clinician and the two assistants pull the chair upward by rolling the drive wheels up and over the step (Figure 13-29). This procedure is repeated one step at a time until the stop step is reached (Figures 13-30 through 13-35), at which point the wheelchair is rolled backward until the casters are clearly beyond the steps before being slowly lowered in a controlled manner (Figure 13-36).

▶ *Assisted navigation descending steps moving forward.* This task requires two to three transporters and should

427

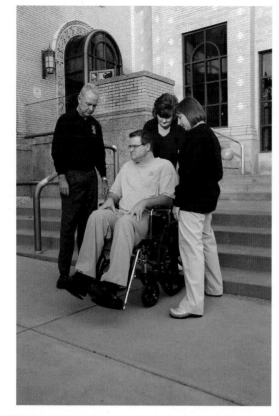

FIGURE 13-27 Wheelchair positioned at bottom of steps

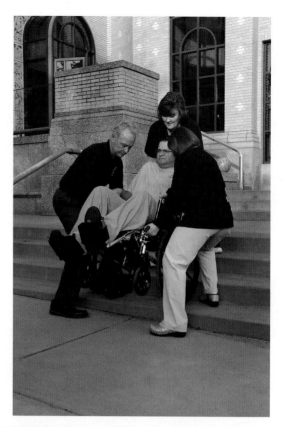

FIGURE 13-29 Wheelchair is moved up to the first step

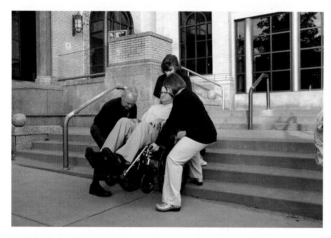

FIGURE 13-28 Wheelchair is tilted back in preparation

only be attempted when absolutely necessary. Normally, the strongest clinician is positioned behind the wheelchair and leads the activity while the other assistants help from the sides. However, if the assistants are both strong, having the strongest clinician behind the wheelchair is not as important. The chair is positioned facing forward near the edge of the top step, and the wheelchair locks are disengaged. The clinician tips the wheelchair back into a wheelie position, elevating the casters, and then slowly and carefully rolls the wheelchair forward until the drive wheels are at the edge of the top step (Figure 13-37). This tipped position is maintained throughout the task. On the count of "three," the clinician and the two assistants control the motion of the rear wheels down to the next step (Figures 13-38 and 13-39). The process is repeated

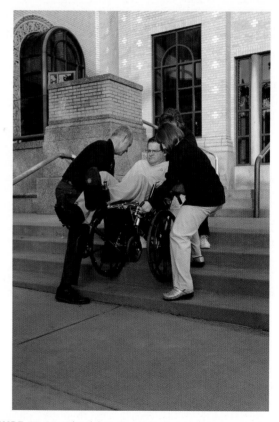

FIGURE 13-30 Wheelchair is gradually moved up one step at a time

one step at a time until the last step is descended (Figures 13-40 through 13-43), at which point the clinician slowly lower the casters to the ground in a controlled manner (Figure 13-44).

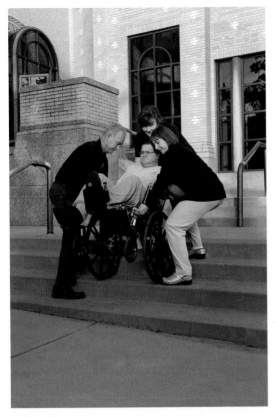

FIGURE 13-31 Wheelchair is gradually moved to the next step

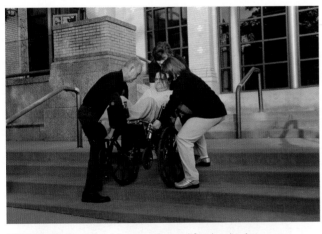

FIGURE 13-32 Wheelchair is prepared for the third step

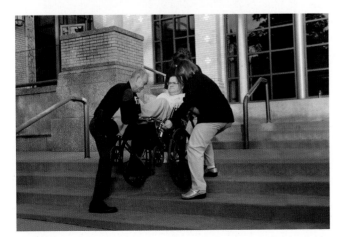

FIGURE 13-33 Wheelchair is gradually moved onto the third step

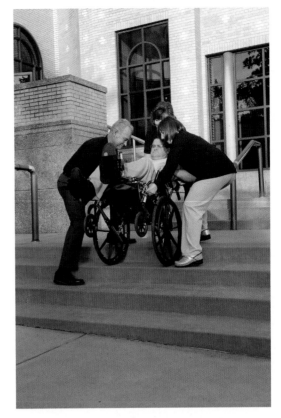

FIGURE 13-34 Wheelchair is prepared for the final step

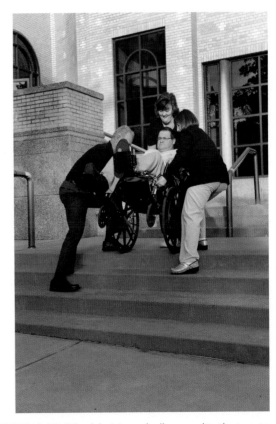

FIGURE 13-35 Wheelchair is gradually moved to the top step

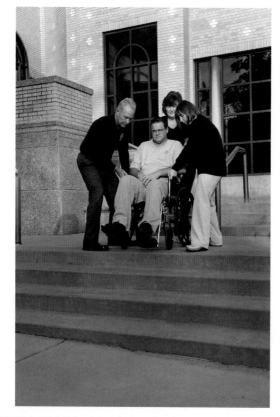

FIGURE 13-36 Wheelchair lowered at the top of the steps

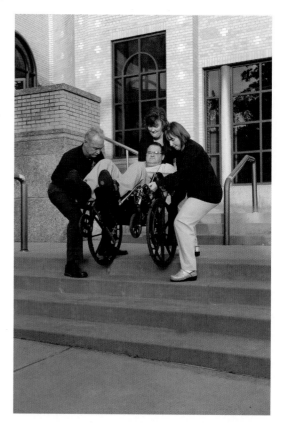

FIGURE 13-38 Wheelchair is lowered down the first step

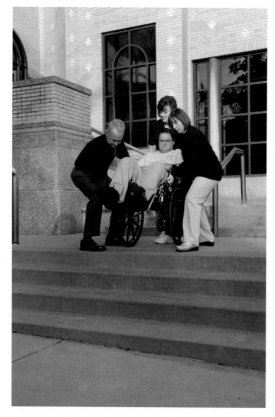

FIGURE 13-37 Wheelchair is tilted back in preparation

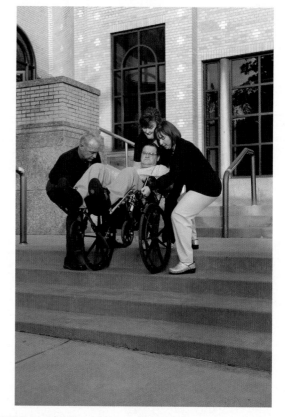

FIGURE 13-39 Wheelchair arrives at the first step

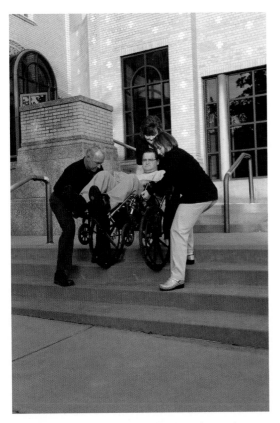

FIGURE 13-40 Wheelchair is gradually moved onto the next step

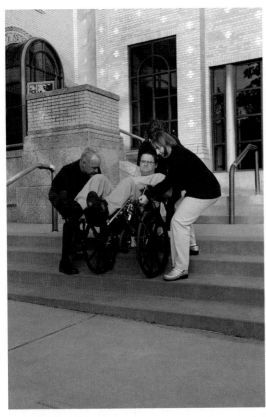

FIGURE 13-41 Wheelchair is lowered onto the next step down

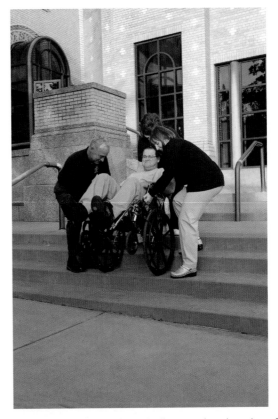

FIGURE 13-42 Wheelchair is gradually moved to the edge of the next step

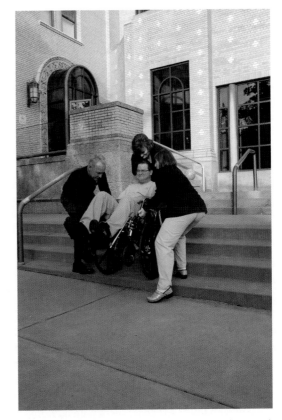

FIGURE 13-43 Wheelchair is gradually moved to the penultimate step

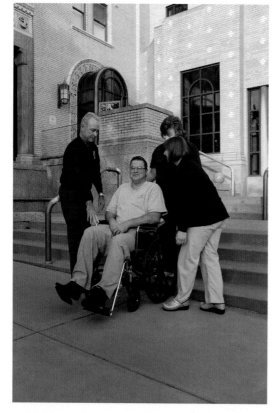

FIGURE 13-44 Casters of the wheelchair are returned to the ground

Independent Propulsion

Depending on functional level, the patient is instructed on how to:

- Operate the wheel locks, foot supports, and armrests, and to use the mechanisms safely without tipping forward or sideways out of the chair seat.

- Transfer in and out of the chair with the least possible assistance (see Patient Transfer section). This may involve transfer training from the wheelchair to a car seat. To transfer from a wheelchair to a car seat, the patient applies the same principles as in a bed-to-chair a transfer. Correct positioning of the wheelchair is critical. The wheelchair armrest and leg rest nearest to the car seat are removed, and the wheelchair is positioned so that it is facing forward between the open door and the car seat, before locking the wheels. Any hand placement during a car transfer must be on a secure surface.

- Propel the wheelchair in all directions and around corners.

- *Propelling forward.* The patient grasps both pushrims simultaneously behind the apex of the wheel at approximately 10 o'clock position and then pushes forward with a long, smooth stroke, releasing the pushrim at about the 2 or 3 o'clock position on the wheels. As the hands are returned to the start position, they remain below the pushrim. This semicircular pattern has been associated with lower stroke frequency, greater time spent in the push phase relative to the recovery phase, less angular joint velocity and acceleration, and increased efficiency.[2–4]

- *Propelling backward.* The patient grasps both pushrims simultaneously at about the 2 or 3 o'clock position on the wheels and then pulls the wheels posteriorly.

- *Turning to the left.* To turn to the left, the patient holds the left pushrim while pushing on the right.

- *Turning to the right.* To turn to the right, the patient holds the right pushrim while pushing on the left.

More advanced users can benefit from the results of a number of biomechanical studies[2–8] about the patient's position within the wheelchair during propulsion:

- To increase efficiency, the axis of the patient's shoulder should be slightly anterior to the rear wheel axle.

- The most efficient push angle can be achieved with a seat alignment that allows 100° to 120° of elbow flexion relative to the apex of the wheel.

Although the most common way to maneuver a wheelchair is to use both upper extremities, the wheelchair can also be propelled using the feet, or a combination of the feet and hands.

- If using the feet to propel a wheelchair, the wheelchair footplates are raised and, if possible, the leg rest is moved out of the way. Using shoes with a good grip, the patient places one foot out in front of the chair, pushes down with the foot, and flexes the knee to move the wheelchair forward. To move the wheelchair backward, the patient places one foot slightly underneath the chair, pushes down on the floor, and extends the knee. If the patient is only able to use one leg, the same technique is used.

- A patient may need to use the hands and feet to propel a wheelchair. For example a patient with one-sided weakness may propel a wheelchair using the arm and leg on the same side.

Once the patient has demonstrated that he or she can maneuver in all directions independently, the clinician must advance the complexity of the navigational tasks as appropriate.

- *Navigating through a doorway.* The patient must determine the type of door (automatic or manual), and in which direction the door opens (away or toward). If the door is automatic, the clinician must be familiar with the speed and closing force of the door. If the door is manual, the method used will depend on the direction in which the door opens, the amount of available space for maneuvering in front of the door, and the patient's abilities.

- *Door opening toward.* The patient approaches the door at the latch side and grasps the door handle, pulls the door open extra wide, and then uses the front rigging of the wheelchair, or a hand, to block the door open. Once the door is blocked open, the patient propels the wheelchair forward through the doorway being careful to avoid pinching the fingers between the wheelchair and the closing door.

- *Door opening away.* The patient approaches the door at the latch side, grasps the door handle, and pushes the door open extra wide. Once the door is open completely, the patient propels the wheelchair quickly through the doorway. Alternatively, the patient can use the front rigging

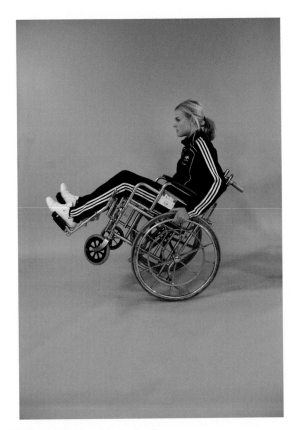

FIGURE 13-45 Wheelchair wheelie

or hand to block the open door while propelling the wheelchair forward until the wheelchair is clear of the door.

▶ *Perform more advanced techniques as necessary or appropriate.* Advanced techniques are necessary when a patient has to negotiate obstacles independently using a wheelie (Figure 13-45). Wheelies are important for patients who need to go up and down curbs independently when there are no curb ramps. A wheelie is performed by balancing on the rear wheels of a wheelchair while the caster wheels are in the air. Initially the clinician must be positioned behind the chair and move with the chair, with the hands held beneath the wheelchair handles, ready to catch the wheelchair if it tilts too far backward. To perform a wheelie, the patient is asked to place the hands at 11 o'clock on the wheels, then lean forward and arch the back. Initially the patient practices bouncing the body off the back of the chair and leaning back while holding the hands still—the front of the chair is raised by pushing backward on the back of the chair. The patient practices until he or she can actually bounce the front end off the ground. By changing the COG (by pushing the chair forward while the body is going backward), the patient will achieve a point of equilibrium. Once the patient is able to bounce the front end off the ground and is able to find a point of equilibrium, he or she can progress to reaching back and placing the hands at about 10 o'clock on the wheels. From this point, the patient leans forward, arches the back, and then begins to push forward quickly while letting the body come back against the chair (when the back hits the chair, the hands should be in the 12 o'clock position). By continuing to

lean back and while pushing the chair forward, the front end should start to leave the ground, and by the time the hands get to the 2 o'clock position, the front end should feel weightless, as the chair balances on the rear axle. To maintain equilibrium, the patient will need to be able to move the chair forward if the front end begins to fall down or backward if the chair begins to fall backward. This may be accomplished by sliding the hands back to about the 1 o'clock position, without taking the hands off the wheels. Once the chair is up and balanced, the patient will need to keep just a fraction of weight on the front end, so that if balance is lost the chair will fall forward, not backward.

Once the patient is ready to try a wheelie independently, a good place to begin practicing is on carpeting, grass, or sand. As part of the wheelie training, the patient should be taught how to fall in a controlled manner.

▶ *Falling backward.* This is probably the most common direction of falling. The patient should be taught on how to tuck the head into the chest if falling backward, so that the back of the head is not hit. In addition, applying a slight braking force to the drive wheels can prevent the wheelchair from sliding too far forward and catching the lower extremities.

▶ *Falling forward.* The patient should be taught on how to land as far forward of the chair as possible by extending the arms and trunk to prevent the upper body from landing on the patient's legs.

▶ *Falling sideways.* The patient should be told to tuck the arms close to the chest and to round the shoulder on the side of the fall while side flexing the head away from the ground.

Finally, the patient should be taught how to use his or her wheelie skills to:

▶ Ascend a curb forward

▶ Descend a curb forward

REFERENCES

1. Edelstein JE: Prosthetics, in O'Sullivan SB, Schmitz TJ (eds): Physical Rehabilitation (ed 5). Philadelphia, FA Davis, 2007, pp 1251-1286.
2. Rankin JW, Kwarciak AM, Richter WM, et al: The influence of wheelchair propulsion technique on upper extremity muscle demand: a simulation study. Clin Biomech (Bristol, Avon) 27(9):879-886, 2012.
3. Kwarciak AM, Turner JT, Guo L, et al: The effects of four different stroke patterns on manual wheelchair propulsion and upper limb muscle strain. Disabil Rehabil Assist Technol 7(6):459-463, 2012.
4. Boninger ML, Souza AL, Cooper RA, et al: Propulsion patterns and pushrim biomechanics in manual wheelchair propulsion. Arch Phys Med Rehabil 83:718-723, 2002.
5. Coutts KD: Kinematics of sport wheelchair propulsion. J Rehabil Res Dev 27:21-26, 1990.
6. Cowan RE, Nash MS, Collinger JL, et al: Impact of surface type, wheelchair weight, and axle position on wheelchair propulsion by novice older adults. Arch Phys Med Rehabil 90:1076-1083, 2009.
7. Desroches G, Dumas R, Pradon D, et al: Upper limb joint dynamics during manual wheelchair propulsion. Clin Biomech (Bristol, Avon) 25:299-306, 2010.
8. Gorce P, Louis N: Wheelchair propulsion kinematics in beginners and expert users: influence of wheelchair settings. Clin Biomech (Bristol, Avon) 27:7-15, 2012.

Gait Training

CHAPTER 14

CHAPTER OBJECTIVES

At the completion of this chapter,
the reader will be able to:

1. Describe the various gait parameters

2. Describe the characteristics of normal gait

3. Discuss how to use the various pieces of pre-ambulation equipment, including the tilt table and parallel bars

4. Describe the various types of weight-bearing status and the functions of each

5. Describe the various methods to monitor weight-bearing status

6. Make a clinical decision as to which assistive device is the most appropriate for a patient

7. Be able to fit a patient for an assistive device

8. Discuss the importance of patient safety during gait or ambulation activities

9. Provide training to the patient on how to use an assistive device during various transfers

10. Teacher patient how to use an assistive device with varying gait patterns, during stair negotiation, and ambulation in the community

OVERVIEW

The lower kinetic chain has two main functions: to provide a stable base of support (BOS) in standing and to propel the body through space with gait. Whereas the objective in standing is to maintain a static equilibrium of forces, the objective with mobility is to create and control dynamic, unbalanced forces to produce movement.[1] Gait is thus an example of controlled instability. It is not clear whether gait is learned or is preprogrammed at the spinal cord level. However, once mastered, gait allows us to move around our environment in an efficient manner, requiring little in the way of conscious thought, at least in familiar surroundings. Bipedal gait has allowed the arms and hands to be free for exploration of the environment. Although gait appears to be a simple process, it is prone to breakdown. Although individual gait patterns are characterized by significant variation, three essential requirements have been identified for locomotion: progression, postural control and adaptation[2]:

► *Progression.* Progression of the head, arms, and trunk is initiated and terminated in the brainstem through a spinal cord central pattern generator (CPG). The locomotor CPG produces self-sustaining patterns of stereotype motor output resulting in gaitlike movements. The fall that occurs at the initiation of gait so that an individual must take the first step is controlled by the central nervous system (CNS).[3] The CNS computes in advance the required size and direction of this fall toward the supporting foot. In addition, gait relies on the control of the limb movements by reflexes. Two such reflexes include the stretch reflex and the extensor thrust. The stretch reflex is involved in the extremes of joint motion, whereas the extensor thrust may facilitate the extensor muscles of the lower extremity during weight bearing.[4] Both the CPG and the reflexes that mediate afferent input to the spinal cord are under the control of the brainstem and are therefore subconscious.[5] This would tend to indicate that verbal coaching (i.e., feedback that is processed in the cortex) regarding an aberrant gait pattern might be less effective than a sensory input that will elicit a brainstem-mediated postural response.[1]

► *Postural control.* Postural control is dynamically maintained to appropriately position the body for efficient gait.

► *Adaptation.* Although central pattern generation occurs independent of sensory input, afferent information from the periphery can influence the central pattern. Adaptation is achieved by adjusting the central pattern generated to meet task demands and environmental demands.

Gait, therefore, is generated grossly in the spinal cord and fine tuned from higher brain centers.[1] In patients who have developed dysfunctional gait patterns, physical therapy can help to restore this exquisite evolutionary gift.[6] Pain, weakness, and disease can all cause a disturbance in the normal rhythm of gait. However, except in obvious cases, abnormal gait does not always equate with impairment.

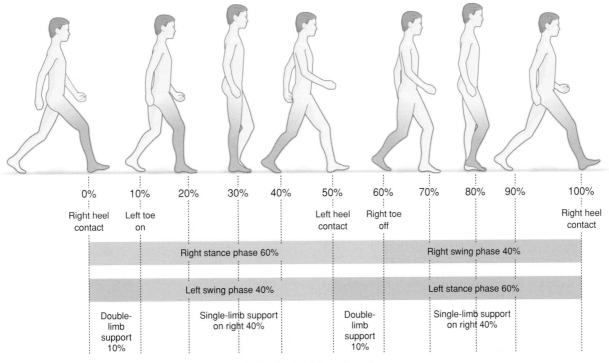

| 0% | 10% | 20% | 30% | 40% | 50% | 60% | 70% | 80% | 90% | 100% |

Right heel contact | Left toe on | | | | Left heel contact | Right toe off | | | | Right heel contact

FIGURE 14-1 The gait cycle

Normal human gait involves a complex synchronization of the cardiopulmonary and neuromuscular systems. The energy required for gait is largely a factor of the health of the cardiopulmonary systems.

Walking involves the alternating action of the two lower extremities. The walking pattern is studied as a gait cycle. The *gait cycle* is defined as the interval of time between any of the repetitive events of walking, such as from the point when the foot first contacts the ground, to the point when the same foot contacts the ground again.[7] The gait cycle consists of two phases (Figure 14-1):

1. *Stance.* This phase constitutes approximately 60% to 65% of the gait cycle[8,9] and describes the entire time the foot is in contact with the ground and the limb is bearing weight. The stance phase begins when the foot makes contact on the ground and concludes when the ipsilateral foot leaves the ground. The stance phase takes about 0.6 seconds at an average walking speed.

2. *Swing.* The swing phase constitutes approximately 35% to 40% of the gait cycle[8,9] and describes the phase when the foot is not in contact with the ground. The swing phase begins as the foot is lifted from the ground and ends when the ipsilateral foot makes contact with the ground again.[7]

CLINICAL PEARL

In terms of energy expenditure, the swing phase requires relatively little, relying heavily on passive soft tissue tension, gravity, and momentum to accelerate and decelerate individual segments.[1] In contrast, stance requires more dynamic activity, with muscles in the stance limb supporting the body and propelling it forward.

GAIT PARAMETERS

A normal gait pattern is a factor of a number of parameters.

Base (Step) Width. The base width is the lateral distance between both feet. The normal BOS is considered to be between 5 and 10 cm (2 to 4 inches). The size of the BOS and its relation to the center of gravity (COG*) are important factors in the maintenance of balance and, thus, the stability of an object. The COG must be maintained over the BOS, if equilibrium is to be maintained. The BOS includes the part of the body in contact with the supporting surface and the intervening area.[10] As the COG moves forward with each step, it briefly passes beyond the anterior margin of the BOS, resulting in a temporary loss of balance.[10] This temporary loss of equilibrium is counteracted by the advancing foot at initial contact, which establishes a new BOS. Larger than normal bases of support are observed in individuals who have muscle imbalances of the lower limbs and trunk, as well as those who have problems with overall static dynamic balance.[11] The base width should decrease to around zero with increased speed. If the base width decreases to a point below zero, crossover occurs, whereby one foot lands where the other should, and vice versa.[12] Assistive devices, such as crutches or walkers, can be prescribed to increase the BOS and, therefore, enhance stability.

Step Length. Step length is measured as the distance between the same part of one foot on successive footprints (ipsilateral to the contralateral foot fall). The average step length is about 72 cm (28 inches). The measurement should be equal for both legs.

Stride Length. Stride length is the distance between successive points of foot-to-floor contact of the same foot. A stride

---
*The COG of the body is located approximately at midline in the frontal plane and slightly anterior (5 cm or 2 inches) to the second sacral vertebra in the sagittal plane.

is one full lower extremity cycle. Two step lengths added together make the stride length. The average stride length for normal individuals is 144 cm (56 inches).[13]

Typically, the step and stride lengths do not vary more than a few centimeters between tall and short individuals. Men typically have longer step and stride lengths than women. Step and stride lengths decrease with age, pain, disease, and fatigue.[14] They also decrease as the speed of gait increases.[15] A decrease in step or stride length may also result from a forward head posture, a stiff hip, or a decrease in the availability of motion at the lumbar spine. The decrease in step and stride length that occurs with aging is thought to be the result of the increased likelihood of falling during the swing phase of ambulation, caused by diminished control of the hip musculature.[16] This lack of control prevents the aged person from being able to intermittently lose and recover the same amount of balance that the younger adult can lose and recover.[16]

Cadence. Cadence is defined as the number of separate steps taken in a certain time. Normal cadence is between 90 and 120 steps per minute.[17,18] The cadence of women is usually 6 to 9 steps per minute slower than that of men.[14] Cadence is also affected by age, decreasing from the age of 4 to the age of 7 years, and then again in advancing years.[19]

CLINICAL PEARL

Compared with men, women generally have narrower shoulders, greater valgus at the elbow, greater varus at the hip, and greater valgus at the knee.[20] Women also have a smaller Achilles tendon, a narrower heel in relationship to the forefoot, and a foot that is narrower than a man's. On average, women walk at a higher cadence than men (6 to 9 steps higher), but at lower speeds.[21–25] Women also have slightly shorter stride lengths,[21,22,24–28] although when normalized for height, women tend to have the same or slightly greater stride lengths.[25–27]

Velocity. The primary determinants of gait velocity are the repetition rate (cadence), physical conditioning, and the length of the person's stride.[13]

CLINICAL PEARL

A mathematical relationship exists between cadence, stride length, and velocity, such that if two of them are directly measured, the third may be derived by calculation[7].

Cadence (steps/min) = velocity (m/s) × 120/stride length (m)

Stride length (m) = velocity (m/s) × 120/cadence (steps/min)

Velocity (m/s) = cadence (steps/min) × stride length (m)/120

Vertical Ground Reaction Forces. Newton's third law states that for every action there is an equal and opposite reaction. During gait, vertical ground reaction forces are created by a combination of gravity, body weight, and the firmness of the ground. Under normal conditions, we are mostly unaware of these forces. However, in the presence of joint inflammation or tissue injury, the significance of these forces becomes apparent. Vertical ground reaction force begins with an impact peak of less than body weight and then exceeds body weight

at the end of the initial contact interval, dropping during midstance, and rising again to exceed body weight, reaching its highest peak during the terminal stance interval. Thus, there are two peaks of ground reaction force during the gait cycle: the first at maximum limb loading during the loading response, and the second during terminal stance.

The ground reaction force vector is anterior to the hip joint at initial contact, then migrates progressively posteriorly until late stance, when the ground reaction force is posterior to the hip.[29,30] Peak flexion torque occurs at initial contact but gradually declines, changing to an extension torque in midstance. The extension torque remains until terminal stance.[29,30]

During the gait cycle, the tibiofemoral joint reaction force has two peaks, the first immediately following initial contact (two to three times body weight) and the second during preswing (three to four times body weight).[31] Tibiofemoral joint reaction forces increase to five to six times body weight during running and stair climbing, and eight times body weight with downhill walking.[31–33]

It is well established that joint angles and ground reaction force components increase with walking speed.[34] This is not surprising, because the dynamic force components must increase as the body is subject to increasing deceleration and acceleration forces when walking speed increases.

CLINICAL PEARL

Because leg length in women is 51.2% of total body height compared with 56% in men, women must strike the ground more often to cover the same distance.[35] Furthermore, because their feet are shorter, women complete the heel-to-toe gait in a shorter time than men do. Therefore, the cumulative ground reaction forces may be greater in women.[20]

Mediolateral Shear Forces. Mediolateral shear in walking gait begins with an initial medial shear (occasionally lateral) after initial contact, followed by lateral shear for the remainder of the stance phase.[29,30] At the end of the stance phase, the shear shifts to a medial direction because of propulsion forces.

Anteroposterior Shear Forces. Anteroposterior shear forces in gait begin with an anterior shear force at initial contact and the loading response intervals, and a posterior shear at the end of the terminal stance interval.

CHARACTERISTICS OF NORMAL GAIT

Much has been written about the criteria for normal and abnormal gait.[7,9,21,29,36–41] Although the presence of symmetry in gait appears to be important, asymmetry in itself does not guarantee impairment. It must be remembered that the definition of what constitutes the so-called normal gait is elusive. Unlike posture, which is a static event, gait is dynamic and as such is protean.

CLINICAL PEARL

Good alignment of the weight-bearing segments of the body:

▶ Reduces the likelihood of strain and injury by reducing joint friction and tension in the soft tissues.

> ▸ Improves the stability of the weight-bearing limb and the balance of the trunk. The stability of the body is directly related to the size of the BOS. In order to be stable, the intersection of the line of gravity with the BOS should be close to the geometric center of the base.[42]
>
> ▸ Reduces excess energy expenditure.

Gait involves the displacement of body weight in a desired direction, using a coordinated effort between the joints of the trunk and extremities and the muscles that control or produce these motions. Any interference that alters this relationship may result in a deviation or disturbance of the normal gait pattern. This, in turn, may result in increased energy expenditure or functional impairment.

Perry[17] lists four *priorities* of normal gait:

1. Stability of the weight-bearing foot throughout the stance phase
2. Clearance of the non–weight-bearing foot during the swing phase
3. Appropriate prepositioning (during terminal swing) of the foot for the next gait cycle
4. Adequate step length

Gage[19] added a fifth priority, energy conservation. The typical energy expended in normal gait (2.5 kcal/min) is less than twice that spent while sitting or standing (1.5 kcal/min).[19] Two-dimensional kinetic data have revealed that approximately 85% of the energy for normal walking comes from the plantarflexors of the ankle, and 15% from the flexors of the hip.[43] It has been proposed that the type of gait selected is based on metabolic energy considerations.[44] Current commonly used parameters used to measure walking efficiency include oxygen consumption, heart rate, and comfortable speed of walking.[45–47] Economy of mobility is a measurement of submaximal oxygen uptake (submax VO_2) for a given speed.[48,49] A decline in functional performance may be evidenced by an increase in submax VO_2 for walking.[50] This change in economy of mobility may be indicative of an abnormal gait pattern.[50] Some researchers have reported no gender differences for economy of mobility,[51–53] whereas others suggest that men are more economical or have lower energy costs than women at the same absolute work.[54–56] Age-related declines in economy of mobility also have been reported in the literature, with differing results. Some researchers reported that older adults were less economical than younger adults while walking at various speeds.[48,57,58] Conversely, economy of mobility appears to be unaffected by aging for individuals who maintain higher levels of physical activity.[59–61]

Some authors have claimed that a limb-length discrepancy leads to mechanical and functional changes in gait[62] and increased energy expenditure.[63] Intervention has been advocated for discrepancies of less than 1 cm to discrepancies greater than 5 cm,[62–64] but the rationale for these recommendations has not been well defined, and the literature contains little substantive information regarding the functional significance of these discrepancies.[65] For example, Gross found no noticeable functional or cosmetic problems in a study of 74 adults who had less than 2 cm of discrepancy and 35 marathon runners who had as much as 2.5 cm of discrepancy.[64]

For gait to be efficient and to conserve energy, the COG must undergo minimal displacement:

▸ Any displacement that elevates, depresses, or moves the COG beyond normal maximum excursion limits wastes energy.

▸ Any abrupt or irregular movement will waste energy even when that movement does not exceed the normal maximum displacement limits of the COG.

To minimize the energy costs of walking, the body uses a number of biomechanical mechanisms. In 1953, Saunders, Inman, and Eberhart[68] proposed that six kinematic features—the Six Determinants—have the potential to reduce the energetic cost of human walking. The six determinants are[68]:

▸ *Lateral displacement of the pelvis:* To avoid significant muscular and balancing demands, the pelvis shifts side to side (approximately 2.5 to 5 cm or 1 to 2 inches) during walking in order to center the weight of the body over the stance leg.[69] If the lower extremities dropped directly vertical from the hip joint, the center of mass would be required to shift 3 to 4 inches to each side to be positioned effectively over the supporting foot. The combination of femoral varus and anatomical valgum at the knee permits a vertical tibial posture with both tibias in close proximity to each other. This narrows the walking base to 5 to 10 cm (2 to 4 inches) from heel center to heel center, thereby reducing the lateral shift required of the COG toward either side.

▸ *Pelvic rotation:* The rotation of the pelvis normally occurs about a vertical axis in the transverse plane toward the weight-bearing limb. The total pelvic rotation is approximately 4° to each side.[19] Forward rotation of the pelvis on the swing side prevents an excessive drop in the body's COG. The pelvic rotation also results in a relative lengthening of the femur by lessening the angle of the femur with the floor, and thus step length, during the termination of the swing period.[70]

▸ Vertical displacement of the pelvis: vertical pelvic shifting keeps the COG from moving superiorly and inferiorly more than 5 cm (2 inches) during normal

gait. Because of the shift, the high point occurs during midstance, and the low point occurs during initial contact. The amount of vertical displacement of the pelvis may be accentuated in the presence of a leg-length discrepancy, fusion of the knee, or hip abductor weakness, the last of which results in a Trendelenburg sign. The Trendelenburg sign is said to be positive if, when standing on one leg, the pelvis drops on the side opposite to the stance leg. The weakness is present on the side of the stance leg—the gluteus medius is not able to maintain the COG on
the side of the stance leg.

▶ *Knee flexion in stance:* Knee motion is intrinsically associated with foot and ankle motion. At initial contact, before the ankle moves into a plantarflexed position and thus is relatively more elevated, the knee is in relative extension. Responding to a plantarflexed posture at loading response, the knee flexes. Midstance knee flexion prevents an excessive rise in the body's COG during that period of the gait cycle. If not for the midstance knee flexion, the COG's rise during midstance would be larger, as would its total vertical displacement. Passing through midstance as the ankle remains stationary with the foot flat on the floor, the knee again reverses its direction to one of extension. As the heel comes off the floor in terminal stance, the heel begins to rise as the ankle plantarflexes, and the knee flexes. In preswing, as the forefoot rolls over the metatarsal heads, the heel elevates even more as further plantarflexion occurs and flexion of the knee increases.

▶ *Ankle mechanism:* For normal foot function and human ambulation the amount of ankle joint motion required is approximately 10° of dorsiflexion (to complete midstance and begin terminal stance) and 20° of plantarflexion (for full push-off in preswing). At initial contact, the foot is in relative dorsiflexion due to the muscle action of the pretibial muscles and the triceps surae. This muscle action produces a relative lengthening of the leg, resulting in a smoothing of the pathway of the COG during stance phase.

▶ *Foot mechanism:* The controlled lever arm of the forefoot at preswing is particularly helpful as it rounds out the sharp downward reversal of the COG. Thus it does not reduce a peak displacement period of the COG as the earlier determinants did, but rather smooths the pathway. An adaptively shortened gastrocnemius muscle may produce movement impairment by restricting normal dorsiflexion of the ankle from occurring during the midstance-to-heel-raise portion of the gait cycle. This motion is compensated for by increased pronation of the subtalar joint, increased internal rotation of the tibia, and resultant stresses to the knee joint complex.

CLINICAL PEARL

A decrease in flexibility or joint motion, or both, may result in an increase in both "internal resistance" and the energy expenditure required.

PRE-AMBULATION EQUIPMENT

Tilt Table

A tilt table, which consists of a padded table with a footplate and restraint straps, can be considered a form of positioning. The tilt table is used to evaluate how a patient regulates his or her vital signs in response to simple stresses, including gravity, while being slowly tilted toward a vertical position (approximately 80–90°) or down toward a horizontal position (0°). The tilt table was originally designed to evaluate patients with fainting spells (syncope), but is now used for a wide variety of patient diagnoses including orthostatic hypotension, pulmonary ventilation dysfunction, dizziness, as well as for patients with weight-bearing restrictions. The tilt table is contraindicated for use with patients who have unstable spinal cord injuries, unstable or erratic blood pressure, or poor cardiac responses to cardiovascular challenges. The speed with which the table is elevated is based on patient response, but it is usually elevated in increments of about 15° about every 15 to 20 minutes. Adverse reactions include excessive changes in blood pressure, heart rate, or oxygen saturation, or patient complaints of dizziness, nausea, and changes in the level of consciousness. A typical tilt table procedure follows.

▶ The patient is transferred or asked to lie supine on the tilt table with his or her feet flat on the footplate, and is then secured by a series of straps or belts around the hips, knees, and trunk (Figure 14-2) based on the level of control that the patient has over the trunk and lower extremities.

▶ Baseline data are recorded, including resting pulse rate, blood pressure, oxygen saturation, and subjective reports.

▶ The table is raised up to a 15° to 30° angle, or in accordance with the physician's orders (Figure 14-3). The patient is maintained in this position for about 15 to 20 minutes while the baseline data are recorded. The table is lowered as indicated if there are negative changes in the patient's condition.

▶ If the patient experienced no adverse effects at 15° to 30°, the tilt table is raised a further 15° to 30° (Figure 14-4). The amount of elevation and the time spent at each

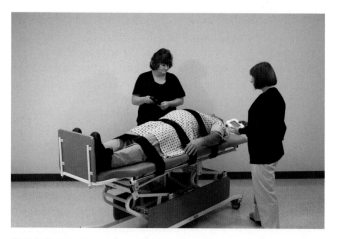

FIGURE 14-2 Tilt table—patient setup

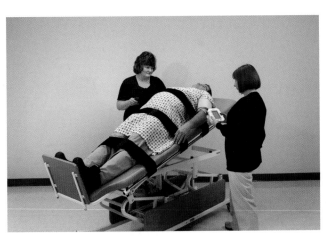

FIGURE 14-3 Tilt table at approximately 30°

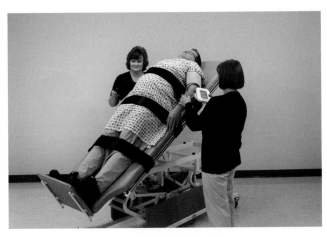

FIGURE 14-4 Tilt table at approximately 60°

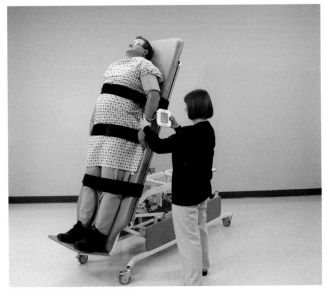

FIGURE 14-5 Tilt table at approximately 80°

elevation depends on the patient's response and the plan of care. The amount of tilt used is based on the goal of the treatment. If the goal is for the patient to ambulate, the table is raised up to near vertical (Figure 14-5), and then to vertical.

At the end of the session, the tilt table is lowered to the horizontal position, the straps are removed, and the patient is transferred from the tilt table. Over a period of time, or series of sessions, the tilt table is raised farther while monitoring both vital signs and subjective reports.

Parallel Bars

Parallel bars can be used to provide maximum stability and security for patients during the beginning stages of ambulation or standing. The correct height of the bar should allow for 20° to 30° of elbow flexion while grasping on the bars approximately 4 to 6 inches in front of the body.

CLINICAL PEARL

Parallel bars should be set at approximate the level of the greater trochanter, wrist crease, or ulnar styloid process of the standing patient, so that when the patient's hands are placed on the bars about 4 to 6 inches anterior to the hips, the elbows should be flexed to approximately 20° to 30°.

The goal is to progress the patient out of the bars as quickly as possible to increase overall mobility and decrease dependence on the parallel bars.

CLINICAL PEARL

Pre-ambulatory training within the parallel bars can include:

▶ Development of standing balance and tolerance
▶ Weight shifting
▶ Proper stance and foot placement
▶ Proper gait pattern training

A typical sequence of gait training using the parallel bars follows.

1. The patient is transported in a wheelchair to the end of the parallel bars, and the clinician makes sure that the patient is wearing a gait belt (Figure 14-6).
2. The wheels of the wheelchair are locked (Figure 14-7).
3. The leg rests of the wheelchair are removed (Figure 14-8).

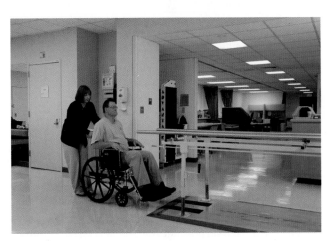

FIGURE 14-6 Wheelchair transport to parallel bars

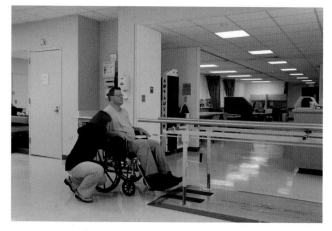

FIGURE 14-7 The wheelchair is locked

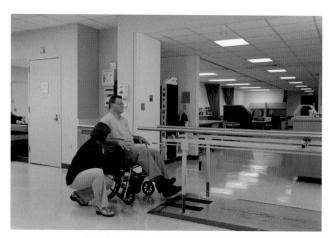

FIGURE 14-8 The leg rests are removed

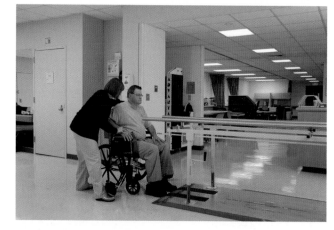

FIGURE 14-9 The patient is asked to place the hands on the armrests and to slide forward in the wheelchair

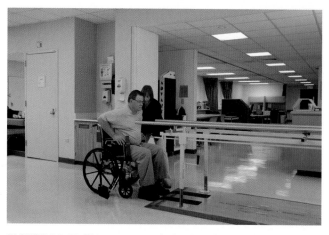

FIGURE 14-10 The patient is asked to lean forward in the chair

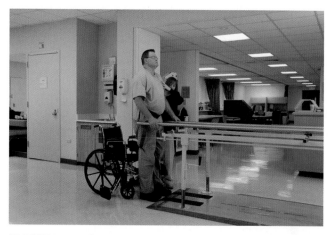

FIGURE 14-11 Once in a standing position, the patient is asked to grasp the parallel bars

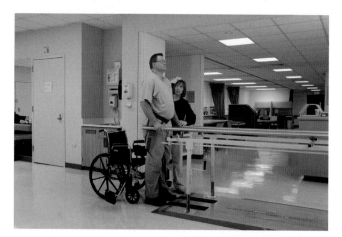

FIGURE 14-12 The clinician asks the patient how he feels

4. The patient is asked to place the hands on the armrests and to slide forward in the wheelchair (Figure 14-9).

5. The patient is asked to lean forward in the chair and, when ready to stand, to push up from the arm rests (Figure 14-10). The patient should be instructed not to pull himself or herself up using the parallel bars.

6. Once in a standing position, the patient is asked to grasp the parallel bars (Figure 14-11), and the clinician asks

the patient how he or she feels (weak, dizzy, nauseated, etc.) (Figure 14-12) before proceeding. At this point, depending on the patient's status and ability, the clinician may choose to ask the patient to shift his or her body from side to side and forward and backward while maintaining the correct weight-bearing status. In addition, the clinician may ask the patient to lift the hands from the bars to challenge the balance, or to step in place depending on

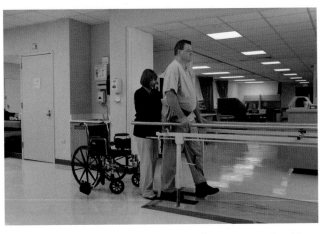

FIGURE 14-13 The clinician adjusts his or her position to be able to grasp the gait belt and to provide manual cues for the patient

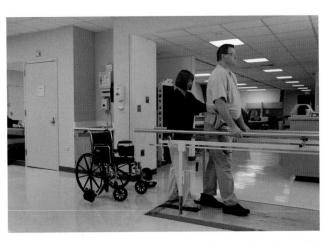

FIGURE 14-15 The patient takes a series of steps within the parallel bars

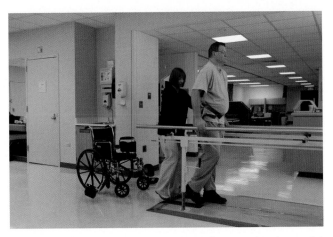

FIGURE 14-14 The patient takes a series of steps within the parallel bars

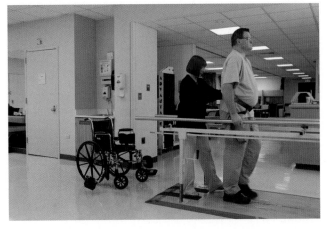

FIGURE 14-16 The patient takes a series of steps within the parallel bars

the weight-bearing status. Parallel bars enable a patient to practice a particular gait pattern in a safe environment. If necessary, an appropriate assistive device can also be used by the patient within the parallel bars.

7. The clinician adjusts his or her position to be able to grasp the gait belt and to provide manual cues for the patient (Figure 14-13). Whenever possible, the clinician should remain inside the bars with the patient to enhance control and safety. When the clinician and patient are both ready, the patient is asked to take a step (see Figure 14-13). The choice to stand in front of or behind the patient is based on whether the clinician wants to watch the patient's face and eyes for signs of distress or possible fainting, and whether the plan is for the patient to turn within the parallel bars.

8. As the patient continues to take steps within the parallel bars, the clinician follows closely, asking questions about the patient's status (Figures 14-14 through 14-17).

9. If the clinician decides that the patient is to turn within the parallel bars, the patient is asked to stand still, and then to turn in the chosen direction (Figures 14-18 through 14-20) until he or she is facing the clinician. Turning within the bars involves asking the patient to turn toward the stronger side.

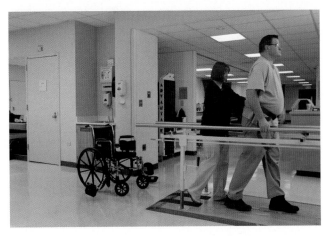

FIGURE 14-17 The patient takes a series of steps within the parallel bars

10. Once the turn is completed, the clinician asks the patient how he or she is feeling (Figure 14-21). This is important after any turning activities as these can provoke dizziness.

11. Once the patient reports having no problems, he or she is asked to begin walking toward the clinician (Figures 14-22 through 14-25).

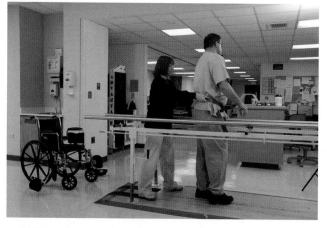

FIGURE 14-18 The patient begins to turn to the left

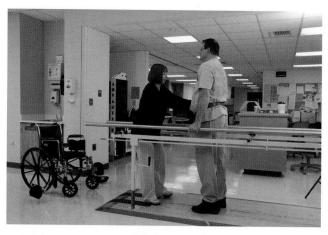

FIGURE 14-21 The clinician asks the patient how he feels

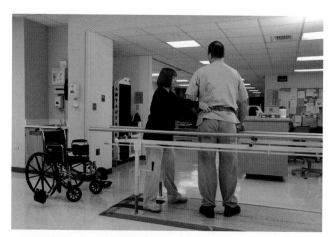

FIGURE 14-19 The patient continues turn to the left

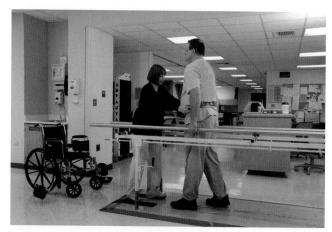

FIGURE 14-22 The patient begins walking toward the clinician

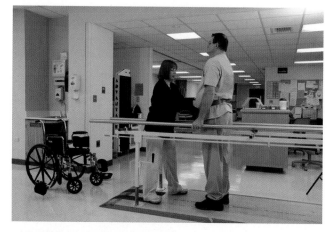

FIGURE 14-20 The patient completes the turn

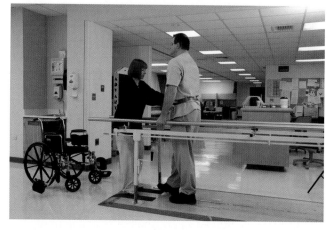

FIGURE 14-23 The patient begins walking toward the clinician

12. At the end of the parallel bars (Figure 14-26), the patient is again asked to turn (Figures 14-27 and 14-28), and a wheelchair is positioned appropriately.

13. The patient is asked to shuffle backward until he or she can feel the seat of the wheelchair against the back of the legs (Figure 14-29). At this point, the patient is asked to reach back for the chair using the hands (Figure 14-30), and then to slowly lower himself or herself into the chair in a controlled manner (Figures 14-31 and 14-32).

Video Description

Video 14-1

There are a number of points to note in the video demonstrating gait within the parallel bars:

► The clinician is constantly aware of patient safety. For example, when the wheelchair is brought to the parallel bars, the clinician makes sure that the wheels are locked and that any obstructions, such as the leg rests, are

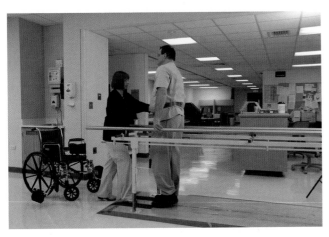

FIGURE 14-24 The patient begins walking toward the clinician

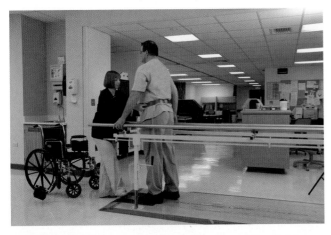

FIGURE 14-25 The patient begins walking toward the clinician

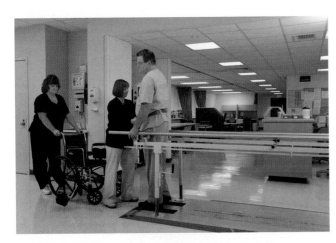

FIGURE 14-26 Patient reaches the end of the parallel bars

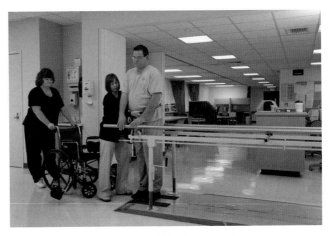

FIGURE 14-27 Patient turns within the parallel bars

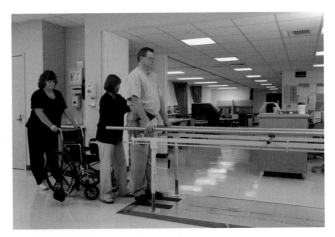

FIGURE 14-28 Patient completes turn within the parallel bars

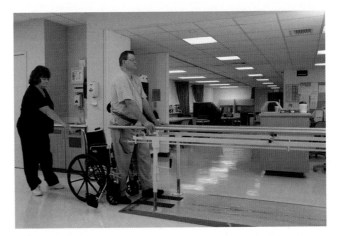

FIGURE 14-29 Patient backs up until he can feel the seat of the wheelchair against the back of his legs

removed. In addition, the patient is wearing a gait belt and the clinician repetitively asks how the patient is feeling, especially at times when the patient has changed position or has turned.

► The clinician prepares the patient to stand up in the wheelchair by emphasizing the importance of moving forward in the chair, leaning forward, and pushing up with the arms.

► When the patient is turning, he always has at least one hand in contact with a bar (Figure 14-33 through 14-36).

► The clinician asks for assistance for positioning of the wheelchair, thus avoiding having to leave the patient unattended.

► The patient is instructed to lower himself slowly into the chair. This reduces the chance of the chair sliding away or the patient injuring himself.

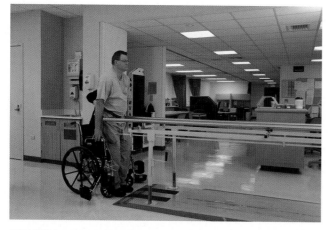

FIGURE 14-30 Patient reaches back with hands

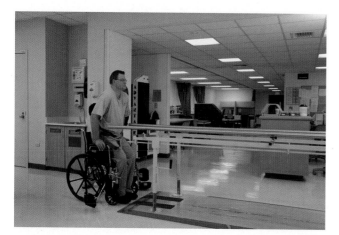

FIGURE 14-31 Patient slowly lowers himself into the chair

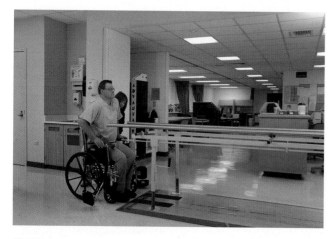

FIGURE 14-32 Patient slowly lowers himself into the chair

Although parallel bars are frequently used for weight-shifting exercises and for gait training, they can also be used to perform exercises. These can be strengthening exercises, such as performing a push-up using the bars, or balance and coordination exercises that reduce the patient's BOS.

WEIGHT-BEARING STATUS

The selection of the proper gait pattern to instruct the patient is dependent on the patient's balance, strength,

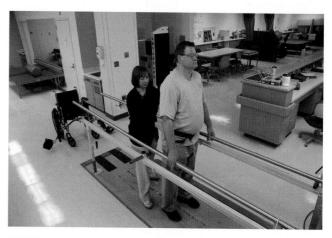

FIGURE 14-33 Detailed view of patient turning to show hand positions

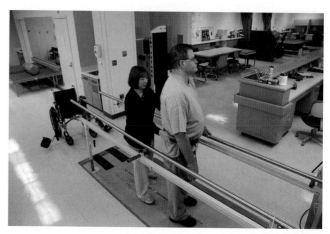

FIGURE 14-34 Detailed view of patient turning to show hand positions

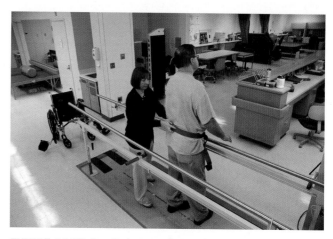

FIGURE 14-35 Detailed view of patient turning to show hand positions

cardiovascular status, coordination, functional needs, and weight-bearing (WB) status. One of the major reasons for using an assistive device is because a physician/surgeon has imposed some form of WB restriction. This restriction is listed in the patient's medical record or, in the case of a patient visiting an outpatient facility, a prescription.

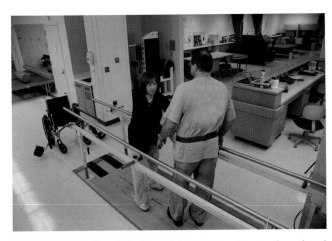

FIGURE 14-36 Detailed view of patient turning to show hand positions

Four terms are commonly used to describe the various types of WB restrictions:

▶ *Non–weight bearing (NWB):* The patient is not permitted to bear any weight through the involved limb (**VIDEO 14-2**). Even though the patient is not bearing weight through the limb, there are number of internal forces at work. These include stretching of the soft tissues around the joint and joint compression forces. Ironically, it has been reported that forces acting on the hip may be greater during NWB gait than they are during ambulation with touchdown weight bearing (see later).[71]

▶ *Touch-down weight bearing (TDWB)/toe-touch weight bearing (TTWB):* The patient is permitted minimal contact of the injured limb with the ground for balance. Of the four terms, this one causes the most confusion because of the various definitions attributed to it. For example, the APTA defines it as contact for balance purposes only, but it is also defined as 10 to 15 kg of weight, and up to 20% of body weight. The expression most commonly used to help the patient understand is "imagine as though you are walking on eggshells."

▶ *Partial weight-bearing (PWB):* The patient is permitted to bear a portion of his or her weight through the injured limb. This portion is typically described as a percentage (25%, 50%, etc.). However, it is important remember that 25% of body weight for a person weighing 150 pounds and 25% of body weight for a person who weighs 350 pounds is significantly different.

▶ *Weight bearing as tolerated (WBAT):* The patient is permitted to bear as much weight through the involved limb as can be moderately tolerated.

Despite the preceding definitions, there are a number of variables that the clinician must consider when determining the actual amount of weight bearing that is occurring. For example, the amount of force exerted on the joint varies depending on the point in the gait cycle as each joint in the lower extremity undergoes different forces throughout the cycle.

Monitoring Weight-Bearing Status

Although the NWB and the WBAT weight-bearing restrictions are relatively straightforward to describe to a patient, it is more difficult for the clinician to describe the PWB and the TDWB/TTWB to the patient. It is also difficult for many patients to perceive their own weight bearing during ambulation based on verbal instructions or objective measurement of their weight bearing. Indeed, one report[72] found that the relationship between the prescribed weight bearing and the actual weight bearing performed by healthy volunteers or by patients with recent lower extremity injury or surgery varied significantly. In fact, another study[73] that used physicians, nurses, physical therapist, and occupational therapist as subjects found that the subjects exceeded the PWB limit by 4 to 13 kg.

Perhaps the most commonly used clinical method to demonstrate weight bearing to a patient is to use two simple bathroom scales. The patient is asked to place each foot on two separate bathroom scales and then to shift the body weight from the involved extremity until the designated amount is reached. This exercise is repeated a number of times until the patient develops a better sense of what the restriction feels like. However, it is one thing to weight shift in a controlled and static environment; it is another to control weight bearing during the more dynamic task of ambulation.

Limb load monitors (LLMs), which are relatively inexpensive, have been used to dynamically monitor weight-bearing status during gait. The patient wears a lightweight boot over the foot of the involved extremity, which is fitted with a strain gauge built into the sole of the boot (Figure 14-37).[74-76] During ambulation, the patient is provided with an auditory feedback signal when the weight-bearing limits are reached or exceeded.

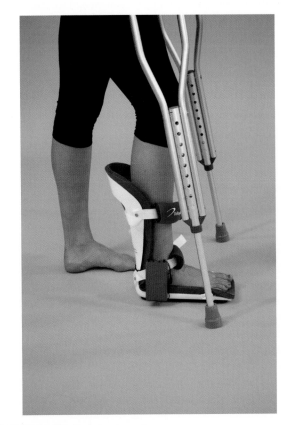

FIGURE 14-37 Limb-load monitor

More recently, computer technology has been used to monitor weight bearing during gait. The computerized air-insole auditory biofeedback system (CAIBS) is a portable system that senses the amount of load and provides auditory feedback in addition to using a wireless receiver connected to a computer. The CAIBS has been found to be a valid and reliable system[77] and has also been shown to increase compliance in subjects with weight-bearing restrictions during gait compared to those provided only with verbal instructions.[78]

ASSISTIVE DEVICES

The most common cause for the breakdown of the normal gait cycle is an injury to one or both of the lower extremities. Such an injury usually results in an antalgic gait. If the injury is severe enough, or if a particular body part requires protection, an assistive device is prescribed. Assistive devices are designed to make ambulation as safe and as painless as possible. In essence, an assistive device is an extension of the upper extremity, used to provide support, balance, and weight bearing normally provided by an intact functioning lower extremity.[79] Assistive devices function to reduce ground reaction forces, with the size of the BOS that they provide being proportional to the amount of reduction in these forces. The indications for using an assistive device include[80]:

▶ Decreased ability to bear weight through the lower extremities

▶ Muscle weakness or paralysis of the trunk or lower extremities

▶ Structural deformity, amputation, injury, or disease resulting in decreased ability to bear weight through a lower extremity

▶ Decreased balance and proprioception in the upright posture

▶ Decreased sensation

▶ Limited passive range of motion

▶ Joint instability and excessive skeletal loading

▶ Fatigue or pain

▶ Fear of falling or history of falling

Choosing a Device

In addition to the weight-bearing restriction, the clinician must consider a number of factors when determining the most suitable assistive device for a patient. These factors include:

▶ *Amount of support required.* This is a factor of the weight-bearing restriction (Table 14-1). The only assistive devices that allow a person to put their full weight through both arms simultaneously are parallel bars, walkers (standard, wheeled, or folding), and bilateral crutches (axillary, or forearm [Lofstrand]), so these devices would be appropriate for a patient with a NWB, TTWB/TDWB, PWB (depending on the percentage allowed), or WBAT (depending on the level of pain) restriction in one lower extremity. Devices such as hemi-walkers (Figure 14-38) and canes are more suitable for patients with a WBAT restriction.

TABLE 14-1	Appropriate Devices Based on Weight-Bearing Restriction
Weight-Bearing Restriction	**Appropriate Device**
Non–weight-bearing (NWB)	Parallel bars Walker Bilateral crutches
Partial weight-bearing (PWB)	Parallel bars Walker Axillary crutches (one or two) Cane (one or two) Lofstrand crutches

CLINICAL PEARL

A NWB, TTWB, and PWB restriction limits the selection of an assistive device to either a walker or bilateral crutches.

A WBAT restriction allows for any unilateral or bilateral device that provides the necessary support.

▶ *Amount of stability required.* Generally speaking, the more mobility a device provides, the less stability it provides, and vice versa. Any device that has a large BOS, such as a standard walker or a platform-style walker (Figure 14-39) with four points of contact, will provide the most stability. Assistive devices, in order of the stability they provide, include parallel bars, platform-style walker, standard walker, bilateral axillary crutches, bilateral forearm crutches, bilateral canes, hemi-walker, quad cane, straight cane, and bent cane.

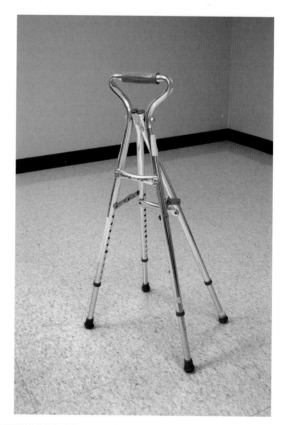

FIGURE 14-38 A hemi-walker

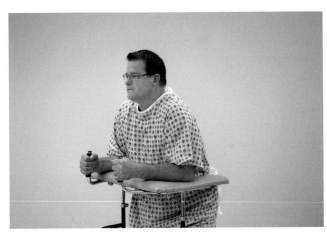

FIGURE 14-39 Modified walker with platform attachment

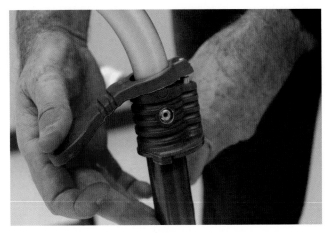

FIGURE 14-40 Folding mechanism on walker

▶ *Patient strength.* Any of the assistive devices that use a handgrip require that the patient have good strength in the wrist stabilizers, elbow extensors, and shoulder depressors.

▶ *Patient endurance.* It is worth remembering that there is an energy cost associated with using each of the various assistive devices (Table 14-2).

▶ *Patient coordination.* The list of assistive devices, ordered from those requiring the least coordination by a patient to those requiring the most, is as follows: parallel bars, platform-style walker, one cane, two canes, axillary crutches, forearm (Lofstrand) crutches.

Description of Devices

▶ *Parallel bars.* Parallel bars (see Pre-Ambulation Equipment) provide the greatest amount of stability of any assistive device, but the least amount of functional carryover.

▶ *Walkers.* Walkers can be used with all levels of weight bearing and offer a significant BOS and good anterior and lateral stability. Consequently, walkers are often used with patients who have poor balance and coordination or decreased weight bearing on one or two lower extremities, and they are also the most commonly prescribed assistive device for the elderly.

Attachments include:

▶ *Glides:* these are small, plastic attachments that replace the rubber tips on the bottom of walker legs that enable patients who are unable to lift and advance a standard walker to glide the walker on a smooth surface.

▶ *Platform (forearm) attachments:* these are used when weight bearing through the wrist or hand is contraindicated. The attachments are fitted to the side of the walker, allowing the forearm to rest in a padded trough, held in place with Velcro straps, and include handle grips with a vertical handle.

▶ *Carrying basket:* these are attached to the front of the walker to provide storage for frequently needed items.

▶ *Fold-down seats:* as the name suggests, these attachments allow a patient to sit down using the walker.

The standard walker has many variations, including:

▶ *Folding (collapsible) (Figures 14-40 and 14-41):* facilitate mobility and travel in the community as they are easier to fit in an automobile or other storage space.

▶ *Rolling (wheeled) (Figure 14-42):* available in either two wheels (one wheel on each of the front legs) or four wheels (one wheel on all four of the legs). The latter type requires a hand brake to provide added stability in stopping, which

TABLE 14-2	Energy Costs Associated with Various Assistive Devices
Assistive Device	**Energy Cost**
Crutches	Energy demand increased 13% to 80%, in part because of increased demands placed on arms and shoulder-girdle muscles
Standard walker	Oxygen consumption increased >200%
Front-wheeled walker	Lesser impact compared with standard walker
Cane	No significant energy cost

Data from Powers CM, Burnfield JM: Normal and pathologic gait, in Placzek JD, Boyce DA (eds): Orthopaedic Physical Therapy Secrets. Philadelphia, Hanley & Belfus, 2001, pp 98-103.

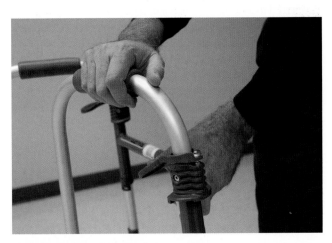

FIGURE 14-41 A folded walker

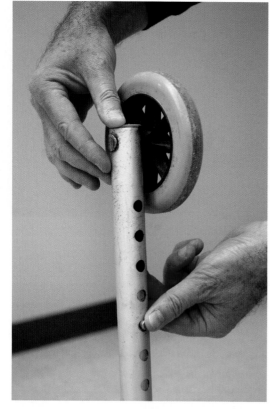

FIGURE 14-42 The wheel of a walker with adjustable height

means that the patient must have sufficient grip strength. The advantage of this type of walker is that it requires less energy to use and facilitates walking as a continuous movement sequence. The disadvantage of this type of walker is that it provides less stability.

▶ *Posterior (reverse):* these have the crossbar positioned behind the patient rather than in front of the patient. This type of walker is often used by children who have cerebral palsy to promote a more upright posture.

▶ *Stair climbing:* fitted with two posterior extensions and additional handgrips off of the rear legs for use on stairs.

▶ *Reciprocal:* fitted with hinges that allow advancement of one side of the walker at a time, thereby facilitating any reciprocal gait pattern.

▶ *Hemi:* this type of walker (see Figure 14-38), sometimes referred to as a walk-cane, is a unilateral assistive device with four legs modified for use with one hand only. It is used in cases when more stability is needed that a single-point or quad cane, but when only one upper extremity can be used.

CLINICAL PEARL

Common problems to look out for during gait training with a walker include:

▶ Patient ambulates with excessively flexed posture. This could indicate that either the assistive device is too short or the patient is subconsciously lowering the COG to improve balance.

▶ The patient looks down instead of ahead. This could indicate that the assistive device is too short or the patient

is relying too heavily on visual input rather than proprioceptive input.

▶ Subjective complaints of pain and numbness of the hand. This could indicate that the patient is leaning too heavily on the walker.

▶ Excessive gripping. The most common cause for this is fear of falling.

▶ The patient rocks the walker. This occurs when the patient makes initial contact with only the rear two legs of the walker instead of placing all four legs down on the floor at the same time.

▶ *Axillary crutches.* Axillary crutches (regular or standard), typically used bilaterally, are made from wood or aluminum and are prescribed for patients who need to partially or fully decrease weight bearing on one of the lower extremities. Axillary crutches provide an increased BOS and a moderate degree of lateral stability, and they can be used with all levels of weight bearing. They can also be used for stair climbing. However, crutches are less stable and require more upper extremity strength, some trunk support, and a higher level of coordination than walkers; are awkward in small areas; and can cause pressure at the radial groove (spiral groove) of the humerus, creating a situation of potential damage to the radial nerve as well as to adjacent vascular structures in the axilla.[81]

CLINICAL PEARL

Crutch palsy, a radial nerve neuropathy, can result from poorly fitted axillary crutches, or if the patient rests on the axillary bars of the crutch.

▶ *Lofstrand (forearm or Canadian) crutches.* This type of crutch, which is generally constructed of aluminum, can be used at all levels of weight bearing, provide increased ease of movement, and, because of the presence of a forearm cuff, allow the wearer to use the hands without dropping the crutches. In addition, the absence of an axillary portion of the crutch allows for more stair-climbing options. However, this type of crutch is slightly more difficult to use than standard crutches, requires good trunk strength, and requires the highest level of coordination for proper use.

▶ *Straight canes.* Using a straight cane to aid walking is perhaps as old as the history of humankind. In ancient times, straight canes were used for support, defense, and the procurement of food.[82] Later, canes became a symbol of power and aristocracy.[83] Currently, straight canes are prescribed for patients with slight weakness of the lower extremity/extremities, to provide support and protection, to reduce pain in the lower extremities, and to improve balance during ambulation.[84]

Canes are usually made out of wood, plastic, or aluminum (adjustable with a pushpin lock—Figure 14-43). The function of a straight cane is to widen the BOS and improve balance. However, because straight canes provide minimal stability and support for patients during ambulation activities, they are not intended for use with restricted weight-bearing gaits.

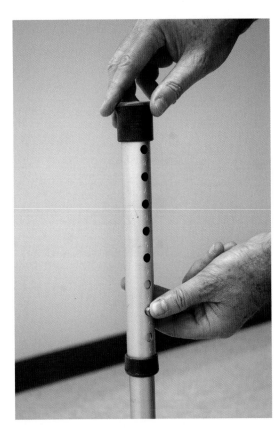

FIGURE 14-43 Adjustable cane

CLINICAL PEARL

Weight limits on standard walkers, canes, and crutches are approximately 300 pounds. Special bariatric gait devices can support 500 pounds or more.

Fitting the Device

Correct fitting of an assistive device is important to ensure for the safety of the patient, to maintain good posture, and to allow for minimal energy expenditure. For correct fitting, the patient is positioned in bilateral support stance, wearing the footwear that he or she will typically wear for ambulation, with the toes slightly out, the ankle in neutral, the knee in neutral extension, and the hip in neutral extension. The upper extremity should be positioned so that the elbows and the shoulders are relaxed and level.

CLINICAL PEARL

The bony landmark in the lower extremities used for the correct fitting of an assistive device is the greater trochanter.

The bony landmarks in the upper extremities used for the correct fitting of an assistive device is the ulnar styloid.

Once fitted, the patient should be taught the correct walking technique with the device. The fitting depends on the device chosen:

▶ *Walkers, hemi-walkers, quad canes, and standard canes.* The height of the device handle should be adjusted to the level of the greater trochanter of the patient's hip, or at the ulnar styloid of the upper extremity (Figures 14-44 and 14-45).

CLINICAL PEARL

Patients are typically instructed to hold a straight cane in the hand opposite the involved extremity. The cane and involved extremity are advanced together, followed by the uninvolved extremity. The use of a cane in the contralateral hand helps preserve reciprocal motion and a more normal pathway for the COG.[85] Use of a cane in this fashion also helps in reducing forces created by the abductor muscles acting at the hip, as estimated by external kinematics and kinetics.[86–89] Use of a cane can transmit 20% to 25% of body weight away from the lower extremities.[90,91] Holding the cane in the hand opposite the involved extremity also widens the BOS with less lateral shifting of the COG.

In addition to the straight cane, canes come in a variety of designs:

▶ *Quad cane:* this type of cane provides a very broad base with four points of floor contact. The legs farther from the patient's body are angled to maintain floor contact and to improve stability. Walk canes fold flat and are adjustable in height. However, this type of cane cannot be used on most stairs and require use of a slow forward progression.

▶ *Rolling cane:* provide a wide wheeled base allowing uninterrupted forward progression. A pressure-sensitive break is built into the handle and can be engaged using pressure from the base of the hand. This type of cane allows weight to be continuously applied because the need to lift and place the cane forward is eliminated, allowing for a faster forward progression.

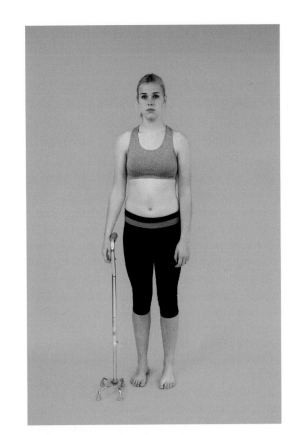

FIGURE 14-44 Measurement for a quad cane

449

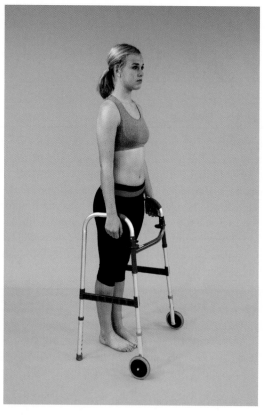

FIGURE 14-45 Measurement for a walker

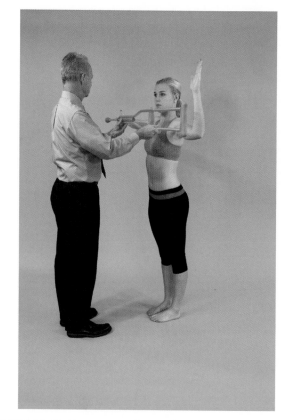

FIGURE 14-46 Measurement for crutches

If measuring for a standard cane, the cane tip should be approximately 3 to 4 inches anterior to the foot at a 45° angle.

► *Standard crutches.* A number of methods can be used for determining the correct crutch length for axillary crutches:

- Ask for a patient's height and then adjust according to the height markings on the crutch.
- Calculate 77% of the patient's height.
- Subtract 16 inches from an adult patient's height.
- Take a measurement from the patient's axillary fold to a point 6 to 8 inches lateral to the bottom of the heel (including footwear).
- Have the patient stand or sit with both arms abducted to 90°. Ask the patient to flex one of the elbows to 90°. The measurement is then taken from the olecranon process of the patient's flexed elbow to the tip of the long finger of the opposite hand (Figure 14-46).
- When the crutches are fitted correctly, there is a 5- to 8-cm (2- to 3-inch) gap between the tops of the axillary pads and the patient's axilla (Figure 14-47) when the crutch tip is vertical to the ground and positioned approximately 5 cm (2 inches) lateral to and 15 cm (6 inches) at a 45° angle anterior to the patient's foot. The handgrips of the crutch are adjusted to the height of the greater trochanter of the hip of the patient, or at the ulnar styloid of the upper extremity with the elbow flexed 20° to 30°.

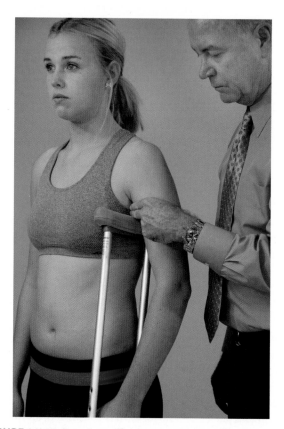

FIGURE 14-47 Ensuring sufficient space in the axilla

▶ *Forearm/Lofstrand crutches.* The crutch is adjusted so that the handgrip is level with the greater trochanter of the patient's hip and the top of the forearm cuff just distal to the elbow.

Patient Instructions

When providing gait training, it is important that the patient receive verbal and illustrated instructions. Patient instruction should initially be provided in a safe environment that is free from distraction so that the patient can concentrate. Ideally, the clinician should demonstrate how to use the assistive device before asking the patient to do so. The patient should be encouraged to look ahead rather than down to help with proprioceptive training. The training should be initiated on level surfaces and then advanced to include negotiation of curbs and stairs, ambulating in busy corridors, and sit-to-stand/stand-to-sit transfers from different surfaces. These instructions should also include any weight-bearing precautions pertinent to the patient, the appropriate gait sequence, and a contact number at which to reach the clinician if questions arise. Finally, the patient should be educated on how to create a safe home environment to prevent falls and on the care and maintenance of the device (replacing rubber tips as needed, tightening any loose fasteners, etc.). The more common methods to prevent falling are outlined in Table 14-3.

Guarding the Patient

The clinician must always provide adequate physical support and instruction while working with a patient using an assistive gait device. Guarding is the process of protecting a patient from excessive weight bearing, incorrect gait pattern, loss of balance, or falling. Proper guarding requires the use of a gait belt fitted around the patient's waist to enable the clinician to assist the patient.

When guarding a patient during gait training, the clinician should be positioned with feet in stride, at a 45° angle slightly to the side and behind the patient. The key is to minimize the distance between the patient's COG and the clinician's COG. Normally, the clinician positions himself or herself slightly posteriorly on the side where the patient will most likely have difficulty. Most frequently, this is the involved side of the patient, although in some cases, the patient may have a tendency

TABLE 14-3	Preventing Falls in the Home	
All Living Spaces	**Bathrooms**	**Outdoors**
_____ Remove throw rugs.	_____ Install grab bars in the bathtub or shower and by the toilet.	_____ Repair cracked sidewalks.
_____ Secure carpet edges.	_____ Use rubber mats in the bathtub or shower.	_____ Install handrails on stairs and steps.
_____ Remove low furniture and objects on the floor.	_____ Take up floor mats when the bathtub or shower is not in use.	_____ Trim shrubbery along the pathway to the home.
_____ Reduce clutter.	_____ Install a raised toilet seat.	_____ Install adequate lighting by doorways and along walkways leading to doors.
_____ Remove cords and wires on the floor.		
_____ Check lighting for adequate illumination at night (especially in the pathway to the bathroom). This can include changing the wattage of a bulb.		
_____ Secure carpet or treads on stairs.		
_____ Install handrail or additional handrail on staircases.		
_____ Eliminate chairs that are too low to sit in and get out of easily.		
_____ Avoid floor wax (or use nonskid wax).		
_____ Ensure that the telephone can be reached from the floor.		
_____ Have medications reviewed by appropriate healthcare professional.		
_____ Have regular vision examinations by appropriate healthcare professional.		

to fall toward the uninvolved side. If using a gait belt, the clinician should grasp it using a supinated forearm position with the palm facing the ceiling, as this provides a stronger and more reliable grip than using a pronated forearm. A common mistake for the novice clinician is to overguard the patient. This typically includes holding the patient back by pulling too hard on the gait belt or at the patient shoulder (**VIDEO 14-3**). Not only is this very frustrating for the patient, it can also introduce a number of safety concerns as it can cause the patient to lose his or her balance.

> ## CLINICAL PEARL
>
> Two types of falls are recognized:
>
> ▸ *Angular:* occurs when the COG moves too far beyond the BOS in any direction for the patient to control.
> ▸ *Collapsing:* occurs when there is a loss of support from either the patient's lower extremities or an assistive device.

Whatever side is chosen, if the patient falls forward, backward, or to either side, the aim is to return the combined COG of the patient and the clinician within the BOS of the clinician, with only a shift of the clinician's weight, and with no large foot movements by the clinician. Thus, the BOS of the clinician must be large enough to support such shifts in the COG should the patient start to fall. The closer the clinician is to the patient, the easier this is to maintain. Although falls typically occur in one direction, the clinician must remember that sometimes the patient's lower extremities can give way, resulting in a collapsing fall. In such instances, the clinician should move closer to the patient and lift on the gait belt to provide time for the patient to regain support.

> ## CLINICAL PEARL
>
> As the COG of most patients is in the lower trunk, the best way to control a patient and thereby prevent a fall is through a gait belt placed around the patient's hip girdle. Because the gait belt is typically fitted when the patient is sitting, the clinician should recheck the belt after the patient stands up to ensure that it still fits snugly.

To prevent any unencumbered weight shifting or foot movement in the event of a fall, the clinician's knee should be slightly bent and feet should not be crossed during gait training, nor should they become entangled with the patient's feet or ambulatory equipment. Hand placement is also important. The clinician should try to keep the upper extremity that is holding the gait belt such that the forearm is horizontal to the level of the patient's COG, with the other hand, if necessary, on the superior anterior aspect of the patient's shoulder.

> ## CLINICAL PEARL
>
> If a patient starts to fall, the clinician must decide whether to try to maintain the patient in an upright position, or permit a controlled descent of the patient. Either the clinician can adopt a stride stance so that the patient can temporarily rest on the clinician's thigh (**VIDEO 14-4**), or the clinician can

help guide the patient to the floor in a manner that will prevent injury to the patient and the clinician (**VIDEO 14-5**). The latter option involves keeping the patient's body close to the clinician while maintaining good body mechanics.

Falling

Although every effort is made to prevent a patient from falling while they are in the clinic, it is not uncommon for a patient to fall outside of the clinic, whether at home or in the community, even if he or she has been provided with instructions on prevention. Most falls occur when a patient is using axillary crutches. The clinician can help train the patient to fall safely with crutches by practicing on a cushioned surface placed on the floor and by slowing down the motion of the fall in the initial stages by using a gait belt. The clinician can also help train the patient to get up from the floor following a fall using the crutches.

Falling Safely

As the patient starts to fall, he or she casts the crutches to the side, far enough out of the way to prevent landing on them, but near enough to be reached to rise back into a standing position. The patient attempts to break the fall by landing on the palms of the hands with the elbows flexed while simultaneously turning the head to one side to minimize the risk of facial injury.

Getting Up from the Floor

The easiest way for a patient to get up from the floor is to crawl to a nearby chair, or other sturdy object, and use it to pull up to a sitting or standing position. If no such object is available, the patient collects both crutches and moves into a quadruped position. From there, the patient moves into a tall kneeling position and stands both crutches on the involved side, holding both handgrips with one hand. The patient then moves into a partial kneeling position with the stronger lower extremity forward and then pushes down through the handgrips and the forward leg to achieve a standing position. Once standing, the patient repositions the crutches, with one crutch under each arm.

GAIT TRAINING WITH ASSISTIVE DEVICES

It is important that a patient wears adequate footwear for gait training. At minimum, the patient should receive gait training for use of the assistive gait device on level surfaces and, as appropriate, to negotiate stairs, curbs, ramps, doors, and transfers.

> ## CLINICAL PEARL
>
> The most important difference between ambulation and gait training is that gait training requires skill on the clinician's part to improve the gait pattern.

Gait training includes:

▸ An initial assessment of any abnormality or deviation of a patient's gait
▸ A plan to address the abnormality or deviation

- Teaching the patient how to establish a normal gait pattern
- Gait training in various environments (different surfaces, different lighting, etc.)

Gait training with assistive devices usually begins in the parallel bars, as they provide maximum stability while requiring the least amount of coordination from the patient. The parallel bars can also be used to measure an assistive device while the patient stands within the bars (see Pre-Ambulation Equipment).

Sit-to-Stand Transfers

When observing a patient moving from a sitting position to a standing position, the clinician should note the biomechanics challenges behind such a move. If the patient remains seated at the back of the wheelchair, the COG remains outside of the BOS created by the feet. If the patient slides forward in the wheelchair, the COG is brought within the BOS. As the patient assumes a standing position, there are a number of forces that must be overcome:

- Gravity is attempting to force the knees into flexion.
- Gravity is attempting to force the ankles into dorsiflexion.

If the patient does not have sufficient strength, a number of incorrect compensations can occur (see Clinical Pearl). The correct technique involves asking the patient to lean the trunk over the knees, which ultimately creates an extensor moment at the knee.

Before the patient can begin gait training, he or she must first learn to safely transfer from a sitting position to a standing position. The following procedure is recommended.

- The wheels of the bed or wheelchair are locked, and the patient is reminded of any weight-bearing restrictions.
- The patient is asked to slide to the front edge of the chair or bed, and the weight-bearing foot is placed underneath the body, with the knees flexed to approximately 110° and the ankles in slight dorsiflexion, so that the COG is closer to the BOS, which will make it easier for the patient to stand. The other lower extremity is positioned appropriately (usually with the knee extended) depending on the weight-bearing status and whether it has been immobilized by a brace.
- The patient is then instructed to lean forward from the hips, which brings the patient's COG over the BOS, and to push up with the hands from the bed or armrests of the wheelchair and extend the elbows, while simultaneously extending the legs and standing erect.
- If the patient is being instructed on the use of a walker, he or she should grasp the handgrips of the walker only after becoming upright (VIDEO 14-6). The patient should not be permitted to try to pull up to a standing position using the walker (VIDEO 14-7), because this can cause the walker to tip over and increase the potential for falls (VIDEO 14-8).

- If the patient is using crutches, he or she is instructed to hold both crutches with the hand on the same side as the involved lower extremity (VIDEO 14-9). The patient then presses down on the handgrips of the crutches, the armrest, or bed and with the uninvolved lower extremity to stand. Once standing, and with adequate balance, the patient moves the crutches into position and begins to ambulate (VIDEO 14-10).
- If the patient is using one or two canes, he or she is instructed to push up with the hands from the bed or armrests (VIDEO 14-11). Once standing, the patient should grasp the handgrip(s) of the cane(s) with the appropriate hand and begin to ambulate (VIDEO 14-12).
- A hemi-walker can be used in a similar fashion to one cane (VIDEO 14-13), but it can also be used for a specific purpose (VIDEO 14-14).

Stand-to-Sit Transfer

The stand-to-sit transfer is essentially the reverse of the sit-to-stand transfer. Normally, in order to return to the chair or bed, the patient has to turn 180°. To enhance safety, the patient should be encouraged to turn using multiple small steps, as these provide increased stability because double contact time is at its highest. Before the patient sits, the clinician must ensure that the bed or wheelchair is locked. To sit down using an assistive device, the patient must first back up against the edge of the bed or chair so that the back of the patient's legs are touching it. If the patient has weight-bearing restrictions of the involved lower extremity, or is unable to flex the knee, he or she is instructed to slowly advance this lower extremity forward. Once in position:

▶ The patient using a walker reaches for the bed or armrest with both hands, flexes the trunk forward, and slowly sits down.

▶ The patient using crutches moves both crutches to the hand on the side of the involved lower extremity. With that hand holding onto both handgrips of the crutches, the patient reaches back for the bed or armrest with the other hand and flexes the trunk forward before slowly sitting down.

▶ The patient using one or two canes places the handgrip of the cane(s) against the edge of the chair or bed. Next, the patient reaches back for the bed or armrest and slowly sits down.

Turning

Making changes in direction can prove challenging for many patients. Common findings include hesitancy, decreased speed, multiple steps, and multiple stops during the turn. Generally speaking, it is easier for the patient to turn toward the stronger side than the weaker side. This is also important for patients who have undergone a posterolateral approach hip arthroplasty to minimize the risk of internal rotation of the involved hip and lower extremity.

Gait Patterns

Several gait patterns are recognized, the most common of which are described here.

Two-Point Pattern

The two-point gait pattern, which closely approximates the normal gait pattern (VIDEO 14-15), requires the use of an assistive gait device (canes or crutches) on each side of the body. This pattern requires the patient to move the assistive gait device and the contralateral lower extremity at the same time. This pattern requires coordination and balance. The uninvolved lower extremity can be advanced to a point at which it is parallel to the involved lower extremity (VIDEO 14-16), or it can be advanced ahead of the uninvolved lower extremity.

Two-Point Modified

The two-point modified pattern is the same as the two-point except that it requires only one assistive device, positioned on the opposite side of the involved lower extremity. This pattern cannot be used if there are any weight-bearing restrictions such as PWB or NWB, but it is appropriate for a patient with unilateral weakness or mild balance deficits. The patient is instructed to move the cane and the involved leg simultaneously, and then the uninvolved leg.

Three-Point Gait Pattern

This pattern is used for non–weight bearing—when the patient is permitted to bear weight through only one lower extremity. The three-point gait pattern, which demands a high degree of energy from the patient, involves the use of two crutches or a walker (VIDEO 14-17). It cannot be used with a cane or one crutch. The three-point gait pattern requires good upper body strength, good balance, and good cardiovascular endurance. The pattern is initiated with the forward movement of the assistive gait device. Next, the involved lower extremity is advanced. The patient then presses down on the assistive gait device and advances the uninvolved lower extremity. Two methods of advancing the lower extremity can be used:

▶ *Swing to:* the uninvolved lower extremity is advanced to a point at which it is parallel to the involved lower extremity (see Video 14-17).

▶ *Swing through:* the involved lower extremity is advanced ahead of the uninvolved lower extremity.

Three-Point Modified or 3 Point 1

A modification of the three-point gait pattern requires two crutches or a walker. This pattern is more stable, slower, and requires less strength and energy than the three-point gait pattern. This pattern is used when the patient can bear full weight through one lower extremity but is only allowed PWB through the involved lower extremity. In partial weight bearing, only part of the patient's weight is allowed to be transferred through the involved lower extremity. It must be remembered that most patients have difficulty replicating a prescribed weight-bearing restriction and will need constant reinforcement.[98]

The pattern is initiated with the forward movement of one of the assistive gait devices, and then the involved lower extremity is advanced. The patient presses down on the assistive gait device and advances the uninvolved lower extremity, using either a "swing-to" or a "swing-through" pattern as described for the three-point pattern.

Four-Point Pattern

The four-point gait pattern, which requires the use of an assistive gait device (canes or crutches) on each side of the body, is used when the patient requires maximum assistance with balance and stability. This pattern provides a slow gait speed but requires a low amount of energy to perform. The pattern is initiated with the forward movement of one of the assistive gait devices, and then the contralateral lower extremity, the other assistive gait device, and finally the opposite lower extremity (e.g., right crutch, then left foot; left crutch, then right foot; VIDEO 14-18).

Four-Point Modified

The four-point modified pattern is the same as the four-point except that it requires only one assistive device, positioned on the side opposite the involved lower extremity. This pattern cannot be used if there are any weight-bearing restrictions such as PWB or NWB, but it is appropriate for a patient with unilateral weakness or mild balance deficits. The patient is instructed to move the cane, then the involved leg, and then the uninvolved leg (VIDEO 14-19).

Stair Negotiation

Stair negotiation brings its own set of challenges. In addition to being more strenuous than walking on the level, stair negotiation has more potential risks and requires more coordination and balance by the patient. The three rules to remember for stair negotiation are:

1. "Up with the good and down with the bad." This means that the patient leads with the uninvolved (good) extremity when ascending (VIDEO 14-20), but leads with the involved (bad) extremity when descending (VIDEO 14-21). There appears to be some controversy about using value-laden terms such as *good* and *bad* when referring to a patient's injury. Some prefer to use the phrase "good people go to heaven and bad people go to hell." Whichever phrase is used, it is important that it be easy to remember for the patient.

2. The assistive device remains with the involved extremity. This means that if the assistive device is used to support a weak or unstable lower extremity, it remains with and moves with the involved lower extremity.

3. The clinician always guards the patient from below. This means that the clinician should stand between the patient and the direction toward which the patient is most likely to fall. Thus, the clinician stands behind a patient who is ascending the stairs, but in front of a patient who is descending the stairs. As with gait training on the level, a gait belt should be used, and the clinician should maintain a wide BOS and should control the patient's movement centrally through the patient's pelvis and shoulder girdles. Maintaining a wide BOS on the stairs involves the clinician avoiding having both feet on one step at the same time.

Ascending Stairs

To ascend steps, the patient must first move to the front edge of the step.

▶ To ascend stairs using a standard walker, the walker will have to be turned toward the opposite side of the handrail or wall. Ascending more than two to three stairs with a standard walker is not recommended. The patient is instructed to grasp the stair handrail with one hand and to turn the walker sideways so that the two front legs of the walker are placed on the first step. When ready, the patient pushes down on the walker handgrip and the handrail and advances the uninvolved lower extremity onto the first step. The patient then advances the uninvolved lower extremity to the first step and moves the legs of the walker to the next step. This process is repeated as the patient moves up the steps.

CLINICAL PEARL

Walkers that are specifically designed for stair negotiation exist but are not common.

▶ To ascend steps or stairs with crutches, the patient should grasp the stair handrail with one hand and grasp both crutches by the handgrips with the other hand (Video 14-20). If the patient is unable to grasp both crutches with one hand, or if the handrail is not stable or available, then the patient should use both crutches only, although this is not recommended if there are more than two to three steps. When in the correct position at the front edge of the step, the patient pushes down on the crutches and handrail, if applicable, and advances the uninvolved lower extremity to the first step. The patient then advances the involved lower extremity, and finally the crutches. This process is repeated for the remaining steps.

▶ To ascend steps or stairs with one or two canes, the patient should use the handrail and the cane(s). If the handrail is not stable or available, then the patient should use the cane(s) only. The patient pushes down on the cane(s) or handrail, as applicable, and advances the uninvolved lower extremity to the first step. The patient then advances the involved lower extremity. This process is repeated for the remaining steps.

Descending Stairs

In order to descend steps, the patient must first move to the front edge of the top step.

▶ To descend stairs using a walker, the walker is turned sideways so that the two front legs of the walker are placed on the lower step. Descending more than two to three stairs with a walker is not recommended. One hand is placed on the rear handgrip, and the other hand grasps the stair handrail. When ready, the patient lowers the involved lower extremity down to the first step. Then the patient pushes down on the walker and handrail and advances the uninvolved lower extremity down the first step. This process is repeated as the patient moves down the steps.

▶ To descend steps or stairs with crutches, the patient should use one hand to grasp the stair handrail and the other to grasp both crutches and handrail (Video 14-21). If the patient is unable to grasp both crutches with one hand, or if the handrail is not stable, then the patient should use both crutches only, although this is not recommended if there are more than two to three steps. When ready, the patient lowers the involved lower extremity down to the first step. Next, the patient pushes down on the crutches and handrail, if applicable, and advances the uninvolved lower extremity down to the first step. This process is repeated for the remaining steps.

▶ To descend steps or stairs with one or two canes, the patient should use the cane(s) and handrail. If the handrail is not stable, then the patient should use the cane(s) only. When ready, the patient lowers the involved lower extremity down to the first step. Next, the patient pushes down on the cane(s) and handrail, if applicable, and advances the uninvolved lower extremity down to the first step. This process is repeated for the remaining steps.

CLINICAL PEARL

A number of studies[99–101] have looked at the required degrees of range of motion for stair negotiation at the various lower extremity joints. These approximate ranges are:

Hip flexion: 7° to 65° for ascending; 15° to 40° for descending

Knee flexion: 8° to 94° for ascending; 10° to 92° for descending

Ankle dorsiflexion: 11° to 14° for ascending; 20° to 34° for descending

Ankle plantarflexion: 20° to 31° for ascending; 22° to 40° for descending

Opening Doors

Most doors open in one of two directions—inward or outward.

Door Opens Outward Toward the Patient

The patient is instructed to stand close to the door, turned slightly to face the door opening (VIDEO 14-22). Using the hand closest to the hinges, the patient pulls the door open, and then shifts the hand to the inside of the door to give the door a push, opening it wider. The patient then uses his or her prescribed gait pattern to walk through the doorway, being careful to avoid the closing door hitting the tip of the assistive device. Alternatively, if the patient is using bilateral axillary crutches, he or she can place the tip of the crutch that is closer to the door in the path of the door so that the door rests against the crutch tip.

Door Opens Inward Away from the Patient

The patient is instructed to stand close to the door, facing the door handle, and then to open and push the door with the hand nearest the door (see Video 14-22). The patient then walks through the doorway using his or her prescribed gait pattern. Alternatively, if the patient is using bilateral axillary crutches, the patient can turn sideways, facing away from the hinges, and then push against the door with the hip so that when the door opens, the patient positions the crutch tip against the bottom edge of the door to prevent it closing.

Video Description

Note the differences in techniques between Video 14-22 and VIDEO 14-23. When the door opens toward the patient, there is a high potential for the door to hit the assistive device, or it can obstruct the assistive device if the door is not opened wide enough. When the door opens away from the patient, there is no problem with the door hitting or obstructing the assistive device. However, the problem arises if the patient has to close the door after passing through, because the assistive device can obstruct the door from closing. Try to determine some strategies that you would provide to the patient to counteract these problems.

Inclines

A number of adaptations need to be made when ambulating up and down on an incline.[102,103] The patient should be instructed to:

▶ Take slightly longer steps when ascending moderate inclines, and take slightly shorter steps when descending inclines

▶ Lean forward when ascending

Different Surfaces

Depending on the treatment environment, sit-to-stand and stand-to-sit transfers can present a number of challenges. Whereas transferring to and from a relatively hard surface provides a high degree of stability for the patient, transferring to and from a soft surface is more difficult. This difficulty results from the patient being unsure on how the push-off surface is going to react. This is best illustrated by viewing VIDEO 14-24.

REFERENCES

1. Rose J: Dynamic lower extremity stability, in Hughes C (ed): Movement Disorders and Neuromuscular Interventions for the Trunk and Extremities—Independent Study Course 18.2.5. La Crosse, Wisc, Orthopaedic Section, APTA, 2008, pp 1-34.
2. Das P, McCollum G: Invariant structure in locomotion. Neuroscience 25:1023-1034, 1988.
3. Mann RA, Hagy JL, White V, et al: The initiation of gait. J Bone Joint Surg 61A:232-239, 1979.
4. Luttgens K, Hamilton N: Locomotion: solid surface, in Luttgens K, Hamilton N (eds): Kinesiology: Scientific Basis of Human Motion (ed 9). Dubuque, Iowa, McGraw-Hill, 1997, pp 519-549.
5. Dobkin BH, Harkema S, Requejo P, et al: Modulation of locomotor-like EMG activity in subjects with complete and incomplete spinal cord injury. J Neurol Rehabil 9:183-190, 1995.
6. Donatelli R, Wilkes R: Lower kinetic chain and human gait. J Back Musculoskel Rehabil 2:1-11, 1992.
7. Levine D, Whittle M: Gait analysis: The lower extremities. La Crosse, Wisc, Orthopaedic Section, APTA, 1992.
8. Mann RA, Hagy J: Biomechanics of walking, running, and sprinting. Am J Sports Med 8:345-350, 1980.
9. Murray MP: Gait as a total pattern of movement. Am J Phys Med 46:290, 1967.
10. Luttgens K, Hamilton N: The center of gravity and stability, in Luttgens K, Hamilton N (eds): Kinesiology: Scientific Basis of Human Motion (ed 9). Dubuque, Iowa, McGraw-Hill, 1997, pp 415-442.
11. Epler M: Gait, in Richardson JK, Iglarsh ZA (eds): Clinical Orthopaedic Physical Therapy. Philadelphia, WB Saunders, 1994, pp 602-625.
12. Subotnick SI: Variations in angles of gait in running. Phys Sportsmed 7:110-114, 1979.
13. Perry J: Stride analysis, in Perry J (ed): Gait Analysis: Normal and Pathological Function. Thorofare, NJ, Slack, 1992, pp 431-441.
14. Ostrosky KM, Van Sweringen JM, Burdett RG, et al: A comparison of gait characteristics in young and old subjects. Phys Ther 74:637-646, 1994.
15. Adelaar RS: The practical biomechanics of running. Am J Sports Med 14:497-500, 1986.
16. Basmajian JV: Therapeutic Exercise (ed 3). Baltimore, Williams & Wilkins, 1979.
17. Perry J: Gait Analysis: Normal and Pathological Function. Thorofare, NJ, Slack, 1992.
18. Rogers MM: Dynamic foot mechanics. J Orthop Sports Phys Ther 21:306-316, 1995.
19. Gage JR, Deluca PA, Renshaw TS: Gait analysis: principles and applications with emphasis on its use with cerebral palsy. Inst Course Lect 45:491-507, 1996.
20. Frey C: Foot health and shoewear for women. Clin Orthop Relat Res 372:32-44, 2000.

21. Oberg T, Karsznia A, Oberg K: Basic gait parameters: reference data for normal subjects, 10-79 years of age. J Rehabil Res Dev 30:210-223, 1993.

22. Molen NH, Rozendal RH, Boon W: Fundamental characteristics of human gait in relation to sex and location. Proceedings of the Koninklijke Nederlandse Akademie van Wetenschappen-Series C. Biol Med Sci 45:215-223, 1972.

23. Finley FR, Cody KA: Locomotive characteristics of urban pedestrians. Arch Phys Med Rehabil 51:423-426, 1970.

24. Sato H, Ishizu K: Gait patterns of Japanese pedestrians. J Hum Ergol (Tokyo) 19:13-22, 1990.

25. Richard R, Weber J, Mejjad O, et al: Spatiotemporal gait parameters measured using the Bessou gait analyzer in 79 healthy subjects: influence of age, stature, and gender. Rev Rhum Engl Ed 62:105-114, 1995.

26. Murray MP, Kory RC, Sepic SB: Walking patterns of normal women. Arch Phys Med Rehabil 51:637-650, 1970.

27. Murray MP, Drought AB, Kory RC: Walking patterns of normal men. J Bone Joint Surg Am 46A:335-360, 1964.

28. Bhambhani Y, Singh M: Metabolic and cinematographic analysis of walking and running in men and women. Med Sci Sports Exerc 17:131-137, 1985.

29. Giannini S, Catani F, Benedetti MG, et al: Terminology, parameterization and normalization in gait analysis, in Gait Analysis: Methodologies and Clinical Applications. Washington, DC, IOS Press, 1994, pp 65-88.

30. Perry J: The hip, in Gait Analysis: Normal and Pathological Function. Thorofare, NJ, Slack, 1992, pp 111-129.

31. Reinking MF: Knee anatomy and biomechanics, in Wadsworth C (ed): Disorders of the Knee—Home Study Course. La Crosse, Wisc, Orthopaedic Section, APTA, 2001.

32. Norkin C, Levangie P: Joint Structure and Function: A Comprehensive Analysis. Philadelphia, FA Davis Company, 1992.

33. Kuster MS, Wood GA, Stachowiak GW, et al: Joint load considerations in total knee replacement. J Bone Joint Surg 79B:109-113, 1997.

34. Andriacchi TP, Ogle JA, Galante JO: Walking speed as a basis for normal and abnormal gait measurements. J Biomech 10:261-268, 1977.

35. Corrigan J, Moore D, Stephens M: The effect of heel height on forefoot loading. Foot Ankle 11:418-422, 1991.

36. Arsenault AB, Winter DA, Marteniuk RG: Is there a "normal" profile of EMG activity in gait? Med Biol Eng Comput 24:337-343, 1986.

37. Berchuck M, Andriacchi TP, Bach BR, et al: Gait adaptations by patients who have a deficient anterior cruciate ligament. J Bone Joint Surg 72-A:871-877, 1990.

38. Boeing DD: Evaluation of a clinical method of gait analysis. Phys Ther 57:795-798, 1977.

39. Dillon P, Updyke W, Allen W: Gait analysis with reference to chondromalacia patellae. J Orthop Sports Phys Ther 5:127-131, 1983.

40. Hunt GC, Brocato RS: Gait and foot pathomechanics, in Hunt GC (ed): Physical Therapy of the Foot and Ankle. Edinburgh, Churchill Livingstone, 1988, pp 39-57.

41. Krebs DE, Robbins CE, Lavine L, et al: Hip biomechanics during gait. J Orthop Sports Phys Ther 28:51-9, 1998.

42. Luttgens K, Hamilton N: The standing posture, in Luttgens K, Hamilton N (eds): Kinesiology: Scientific Basis of Human Motion (ed 9). Dubuque, Iowa, McGraw-Hill, 1997, pp 445-459.

43. Winter DA: Biomechanical motor patterns in normal walking. J Motor Behav 15:302-329, 1983.

44. Hoyt DF, Taylor CF: Gait and the energetics of locomotion in horses. Nature 292:239-240, 1981.

45. Corcoran PJ, Brengelmann G: Oxygen uptake in normal and handicapped subjects in relation to the speed of walking beside a velocity-controlled cart. Arch Phys Med Rehabil 51:78-87, 1970.

46. Gonzalez EG, Corcoran PJ, Reyes RL: Energy expenditure in below-knee amputees: correlation with stump length. Arch Phys Med Rehabil 55:111-119, 1974.

47. Waters RL, Hislop HJ, Perry J, et al: Energetics: application to the study and management of locomotor disabilities. Orthop Clin North Am 9:351-377, 1978.

48. Martin PE, Rothstein DE, Larish DD: Effects of age and physical activity status on the speed-aerobic demand relationship of walking. J Appl Physiol 73:200-206, 1992.

49. Prampero PE: The energy cost of human locomotion on land and in the water. Int J Sports Med 7:55-72, 1986.

50. Davies MJ, Dalsky GP: Economy of mobility in older adults. J Orthop Sports Phys Ther 26:69-72, 1997.

51. Daniels J, Krahenbuhl G, Foster C, et al: Aerobic responses of female distance runners to submaximal and maximal exercise. Ann N Y Acad Sci 301:726-733, 1977.

52. Pate RR, Barnes CG, Miller CA: A physiological comparison of performance-matched female and male distance runners. Res Q Exerc Sport 56:245-250, 1985.

53. Wells CL, Hecht LH, Krahenbuhl GS: Physical characteristics and oxygen utilization of male and female marathon runners. Res Q Exerc Sport 52:281-285, 1981.

54. Bransford DR, Howley ET: Oxygen cost of running in trained and untrained men and women. Med Sci Sports Exerc 9:41-44, 1977.

55. Daniels J, Daniels N: Running economy of elite male and females runners. Med Sci Sports Exerc 24:483-489, 1992.

56. Howley ET, Glover ME: The caloric costs of running and walking one mile for men and women. Med Sci Sports Exerc 6:235-237, 1974.

57. Larish DD, Martin PE, Mungiole M: Characteristic patterns of gait in the healthy old. Ann N Y Acad Sci 515:18-32, 1987.

58. Waters RL, Hislop HJ, Perry J, et al: Comparative cost of walking in young and old adults. J Orthop Res 1:73-76, 1983.

59. Allen W, Seals DR, Hurley BF, et al: Lactate threshold and distance running performance in young and older endurance athletes. J Appl Physiol 58:1281-1284, 1985.

60. Trappe SW, Costill DL, Vukovich MD, et al: Aging among elite distance runners: A 22-year longitudinal study. J Appl Physiol 80:285-290, 1996.

61. Wells CL, Boorman MA, Riggs DM: Effect of age and menopausal status on cardiorespiratory fitness in masters women runners. Med Sci Sports Exerc 24:1147-1154, 1992.

62. Moseley CF: Leg-length discrepancy, in Morrissy RT (ed): Lovell and Winter's Pediatric Orthopaedics (ed 3). Philadelphia, JB Lippincott, 1990, pp 767-813.

63. Beaty JH: Congenital anomalies of lower extremity, in Crenshaw AH (ed): Campbell's Operative Orthopaedics (ed 8). St. Louis, Mosby-Year Book, 1992, pp 2126-2158.

64. Gross RH: Leg length discrepancy: how much is too much? Orthopedics 1:307-310, 1978.

65. Song KM, Halliday SE, Little DG: The effect of limb-length discrepancy on gait. J Bone Joint Surg 79A:1690-8, 1997.

66. Lange GW, Hintermeister RA, Schlegel T, et al: Electromyographic and kinematic analysis of graded treadmill walking and the implications for knee rehabilitation. J Orthop Sports Phys Ther 23:294-301, 1996.

67. Croskey MI, Dawson PM, Luessen AC, et al: The height of the center of gravity in man. Am J Physiol 61:171-185, 1922.

68. Saunders JBD, Inman VT, Eberhart HD: The major determinants in normal and pathological gait. J Bone Joint Surg Am 35:543-558, 1953.

69. Dodd KJ, Morris ME. Lateral pelvic displacement during gait: abnormalities after stroke and changes during the first month of rehabilitation. Arch Phys Med Rehabil. 2003 Aug;84(8):1200-5.

70. Perry J: Gait cycle, in Perry J (ed): Gait Analysis: Normal and Pathological Function. Thorofare, NJ, Slack, 1992, pp 3-7.

71. Givens-Heiss DL, Krebs DE, Riley PO, et al: In vivo acetabular contact pressures during rehabilitation, Part II: Postacute phase. Phys Ther 72:700-705; discussion 706-710, 1992.

72. Dabke HV, Gupta SK, Holt CA, et al: How accurate is partial weightbearing? Clin Orthop Relat Res (421):282-286, 2004.

73. Sutton P, Stedman J, Livesley P: Perception and education of unilateral weightbearing amongst health care professionals. Injury 38:163-164, 2007.

74. Miyazaki S, Ishida A, Iwakura H, et al: Portable limb-load monitor utilizing a thin capacitive transducer. J Biomed Eng 8:67-71, 1986.

75. Gapsis JJ, Grabois M, Borrell RM, et al: Limb load monitor: evaluation of a sensory feedback device for controlled weight bearing. Arch Phys Med Rehabil 63:38-41, 1982.

76. Wannstedt G, Craik RL: Clinical evaluation of a sensory feedback device: the limb load monitor. Bull Prosthet Res :8-49, 1978.

77. Isakov E: Gait rehabilitation: a new biofeedback device for monitoring and enhancing weight-bearing over the affected lower limb. Eura Medicophys 43:21-26, 2007.

78. Hershko E, Tauber C, Carmeli E: Biofeedback versus physiotherapy in patients with partial weight-bearing. Am J Orthop (Belle Mead NJ) 37:E92-E96, 2008.

79. Hoberman M: Crutch and cane exercises and use, in Basmajian JV (ed): Therapeutic Exercise (ed 3). Baltimore, Williams & Wilkins, 1979, pp 228-255.

80. Duesterhaus MA, Duesterhaus S: Patient Care Skills (ed 2). East Norwalk, Conn, Appleton & Lange, 1990.

81. Schmitz TJ: Locomotor training, in O'Sullivan SB, Schmitz TJ (eds): Physical Rehabilitation (ed 5). Philadelphia, FA Davis, 2007, pp 523-560.

82. Lyu SR, Ogata K, Hoshiko I: Effects of a cane on floor reaction force and center of force during gait. Clin Orthop Relat Res 375:313-319, 2000.

83. Blount WP: Don't throw away the cane. J Bone Joint Surg 38A:695-708, 1956.

84. Joyce BM, Kirby RL: Canes, crutches and walkers. Am Fam Phys 43:535-542, 1991.

85. Baxter ML, Allington RO, Koepke GH: Weight-distribution variables in the use of crutches and canes. Phys Ther 49:360-365, 1969.

86. Edwards BG: Contralateral and ipsilateral cane usage by patients with total knee or hip replacement. Arch Phys Med Rehabil 67:734-740, 1986.

87. Oatis CA: Biomechanics of the hip, in Echternach J (ed): Clinics in Physical Therapy: Physical Therapy of the Hip. New York, Churchill Livingstone, 1990, pp 37-50.

88. Olsson EC, Smidt GL: Assistive devices, in Smidt G (ed): Gait in Rehabilitation. New York, Churchill Livingstone, 1990, pp 141-155.

89. Vargo MM, Robinson LR, Nicholas JJ: Contralateral vs. ipsilateral cane use: effects on muscles crossing the knee joint. Am J Phys Med Rehabil 71:170-176, 1992.

90. Jebsen RH: Use and abuse of ambulation aids. JAMA 199:5-10, 1967.

91. Kumar R, Roe MC, Scremin OU: Methods for estimating the proper length of a cane. Arch Phys Med Rehabil 76:1173-1175, 1995.

92. Bauer DM, Finch DC, McGough KP, et al: A comparative analysis of several crutch-length-estimation techniques. Phys Ther 71:294-300, 1991.

93. Barbur JL, Konstantakopoulou E: Changes in color vision with decreasing light level: separating the effects of normal aging from disease. J Opt Soc Am A Opt Image Sci Vis 29:A27-A35, 2012.

94. Owsley C: Aging and vision. Vision Res 51:1610-1622, 2011.

95. Smith SC: Aging and vision. Insight 33:16-20; quiz 21-22, 2008.

96. Wood JM: Aging, driving and vision. Clin Exp Optom 85:214-220, 2002.

97. Kline DW, Kline TJ, Fozard JL, et al: Vision, aging, and driving: the problems of older drivers. J Gerontol 47:P27-P34, 1992.

98. Li S, Armstrong CW, Cipriani D: Three-point gait crutch walking: variability in ground reaction force during weight bearing. Arch Phys Med Rehabil :86-92, 2001.

99. Reeves ND, Spanjaard M, Mohagheghi AA, et al: The demands of stair descent relative to maximum capacities in elderly and young adults. J Electromyogr Kinesiol 18:218-227, 2008.

100. Protopapadaki A, Drechsler WI, Cramp MC, et al: Hip, knee, ankle kinematics and kinetics during stair ascent and descent in healthy young individuals. Clin Biomech (Bristol, Avon) 22:203-210, 2007.

101. Powers CM, Perry J, Hsu A, et al: Are patellofemoral pain and quadriceps femoris muscle torque associated with locomotor function? Phys Ther 77:1063-1075; discussion 1075-1078, 1997.

102. Leroux A, Fung J, Barbeau H: Postural adaptation to walking on inclined surfaces: I. Normal strategies. Gait Posture 15:64-74, 2002.

103. McIntosh AS, Beatty KT, Dwan LN, et al: Gait dynamics on an inclined walkway. J Biomech 39:2491-2502, 2006.

APPENDIX A

Standards of Practice for Physical Therapy

APTA House of Delegates Standard S06-03-09-10

PREAMBLE

The physical therapy profession's commitment to society is to promote optimal health and functioning in individuals by pursuing excellence in practice. The American Physical Therapy Association attests to this commitment by adopting and promoting the following Standards of Practice for Physical Therapy. These Standards are the profession's statement of conditions and performances that are essential for provision of high quality professional service to society, and provide a foundation for assessment of physical therapist practice.

I. ETHICAL/LEGAL CONSIDERATIONS

A. Ethical Considerations

The physical therapist practices according to the *Code of Ethics* of the American Physical Therapy Association.

The physical therapist assistant complies with the *Standards of Ethical Conduct for the Physical Therapist Assistant* of the American Physical Therapy Association.

B. Legal Considerations

The physical therapist complies with all the legal requirements of jurisdictions regulating the practice of physical therapy.

The physical therapist assistant complies with all the legal requirements of jurisdictions regulating the work of the assistant.

II. ADMINISTRATION OF THE PHYSICAL THERAPY SERVICE

A. Statement of Mission, Purposes, and Goals

The physical therapy service has a statement of mission, purposes, and goals that reflects the needs and interests of the patients/clients served, the physical therapy personnel affiliated with the service, and the community.

B. Organizational Plan

The physical therapy service has a written organizational plan.

C. Policies and Procedures

The physical therapy service has written policies and procedures that reflect the operation, mission, purposes, and goals of the service, and are consistent with the association's standards, policies, positions, guidelines, and *Code of Ethics*.

D. Administration

A physical therapist is responsible for the direction of the physical therapy service.

E. Fiscal Management

The director of the physical therapy service, in consultation with physical therapy staff and appropriate administrative personnel, participates in the planning for and allocation of resources. Fiscal planning and management of the service is based on sound accounting principles.

F. Improvement of Quality of Care and Performance

The physical therapy service has a written plan for continuous improvement of quality of care and performance of services.

G. Staffing

The physical therapy personnel affiliated with the physical therapy service have demonstrated competence and are sufficient to achieve the mission, purposes, and goals of the service.

H. Staff Development

The physical therapy service has a written plan that provides for appropriate and ongoing staff development.

I. Physical Setting

The physical setting is designed to provide a safe and accessible environment that facilitates fulfillment of the mission, purposes, and goals of the physical therapy service.

The equipment is safe and sufficient to achieve the purposes and goals of physical therapy.

J. Collaboration

The physical therapy service collaborates with all disciplines as appropriate.

III. PATIENT/CLIENT MANAGEMENT

A. Patient/Client Collaboration

Within the patient/client management process, the physical therapist and the patient/client establish and maintain an ongoing collaborative process of decision making that exists throughout the provision of services.

B. Initial Examination/Evaluation/Diagnosis/Prognosis

The physical therapist performs an initial examination and evaluation to establish a diagnosis and prognosis prior to intervention.

C. Plan of Care

The physical therapist establishes a plan of care and manages the needs of the patient/client based on the examination, evaluation, diagnosis, prognosis, goals, and outcomes of the planned interventions for identified impairments, functional limitations, and disabilities.

The physical therapist involves the patient/client and appropriate others in the planning, implementation, and assessment of the plan of care.

The physical therapist, in consultation with appropriate disciplines, plans for discharge of the patient/client taking into consideration achievement of anticipated goals and expected outcomes, and provides for appropriate follow-up or referral.

D. Intervention

The physical therapist provides or directs and supervises the physical therapy intervention consistent with the results of the examination, evaluation, diagnosis, prognosis, and plan of care.

E. Reexamination

The physical therapist reexamines the patient/client as necessary during an episode of care to evaluate progress or change in patient/client status and modifies the plan of care accordingly or discontinues physical therapy services.

F. Discharge/Discontinuation of Intervention

The physical therapist discharges the patient/client from physical therapy services when the anticipated goals or expected outcomes for the patient/client have been achieved.

The physical therapist discontinues intervention when the patient/client is unable to continue to progress toward goals or when the physical therapist determines that the patient/client will no longer benefit from physical therapy.

G. Communication/Coordination/Documentation

The physical therapist communicates, coordinates, and documents all aspects of patient/client management including the results of the initial examination and evaluation, diagnosis, prognosis, plan of care, interventions, response to interventions, changes in patient/client status relative to the interventions, reexamination, and discharge/discontinuation of intervention and other patient/client management activities.

IV. EDUCATION

The physical therapist is responsible for individual professional development. The physical therapist assistant is responsible for individual career development.

The physical therapist and the physical therapist assistant, under the direction and supervision of the physical therapist, participate in the education of students.

The physical therapist educates and provides consultation to consumers and the general public regarding the purposes and benefits of physical therapy.

The physical therapist educates and provides consultation to consumers and the general public regarding the roles of the physical therapist and the physical therapist assistant.

V. RESEARCH

The physical therapist applies research findings to practice and encourages, participates in, and promotes activities that establish the outcomes of patient/client management provided by the physical therapist.

VI. COMMUNITY RESPONSIBILITY

The physical therapist demonstrates community responsibility by participating in community and community agency activities, educating the public, formulating public policy, or providing pro bono physical therapy services.

Data from American Physical Therapy Association: Today's Physical Therapist: A Comprehensive Review of a 21st-Century Health Care Profession. Alexandria, Va, American Physical Therapy Association, 2011.

APPENDIX B

Criteria for Standards of Practice for Physical Therapy

APTA Board of Directors Standard BOD S03-06-16-38

The Standards of Practice for Physical Therapy are promulgated by APTA's House of Delegates; criteria for the standards are promulgated by APTA's Board of Directors. Criteria are italicized beneath the standards to which they apply.

PREAMBLE

The physical therapy profession's commitment to society is to promote optimal health and function in individuals by pursuing excellence in practice. The American Physical Therapy Association attests to this commitment by adopting and promoting the following Standards of Practice for Physical Therapy. These Standards are the profession's statement of conditions and performances that are essential for provision of high quality professional service to society, and provide a foundation for assessment of physical therapist practice.

I. ETHICAL/LEGAL CONSIDERATIONS

A. Ethical Considerations
   The physical therapist practices according to the Code of Ethics of the American Physical Therapy Association.
   The physical therapist assistant complies with the *Standards of Ethical Conduct for the Physical Therapist Assistant* of the American Physical Therapy Association.

B. Legal Considerations
   The physical therapist complies with all the legal requirements of jurisdictions regulating the practice of physical therapy.
   The physical therapist assistant complies with all the legal requirements of jurisdictions regulating the work of the assistant.

II. ADMINISTRATION OF THE PHYSICAL THERAPY SERVICE

A. Statement of Mission, Purposes, and Goals
   The physical therapy service has a statement of mission, purposes, and goals that reflects the needs and interests of the patients/clients served, the physical therapy personnel affiliated with the service, and the community.

The statement of mission, purposes, and goals:

▸ *Defines the scope and limitations of the physical therapy service.*

▸ *Identifies the goals and objectives of the service.*

▸ *Is reviewed annually.*

B. Organizational Plan
   The physical therapy service has a written organizational plan.

The organizational plan:

▸ *Describes relationships among components within the physical therapy service and, where the service is part of a larger organization, between the service and the other components of that organization.*

▸ *Ensures that the service is directed by a physical therapist.*

▸ *Defines supervisory structures within the service.*

▸ *Reflects current personnel functions.*

C. Policies and Procedures
   The physical therapy service has written policies and procedures that reflect the operation, mission, purposes, and goals of the service, and are consistent with the Association's positions, standards, guidelines, policies, procedures, and Code of Ethics.

The written policies and procedures:

▸ *Are reviewed regularly and revised as necessary.*

▸ *Meet the requirements of federal and state law and external agencies.*

▸ *Apply to, but are not limited to:*
   ▪ *Care of patients/clients, including guidelines*
   ▪ *Clinical education*
   ▪ *Clinical research*
   ▪ *Collaboration*
   ▪ *Collection of patient data*
   ▪ *Competency assessment*
   ▪ *Criteria for access to care*
   ▪ *Criteria for initiation and continuation of care*

461

- *Criteria for referral to other appropriate health care providers*
- *Criteria for termination of care*
- *Documentation*
- *Environmental safety*
- *Equipment maintenance*
- *Fiscal management*
- *Improvement of quality of care and performance of services*
- *Infection control*
- *Job/position descriptions*
- *Medical emergencies*
- *Personnel-related policies*
- *Rights of patients/clients*
- *Staff orientation*

D. Administration

A physical therapist is responsible for the direction of the physical therapy service.

The physical therapist responsible for the direction of the physical therapy service:

- *Ensures compliance with local, state, and federal requirements.*
- *Ensures compliance with current APTA documents, including Standards of Practice for Physical Therapy and the Criteria, Guide to Physical Therapist Practice, Code of Ethics, Guide for Professional Conduct, Standards of Ethical Conduct for the Physical Therapist Assistant, and Guide for Conduct of the Physical Therapist Assistant.*
- *Ensures that services are consistent with the mission, purposes, and goals of the physical therapy service.*
- *Ensures that services are provided in accordance with established policies and procedures.*
- *Ensures that the process for assignment and reassignment of physical therapist staff supports individual physical therapist responsibility to their patients and meets the needs of the patients/clients.*
- *Reviews and updates policies and procedures.*
- *Provides for training of physical therapy support personnel that ensures continued competence for their job description.*
- *Provides for continuous in-service training on safety issues and for periodic safety inspection of equipment by qualified individuals.*

E. Fiscal Management

The director of the physical therapy service, in consultation with physical therapy staff and appropriate administrative personnel participates in planning for, and allocation of, resources. Fiscal planning and management of the service is based on sound accounting principles.

The fiscal management plan:

- *Includes a budget that provides for optimal use of resources.*
- *Ensures accurate recording and reporting of financial information.*
- *Ensures compliance with legal requirements.*

- *Allows for cost-effective utilization of resources.*
- *Uses a fee schedule that is consistent with the cost of physical therapy services and that is within customary norms of fairness and reasonableness.*
- *Considers option of providing pro bono services.*

F. Improvement of Quality of Care and Performance

The physical therapy service has a written plan for continuous improvement of quality of care and performance of services.

The improvement plan:

- *Provides evidence of ongoing review and evaluation of the physical therapy service.*
- *Provides a mechanism for documenting improvement in quality of care and performance.*
- *Is consistent with requirements of external agencies, as applicable.*

G. Staffing

The physical therapy personnel affiliated with the physical therapy service have demonstrated competence and are sufficient to achieve the mission, purposes, and goals of the service.

The physical therapy service:

- *Meets all legal requirements regarding licensure and certification of appropriate personnel.*
- *Ensures that the level of expertise within the service is appropriate to the needs of the patients/clients served.*
- *Provides appropriate professional and support personnel to meet the needs of the patient/client population.*

H. Staff Development

The physical therapy service has a written plan that provides for appropriate and ongoing staff development.

The staff development plan:

- *Includes self-assessment, individual goal setting, and organizational needs in directing continuing education and learning activities.*
- *Includes strategies for lifelong learning and professional and career development.*
- *Includes mechanisms to foster mentorship activities.*
- *Includes knowledge of clinical research methods and analysis.*

I. Physical Setting

The physical setting is designed to provide a safe and accessible environment that facilitates fulfillment of the mission, purposes, and goals of the physical therapy service. The equipment is safe and sufficient to achieve the purposes and goals of physical therapy.

The physical setting:

- *Meets all applicable legal requirements for health and safety.*
- *Meets space needs appropriate for the number and type of patients/clients served.*

The equipment:

▶ *Meets all applicable legal requirements for health and safety.*

▶ *Is inspected routinely.*

J. Collaboration

The physical therapy service collaborates with all disciplines as appropriate.

The collaboration when appropriate:

▶ *Uses a team approach to the care of patients/clients.*

▶ *Provides instruction of patients/clients and families.*

▶ *Ensures professional development and continuing education.*

III. PATIENT/CLIENT MANAGEMENT

A. Patient/Client Collaboration

Within the patient/client management process, the physical therapist and the patient/client establish and maintain an ongoing collaborative process of decision-making that exists throughout the provision of services.

B. Initial Examination/Evaluation/Diagnosis/Prognosis

The physical therapist performs an initial examination and evaluation to establish a diagnosis and prognosis prior to intervention.

The physical therapist examination:

▶ *Is documented, dated, and appropriately authenticated by the physical therapist who performed it.*

▶ *Identifies the physical therapy needs of the patient/client.*

▶ *Incorporates appropriate tests and measures to facilitate outcome measurement.*

▶ *Produces data that are sufficient to allow evaluation, diagnosis, prognosis, and the establishment of a plan of care.*

▶ *May result in recommendations for additional services to meet the needs of the patient/client.*

C. Plan of Care

The physical therapist establishes a plan of care and manages the needs of the patient/client based on the examination, evaluation, diagnosis, prognosis, goals, and outcomes of the planned interventions for identified impairments, functional limitations, and disabilities.

The physical therapist involves the patient/client and appropriate others in the planning, implementation, and assessment of the plan of care.

The physical therapist, in consultation with appropriate disciplines, plans for discharge of the patient/client taking into consideration achievement of anticipated goals and expected outcomes, and provides for appropriate follow-up or referral.

The plan of care:

▶ *Is based on the examination, evaluation, diagnosis, and prognosis.*

▶ *Identifies goals and outcomes.*

▶ *Describes the proposed intervention, including frequency and duration.*

▶ *Includes documentation that is dated and appropriately authenticated by the physical therapist who established the plan of care.*

D. Intervention

The physical therapist provides, or directs and supervises, the physical therapy intervention consistent with the results of the examination, evaluation, diagnosis, prognosis, and plan of care.

The intervention:

▶ *Is based on the examination, evaluation, diagnosis, prognosis, and plan of care.*

▶ *Is provided under the ongoing direction and supervision of the physical therapist.*

▶ *Is provided in such a way that directed and supervised responsibilities are commensurate with the qualifications and the legal limitations of the physical therapist assistant.*

▶ *Is altered in accordance with changes in response or status.*

▶ *Is provided at a level that is consistent with current physical therapy practice.*

▶ *Is interdisciplinary when necessary to meet the needs of the patient/client.*

▶ *Documentation of the intervention is consistent with the Guidelines: Physical Therapy Documentation of Patient/Client Management.*

▶ *Is dated and appropriately authenticated by the physical therapist or, when permissible by law, by the physical therapist assistant.*

E. Reexamination

The physical therapist reexamines the patient/client as necessary during an episode of care to evaluate progress or change in patient/client status and modifies the plan of care accordingly or discontinues physical therapy services.

The physical therapist reexamination:

▶ *Is documented, dated, and appropriately authenticated by the physical therapist who performs it.*

▶ *Includes modifications to the plan of care.*

F. Discharge/Discontinuation of Intervention

The physical therapist discharges the patient/client from physical therapy services when the anticipated goals or expected outcomes for the patient/client have been achieved.

The physical therapist discontinues intervention when the patient/client is unable to continue to progress toward goals or when the physical therapist determines that the patient/client will no longer benefit from physical therapy.

Discharge documentation:

▶ *Includes the status of the patient/client at discharge and the goals and outcomes attained.*

▶ *Is dated and appropriately authenticated by the physical therapist who performed the discharge.*

▶ *Includes, when a patient/client is discharged prior to attainment of goals and outcomes, the status of the patient/client and the rationale for discontinuation.*

G. Communication/Coordination/Documentation

The physical therapist communicates, coordinates and documents all aspects of patient/client management including the results of the initial examination and evaluation, diagnosis, prognosis, plan of care, interventions, response to interventions, changes in patient/client status relative to the interventions, reexamination, and discharge/discontinuation of intervention and other patient/client management activities.

Physical therapist documentation:

▶ *Is dated and appropriately authenticated by the physical therapist who performed the examination and established the plan of care.*

▶ *Is dated and appropriately authenticated by the physical therapist who performed the intervention or, when allowable by law or regulations, by the physical therapist assistant who performed specific components of the intervention as selected by the supervising physical therapist.*

▶ *Is dated and appropriately authenticated by the physical therapist who performed the reexamination, and includes modifications to the plan of care.*

▶ *Is dated and appropriately authenticated by the physical therapist who performed the discharge, and includes the status of the patient/client and the goals and outcomes achieved.*

▶ *Includes, when a patient/client is discharged prior to achievement of goals and outcomes, the status of the patient/client and the rationale for discontinuation.*

▶ *As appropriate, records patient data using a method that allows collective analysis.*

IV. EDUCATION

The physical therapist is responsible for individual professional development. The physical therapist assistant is responsible for individual career development.

The physical therapist, and the physical therapist assistant, under the direction and supervision of the physical therapist, participate in the education of students.

The physical therapist educates and provides consultation to consumers and the general public regarding the purposes and benefits of physical therapy.

The physical therapist educates and provides consultation to consumers and the general public regarding the roles of the physical therapist and the physical therapist assistant.

The physical therapist:

▶ *Educates and provides consultation to consumers and the general public regarding the roles of the physical therapist, the physical therapist assistant, and other support personnel.*

V. RESEARCH

The physical therapist applies research findings to practice and encourages, participates in, and promotes activities that establish the outcomes of patient/client management provided by the physical therapist.

The physical therapist:

▶ *Ensures that their knowledge of research literature related to practice is current.*

▶ *Ensures that the rights of research subjects are protected, and the integrity of research is maintained.*

▶ *Participates in the research process as appropriate to individual education, experience, and expertise.*

▶ *Educates physical therapists, physical therapist assistants, students, other health professionals, and the general public about the outcomes of physical therapist practice.*

VI. COMMUNITY RESPONSIBILITY

The physical therapist demonstrates community responsibility by participating in community and community agency activities, educating the public, formulating public policy, or providing pro bono physical therapy services.

The physical therapist:

▶ *Participates in community and community agency activities.*

▶ *Educates the public, including prevention, education, and health promotion.*

▶ *Helps formulate public policy.*

▶ *Provides pro bono physical therapy services.*

Data from American Physical Therapy Association: Today's Physical Therapist: A Comprehensive Review of a 21st-Century Health Care Profession. Alexandria, Va, American Physical Therapy Association, 2011.

APPENDIX C | Code of Ethics

CODE OF ETHICS HOD S06-09-07-12 [Amended HOD S06-00-12-23; HOD 06-91-05-05; HOD 06-87-11-17; HOD 06-81-06-18; HOD 06-78-06-08; HOD 06-78-06-07; HOD 06-77-18-30; HOD 06-77-17-27; Initial HOD 06-73-13-24] [Standard]

PREAMBLE

The *Code of Ethics for the Physical Therapist* (*Code of Ethics*) delineates the ethical obligations of all physical therapists as determined by the House of Delegates of the American Physical Therapy Association (APTA). The purposes of this *Code of Ethics* are to:

1. Define the ethical principles that form the foundation of physical therapist practice in patient/client management, consultation, education, research, and administration.

2. Provide standards of behavior and performance that form the basis of professional accountability to the public.

3. Provide guidance for physical therapists facing ethical challenges, regardless of their professional roles and responsibilities.

4. Educate physical therapists, students, other health care professionals, regulators, and the public regarding the core values, ethical principles, and standards that guide the professional conduct of the physical therapist.

5. Establish the standards by which the American Physical Therapy Association can determine if a physical therapist has engaged in unethical conduct.

No code of ethics is exhaustive nor can it address every situation. Physical therapists are encouraged to seek additional advice or consultation in instances where the guidance of the *Code of Ethics* may not be definitive.

This *Code of Ethics* is built upon the five roles of the physical therapist (management of patients/clients, consultation, education, research, and administration), the core values of the profession, and the multiple realms of ethical action (individual, organizational, and societal). Physical therapist practice is guided by a set of seven core values: accountability, altruism, compassion/caring, excellence, integrity, professional duty, and social responsibility. Throughout the document the primary core values that support specific principles are indicated in parentheses. Unless a specific role is indicated in the principle, the duties and obligations being delineated pertain to the five roles of the physical therapist. Fundamental to the *Code of Ethics* is the special obligation of physical therapists to empower, educate, and enable those with impairments, activity limitations, participation restrictions, and disabilities to facilitate greater independence, health, wellness, and enhanced quality of life.

PRINCIPLES

Principle #1: Physical therapists shall respect the inherent dignity and rights of all individuals.

(Core Values: Compassion, Integrity)

▶ 1A. Physical therapists shall act in a respectful manner toward each person regardless of age, gender, race, nationality, religion, ethnicity, social or economic status, sexual orientation, health condition, or disability.

▶ 1B. Physical therapists shall recognize their personal biases and shall not discriminate against others in physical therapist practice, consultation, education, research, and administration.

Principle #2: Physical therapists shall be trustworthy and compassionate in addressing the rights and needs of patients/clients.

(Core Values: Altruism, Compassion, Professional Duty)

▶ 2A. Physical therapists shall adhere to the core values of the profession and shall act in the best interests of patients/clients over the interests of the physical therapist.

▶ 2B. Physical therapists shall provide physical therapy services with compassionate and caring behaviors that incorporate the individual and cultural differences of patients/clients.

▶ 2C. Physical therapists shall provide the information necessary to allow patients or their surrogates to make informed decisions about physical therapy care or participation in clinical research.

▶ 2D. Physical therapists shall collaborate with patients/clients to empower them in decisions about their health care.

▶ 2E. Physical therapists shall protect confidential patient/client information and may disclose confidential information to appropriate authorities only when allowed or as required by law.

Principle #3: Physical therapists shall be accountable for making sound professional judgments.

(Core Values: Excellence, Integrity)

▶ 3A. Physical therapists shall demonstrate independent and objective professional judgment in the patient's/client's best interest in all practice settings.

▶ 3B. Physical therapists shall demonstrate professional judgment informed by professional standards, evidence (including current literature and established best practice), practitioner experience, and patient/client values.

▶ 3C. Physical therapists shall make judgments within their scope of practice and level of expertise and shall communicate with, collaborate with, or refer to peers or other health care professionals when necessary.

▶ 3D. Physical therapists shall not engage in conflicts of interest that interfere with professional judgment.

▶ 3E. Physical therapists shall provide appropriate direction of and communication with physical therapist assistants and support personnel.

Principle #4: Physical therapists shall demonstrate integrity in their relationships with patients/clients, families, colleagues, students, research participants, other health care providers, employers, payers, and the public.

(Core Value: Integrity)

▶ 4A. Physical therapists shall provide truthful, accurate, and relevant information and shall not make misleading representations.

▶ 4B. Physical therapists shall not exploit persons over whom they have supervisory, evaluative or other authority (eg, patients/clients, students, supervisees, research participants, or employees).

▶ 4C. Physical therapists shall discourage misconduct by health care professionals and report illegal or unethical acts to the relevant authority, when appropriate.

▶ 4D. Physical therapists shall report suspected cases of abuse involving children or vulnerable adults to the appropriate authority, subject to law.

▶ 4E. Physical therapists shall not engage in any sexual relationship with any of their patients/clients, supervisees, or students.

▶ 4F. Physical therapists shall not harass anyone verbally, physically, emotionally, or sexually.

Principle #5: Physical therapists shall fulfill their legal and professional obligations.

(Core Values: Professional Duty, Accountability)

▶ 5A. Physical therapists shall comply with applicable local, state, and federal laws and regulations.

▶ 5B. Physical therapists shall have primary responsibility for supervision of physical therapist assistants and support personnel.

▶ 5C. Physical therapists involved in research shall abide by accepted standards governing protection of research participants.

▶ 5D. Physical therapists shall encourage colleagues with physical, psychological, or substance related impairments that may adversely impact their professional responsibilities to seek assistance or counsel.

▶ 5E. Physical therapists who have knowledge that a colleague is unable to perform their professional responsibilities with reasonable skill and safety shall report this information to the appropriate authority.

▶ 5F. Physical therapists shall provide notice and information about alternatives for obtaining care in the event the physical therapist terminates the provider relationship while the patient/client continues to need physical therapy services.

Principle #6: Physical therapists shall enhance their expertise through the lifelong acquisition and refinement of knowledge, skills, abilities, and professional behaviors.

(Core Value: Excellence)

▶ 6A. Physical therapists shall achieve and maintain professional competence.

▶ 6B. Physical therapists shall take responsibility for their professional development based on critical self-assessment and reflection on changes in physical therapist practice, education, health care delivery, and technology.

▶ 6C. Physical therapists shall evaluate the strength of evidence and applicability of content presented during professional development activities before integrating the content or techniques into practice.

▶ 6D. Physical therapists shall cultivate practice environments that support professional development, lifelong learning, and excellence.

Principle #7: Physical therapists shall promote organizational behaviors and business practices that benefit patients/clients and society.

(Core Values: Integrity, Accountability)

▶ 7A. Physical therapists shall promote practice environments that support autonomous and accountable professional judgments.

▶ 7B. Physical therapists shall seek remuneration as is deserved and reasonable for physical therapist services.

▶ 7C. Physical therapists shall not accept gifts or other considerations that influence or give an appearance of influencing their professional judgment.

▶ 7D. Physical therapists shall fully disclose any financial interest they have in products or services that they recommend to patients/clients.

▶ 7E. Physical therapists shall be aware of charges and shall ensure that documentation and coding for physical therapy services accurately reflect the nature and extent of the services provided.

▶ 7F. Physical therapists shall refrain from employment arrangements, or other arrangements, that prevent physical therapists from fulfilling professional obligations to patients/clients.

Principle #8: Physical therapists shall participate in efforts to meet the health needs of people locally, nationally, or globally.

(Core Values: Social Responsibility)

▶ 8A. Physical therapists shall provide *pro bono* physical therapy services or support organizations that meet the health needs of people who are economically disadvantaged, uninsured, and underinsured.

▶ 8B. Physical therapists shall advocate to reduce health disparities and health care inequities, improve access to health care services, and address the health, wellness, and preventive health care needs of people.

▶ 8C. Physical therapists shall be responsible stewards of health care resources and shall avoid over-utilization or under-utilization of physical therapy services.

▶ 8D. Physical therapists shall educate members of the public about the benefits of physical therapy and the unique role of the physical therapist.

Standards of Ethical Conduct for the Physical Therapist Assistant

APPENDIX D

HOD S06-09-20-18 [Amended HOD S06-00-13-24; HOD 06-91-06-07; Initial HOD 06-82-04-08] [Standard]

PREAMBLE

The *Standards of Ethical Conduct for the Physical Therapist Assistant* (*Standards of Ethical Conduct*) delineate the ethical obligations of all physical therapist assistants as determined by the House of Delegates of the American Physical Therapy Association (APTA). The *Standards of Ethical Conduct* provide a foundation for conduct to which all physical therapist assistants shall adhere. Fundamental to the *Standards of Ethical Conduct* is the special obligation of physical therapist assistants to enable patients/clients to achieve greater independence, health and wellness, and enhanced quality of life.

No document that delineates ethical standards can address every situation. Physical therapist assistants are encouraged to seek additional advice or consultation in instances where the guidance of the *Standards of Ethical Conduct* may not be definitive.

STANDARDS

Standard #1: Physical therapist assistants shall respect the inherent dignity, and rights, of all individuals.

▶ 1A. Physical therapist assistants shall act in a respectful manner toward each person regardless of age, gender, race, nationality, religion, ethnicity, social or economic status, sexual orientation, health condition, or disability.

▶ 1B. Physical therapist assistants shall recognize their personal biases and shall not discriminate against others in the provision of physical therapy services.

Standard #2: Physical therapist assistants shall be trustworthy and compassionate in addressing the rights and needs of patients/clients.

▶ 2A. Physical therapist assistants shall act in the best interests of patients/clients over the interests of the physical therapist assistant.

▶ 2B. Physical therapist assistants shall provide physical therapy interventions with compassionate and caring behaviors that incorporate the individual and cultural differences of patients/clients.

▶ 2C. Physical therapist assistants shall provide patients/clients with information regarding the interventions they provide.

▶ 2D. Physical therapist assistants shall protect confidential patient/client information and, in collaboration with the physical therapist, may disclose confidential information to appropriate authorities only when allowed or as required by law.

Standard #3: Physical therapist assistants shall make sound decisions in collaboration with the physical therapist and within the boundaries established by laws and regulations.

▶ 3A. Physical therapist assistants shall make objective decisions in the patient's/client's best interest in all practice settings.

▶ 3B. Physical therapist assistants shall be guided by information about best practice regarding physical therapy interventions.

▶ 3C. Physical therapist assistants shall make decisions based upon their level of competence and consistent with patient/client values.

▶ 3D. Physical therapist assistants shall not engage in conflicts of interest that interfere with making sound decisions.

▶ 3E. Physical therapist assistants shall provide physical therapy services under the direction and supervision of a physical therapist and shall communicate with the physical therapist when patient/client status requires modifications to the established plan of care.

Standard #4: Physical therapist assistants shall demonstrate integrity in their relationships with patients/clients, families, colleagues, students, other health care providers, employers, payers, and the public.

▶ 4A. Physical therapist assistants shall provide truthful, accurate, and relevant information and shall not make misleading representations.

▶ 4B. Physical therapist assistants shall not exploit persons over whom they have supervisory, evaluative or other authority (eg, patients/clients, students, supervisees, research participants, or employees).

▶ 4C. Physical therapist assistants shall discourage misconduct by health care professionals and report illegal or unethical acts to the relevant authority, when appropriate.

▶ 4D. Physical therapist assistants shall report suspected cases of abuse involving children or vulnerable adults to the supervising physical therapist and the appropriate authority, subject to law.

▶ 4E. Physical therapist assistants shall not engage in any sexual relationship with any of their patients/clients, supervisees, or students.

▶ 4F. Physical therapist assistants shall not harass anyone verbally, physically, emotionally, or sexually.

Standard #5: Physical therapist assistants shall fulfill their legal and ethical obligations.

▶ 5A. Physical therapist assistants shall comply with applicable local, state, and federal laws and regulations.

▶ 5B. Physical therapist assistants shall support the supervisory role of the physical therapist to ensure quality care and promote patient/client safety.

▶ 5C. Physical therapist assistants involved in research shall abide by accepted standards governing protection of research participants.

▶ 5D. Physical therapist assistants shall encourage colleagues with physical, psychological, or substance related impairments that may adversely impact their professional responsibilities to seek assistance or counsel.

▶ 5E. Physical therapist assistants who have knowledge that a colleague is unable to perform their professional responsibilities with reasonable skill and safety shall report this information to the appropriate authority.

Standard #6: Physical therapist assistants shall enhance their competence through the lifelong acquisition and refinement of knowledge, skills, and abilities.

▶ 6A. Physical therapist assistants shall achieve and maintain clinical competence.

▶ 6B. Physical therapist assistants shall engage in lifelong learning consistent with changes in their roles and responsibilities and advances in the practice of physical therapy.

▶ 6C. Physical therapist assistants shall support practice environments that support career development and lifelong learning.

Standard #7: Physical therapist assistants shall support organizational behaviors and business practices that benefit patients/clients and society.

▶ 7A. Physical therapist assistants shall promote work environments that support ethical and accountable decision-making.

▶ 7B. Physical therapist assistants shall not accept gifts or other considerations that influence or give an appearance of influencing their decisions.

▶ 7C. Physical therapist assistants shall fully disclose any financial interest they have in products or services that they recommend to patients/clients.

▶ 7D. Physical therapist assistants shall ensure that documentation for their interventions accurately reflects the nature and extent of the services provided.

▶ 7E. Physical therapist assistants shall refrain from employment arrangements, or other arrangements, that prevent physical therapist assistants from fulfilling ethical obligations to patients/clients.

Standard #8: Physical therapist assistants shall participate in efforts to meet the health needs of people locally, nationally, or globally.

▶ 8A. Physical therapist assistants shall support organizations that meet the health needs of people who are economically disadvantaged, uninsured, and underinsured.

▶ 8B. Physical therapist assistants shall advocate for people with impairments, activity limitations, participation restrictions, and disabilities in order to promote their participation in community and society.

▶ 8C. Physical therapist assistants shall be responsible stewards of health care resources by collaborating with physical therapists in order to avoid over-utilization or under-utilization of physical therapy services.

▶ 8D. Physical therapist assistants shall educate members of the public about the benefits of physical therapy.

Index

Note: Page numbers followed by *f* and *t* indicate figure and table, respectively.

INDEX